DOSAGE AND SOLUTIONS CALCULATIONS
The Dimensional Analysis Way

DOSAGE AND SOLUTIONS CALCULATIONS

The Dimensional Analysis Way

ALICE J. SMITH, M.S., R.N.

Formerly Assistant Professor of Nursing,
Texas Christian University, Harris College of Nursing;
Retired Major, United States Air Force Nurse Corps

Illustrated

The C.V. Mosby Company

ST. LOUIS • BALTIMORE • PHILADELPHIA • TORONTO   1989

Acquisitions editor: Nancy L. Coon
Developmental editor: Susan Epstein
Project manager: Carlotta Seely
Book design: Susan E. Lane
Cover design: Elise A. Stimac
Production editing: Publication Services, Inc.

The authors and publisher have exerted every effort to ensure that drug selection and dosage used in this text are in accord with current practice. In view of the ongoing changes in drug therapy, however, the reader is cautioned to check package inserts for changes in recommended dosage and for warnings and precautions.

The C.V. Mosby Company
11830 Westline Industrial Drive, St. Louis, Missouri 63146

Library of Congress Cataloging in Publication Data

Smith, Alice J.
  Dosage and solutions calculations.

  Includes index.
  1. Pharmaceutical arithmetic. 2. Nursing.
I. Title. [DNLM: 1. Drugs—administration & dosage—
problems. 2. Mathematics—problems. 3. Solutions—
problems. QV 18 S642d]
RS57.S55 1989   615.5'8   88–34541
ISBN 0-8016-5146-8

PS/VHP/VHP   9 8 7 6 5 4 3 2 1

Preface

This dosage and solutions calculation workbook is designed as a text for beginning and advanced nursing students and as a reference for nurses in clinical practice. Problems originating in all areas of nursing practice are included. Some calculations are pertinent to any clinical nursing situation, while others are used primarily in specialty situations such as critical care, pediatrics, or community health.

This workbook may be used for independent study since the format is intended to guide students. Material is presented in small segments, explained very clearly, and followed by practice problems. Answers to problems include all steps so that students can find their own errors. A self-assessment posttest including all content presented concludes each chapter.

Many students are introduced to the dimensional analysis (factor-labeling) method in a chemistry or other physical science class. There are no formulas to learn and no advanced mathematical skills are required. Most problems can be set up in one equation, rather than several as in the traditional ratio-proportion method. There are various ways to set up dimensional analysis equations. In this workbook each equation is set up in the same logical sequence, beginning with the unit of the answer. Students learning this method can solve any type of problem. The dimensional analysis method is easier and less frustrating for students than either the formula or ratio-proportion methods.

This workbook is divided into three sections. The foundations of dimensional analysis section includes a mathematics pretest to help students assess their math skills; this is followed by a comprehensive math review. The introduction to the dimensional analysis method explains the problem-solving process used throughout the workbook. Included in this unit is a section to help students learn to check the accuracy of their own answers.

The second section contains content normally found in basic dosage and solutions calculation courses. Included in this section are units covering conversions among measurement systems and calculation of oral and parenteral dosages and dosages based on weight. Some unique inclusions in this section are interpretation of medication orders and recommended dosages. Each type of problem is presented with a word equation followed by several sample problems and practice problems. Actual medication labels are used to help students visualize problems originating in clinical situations. In addition to the self-assessment chapter posttests, each unit in this section has three posttests that may be used for extra practice or mastery testing purposes. Subsequent units in this section include calculations of solutions and intravenous fluids. The student may bypass either unit without having difficulty understanding subsequent units. Word equations are repeated periodically for reinforcement of learning and to alleviate the need to refer to previous portions of the workbook. There are more than 250 practice problems in this section alone, plus exercises in interpretation of orders and reading labels and syringes. An additional 350 problems are in this section's chapter and unit posttests. Students are encouraged to show all calculations for each of the various problems. In some instances this may require the use of additional paper.

Calculations used in specialty areas are covered in the third section. The comprehensive intravenous medications unit is an excellent reference for any critical care unit. The pediatric section includes medication and intravenous infusion calculations. Other pediatric calculations are in the appendix.

The glossary provides a quick reference for terminology used throughout the workbook. Calculation of kilocalories, temperature conversion, and conversions between standard and military time are included in the appendix.

Acknowledgments

I wish to thank the faculty of Texas Christian University, Harris College of Nursing, who encouraged me during the writing of this workbook. I especially want to thank Dr. Alice Gaul, who encouraged me to publish the material and suggested some critical care problems; Marla Buckles, who brought actual clinical problems to me, offered support, and listened to me; Allene Jones, for her support, encouragement, and suggestions, and for letting me guest lecture on this content.

This workbook would not have been written if I had not been forced to learn the dimensional analysis method to correct several students' dosage and solutions calculation tests. A special thanks goes to Cynthia Wagnon, who, in the summer of 1982, showed some non-math–minded classmates how to pass the dosage and solutions calculation requirements. Her method proved more effective than my ratio-proportion method. I owe the TCU-HCN students many thanks for their feedback and support during the evolution of the sequence for equation set-up used in this workbook. I also wish to thank those students who brought problems from clinical practice to my attention. It is to these wonderful nursing students—past, present, and future—of Texas Christian University, Harris College of Nursing, that this workbook is dedicated.

Special thanks to the reviewers: Shirley Horstman, R.N., M.S.N.; Marcile Lewis, R.N.; Jane T. Scott, R.N.; and Paula Broussard, R.N., M.N. Their comments and suggestions were invaluable during the preparation of this workbook.

Thanks to Fort Worth Osteopathic Medical Center for permission to reproduce their inpatient record forms. Thanks also to the following pharmaceutical companies for permission to reproduce their drug labels in this workbook: Abbott Laboratories; Adria Laboratories; Biocraft Laboratories; Boots-Flint, Inc.; Bristol-Myers U.S. Pharmaceutical and Nutritional Group; Burroughs Wellcome Company; DuPont Pharmaceuticals; Elkins-Sinn, Inc.; Hoechst-Rousel Pharmaceuticals; Knoll Pharmaceuticals; Lederle Laboratories; Eli Lilly and Company; Marion Laboratories, Inc.; McNeil Pharmaceutical; Merck Sharp and Dohme; Norwich Eaton Pharmaceuticals; Parke-Davis and Company; Pfizer Pharmaceuticals; A.H. Robins Company; Roche Laboratories; Roxane Laboratories, Inc.; Smith Kline and French Laboratories; E.R. Squibb and Sons, Inc.; Stuart Pharmaceuticals; The Upjohn Company; Winthrop-Breon Laboratories; and Wyeth Laboratories.

Contents

THE FOUNDATIONS
OF DIMENSIONAL ANALYSIS

UNIT I

Mathematical Knowledge Base

OBJECTIVES *Upon completion of this unit, the student will demonstrate the ability to correctly:*

- Interpret and write roman numerals.

- Compare the value of fractions, decimals, and percentages.

- Add, subtract, multiply, and divide fractions, including improper fractions and mixed numbers.

- Reduce fractions to their lowest denominators.

- Convert from fractions to decimals and from decimals to fractions.

- Add, subtract, multiply, and divide decimals.

- Convert decimals and fractions to percentages.

- Multiply numbers by percentages.

- Determine percentage.

- Solve equations written as fractions.

A basic understanding of mathematics is essential for the calculation of dosage and solution, regardless of the problem-solving method used. The student must know how to perform basic addition, subtraction, multiplication, and division using whole numbers, decimals, and fractions. A basic knowledge of roman numerals and percentages is also a prerequisite. A pretest is provided to assess math skills. This pretest should identify areas in which the student is weak.

If areas of weakness are identified by the pretest, the student is expected to review those areas. Any basic math book can be used to review addition, subtraction, multiplication, and division of whole numbers. This workbook contains a review of roman numerals, fractions, decimals, percentages, and equations set up as fractions.

SELF-ASSESSMENT MATHEMATICS PRETEST

Whole Numbers

Show all your work. (Check your answers on page 6.)

1. Add 67, 312, 1005, and 36.

2. Subtract 198 from 272.

3. $25 \times 40 \times 20 =$

4. $400 \overline{)\,125000}$

5. $400 \div 25 =$

Roman Numerals

Write arabic numerals for the following roman numerals.

6. II

7. vii

8. XV

9. XIX

10. iv

11. XXIX

Write roman numerals for the following arabic numerals.

12. 21

13. 6

14. 34

15. 18

Fractions

Write the following as fractions.

16. Seven-sixteenths.

17. Four and nine-thousandths.

18. Three-hundredths.

19. Three-thousandths.

Solve the following fraction problems. Reduce all fractions to their lowest terms.

20. $\begin{aligned} & 2\frac{5}{12} \\ & 3\frac{5}{6} \\ & 1\frac{1}{4} \\ +\,& 2\frac{1}{2} \\ \hline \end{aligned}$

23. $\frac{3}{8} \times 4 =$

21. $2\frac{3}{4}$
     $-1\frac{7}{8}$

24. $\frac{3}{4} \div \frac{3}{4} =$

22. $\frac{3}{4} \times \frac{3}{4} =$

25. $\frac{3}{8} \div 4 =$

Decimals

Write the following as decimals.

26. Three-hundredths.

27. Six and four-thousandths.

Convert the following fractions to decimals.

28. $\frac{27}{40}$

29. $\frac{3}{20}$

Solve the following.

30. $4.108 + 6.08 + 5.40 =$

33. Multiply 0.65 by 1.02.

31. 2.68
     -1.89

34. $1.7\overline{)51}$

32. 2.014
     $\times\ 20.5$

35. $48.48 \div 1.6 =$

Percentages

Write the following as percentages.

36. Four-hundredths

38. Thirty-eight hundredths

37. Four ten-thousandths

39. Thirteen-thousandths

Write the following as a fraction.

40. 9% =   41. 0.5% =

Write the following as a decimal.

42. 9%   43. 0.7%

Convert the following fractions to percentage.

44. $\frac{12}{25}$ 45. $\frac{7}{20}$

Equations

46. $\dfrac{1000 \times 20}{12 \times 60} =$

49. $\dfrac{5\frac{7}{16} \times \ 1 \times 21}{1 \times 2.2 \times \ 1} =$

47. $\dfrac{1\frac{1}{4} \times \ 1 \times \ 2}{1 \times 60 \times 0.8} =$

50. $\dfrac{1 \times 1000 \times 60}{60 \times \ 10 \times \ 1} =$

48. $\dfrac{1\frac{3}{8} \times 0.4 \times 20}{1 \times 2.2 \times \ \frac{1}{2}} =$

Self-Assessment Mathematics Pretest Answers
Whole Numbers
(Refer to basic mathematics book if errors were made in this section.)

1. 1420   3. 20,000   4. 312.5 or $312\frac{1}{2}$ 5. 16
2. 74

Roman Numerals
(Refer to page 8 if errors were made in this section.)
Roman numerals to arabic numerals.

6. 2   8. 15   10. 4   11. 29
7. 7   9. 19

Arabic numerals to roman numerals.

12. XXI   13. VI   14. XXXIV   15. XVIII

Fractions
(Refer to page 11 if errors were made in this section.)

16. $\frac{7}{16}$ 17. $4\frac{9}{1000}$ 18. $\frac{3}{100}$ 19. $\frac{3}{1000}$

Addition, subtraction, multiplication, and division of fractions.

20. 10   22. $\frac{9}{16}$ 24. 1   25. $\frac{3}{32}$
21. $\frac{7}{8}$ 23. $1\frac{1}{2}$

Decimals
(Refer to page 30 if errors were made in this section.)
Written fractions to decimals.

26. 0.03   27. 6.004

Converting fractions to decimals.

28. 0.675   29. 0.15

Addition, subtraction, multiplication, and division of decimals.

30. 15.588   32. 41.2870   34. 30   35. 30.3
31. 0.79   33. 0.6630 or 0.663

Percentages
(Refer to page 42 if errors were made in this section.)
Written decimals to percentage.

36. 4%   37. 0.04%   38. 38%   39. 1.3%

Percentage to fractions.

40. $\frac{9}{100}$ 41. $\frac{5}{1000}$

Percentage to decimal.

42. 0.09   43. 0.007

Converting fractions to percents.

44. 48%   45. 35%

Equations
(Refer to page 49 if errors were made in this section.)

46. 27.77   48. 10   49. 51.90 or 51.9   50. 100
47. 0.052

Chapter 1

Roman Numerals

Arabic numerals, such as 1, 2, 3, etc., are used universally to indicate quantities. They are easy to read and less likely to be confused than roman numerals. Roman numerals are always converted to arabic numerals for problem solving.

Roman numerals are used with the apothecary system of measurement. Any whole-numbered quantity in a technically correct apothecary measurement order is written in roman numerals. Roman numerals are not used with the household or metric measurement systems.

Technically, lowercase roman numerals are to be used in apothecary orders. In practice, however, both uppercase and lowercase are used. In addition, lowercase roman numerals are often written with a line above the numeral. A 1 could be written as I, $\bar{\text{i}}$ or i.

The value of roman numerals is as follows:

I or i = 1	L = 50	D = 500
V or v = 5	C = 100	M = 1000
X or x = 10		

Only the roman numerals in the left column are used by health care providers. The others—L, C, D, and M—are not used because they easily could be confused with abbreviations commonly used by health care professionals.

RULES GOVERNING ROMAN NUMERALS

1. Roman numerals of lesser value following one of greater value are added together.

    Example: VII (vii) = 5 + 1 + 1 = 7

2. A roman numeral of lesser value preceding one of greater value is subtracted from the greater value numeral.

    Example: IV (iv) = 5 − 1 = 4

3. Roman numerals of the same value are written in sequence unless to do so would change the value of the number to be written.

    Example: XXX(xxx) = 10 + 10 + 10 = 30
    However, 29 is written XXIX rather than XXXI,
    which would be 31, a change in value.

4. Roman numerals are usually written using the largest value numerals possible.

    Example: 20 is written as XX (xx) rather than VVVV.
    9 is written as IX (ix) instead of VIIII.

Roman numerals are often combined with the abbreviation for one half, ss, in doctors' orders and nursing notes. The abbreviation is always at the end of the roman numeral. Almost always, roman numerals are written in lowercase when using ss to indicate the fraction $\frac{1}{2}$.

$$\text{Example:} \quad iss = 1\frac{1}{2}.$$

Roman numerals are not used when there is a fraction other than $\frac{1}{2}$ following a whole number. Arabic numerals are used when whole numbers are coupled with fractions other than $\frac{1}{2}$.

$$\text{Example:} \quad 7\frac{3}{8} \text{ is never written VII } \frac{3}{8}$$

PRACTICE PROBLEMS

Roman Numerals

Write arabic numerals for the following roman numerals. Show all your work. (Check your answers on page 312.)

1. XXV
2. iiss
3. XIV

4. XXXVI
5. viiss

Write roman numerals for the following arabic numbers.

6. $14\frac{1}{2}$
7. $9\frac{1}{2}$
8. 15

9. 29
10. 4

SELF-ASSESSMENT POSTTEST

Roman Numerals

Write arabic numerals for these roman numerals. Show all your work. (Check your answers on page 349.)

1. XIX
2. xxivss
3. xxiii
4. xvi
5. XV

6. ivss
7. VII
8. iiiss
9. XXIX
10. XXXVI

Write Roman numerals for these Arabic numerals.

11. 25
12. 12
13. 26

14. 8
15. $7\frac{1}{2}$

17. 34

18. $2\frac{1}{2}$

19. 39

20. 18

Chapter 2

Common Fractions

Knowledge of the definition of mathematical terms is essential prior to solving problems. The box below lists terms for mathematical processes used in this chapter.

TERMS FOR MATHEMATICAL PROCESSES

Addends: the numbers to be added.
Difference: the answer in subtraction.
Dividend: the number to be divided.
Divisor: the number by which the dividend is divided.
Function sign: mathematical sign showing addition (+), subtraction (−), multiplication (×, ·), or division (÷).
Minuend: The number from which the subtrahend is subtracted.
Multiplicand: the number which is being multiplied.
Multiplier: the number(s) by which the multiplicand is multiplied.
Product: the results or answer of the multiplication.
Quotient: the number or answer resulting from the division of one quantity by another.
Subtrahend: the number that is subtracted from the minued.
Sum: the answer in addition.
Total: the process of addition; the answer in addition is sometimes called the total.

The whole of a thing is always one (1). The whole of a pie is one pie. The whole of a dollar is one dollar. The parts of the whole, when added together, always equal 1. A part of the whole may be written as a common fraction, a decimal fraction, or a percentage of the whole. Throughout this workbook, common fractions will be called fractions and decimal fractions will be called decimals.

Wholes are frequently depicted as circles. Figure 2-1 shows three circles, each representing a whole: the corresponding parts of each are designated by fractions, decimals, and percentages. It is obvious that the corresponding parts ($\frac{1}{2}$, 0.5, and 50%) occupy the same amount of space on the whole circle; they are equal. Similarly, $\frac{1}{4}$, 0.25, and 25% are equal. The methods for changing fractions to decimals and percentages are discussed in later chapters of this unit.

COMMON FRACTION KNOWLEDGE BASE

Common fractions are occasionally used by health care professionals. Medications ordered in the apothecary system of measurement are sometimes ordered as fractions. The use of fractions with household measurements is appropriate. It is never appropriate to use common fractions when using the metric system of measurement. A basic understanding of fractions is necessary for using this workbook, as the dimensional analysis equations are set up and solved as though they are large fractions.

A fraction must have a *numerator* (the top number) and a *denominator* (the bottom

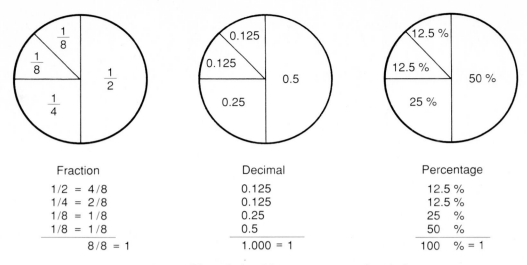

Fraction	Decimal	Percentage
1/2 = 4/8	0.125	12.5 %
1/4 = 2/8	0.125	12.5 %
1/8 = 1/8	0.25	25 %
1/8 = 1/8	0.5	50 %
8/8 = 1	1.000 = 1	100 % = 1

FIGURE 2-1. The relationship among parts of a whole

number), separated by a line. Fractions such as $\frac{1}{2}$ and $\frac{1}{8}$ are read as one-half and one-eighth, and $\frac{3}{1000}$ is three-thousandths.

Fractions mixed with whole numbers are read as the whole number and the fraction—so $2\frac{1}{5}$ is read as two and one-fifth.

Fractions are sometimes read as the numerator over the denominator, such as the fraction $\frac{1}{2}$ might be read as 1 over 2. The fraction $\frac{8}{10}$ could be 8 over 10. Frequently used in this chapter are the words "a number over itself." This refers to any fraction in which the numerator and the denominator are the same number, such as $\frac{3}{3}$ or $\frac{10}{10}$. A fraction also can be read as the numerator divided by the denominator.

There are four types of common fractions: *proper, improper, complex fractions* and *mixed numbers*. These fraction types are defined as follows:

1. In proper fractions the numerator is smaller than the denominator.

Example: $\frac{1}{4}$

2. In improper fractions the numerator is larger than the denominator.

Example: $\frac{5}{4}$

3. Complex fractions feature fractions in the numerator and/or the denominator.

Example: $\frac{1/4}{1/2}$

4. Mixed numbers combine a whole number and a fraction.

Example: $1\frac{1}{4}$

Improper fractions and mixed numbers always are equal to or greater than 1 in value, whereas proper fractions are always less than 1. An improper fraction can never be a final answer; it must be reduced to a whole or mixed number.

It is necessary to know four rules before solving fraction problems:

Rule 1: Any number multiplied or divided by 1 is the original number.

Example: 2 divided by 1 is 2.

Rule 2: Any fraction consisting of a number over itself has the value of 1.

Example: $\frac{2}{2} = 1$

Divide both the numerator and denominator of the fraction $\frac{2}{2}$ by 2.
Multiplying or dividing by 2 over 2 ($\frac{2}{2}$) is the same as multiplying or dividing by 1.
$\frac{2}{2}$ divided by $\frac{2}{2}$ equals $\frac{1}{1}$ or 1.

Rule 3: The value of a fraction does not change when both the numerator and the denominator are subjected to the same multiplication or division process.

Example: Multiply both the numerator and the denominator of the fraction $\frac{3}{5}$ by 2.

$$\frac{3 \times 2}{5 \times 2} = \frac{6}{10}$$

The new fraction is $\frac{6}{10}$. The value does not change because multiplying both the numerator and denominator by $\frac{2}{2}$ is the same as multiplying the fraction by 1. Any number over itself is 1. Therefore, $\frac{3}{5}$ and $\frac{6}{10}$ are of equal value.

Rule 4: A whole number may be written as a numerator over a denominator of 1. The 1 in the denominator can be implied in any whole number.

Example: $2 = \frac{2}{1}$

Fractions are sometimes written in the form of *ratios*. A ratio consists of two numbers, the numerator and denominator, separated by a colon. The first number is always the numerator, just as the top number of the fraction is always the numerator. The fraction $\frac{1}{2}$ written as a ratio is 1:2. Any fraction can be written as a ratio. Conversely, any ratio can be written as a fraction.

LEAST COMMON DENOMINATOR

The least common denominator is used when comparing values of fractions and when adding or subtracting fractions. The rules presented above are involved in finding it.

The least common denominator has to be evenly divisible by all of the original denominators. Evenly divisible means that one number divided by a second number produces a quotient that is a whole number with no fractional parts remaining.

Examples: 10 is evenly divisible by 5 because the quotient is 2 with no remainder.
10 is not evenly divisible by 3 because the quotient is $3\frac{1}{3}$ or 3 with one remaining fractional part.

The least common denominator is the smallest number that is evenly divisible by all the denominators. Therefore, this least common denominator cannot be smaller than the largest denominator. For example, of the fractions $\frac{1}{2}$, $\frac{1}{3}$, and $\frac{1}{6}$, the smallest possible common denominator is 6 because 2 and 3 are not divisible by 6. Some helpful division hints are provided below.

HELPFUL HINTS FOR DIVISION

Only even numbers are evenly divisible by even numbers.
Only numbers ending in 0 or 5 are evenly divisible by 5.
A number is evenly divisible by 3 if the sum of the digits equals 3 or multiples of three.

Example: 111 $1 + 1 + 1 = 3$
81     $8 + 1 = 9$

A number is evenly divisible by nine if the sum of the digits equals 9 or multiples of 9.

Example: 72 $7 + 2 = 9$
108     $1 + 0 + 8 = 9$

Least common denominators may be found in three ways:

1. Converting the smaller denominator numerals to the largest denominator numeral. This can be done only when the largest denominator is evenly divisible by the rest of the denominators.

SAMPLE PROBLEM   **Find the least common denominator of the following fractions: $\frac{1}{2}, \frac{1}{4}, \frac{1}{8}$.**

The least common denominator is 8 because 8 is evenly divisible by 2, 4, and 8.

2. Multiplying the numbers of the denominators together.

SAMPLE PROBLEM   **Find the least common denominator of the following fractions: $\frac{1}{5}, \frac{3}{4}$, and $\frac{2}{3}$.**

None of the denominators are evenly divisible by
the others.

Multiply 5 by 4 and by 3: $\qquad\qquad\qquad\qquad\qquad 5 \times 4 = 20 \times 3 = 60$

60 is the least common denominator.

3. Sometimes the least common denominator is less than the multiplication of all
   denominators. In this instance, find a different number that is evenly divisible by
   the denominators. That number is the multiple of several of the denominators.
   Always start by multiplying the smaller values first.

SAMPLE PROBLEM   **Find the least common denominator of the following fractions: $\frac{1}{2}, \frac{1}{4}$, and $\frac{1}{6}$.**

6 is divisible by 2 and 6 but not by 4.

Multiply 2 by 4: $\qquad\qquad\qquad\qquad\qquad\qquad 2 \times 4 = 8$

8 is divisible by 2 and 4 but not by 6.

Multiply 2 by 6: $\qquad\qquad\qquad\qquad\qquad\qquad 2 \times 6 = 12$

12 is divisible by 2, 4, and 6. Therefore, the least common denominator is 12.

PRACTICE PROBLEMS

Least Common Denominator

Find the least common denominator of the following fractions. Show all your work. (Check
your answers on page 312.)

1. $\frac{1}{4}, \frac{1}{5}, \frac{1}{6}$

4. $\frac{3}{8}, \frac{5}{6}, \frac{7}{12}$

2. $\frac{1}{3}, \frac{1}{6}, \frac{2}{9}$

5. $\frac{1}{2}, \frac{2}{3}, \frac{3}{4}$

3. $\frac{1}{8}, \frac{2}{5}, \frac{1}{4}$

CONVERSION OF FRACTIONS USING THE LEAST COMMON DENOMINATOR

After the least common denominator is found, the fraction can be converted to one of equal value. Conversion is accomplished in three steps:

(1) Find the least common denominator.

(2) Divide the least common denominator by the denominator of the fraction being converted.

(3) Multiply both the numerator and the denominator by the quotient obtained in step 2.

These steps are identified in the following sample problem.

SAMPLE PROBLEM   **Convert the following fractions to least common denominator: $\frac{1}{2}$, $\frac{1}{4}$, $\frac{1}{8}$.**

(1) The least common denominator is 8.

To convert $\frac{1}{2}$ to eighths:

(2) Divide the least common denominator (8) by 2:

$$8 \div 2 = 4$$

(3) Multiply both the numerator and denominator by the quotient (4):

$$\frac{1 \times 4}{2 \times 4} = \frac{4}{8}$$

To change $\frac{1}{4}$ to eighths:

(2) Divide the least common denominator (8) by 4:

$$8 \div 4 = 2$$

(3) Multiply both the numerator and denominator by the quotient (2):

$$\frac{1 \times 2}{2 \times 2} = \frac{2}{8}$$

Of course, $\frac{1}{8}$ is already in the form of the least common denominator.

PRACTICE PROBLEMS

Conversion of Fractions Using Least Common Denominators

Convert the following fractions to their least common denominators. (These fractions are the same fractions as in the previous practice problems.) Show all your work. (Check your answers on page 312.)

6. $\frac{1}{4}$, $\frac{1}{5}$, $\frac{1}{6}$

9. $\frac{3}{8}$, $\frac{5}{6}$, $\frac{7}{12}$

7. $\frac{1}{3}$, $\frac{1}{6}$, $\frac{2}{9}$

10. $\frac{1}{2}$, $\frac{2}{3}$, $\frac{3}{4}$

8. $\frac{1}{8}$, $\frac{2}{5}$, $\frac{1}{4}$

COMPARISON OF VALUE OF FRACTIONS

It is sometimes necessary to determine which of several fractions is larger, smaller, or of the same value. Several rules apply when comparing the values of fractions.

1. If the numerators of several fractions are constant (the same number), the larger the denominator, the smaller the value of the fraction.

SAMPLE PROBLEM   **Compare $\frac{1}{2}$ to $\frac{1}{4}$.**

The numerator is constant. In the denominators, 2 is smaller than 4. Therefore, $\frac{1}{2}$ is larger than $\frac{1}{4}$. Figure 2-2 depicts this relationship and may be written as follows:

$$\frac{1}{2} > \frac{1}{4}$$

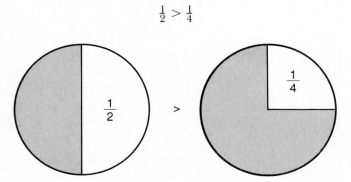

FIGURE 2-2. The relationship between $\frac{1}{2}$ and $\frac{1}{4}$

2. If the denominators of two or more fractions are constant, the larger the numerator, the greater the value of the fraction.

SAMPLE PROBLEM   **Compare $\frac{1}{4}$ to $\frac{3}{4}$.**

The denominator, 4, is constant. The 1 in the first numerator is smaller than the 3 in the second numerator. Therefore, $\frac{1}{4}$ is smaller than $\frac{3}{4}$. This relationship is depicted in Figure 2-3 and may be written as:

$$\frac{1}{4} < \frac{3}{4}$$

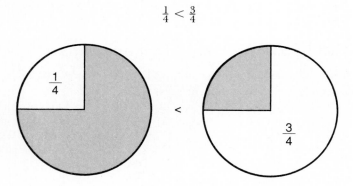

FIGURE 2-3. The relationship between $\frac{1}{4}$ and $\frac{3}{4}$

3. When neither the numerators nor the denominators are constant, common denominators must be calculated in order to compare the values of the fractions.

SAMPLE PROBLEM   **Compare $\frac{3}{4}$ to $\frac{5}{8}$.**

Neither the numerators nor the denominators are constant.

Find the least common denominator.   8

To change $\frac{3}{4}$ to $\frac{?}{8}$:

Divide the least common denominator by 4: $8 \div 4 = 2$

Multiply both the numerator and the denominator by the quotient, 2: $\frac{3 \times 2}{4 \times 2} = \frac{6}{8}$

Figure 2-4 shows the equality of $\frac{3}{4}$ and $\frac{6}{8}$.
Now, rule 2 applies because the denominators are constant. Six is greater than 5, so $\frac{6}{8}$ is greater than $\frac{5}{8}$. Therefore, $\frac{3}{4}$ is greater than $\frac{5}{8}$.

This relationship is shown in Figure 2-5. $\frac{3}{4} > \frac{5}{8}$

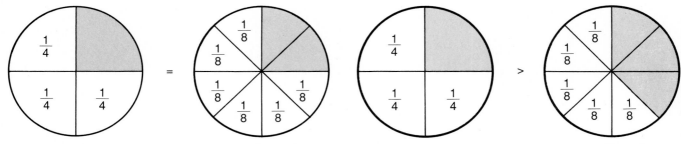

FIGURE 2-4. The relationship between $\frac{3}{4}$ and $\frac{6}{8}$ **FIGURE 2-5.** The relationship between $\frac{3}{4}$ and $\frac{5}{8}$

REDUCTION OF FRACTIONS

Fractions are always reduced to their lowest terms for the final answer. Proper fractions are reduced to fractions with the smallest possible numerators and denominators, or lowest terms. Improper fractions are reduced to whole numbers or mixed numbers with the fraction portions reduced to the lowest terms. Mixed numbers with improper fractions are reduced to larger numerals with the fraction portions reduced to their lowest terms.

A proper fraction can be reduced if both the numerator and the denominator are evenly divisible by the same number. Remember, the value of a fraction does not change when the numerator and the denominator are subjected to the same multiplication or division process.

SAMPLE PROBLEM   **Reduce the fraction $\frac{6}{8}$.**

Both 6 and 8 are evenly divisible by 2. $\frac{6}{8} \div \frac{2}{2} = \frac{3}{4}$

Sometimes reducing fractions is easier to accomplish when done in steps. The following example shows a fraction in which both the numerator and denominator are evenly divisible by 16. This is not easily apparent, however. What is apparent is that the number is divisible by 2 because any even number is divisible by 2. Also, dividing by 16 is harder than dividing by one-digit numbers, which often can be done without the long-division process.

SAMPLE PROBLEM   **Reduce the fraction $\frac{112}{192}$.**

Both 112 and 192 are divisible by 2.

$$\frac{112}{192} \div \frac{2}{2} = \frac{56}{96}$$

Both 56 and 96 are divisible by 2.

$$\frac{56}{96} \div \frac{2}{2} = \frac{28}{48}$$

Both 28 and 48 are divisible by 2.

$$\frac{28}{48} \div \frac{2}{2} = \frac{14}{24}$$

Both 14 and 24 are divisible by 2.

$$\frac{14}{24} \div \frac{2}{2} = \frac{7}{12}$$

Seven and 12 are not both evenly divisible by the same number. Therefore $\frac{112}{192}$, reduced to its lowest terms, is $\frac{7}{12}$.

This process of dividing the numerator and the denominator by the same number is called *cancellation*. This can be accomplished only if the numerator and denominator numerals are evenly divisible by the same divisor. Canceling is shown by making a slash through the numbers in the numerator and denominator and writing the quotients of the division above the numerator and below the denominator. In the example on the left, each slash represents division by 2. That slash also could represent division by other numbers. In the example on the right, each slash represents division by 4.

Examples:

$$\frac{\overset{7}{\cancel{14}}\,\cancel{56}\,\cancel{112}}{\cancel{192}\,\cancel{96}\,\underset{12}{\cancel{48}\,\cancel{24}}}\qquad\qquad\frac{\overset{7}{\cancel{28}}\,\cancel{112}}{\cancel{192}\,\underset{12}{\cancel{48}}}$$

To reduce an improper fraction, divide the numerator by the denominator. The resulting quotient becomes a whole number and the remainder is written as a fraction. Remember, an improper fraction is always greater than 1.

SAMPLE PROBLEM   **Reduce $\frac{56}{32}$.**

Divide the numerator by the denominator:

$$\begin{array}{r} 1\frac{24}{32} \\ 32\overline{)56} \\ \underline{32} \\ 24 \end{array}$$

The answer is $1\frac{24}{32}$. 24 and 32 are both divisible by 8. The parentheses indicate that only the fraction is to be divided by $\frac{8}{8}$.

$$1\left(\frac{24}{32} \div \frac{8}{8}\right) = 1\frac{3}{4}$$

Sometimes it is easier to reduce the fraction by canceling prior to dividing the numerator by the denominator. It is always easier to divide small numbers than large ones.

Example:

$$\frac{\overset{7}{\cancel{56}}}{\underset{4}{\cancel{32}}} = \frac{7}{4}$$

Divide the numerator by the denominator.

$$\begin{array}{r} 1\frac{3}{4} \\ 4\overline{)7} \\ \underline{4} \\ 3 \end{array}$$

Mixed numbers containing improper fractions are reduced in the same way as improper fractions except that the quotient is added to the existing whole number.

SAMPLE PROBLEM   **Reduce $2\frac{21}{4}$.**

Divide the fraction numerator by the denominator:

$$2 + (21 \div 4) = 2 + 5\frac{1}{4} = 7\frac{1}{4}$$

$$\begin{array}{r} 5\frac{1}{4} \\ 4{\overline{)21}} \\ \underline{20} \\ 1 \end{array}$$

PRACTICE PROBLEMS

Reduction of Fractions

Reduce the following. Show all your work. (Check your answers on page 312.)

11. $\frac{19}{6}$

14. $\frac{8}{20}$

12. $2\frac{20}{5}$

15. $5\frac{5}{4}$

13. $\frac{43}{8}$

CREATION OF IMPROPER FRACTIONS

Mixed numbers can be multiplied and divided only after they are converted to improper fractions. Mixed numbers including improper fractions often are necessary when subtracting fractions.

To create the numerator of an improper fraction from a mixed number, multiply the whole number by the denominator and add the product to the existing numerator. The denominator remains the same. This could be written mathematically as follows:

$$\frac{(\text{whole number} \times \text{denominator}) + \text{existing numerator}}{\text{denominator}} = \text{improper fraction}$$

The parentheses indicate that the function within the parentheses is completed before doing anything else. Therefore, the whole number and denominator are multiplied before adding the existing numerator.

SAMPLE PROBLEM   **Create an improper fraction from the mixed number $2\frac{3}{8}$.**

Multiply the whole number by the denominator: $\dfrac{(2 \times 8) + 3}{8} = \dfrac{16 + 3}{8}$

Add the product to the existing numerator: $\dfrac{16 + 3}{8} = \dfrac{19}{8}$

The improper fraction of $2\frac{3}{8}$ is $\frac{19}{8}$.

A mixed number with an improper fraction may be necessary when subtracting fractions. To create a mixed number with an improper fraction from a mixed number, borrow 1 from the whole number and create an improper fraction of this number and the existing fraction.

Whole number $- 1\dfrac{(1 \times \text{denominator}) + \text{existing numerator}}{\text{denominator}} = $ mixed number with improper fraction

SAMPLE PROBLEM   **Create a mixed number with an improper fraction from the mixed number $4\frac{7}{9}$.**

Borrow 1 from the whole number for the improper fraction: $4\frac{7}{9} = 3 + 1\frac{7}{9}$

Multiply the borrowed 1 by the denominator: $3 + \dfrac{(1 \times 9) + 7}{9}$

Add the product to the existing numerator: $3 + \dfrac{9 + 7}{9} = 3 + \dfrac{16}{9}$

The mixed number with an improper fraction is $3\frac{16}{9}$.

PRACTICE PROBLEMS

Creation of Improper Fractions

Make improper fractions of the following mixed numbers. Show all your work. (Check your answers on page 312.)

16. $5\frac{3}{4}$ 18. $8\frac{1}{2}$

17. $2\frac{1}{3}$

Make mixed numbers with improper fractions from the following mixed numbers.

19. $5\frac{3}{4}$ 20. $2\frac{1}{3}$

ADDITION OF FRACTIONS

Fractions can be added together only when they have common denominators. After conversion to the least common denominator, the numerators are added. The common denominator remains the same.

SAMPLE PROBLEM   **Add the following fractions: $\frac{1}{2}$, $\frac{1}{3}$, $\frac{3}{4}$, $\frac{5}{6}$.**

Find the least common denominator:
(12 is evenly divisible by 2, 3, 4, and 6)

$$12$$

Convert the fractions to their common denominator:

$$\frac{1 \times 6}{2 \times 6} = \frac{6}{12}$$

$$\frac{1 \times 4}{3 \times 4} = \frac{4}{12}$$

$$\frac{3 \times 3}{4 \times 3} = \frac{9}{12}$$

$$\frac{5 \times 2}{6 \times 2} = \frac{10}{12}$$

The denominator is the same. Add the numerators together:

$$\frac{6 + 4 + 9 + 10}{12} = \frac{29}{12}$$

Reduce the improper fraction to a mixed number:

$$\begin{array}{r} 2\frac{5}{12} \\ 12\overline{)29} \\ \underline{24} \\ 5 \end{array}$$

The sum of $\frac{1}{2}$, $\frac{1}{3}$, $\frac{3}{4}$ and $\frac{5}{6}$ is $2\frac{5}{12}$.

   Addition of mixed numbers is accomplished by adding the whole numbers, then adding the numerators of the fractions. The denominator remains the same.

SAMPLE PROBLEM   **Add the following mixed numbers: $1\frac{1}{2}$, $2\frac{1}{4}$, $3\frac{1}{8}$, $3\frac{5}{8}$.**

Find the least common denominator:

$$8$$

Convert the fractions to common denominators:

$$1\frac{1 \times 4}{2 \times 4} = 1\frac{4}{8}$$

$$2\frac{1 \times 2}{4 \times 2} = 2\frac{2}{8}$$

$$3\frac{1}{8}$$

$$+3\frac{5}{8}$$

Add the whole numbers and the numerators together; The denominator remains the same.

$$9\frac{12}{8}$$

Reduce the improper fraction by canceling ($\div$ 4):

$$9\frac{\cancel{12}^{3}}{\cancel{8}_{2}}$$

Divide the fraction numerator by the denominator:

$$9 + (3 \div 2) = 9 + 1\frac{1}{2}$$

Add the quotient to the whole number:

$$9 + 1\frac{1}{2} = 10\frac{1}{2}$$

PRACTICE PROBLEMS

Addition of Fractions

Add the following fractions and mixed numbers. Reduce all fractions to their lowest terms. Show all your work. (Check your answers on page 312.)

21. $\frac{1}{8}$, $\frac{11}{12}$, $\frac{5}{6}$, $\frac{3}{4}$

24. $2\frac{9}{10}$, $1\frac{4}{5}$, $3\frac{1}{4}$

22. $\frac{1}{6}$, $\frac{1}{10}$, $\frac{3}{5}$

25. $\frac{1}{3}$, $\frac{1}{7}$, $\frac{1}{9}$

23. $\frac{8}{9}$, $\frac{2}{3}$, $\frac{1}{2}$

SUBTRACTION OF FRACTIONS

The terms of subtraction are minuend, subtrahend, and difference.

$$\begin{array}{r} \text{minuend} \\ -\ \text{subtrahend} \\ \hline \text{difference} \end{array}$$

The subtraction of fractions can be accomplished only when the fractions have common denominators. Therefore, fractions with unlike denominators must be converted to fractions with common denominators. Then subtract the subtrahend numerator from the minuend numerator. The denominators remain the same.

SAMPLE PROBLEM $\frac{3}{4} - \frac{5}{8}$

Find the least common denominator: 8

Convert the fractions to their common denominators: $\dfrac{3 \times 2}{4 \times 2} = \dfrac{6}{8}$

$$-\ \frac{5}{8}$$

Subtract the subtrahend numerator; the denominator remains the same. $\dfrac{1}{8}$

The difference between the fractions $\frac{3}{4}$ and $\frac{5}{8}$ is $\frac{1}{8}$.

Subtracting fractions or mixed numbers from mixed numbers often involves borrowing 1 from the whole number and converting it to an improper fraction.

SAMPLE PROBLEM $3\frac{3}{4} - 1\frac{4}{5}$

Find the least common denominator: 20

Convert the fractions to common denominators:

$$3\frac{3 \times 5}{4 \times 5} = 3\frac{15}{20}$$

$$1\frac{4 \times 4}{5 \times 4} = 1\frac{16}{20}$$

Borrow 1 from the 3 of the fraction $3\frac{3}{4}$: $3\frac{15}{20} = 2 + 1\frac{15}{20}$

Multiply the borrowed 1 by the denominator: $2 + \dfrac{(1 \times 20) + 15}{20}$

Add the product to the existing numerator: $2 + \dfrac{20 + 15}{20} = 2\frac{35}{20}$

Subtract the whole numbers and numerators; the denominator remains the same. $-1\frac{16}{20}$

The difference between $3\frac{3}{4}$ and $1\frac{4}{5}$ is $1\frac{19}{20}$. $1\frac{19}{20}$

Sometimes proper fractions or mixed numbers are subtracted from whole numbers. Then it is necessary to borrow 1 from the whole number and make a fraction of a number over itself, consistent with the denominator of the fraction in the subtrahend. Remember, any number over itself is equal to 1.

SAMPLE PROBLEM $4 - 2\frac{1}{3}$

Borrow 1 from 4 and convert it to thirds: $4 - 1 = 3\frac{3}{3}$

$-2\frac{1}{3}$

Subtract the whole number and numerators; the denominator remains the same. $1\frac{2}{3}$

The difference between 4 and $2\frac{1}{3}$ is $1\frac{2}{3}$.

PRACTICE PROBLEMS

Subtraction of Fractions

Subtract the following fractions and mixed numbers. Reduce fractions to their lowest terms. Show all your work. (Check your answers on page 313.)

26. $2\frac{5}{8} - 1\frac{3}{8}$

29. $4 - 3\frac{15}{16}$

27. $5\frac{3}{16} - 2\frac{7}{8}$

30. $5\frac{1}{4} - 3\frac{15}{16}$

28. $2\frac{5}{6} - 1\frac{2}{3}$

MULTIPLICATION OF FRACTIONS

Prior to any discussion about multiplication, it is important to understand the terminology of multiplication.

Remember: The multiplicand $\times$ the multiplier(s) = product

---

Example: $\frac{1}{2} \times \frac{1}{5} \times \frac{1}{6} = \frac{1}{60}$

In this example, the multiplicand is $\frac{1}{2}$; the multipliers are $\frac{1}{5}$ and $\frac{1}{6}$. The product is $\frac{1}{60}$.

Multiplication of fractions is accomplished by multiplying the numerators together and then multiplying the denominators together. This could be written as:

$$\frac{\text{multiplication of all numerators}}{\text{multiplication of all denominators}} = \text{product}$$

When multiplying, the fractions may be set up individually, as in the example above, or as one long fraction.

Example: $\frac{1 \times 1 \times 1}{2 \times 5 \times 6} = \frac{1}{60}$

Either method is correct. Equations in later chapters of this workbook are set up as one long fraction. Multiplication of proper fractions will result in a product that is smaller in value than any of the fractions being multiplied.

SAMPLE PROBLEM $\frac{3}{4} \times \frac{4}{5} \times \frac{1}{2}$

Multiply the numerators:
Multiply the denominators:

$$\frac{3 \times 4 \times 1}{4 \times 5 \times 2} = \frac{12}{40}$$

Reduce the product:

$$\frac{\overset{3}{\cancel{12}}}{\underset{10}{\cancel{40}}} = \frac{3}{10}$$

$\frac{3}{10}$ $(\frac{12}{40})$ is less than $\frac{1}{2}$ $(\frac{20}{40})$, $\frac{4}{5}$ $(\frac{32}{40})$, or $\frac{3}{4}$ $(\frac{30}{40})$.

Mixed numbers cannot be multiplied until they are converted to improper fractions. Remember, to convert mixed numbers to improper fractions, multiply the whole number by the denominator and add the existing numerator. This becomes the new numerator. The denominator remains the same. Once the mixed numbers are converted to improper fractions, multiply the numerators and then the denominators. Always reduce the fractions.

SAMPLE PROBLEM $2\frac{1}{2} \times 1\frac{3}{4} \times 3\frac{1}{3}$

Convert the whole numbers to improper fractions:

$$\frac{(2 \times 2) + 1}{2} = \frac{5}{2}$$

$$\frac{(1 \times 4) + 3}{4} = \frac{7}{4}$$

$$\frac{(3 \times 3) + 1}{3} = \frac{10}{3}$$

Substitute the improper fractions for the mixed numbers:

$$\frac{5 \times 7 \times 10}{2 \times 4 \times 3}$$

Multiply the numerators:
Multiply the denominators:

$$\frac{5 \times 7 \times 10}{2 \times 4 \times 3} = \frac{350}{24}$$

Reduce the improper fraction:

$$\frac{\overset{175}{\cancel{350}}}{\underset{12}{\cancel{24}}}$$

$$\begin{array}{r} 14\frac{7}{12} \\ 12\overline{)175} \\ \underline{12} \\ 55 \\ \underline{48} \\ 7 \end{array}$$

Before multiplying whole numbers by fractions, the whole numbers must be converted into fractions. Remember, a whole number can be written over the implied 1 without changing its value.

SAMPLE PROBLEM $2 \times \frac{3}{10}$

Convert the 2 to $\frac{2}{1}$:

$$\frac{2 \times 3}{1 \times 10}$$

Multiply the numerators:
Multiply the denominators:

$$\frac{2 \times 3}{1 \times 10} = \frac{6}{10}$$

Reduce the fraction:

$$\frac{\overset{3}{\cancel{6}}}{\underset{5}{\cancel{10}}} = \frac{3}{5}$$

Often, multiplication is easier when canceling is done first. The larger the numbers being multiplied, the greater the chance of error. Canceling reduces the size of the numbers, but does not change the value.

SAMPLE PROBLEM $2\frac{1}{2} \times \frac{3}{5} \times \frac{2}{9} \times 2\frac{1}{4}$

Convert the mixed numbers to improper fractions:

$$\frac{(2 \times 2) + 1}{2} = \frac{5}{2}$$

$$\frac{(2 \times 4) + 1}{4} = \frac{9}{4}$$

Substitute the improper fractions for the mixed numbers and set up the equation:

$$\frac{5 \times 3 \times 2 \times 9}{2 \times 5 \times 9 \times 4}$$

Cancel by dividing both the numerator and denominator by 5 (marked with the right-to-left diagonal slash), then by 2 (left-to-right diagonal slash), and finally by 9 (horizontal slash).

$$\frac{\overset{1}{\cancel{5}} \times 3 \times \overset{1}{\cancel{2}} \times \overset{1}{\cancel{9}}}{\underset{1}{\cancel{2}} \times \underset{1}{\cancel{5}} \times \underset{1}{\cancel{9}} \times 4}$$

Multiply the new numerators:
Multiply the new denominators:

$$\frac{1 \times 3 \times 1 \times 1}{1 \times 1 \times 1 \times 4} = \frac{3}{4}$$

Multiplication prior to canceling would have resulted in the fraction $\frac{270}{360}$. Solving the problem either way is correct. Some people are confused by canceling; others find it easier than the long-multiplication process.

PRACTICE PROBLEMS

Multiplication of Fractions

Multiply the following whole numbers, fractions, and mixed numbers. Reduce the products to their lowest terms. Show all your work. (Check your answers on page 313.)

31. $\frac{1}{4} \times \frac{3}{5} \times \frac{1}{3}$

34. $3\frac{1}{4} \times \frac{2}{5} \times 4$

32. $2\frac{1}{2} \times 1\frac{3}{8} \times 6\frac{1}{3}$

35. $\frac{1}{3} \times \frac{1}{3} \times \frac{1}{3}$

33. $3 \times \frac{1}{3} \times 1\frac{3}{16}$

DIVISION OF FRACTIONS

Before discussing division of fractions, it is important to understand the terminology of division.

> Remember: The dividend ÷ the divisor = the quotient
>
> $$\text{divisor}\,\overline{)\,\text{dividend}}^{\,\text{quotient}} \qquad \text{or} \qquad \frac{\text{dividend}}{\text{divisor}} = \text{quotient}$$

Note that in the example on the right, the dividend is the numerator and the divisor is the denominator.

Division is accomplished by inverting the divisor. This means that the numerator and denominator of the divisor are transposed. Then the numerators are multiplied and the denominators are multiplied.

$$\frac{\text{numerator of dividend}}{\text{denominator of dividend}} \div \frac{\text{numerator of divisor}}{\text{denominator of divisor}} = \frac{\text{numerator of dividend}}{\text{denominator of dividend}} \times \frac{\text{denominator of divisor}}{\text{numerator of divisor}}$$

SAMPLE PROBLEM $\quad \frac{1}{3} \div \frac{2}{3}$

Invert the numerator and denominator of divisor:

$$\frac{2}{3} \text{ becomes } \frac{3}{2}$$

Change the function sign (from ÷ to ×):

$$\frac{1}{3} \times \frac{3}{2}$$

Multiply the numerators:
Multiply the denominators:

$$\frac{1 \times 3}{3 \times 2} = \frac{3}{6}$$

Reduce the fraction:

$$\frac{\overset{1}{\cancel{3}}}{\underset{2}{\cancel{6}}} = \frac{1}{2}$$

Mixed numbers cannot be divided until they are converted to improper fractions. Remember, to find the numerator of the improper fraction, multiply the whole number by the denominator and add the existing numerator. The denominator remains the same.

SAMPLE PROBLEM $\quad 1\frac{1}{2} \div \frac{3}{8}$

Convert the mixed number to improper fraction:

$$\frac{(1 \times 2) + 1}{2} = \frac{3}{2}$$

Invert the divisor fraction:

$$\frac{3}{8} \text{ becomes } \frac{8}{3}$$

Change the function sign to multiply:

$$\frac{3}{2} \times \frac{8}{3}$$

Multiply the numerators:
Multiply the denominators:

$$\frac{3 \times 8}{2 \times 3} = \frac{24}{6}$$

Reduce the fraction:

$$\frac{\overset{4}{\cancel{24}}}{\underset{1}{\cancel{6}}} = 4$$

Before dividing whole numbers by fractions or fractions by whole numbers, the whole numbers must be converted to fractions. Remember, a whole number can be expressed as a fraction by writing it over the implied 1.

SAMPLE PROBLEM $2 \div \frac{2}{5}$

Convert the whole number to a fraction: $2 = \frac{2}{1}$

Invert the divisor fraction: $\frac{2}{5}$ becomes $\frac{5}{2}$

Change the function sign to multiply: $\frac{2}{1} \times \frac{5}{2}$

Multiply the numerators:
Multiply the denominators: $\dfrac{2 \times 5}{1 \times 2} = \dfrac{10}{2}$

Reduce the fraction: $\dfrac{10}{2} = 5$

This problem could have been solved by canceling after the divisor was inverted and the func-
tion sign changed. $\dfrac{\overset{1}{\cancel{2}} \times 5}{1 \times \cancel{2}} = \dfrac{5}{1} = 5$

PRACTICE PROBLEMS

Division of Fractions

Divide the following fractions, whole numbers, and mixed numbers. Reduce the quotients to
their lowest terms. Show all your work. (Check your answers on page 313.)

36. $2\frac{1}{3} \div \frac{6}{7}$ 39. $\frac{3}{8} \div 1\frac{1}{3}$

37. $\frac{1}{3} \div \frac{1}{3}$ 40. $\frac{3}{7} \div 3$

38. $6 \div \frac{1}{8}$

SELF-ASSESSMENT POSTTEST

Fractions

Show all your work. (Check your answers on page 349.)
Write the following as common fractions.

1. Two and thirty-eight seventy-fifths   3. Sixty-seven thousandths

2. Three twenty-fifths   4. 1:5

Find the least common denominators for these fractions.

5. $\frac{1}{7}, \frac{1}{8}, \frac{1}{4}$

6. $\frac{7}{10}, \frac{4}{5}, \frac{3}{4}$

Add the following fractions and mixed numbers. Reduce answers to their lowest terms.

7. $3\frac{1}{4} + 1\frac{1}{2} + 4\frac{2}{3} + 1\frac{5}{6}$

8. $\frac{5}{8} + \frac{3}{4} + \frac{7}{16} + \frac{1}{2}$

Subtract the following fractions and mixed numbers. Reduce answers to their lowest terms.

9. $\frac{8}{9} - \frac{1}{2}$

11. $3\frac{1}{8} - 1\frac{1}{2}$

10. $5\frac{5}{7} - 3\frac{20}{21}$

12. $1\frac{5}{8} - \frac{3}{4}$

Multiply the following fractions and mixed numbers. Reduce answers to their lowest terms.

13. $\frac{1}{3} \times \frac{1}{4} \times \frac{2}{3}$

15. $2\frac{1}{2} \times \frac{1}{6} \times 4\frac{1}{3}$

14. $3 \times \frac{2}{3} \times \frac{1}{3}$

16. $\frac{1}{6} \times 1\frac{1}{2} \times 4$

Divide the following fractions and mixed numbers. Reduce answers to their lowest terms.

17. $\frac{1}{4} \div \frac{1}{4}$

19. $6 \div 1\frac{1}{3}$

18. $\frac{1}{4} \div 4$

20. $2\frac{1}{2} \div \frac{1}{6}$

Chapter 3

Decimal Fractions

Americans use decimal fractions every day. Our monetary system is based on the decimal system, and health care professionals encounter decimals when using metric measurements.

A decimal fraction is a part of a whole measured in tenths or powers of tenths, such as hundredths or thousandths. A power of a number means multiplying the number by itself the number of times indicated by the power: 0.1 to the first power (0.1^1) means the number itself, or 0.1, while 0.1 to the second power (0.1^2) means 0.1 multiplied by 0.1, or 0.01. The number 10^2 is 10 times 10.

The decimal fraction is indicated by the decimal point, which separates the whole number from the fractional part. All numbers to the left of the decimal points are read as whole numbers, while the numbers to the right of the decimal point are the decimal fraction. A whole number without a decimal fraction may be written with or without an ending decimal point. The decimal point is implied at the end of any whole number. The whole number also can be followed by a decimal point and several zeroes without changing the number's value.

Examples: One dollar can be written as $1 or as $1.00, and
24 is the same as 24., 24.0 or 24.00.

A decimal fraction without a whole number is usually written with a zero preceding the decimal point. It is not incorrect to omit the zero, but less confusion results if the zero precedes the decimal point, especially when writing decimal fractions by hand.

Examples: 0.25 $0.25

Zeroes at the end of a decimal fraction have no value and may be dropped without affecting the value of the decimal fraction. Zeroes to the right of the decimal point followed by a numeral may not be dropped because doing so changes the value of the decimal fraction.

Examples: 0.00200 is the same as 0.002 or 0.0020.
0.002 is not the same as 0.02 or 0.2.

The number to the immediate right of the decimal point is in the tenths position. The second position to the right of the decimal point is the hundredths position. This is depicted graphically on the scale in Figure 3-1.

A decimal fraction is read as the number followed by the position of the last number in the decimal. Therefore, the decimal 0.0005, in which the last number is in the ten-thousandths position, is read as five ten-thousandths. Sometimes the word *point* is used to indicate the decimal, and the decimal fraction numerals are read. In this case, 0.0005 might be read as zero point zero zero zero five.

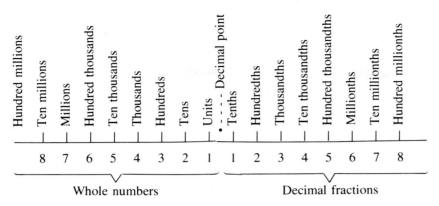

FIGURE 3-1. Decimal fractions scale. (*From Verovoren, T.M., and Oppeneer, J.E.: Workbook of solutions and dosage of drugs, ed. 12, St. Louis, 1983, The C.V. Mosby Co.*)

Examples: 0.05 is read as five hundredths, five one-hundredths, or zero point zero five. Written as a common fraction, 0.05 is $\frac{5}{100}$ or $\frac{1}{20}$.

0.204 is read as two hundred four thousandths, two hundred four one-thousandths, or zero point two zero four.
Written as a common fraction, 0.204 is $\frac{204}{1000}$ or $\frac{51}{250}$.

To read a mixed decimal number, one containing a whole number and a decimal fraction, the whole number is followed by the word *and*, to indicate the decimal point, and the decimal fraction.

Examples: 12.06 is read as twelve and six-hundredths, twelve and six one-hundredths, or twelve point zero six.

2.246 is read as two and two-hundred-forty-six thousandths, two and two-hundred-forty-six one-thousandths, or two point two four six.

CONVERSIONS BETWEEN COMMON FRACTIONS AND DECIMALS

Remember: $\dfrac{\text{quotient}}{\text{divisor}\,)\,\text{dividend}}$ is the same as $\dfrac{\text{dividend}}{\text{divisor}}$ or $\dfrac{\text{numerator}}{\text{denominator}} = \text{quotient}$

To change a common fraction into a decimal, divide the numerator by the denominator. Conversion of a proper fraction will result in a number less than one, while conversion of an improper fraction will result in a number greater than 1.

Converting a common fraction to a decimal fraction = the numerator ÷ the denominator.

SAMPLE PROBLEM   **Change $\frac{1}{4}$ to a decimal fraction.**

Divide the numerator by the denominator: $4\overline{)\,1}$

Add the decimal point following the dividend: $4\overline{)\,1.}$

Place a decimal point in the quotient above the
decimal point in the dividend: $4\overline{)\,\overset{.}{1.}}$

Divide. Add zeros to the dividend as needed.

$$
\begin{array}{r}
0.25 \\
4\,\overline{)\,1.00} \\
\underline{8} \\
20 \\
20 \\
0
\end{array}
$$

Therefore, $\frac{1}{4}$ is equal to 0.25, as depicted in Figure 3-2.

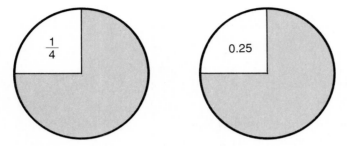

FIGURE 3-2. The relationship between $\frac{1}{4}$ and 0.25

SAMPLE PROBLEM   **Change $\frac{92}{15}$ to a mixed decimal fraction.**

Divide the numerator by the denominator:

$$
\begin{array}{r}
6.1\overline{3} \\
15\,\overline{)\,92.00} \\
\underline{90} \\
2\,0 \\
\underline{1\,5} \\
50 \\
\underline{45} \\
5
\end{array}
$$

The line above the three in the decimal indicates that the 3 is a repeating number. The remainder when dividing 50 by 15 is 5, which will become 50 when the zero is brought down. This could happen ad infinitim, or indefinitely. The line above a repeating number is used only with decimal fractions, never with whole numbers.

To change mixed numbers to decimal fractions, only the fraction portion of the mixed number is changed. The fraction is converted to a decimal, and its quotient is added to the whole number.

Conversion of mixed number to decimal fraction	=	existing whole number	+	quotient of the conversion of the fraction to a decimal

The fraction $\frac{1}{4}$ was changed to 0.25 in the first sample problem in this chapter.

SAMPLE PROBLEM   **Change $1\frac{1}{4}$ to a decimal.**

The whole number remains the same and the $\frac{1}{4}$ is changed to a decimal.

$$1 + 0.25 = 1.25$$

To change a mixed number with an improper fraction to a decimal mixed number, add the existing whole number to the quotient obtained from converting the improper fraction to a decimal. The improper fraction $\frac{92}{15}$ was changed to 6.13 in the second sample problem.

SAMPLE PROBLEM   **Convert $5\frac{92}{15}$ to decimal.**

Add the whole number to the quotient obtained
from conversion of the fraction: $5 + 6.13 = 11.13$

Changing common fractions with denominators of 10 or powers of 10, such as
100 or 1000, to decimal fractions is very easy. To divide the numerator by the
denominator of 10 or any power of 10, move the decimal point in the numerator
one place to the left for each zero in the denominator. A place is the space between
the numbers and includes the space occupied by the decimal point. Simply write
the number of the numerator followed by the decimal point, then move the decimal
point the correct number of places to the left.

MULTIPLICATION AND DIVISION BY POWERS OF TEN

Multiplication: Numbers get larger as the decimal point is moved to the right.
Move the decimal point one place to the right for every zero in
the multiplier.

Division: Numbers get smaller as the decimal point is moved to left.
Move the decimal point one place to the left for each zero in
the divisor.

SAMPLE PROBLEM   **Change $\frac{62}{100}$ to a decimal fraction.**

Write the numerator with the implied decimal
point at the end of the number: 62.

The denominator 100 has two zeroes.

Move the decimal point two places to the left.   0.6 2.
                                                                    2 1

Therefore, $\frac{62}{100}$ is 0.62.

SAMPLE PROBLEM   **Convert $\frac{7}{1000}$ to a decimal.**

There are three zeroes in 1000. Move the decimal
point three spaces to the left.

To do this, zeroes must be placed in front of the   0.0 0 7.
seven.   3 2 1

Therefore, $\frac{7}{1000}$ is 0.007.

The caret (∧) is usually used to indicate the new position of the decimal point. The
previous decimal fraction would be expressed as:

0∧007.

When recording the conversion of common fractions to decimal fractions, however,
use the decimal point rather than the caret.

Decimals are often rounded to a particular position, such as the nearest hundredths. To round off a decimal to the nearest hundredths, consider the numeral
following the hundredths position, i.e., the thousandths position numeral. If the
numeral in the thousandths position is 5 or greater than 5, add 1 to the hundredths
numeral. If the numeral in the thousandths position is less than 5, nothing is added
to the hundredths numeral.

SAMPLE PROBLEM   **The answer to a problem is 6.1333333. Round off the decimal to the nearest thousandths.**

The Answer: 6.1333333

Identify the number in the ten-thousandths position:

3

3 is less than 5.

3 < 5

The number in the hundredths position is not changed if the number in the thousandths position number is less than 5.

6.133

Therefore, 6.1333333 rounded off to the nearest thousandth is 6.133.

SAMPLE PROBLEM   **The answer to a decimal problem is 3.05648. Round this to the nearest hundredth.**

The Answer: 3.05648

Identify the numeral in the thousandths place:

6

6 is greater than 5.

6 > 5

Add 1 to the hundredths position numeral:

3.05 + 0.01 = 3.06

Therefore, 3.05648 rounded to the nearest hundredths is 3.06.

Converting a decimal to a common fraction is very easy. Find the position of the last number of the decimal. That position (e.g., hundredths) is the denominator. The numeral becomes the numerator. Reduce the fraction to its lowest terms.

SAMPLE PROBLEM   **Convert 0.6875 to a common fraction.**

Write the numerals of the decimal in the numerator:

6875

The last numeral of the decimal is in the ten-thousandths position. Make this the denominator:

$\overline{10,000}$

Therefore, 0.6875 written as a fraction is $\frac{6875}{10,000}$.

$\frac{6875}{10,000}$

Reduce the fraction. Cancel with a series of fives:

11
$\cancel{55}$
$\cancel{275}$
$\cancel{1375}$
$\cancel{6875}$
$\cancel{10,000}$
$\cancel{2000}$
$\cancel{400}$
$\cancel{80}$
16

SAMPLE PROBLEM   **Convert 0.033 to a fraction.**

Write the numerals of the decimal in the
numerator: 33

Identify the position of the last numeral of the
decimal for the denominator: ‾‾‾‾
                                                       1000

Therefore, 0.033 is $\frac{33}{1000}$, which cannot be
reduced. $\frac{33}{1000}$

PRACTICE PROBLEMS

Conversion between Common Fractions and Decimal Fractions

Change the following common fractions to decimal fractions. Round the answers to the nearest thousandths. Show all your work. (Check your answers on page 313.)

1. $\frac{3}{12}$

3. $2\frac{4}{9}$

2. $\frac{4}{1000}$

Convert the following decimals to fractions.

4. 0.326

5. 0.15

ADDITION OF DECIMALS

Adding decimals requires that the decimals be written so that each decimal point is in line with the one below it. Addition is then accomplished as for whole numbers.

SAMPLE PROBLEM   **Add 25 + 2.05 + 2.005 + 200.50.**

25.	25.000
2.05	2.050
2.005	2.005
200.50	200.500
229.555	229.555

The example at the right is the same as the one on the left. Writing zeroes at the end of the decimals helps keep the columns straight and makes addition easier.

PRACTICE PROBLEMS

Addition of Decimals

Show all your work. (Check your answers on page 314.)

6. $102 + 1.02 + 10.2$

9. $1.03 + 5.2 + 3.13$

7. $1.05 + 10 + 10.30$

10. $13.6 + 18.25 + 2.003$

8. $16.9 + 19.243 + 170.23 + 1.982$

SUBTRACTION OF DECIMALS

Placing the decimal points in line is as important in the subtraction of decimals as in addition. Once the decimals are in line, subtract as with whole numbers.

SAMPLE PROBLEM $204 - 193.004$

$$
\begin{array}{r}
204. \\
-193.004 \\
\hline
10.996
\end{array}
\qquad
\begin{array}{r}
1\ 3\ 99 \\
204.000 \\
-193.004 \\
\hline
10.996
\end{array}
$$

Inserting zeroes after the decimal in the whole number makes subtraction much easier since "borrowing" from the digit to the left is frequently involved. The example on the right shows the borrowing process.

PRACTICE PROBLEMS

Subtraction of Decimals

Show all your work. (Check your answers on page 314.)

11. $214.5 - 138.24$

12. $9.24 - 8.98$

13. 26.0 − 8.3333   15. 32.98 − 3.89

14. 3.1 − 1.0504

MULTIPLICATION OF DECIMALS

Decimals are multiplied in the same way as whole numbers. Once the numbers are multiplied, the decimal spaces are marked off.

Remember: Multiplicand × Multiplier = Product

To place the decimal point in the correct position, count the number of places after the decimal point in the multiplicand and then in the multiplier. A place is the space between the numbers and includes the space occupied by the decimal point. Always start with the decimal number in the far right position.

SAMPLE PROBLEM   **3.0602 × 4.2**

Multiply the numbers:

$$
\begin{array}{r}
3.0602 \\
\times\ 4.2 \\
\hline
61204 \\
122408\ \\
\hline
1285284
\end{array}
$$

Count the decimal spaces after the decimal point: The multiplicand has four places.

3.0 6 0 2
4 3 2 1

The multiplier has one place for a total of five.

4.2
5

Place the decimal in the fifth space from the right in the answer.

12.8 5 2 8 4
5 4 3 2 1

The product of 3.0602 × 4.2 is 12.85284

PRACTICE PROBLEMS

Multiplication of Decimals

Show all your work. (Check your answers on page 314.)

16. 22.9 × 15   17. 4.0005 × 4.005

18. 6.000×0.34 20. 0.98×9.8

19. 1.02×25.2

DIVISION OF DECIMALS

Remember: $\text{divisor} \overline{)\text{dividend}}^{\text{quotient}}$ is the same as $\dfrac{\text{dividend}}{\text{divisor}}$ or $\dfrac{\text{numerator}}{\text{denominator}} = \text{quotient}$

Division of decimals is different from plain division when the divisor contains a decimal fraction. Prior to dividing, the divisor must be converted to a whole number by multiplying it by the power of 10 indicated by the position of the last decimal number. The same number is used to multiply the dividend so as not to change the value of the two numbers. Remember, the value of a fraction does not change when both the numerator (dividend) and denominator (divisor) are subjected to the same multiplication process.

To multiply by 10 or powers of 10, the decimal point is moved one place to the right for each zero in the multiplier.

Use the caret ($\wedge$) to indicate the new position of the decimal point.

SAMPLE PROBLEM   **Divide 26 by 2.006.**

Identify the position of the last digit in the decimal:

1000th position

Multiply the dividend by 1000:   2 6.0 0 0$_\wedge$

Multiply the divisor by 1000:   2.0 0 6$_\wedge$

$2.006_\wedge \overline{)2\,6.0\,0\,0_\wedge}$

Place the decimal point in the quotient:

$2006. \overline{)26000.}$

Divide, adding zeroes after decimal point as needed:

$$
\begin{array}{r}
12.961 \\
2006. \overline{)26000.000} \\
\underline{2006} \\
5940 \\
\underline{4012} \\
1928\,0 \\
\underline{1805\,4} \\
122\,60 \\
\underline{120\,36} \\
2\,240 \\
\underline{2\,006} \\
234
\end{array}
$$

The quotient is 12.961, or 12.96 if the divisor decimal is rounded off to the nearest hundredth.

SAMPLE PROBLEM   **Divide 162.058 by 2.81.**

Identify the position of the last digit in the divisor decimal: 100th position

Multiply the dividend by 100:   1 6 2.0 5ₐ8

Multiply the divisor by 100:   2.8 1ₐ   2.8 1ₐ$\overline{)\,1\ 6\ 2.0\ 5_\wedge 8}$

Place the decimal point in the quotient: 281.$\overline{)\,16205.8}$

Divide the problem:

$$
\begin{array}{r}
57.67 \\
281.\overline{)\,16205.80} \\
\underline{1405} \\
2155 \\
\underline{1967} \\
188\ 8 \\
\underline{168\ 6} \\
20\ 20 \\
\underline{19\ 67} \\
53
\end{array}
$$

The most common mistakes made in division of decimals:
(1) improper placement of the decimal point,
(2) improper placement of numerals in the quotient, and
(3) omission of necessary zeros in the quotient.

SAMPLE PROBLEM   **Divide 734.5836 by 30.6**

Ensure proper placement of the decimal in the quotient: 30.6ₐ$\overline{)\,734.5_\wedge 836}$

Divide the problem:

734 divided by 306 is 2. Place the 2 over the 4.
1225 divided by 306 is 4. Place the 4 over the 5.
18 divided by 306 is 0; place a 0 over the 8.
183 divided by 306 is 0; place a 0 over the 3.

$$
\begin{array}{r}
2\ 4.006 \\
30.6_\wedge\overline{)\,734.5_\wedge 836} \\
\underline{612} \\
122\ 5 \\
\underline{122\ 4} \\
1\ 8 \\
\underline{0} \\
1\ 83 \\
\underline{0} \\
1\ 836 \\
\underline{1\ 836} \\
0
\end{array}
$$

PRACTICE PROBLEMS

Division of Decimals

Divide the following decimals, rounding to the nearest hundredths. Show all your work. (Check your answers on page 314.)

21. $0.400 \div 0.25$

24. $26.8 \div 18.5$

22. $26.986 \div 15.4$

25. $560 \div 22.08$

23. $823 \div 25.06$

SELF-ASSESSMENT POSTTEST

Decimal Fractions

Write the following written numbers as decimal fractions. Show all your work. (Check your answers on page 350.)

1. Four ten-thousandths

2. Two and three hundredths

Convert the following fractions and mixed numbers to decimal fractions. Round the decimals to the nearest hundredths unless to do so results in a zero in the decimal.

3. $\frac{4}{10}$

5. $1\frac{7}{1000}$

4. $\frac{3}{7}$

6. $\frac{37}{12}$

Convert the following decimals to fractions or mixed numbers. Reduce the fractions to their lowest terms.

7. 0.016

8. 1.13

Add the following decimals.

9. 1.3087 + 1.63 + 4.631 + 4

10. 0.25 + 0.5 + 0.341 + 1.00

Subtract the following decimals.

11. 13.0896 − 6.10556

12. 1 − 0.534

Multiply the following decimals.

13. 2.54 × 3.2

15. 1.98 × 6.2

14. 0.06 × 0.005

16. 33.05 × 0.5

Divide the following decimals, rounding to the nearest thousandths.

17. 26 ÷ 0.05

19. $0.5\overline{)0.63487}$

18. $0.007\overline{)21.08724}$

20. $0.56\overline{)3.40000006}$

Chapter 4

Percentages

The word *percentage* is familiar to everyone. Sales taxes are percentages of the sale price; interest on home mortgages is a percentage of the balance owed. Health care professionals use percentages primarily with solutions.

Percent means hundredths of a whole. One percent is the equivalent of one hundredths or one one-hundredths of the whole. Therefore, 1% is the same as the fraction $\frac{1}{100}$ or the decimal fraction 0.01. Figure 4-1 shows the relationship of parts of a whole in fractions, decimals, and percentages.

The whole of anything is 1 or 100%. Therefore, percentages of less than 100 are parts of a whole and less than 1. Percentages greater than 100 are greater than a whole and greater than 1.

CONVERSION BETWEEN DECIMALS AND PERCENTAGES

To convert a decimal to a percentage, multiply the decimal by 100 and add the percent symbol %. To multiply by 100, move the decimal point two places to the right.

Remember: To multiply by 10 or any power of 10, move the decimal point one place to the right for each zero in the multiplier. To divide by 10 or any power of 10, move the decimal point one place to the left for each zero in the divisor.

SAMPLE PROBLEM   **Change 0.004 to a percentage.**

Multiply the decimal by 100 and add the percent symbol:

$$0.004 \times 100 = 0.4\%$$

Therefore, 0.004 is 0.4%

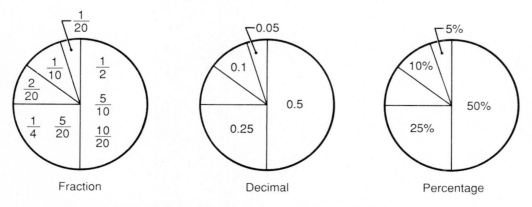

FIGURE 4-1. Relationship among fractions, decimals, and percents

SAMPLE PROBLEM   **Change 0.6 to a percentage.**

Multiply the decimal by 100 and add the percent
symbol:
$$0.6 \times 100 = 60\%$$

Therefore, 0.6 is 60%

Percentages are changed to decimals by dividing the percentage by 100.

SAMPLE PROBLEM   **Change 12.6% to a decimal.**

Divide the percentage by 100:
$$12.6 \div 100 = 0.126$$

Therefore, 12.6% equals 0.126

Sometimes percentages are written using mixed numbers such as $5\frac{1}{2}\%$. Technically this is incorrect; it is seen occasionally in connection with interest. The common fraction must be converted to a decimal fraction to convert percentages to decimals. There is no such thing as $0.05\frac{1}{2}$; it is correctly written 0.055.

Remember: To convert a fraction to a decimal, divide the numerator by the denominator. The decimal point is implied at the end of a whole number.

SAMPLE PROBLEM   **Convert $7\frac{1}{4}\%$ to a decimal.**

Divide the fraction numerator by the denominator and add the decimal fraction to the whole number:

$$7 + \frac{0.25}{4\overline{)1.00}} = 7.25\%$$
$$\underline{8}$$
$$20$$
$$\underline{20}$$
$$0$$

Divide the percentage by 100.
$$7.25 \div 100 = 0.0725$$

Therefore, $7\frac{1}{4}\%$ is equal to 0.0725.

PRACTICE PROBLEMS

Conversion between Decimals and Percentage

Show all your work. (Check your answers on page 315.) Convert the following decimals to percentages:

1. 0.42

3. 0.0275

2. 1.05

Convert the following percentages to decimals:

4. $13\frac{1}{2}\%$

5. $\frac{3}{4}\%$ (be careful!)

CONVERSION BETWEEN FRACTIONS AND PERCENTAGES

Fractions must be converted to decimals before they can be converted to percentages. Therefore, the fraction $\frac{1}{4}$ must be converted to 0.25 prior to converting it to 25%.

SAMPLE PROBLEM   **Convert $\frac{3}{8}$ to a percentage.**

Divide the numerator by the denominator.

$$
\begin{array}{r}
0.375 \\
8\,)\overline{3.000} \\
\underline{2\ 4} \\
60 \\
\underline{56} \\
40 \\
\underline{40} \\
0
\end{array}
$$

Multiply the decimal by 100.

$0.375 \times 100 = 37.5\%$

Therefore, $\frac{3}{8}$ is equal to 37.5%

Fractions with denominators of 100 can be converted by simply substituting the percentage symbol for 100 in the denominator. For example, $\frac{3}{100}$ is equal to 3%.

To convert a percentage to a fraction, substitute $\frac{1}{100}$ for the percent symbol and reduce the fraction. Remember, percent means part of 100.

SAMPLE PROBLEM   **Convert 75% to a fraction.**

Substitute $\frac{1}{100}$ for the percent symbol

$75\% = \frac{75}{100}$

Reduce the fraction to its lowest terms

$\dfrac{\overset{3}{\cancel{75}}}{\underset{4}{\cancel{100}}} = \dfrac{3}{4}$

If there is a decimal within the percentage, divide the percentage by 100 to obtain the decimal. Then write the decimal as a fraction and reduce it to its lowest terms.

SAMPLE PROBLEM   **Convert 7.5% to a fraction.**

Divide the percentage by 100:

$7.5 \div 100 = 0.075$

The last digit of the decimal is in the thousandths position.

$\overline{1000}$

Write the decimal as a fraction:

$0.075 = \dfrac{75}{1000}$

Reduce the fraction to its lowest terms:

$\dfrac{\overset{3}{\cancel{75}}}{\underset{40}{\cancel{1000}}} = \dfrac{3}{40}$

7.5% is equal to $\frac{3}{40}$.

PRACTICE PROBLEMS

Conversion between Fractions and Percentages

Show all your work. (Check your answers on page 315.) Convert the following fractions to percentages.

6. $\frac{6}{7}$

8. $\frac{7}{10}$

7. $\frac{2}{15}$

Convert the following percentages to fractions.

9. 12%

10. 55%

PERCENTAGES OF NUMBERS

Finding the percentage of a number is accomplished by multiplying the number by the percentage. Since percentages cannot be multiplied until they have been converted to decimal fractions, this must be accomplished first. Therefore, convert the percentage to a decimal and multiply the number by the resulting decimal. Thus, 10% of 100 is the same as 100 multiplied by 0.10 or 0.1.

Remember, to correctly place the decimal in the product of multiplication, count the number of decimal places from the right in the multiplicand and in the multiplier. Count the same number of places from the right in the product and insert the decimal.

SAMPLE PROBLEM **Find 3% of 50.**

Convert 3% to a decimal: $3 \div 100 = 0.03$

Multiply the number by the decimal: $50 \times 0.03 = 1.5$

3% of 50 is 1.5

SAMPLE PROBLEM **Find 45% of 278.**

Convert the percentage to a decimal. $45 \div 100 = 0.45$

Multiply the number by the decimal.
$$\begin{array}{r} 278 \\ \times 0.45 \\ \hline 13\ 90 \\ 111\ 2\ \\ \hline 125.10 \end{array}$$

Therefore, 45% of 278 is 125.1

Some problems are expressed with words rather than with numbers alone. Word problems need to be deciphered before they can be solved. First, determine for what the problem asks. Then the problem is examined for those elements needed to calculate the answer.

SAMPLE PROBLEM   **The interest on a savings account is 5.5% per year. What is the yearly interest on a savings account containing $100.00?**

This problem asks for the dollar value of a percentage, 5.5%, of an amount, $100.00. To find this, the percentage, 5.5%, and the original amount, $100.00, are needed.

Convert the percent to a decimal: $5.5 \div 100 = 0.055$

Multiply the amount and the decimal: $\$100 \times 0.055 = \$5.50$

Therefore, 5.5% of $100 is $5.50.

There are some instances in which percentages greater than 100% are used. If productivity increases 25% this would mean that the original rate (100%) plus 25% of the original rate is the new rate of productivity. Another way to say this would be that the new productivity is 125% of the old productivity.

Consider the state sales tax. A 7% sales tax is collected on an item of clothing that costs $9.99. This means that 7% of the cost of this $9.99 article is added to the whole (100%). In other words, the actual cost to the consumer is 107% of $9.99.

SAMPLE PROBLEM   **A company routinely produces 115 cogs per day. If this amount were increased 20%, how many cogs would be produced each day?**

This problem asks for the total number of cogs.
This problem can be solved two ways: (1) Find the percentage of the whole (20% × 115) and add it to the whole (115).

This can be written mathematically as follows: $(115 \times 20\%) + 115 =$ _____ cogs

The parentheses indicate the portion to be solved
first. Convert percentage to a decimal: $20\% \div 100 = 0.20$ or 0.2

Multiply the decimal times the number: $115 \times 0.2 = 23.0$

Add the product to the number: $23 + 115 = 138$ cogs

(2) Add the percent of the whole and the percentage of increase (100% + 20%) and multiply that amount by the whole (115).

This can be written mathematically as follows: $(100\% + 20\%) \times 115 =$ _____ cogs

Add the percentages: $100\% + 20\% = 120\%$

Convert the fraction to a decimal: $120\% \div 100 = 1.2$

Multiply the decimal times the number: $1.2 \times 115 =$ _____ cogs

$$
\begin{array}{r}
115 \\
\times\, 1.2 \\
\hline
23\,0 \\
115 \\
\hline
138.0
\end{array}
$$

A 20% increase in productivity of 115 cogs per day means that 138 cogs are produced daily.

This problem is repeated in the next unit. The dimensional analysis method, a different way to solve the problem, is shown there.

PRACTICE PROBLEMS

Percentages of Numbers

Show all your work. (Check your answers on page 315.) Find the quantities of the following:

11. 20% of 120

13. $12\frac{1}{2}\%$ of 100

12. 2% of 21

Find the quantities of the following word problems:

14. The interest rate of a savings account is 6% per year. The account contains $250.35. What is the new amount after the interest has been added to the account?

15. A company produces 1260 computer parts each week. How many more computer parts need to be produced each week to bring about a 10% increase?

SELF-ASSESSMENT POSTTEST

Percentages

(Answers on page 350.) Convert the following decimals to percentages:

1. 0.27

3. 0.13

2. 1.055

4. 0.44

Convert the following percentages to decimals:

5. 7.5%

6. 28%

Convert the following fractions to percentages:

7. $\frac{27}{100}$

9. $\frac{3}{5}$

8. $\frac{18}{21}$

10. $\frac{11}{20}$

Convert the following percentages to fractions:

11. 16%

12. 18%

Find the quantities of the following:

13. 15% of 200

16. 8% of 150

14. 25% of 15

17. 105% of 400

15. 33% of 60

18. 30% of 6

Find the quantities of the following word problems. Round off the answer to the nearest cent (the same as the nearest hundredth).

19. A blouse costs $19.95. The sales tax is $6\frac{3}{8}$%. What is the amount of sales tax for this garment?

20. What is the total cost of the $19.95 blouse, including the $6\frac{3}{8}$% sales tax?

Chapter 5

Equations Written as Fractions

Equations written as fractions are used to solve problems throughout this workbook. Multiplication of fractions in Chapter 3 was accomplished by writing each individual fraction in a series, using one line to separate the numerators and denominators. In this chapter, the equations include fractions, decimals, whole numbers, and mixed numbers. Equations in this chapter are set up and ready to be solved. In later chapters, the equations need to be set up before being solved.

The use of the fraction form of equation for problem solving aids the visualization of processes peculiar to fractions. The following equation is nothing more than a series of fractions—$\frac{1}{2}$, $\frac{5}{3}$, $\frac{6}{1}$, and $\frac{20}{4}$—that are to be multiplied together.

$$\text{Example:} \quad \frac{1 \times 5 \times 6 \times 20}{2 \times 3 \times 1 \times 4}$$

Once the fractions are written in this long equation, they are treated as a single fraction. The numerator and denominator can be subjected to the same processes as any single fraction.

To solve the equation, the numerators are multiplied together, then the denominators. The last step is the division of the numerator by the denominator. Cancellation can be done prior to the multiplication of the numerators and denominators. Remember, canceling is nothing more than dividing both the numerator and denominator by the same number. The following equation is solved both ways. The direction of the slash marks indicates the individual cancellations.

SAMPLE PROBLEM $\dfrac{1 \times 5 \times 6 \times 20}{2 \times 3 \times 1 \times 4}$

$$\frac{1 \times 5 \times 6 \times 20}{2 \times 3 \times 1 \times 4} = \frac{30 \times 20}{6 \times 4} = \frac{600}{24}$$

$$= 24 \overline{)600} \\ \quad \underline{48} \\ \quad 120 \\ \quad \underline{120} \\ \quad \quad 0$$

$$\frac{1 \times 5 \times \cancel{6} \times \cancel{20}}{\cancel{2} \times \cancel{3} \times 1 \times \cancel{4}} = \frac{25}{1} = 25$$

Cancellation reduces the size of the numbers, making multiplication and division easier. The process of cancellation can be confusing, but it saves a lot of time. Making the slashes in opposite directions as done in the example reduces the confusion. Be careful when multiplying the numerator and denominator after cancellation. It is easy to miss multiplication of one of the numerals. Cancellation also can be done after the numerator and denominator have been multiplied. Practice canceling on these problems.

PRACTICE PROBLEMS

Multiplication Equations

Show all your work. (Check your answers on page 315.)

1. $\dfrac{5 \times 3 \times 6 \times 5}{2 \times 10 \times 5 \times 15}$

4. $\dfrac{8 \times 16 \times 24 \times 9}{6 \times 27 \times 4 \times 5}$

2. $\dfrac{3 \times 12 \times 5 \times 16}{10 \times 4 \times 6 \times 6}$

5. $\dfrac{6 \times 5 \times 120 \times 60}{1 \times 25 \times 45 \times 3}$

3. $\dfrac{2 \times 7 \times 25 \times 9}{6 \times 3 \times 21 \times 20}$

EQUATIONS WITH FRACTIONS IN THE NUMERATORS AND/OR DENOMINATORS

Fractions that have fractions in the numerator and/or the denominator are called *complex fractions*. Some equations have common fractions or mixed numbers in the numerator and/or the denominator. These pose special problems when the equations are written as long fractions. Fractions in the numerator or denominator cannot be canceled easily; therefore, multiplication of the numerators or denominators results in answers that are complex fractions. This means that multiplication and division are done several times before the problem is solved.

SAMPLE PROBLEM $\quad \dfrac{\frac{1}{4} \times 3 \times 12 \times 11}{1 \times 2 \times 13 \times 9}$

Cancel and multiply:

$$\dfrac{\frac{1}{4} \times \overset{1}{\cancel{3}} \times \overset{\overset{2}{\cancel{6}}}{\cancel{12}} \times 11}{1 \times \underset{1}{\cancel{2}} \times 13 \times \underset{\underset{1}{\cancel{3}}}{\cancel{9}}} = \dfrac{\frac{1}{4} \times 1 \times 2 \times 11}{1 \times 1 \times 13 \times 1}$$

Multiply the numerator:
Multiply the denominator:

$$\dfrac{\frac{1 \times 1 \times 2 \times 11}{4 \times 1 \times 1 \times 1}}{1 \times 1 \times 13 \times 1} = \dfrac{\frac{22}{4}}{13} = \dfrac{\frac{11}{2}}{13}$$

Divide the numerator of the fraction by the denominator of the fraction:

$$\frac{11}{2} = 5\frac{1}{2} \text{ or } 5.5$$

Divide the numerator of the equation by the denominator of the equation:

$$\frac{5.5}{13} = \quad 13\overline{)\begin{array}{l} 0.423 \\ 5.500 \end{array}}$$

$$\begin{array}{r} 5\,2 \\ \hline 30 \\ 26 \\ \hline 40 \\ 39 \\ \hline 1 \end{array}$$

This complicated process can be simplified by dropping the denominator of the fraction in the numerator to the denominator of the equation. In other words, the 4 in the denominator of the fraction $\frac{1}{4}$ in the numerator of the previous equation can be dropped to the denominator of the equation fraction. The 4 is then multiplied with the denominator. This saves one division step. The previous equation solved in this manner would be as follows:

$$\frac{1/4 \times 3 \times 12 \times 11}{1 \times 2 \times 13 \times 9} = \frac{1}{4 \times 1 \times 2 \times 13 \times 9} = \frac{1}{1 \times 1 \times 2 \times 13 \times 1} = \frac{11}{26} = 0.423$$

This problem also could have been solved by converting the fraction to a decimal. It is simple to convert $\frac{1}{4}$ to a decimal, but it results in a decimal that is more difficult to multiply than the whole numbers of a fraction. Some fractions are not as easy to convert to decimals because they require longer division or result in quotients that could go on indefinitely. The following problem on the left is solved by converting the fraction to a decimal. The problem on the right is solved by dropping the fraction denominator in the equation numerator into the denominator. It is obvious that the solution on the right is much easier and requires fewer steps.

SAMPLE PROBLEM
$$\frac{3/16 \times 8 \times 4 \times 30}{2 \times 9 \times 5 \times 1}$$

Convert fraction to decimal:
Drop the fraction denominator
in the right equation. Cancel.

$$16\overline{)\begin{array}{l} 0.1875 \\ 3.0000 \end{array}}$$

$$\begin{array}{r} 1\,6 \\ \hline 1\,40 \\ 1\,28 \\ \hline 120 \\ 112 \\ \hline 80 \\ 80 \\ \hline 0 \end{array}$$

$$\frac{3 \times 8 \times 4 \times 30}{16 \times 2 \times 9 \times 5 \times 1}$$

Substitute the decimal for the fraction in the left
equation. Cancel.

$$\frac{0.1875 \times 8 \times 4 \times 30}{2 \times 9 \times 5 \times 1}$$

Multiply the numerators:
Multiply the denominators:

$$\frac{0.1875 \times 4 \times 4 \times 2}{1 \times 3 \times 1 \times 1}$$

$$\frac{1 \times 1 \times 1 \times 2}{1 \times 1 \times 1 \times 1 \times 1 \times 1}$$

$$= \frac{2}{1} = 2$$

$$\begin{array}{r} 0.1875 \\ \times \quad 4 \\ \hline 0.7500 \\ \times \quad 4 \\ \hline 3.00 \end{array} \times 2 = \frac{6}{3} = 2$$

The following problem has a proper fraction in the numerator. The example on the left solves the problem without dropping the fraction denominator into the equation denominator; the one on the right shows the denominator of the fraction dropped into the denominator of the equation prior to cancellation. The solution on the right requires fewer steps and is easier.

SAMPLE PROBLEM $\dfrac{1/4 \times 3 \times 6 \times 2}{1 \times 2 \times 5 \times 9}$

Drop fraction denominator and cancel:

$$\frac{1/4 \times \overset{1}{\cancel{3}} \times \overset{2}{\cancel{6}} \times \overset{1}{\cancel{2}}}{1 \times \underset{1}{\cancel{2}} \times 5 \times \underset{3}{\cancel{9}}}$$

$$\frac{\overset{1}{\cancel{4}} \times \overset{1}{\cancel{}} \times \overset{\overset{1}{\cancel{2}}}{\cancel{3}} \times \overset{2}{\cancel{6}} \times \overset{1}{\cancel{2}}}{\underset{2}{\cancel{4}} \times 1 \times \underset{1}{\cancel{2}} \times 5 \times \underset{3}{\cancel{9}}}$$

Multiply the numerators:
Multiply the denominators:

$$\frac{1/4 \times 1 \times 2 \times 1}{1 \times 1 \times 5 \times 1}$$

$$\frac{1 \times 1 \times 1 \times 1}{2 \times 1 \times 1 \times 5 \times 1} = \frac{1}{10}$$

$$\frac{\frac{1 \times 1 \times 2 \times 1}{4 \times 1 \times 1 \times 1}}{1 \times 1 \times 5 \times 1} = \frac{\frac{2}{4}}{5}$$

$$\frac{\frac{2}{4}}{5} = \frac{\frac{1}{2}}{5} = \frac{0.5}{5}$$

Divide the numerator by the denominator:

$$5\overline{)0.5}^{\,0.1}$$

$$\frac{1}{10} = 0.1$$

The next problem has a mixed number in the numerator. Dropping the fraction denominator to the equation denominator cannot be done directly with mixed numbers. Mixed numbers must be converted into improper fractions before dropping the fraction denominator to the equation denominator.

Remember, to convert a mixed number to an improper fraction, multiply the whole number by the denominator and add the existing numerator. This number becomes the new numerator. The denominator remains the same.

$$\frac{(\text{Whole Number} \times \text{Denominator}) + \text{Existing Numerator}}{\text{Denominator}} = \frac{\text{New Numerator}}{\text{Denominator}}$$

Once the mixed number is converted to the improper fraction, the fraction denominator can be dropped to the equation denominator.

SAMPLE PROBLEM $\dfrac{3\frac{1}{2}\times\ 4\times 6\times 2}{3\times 12\times 8\times 7}$

Convert mixed number to improper fraction.

$$\dfrac{7/2\times\ 4\times 6\times 2}{3\times 12\times 8\times 7}$$

Drop the fraction denominator into the equation denominator. Cancel.

$$\dfrac{\overset{1}{\cancel{7}}\quad\times\ \overset{1}{\cancel{4}}\times\overset{\overset{1}{\cancel{6}}}{\cancel{6}}\times\overset{1}{\cancel{2}}}{\underset{1}{\cancel{2}}\times 3\times\underset{\underset{1}{3}}{\cancel{12}}\times\underset{4}{\cancel{8}}\times\underset{1}{\cancel{7}}}$$

Multiply the numerator:
Multiply the denominator:

$$\dfrac{1\quad\times 1\times 1\times 1}{1\times 3\times 1\times 4\times 1}=\dfrac{1}{12}$$

Divide the numerator by the denominator:

$$\begin{array}{r}0.083\\ 12\overline{)1.000}\end{array}=0.08 \text{ rounded to the nearest hundredth.}$$

$$\begin{array}{r}\underline{0}\\ 1\,00\\ \underline{96}\\ 40\\ \underline{36}\\ 4\end{array}$$

PRACTICE PROBLEMS

Equations with Fractions in Numerator

Show all your work. (Check your answers on page 315.)

6. $\dfrac{\frac{1}{2}\times 5\times 6\times\ 2}{1\times 4\times 7\times 15}$

9. $\dfrac{3/5\times 5\times\ 2\times 9}{1\times 4\times 18\times 1}$

7. $\dfrac{4\frac{2}{3}\times 30\times 9\times 2}{2\times\ 7\times 8\times 1}$

10. $\dfrac{6/7\times\ 5\times 9\times 30}{2\times 25\times 6\times\ 4}$

8. $\dfrac{1\frac{1}{4}\times 2\times 1\times 2}{1\times 3\times 5\times 1}$

EQUATIONS WITH FRACTIONS IN THE DENOMINATOR

Occasionally an equation will have a fraction in the denominator, which can be treated in the same manner as any divisor that is a fraction.

Remember, to divide by a fraction, invert the divisor and multiply.

$$\frac{\text{Numerator of Dividend}}{\text{Denominator of Dividend}} \div \frac{\text{Numerator of Divisor}}{\text{Denominator of Divisor}} = \frac{\text{Numerator of Dividend}}{\text{Denominator of Dividend}} \times \frac{\text{Denominator of Divisor}}{\text{Numerator of Divisor}}$$

For example, if the fraction $\frac{1}{2}$ is in the denominator of the equation fraction, it is inverted and the 2 is placed in the equation numerator.

SAMPLE PROBLEM $\dfrac{3\times\quad7\times16\times5}{8\times1/8\times21\times8}$

Invert the fraction in the denominator. Cancel.

$$\frac{\overset{1}{\cancel{3}}\times\overset{1}{\cancel{7}}\times\overset{\overset{1}{\cancel{2}}}{\cancel{16}}\times5}{\underset{1}{\cancel{8}}\times1/8\times\underset{\underset{1}{\cancel{7}}}{\cancel{21}}\times\underset{4}{\cancel{8}}}$$

$$\frac{\overset{1}{\cancel{3}}\times\overset{1}{\cancel{7}}\times\overset{1}{\cancel{8}}\times\overset{2}{\cancel{16}}\times5}{\underset{1}{\cancel{8}}\times1\times\underset{\underset{1}{\cancel{7}}}{\cancel{21}}\times8}$$

Multiply the numerators:
Multiply the denominators:

$$\frac{1\times1\;\times1\times5}{1\times1/8\times1\times4}=\qquad \frac{1\times1\times1\times2\times5}{1\times\quad1\times1\times1}=$$

$$\frac{\frac{1\times1\times1\times5}{1\times1\times1\times4}}{1\times8\times1\times1}=\frac{5}{4/8} \qquad \frac{10}{1}=10$$

$$=\frac{5}{1/2}=\frac{5}{1}\div\frac{1}{2}=\frac{5\times2}{1\times1}$$

$$=10$$

Mixed numbers must be converted to improper fractions prior to placing the fraction denominator in the equation numerator.

SAMPLE PROBLEM $\dfrac{5\times4\times\quad9\times11}{6\times5\times2\frac{1}{5}\times12}$

Convert the mixed number to an improper fraction:

$$\frac{(2\times5)+1}{5}=\frac{11}{5}$$

$$\frac{5\times4\times\quad9\times11}{6\times5\times11/5\times12}$$

Invert the improper fraction by placing the denominator in the equation numerator. Cancel.

$$\frac{\underset{1}{\cancel{5}}\times\overset{1}{\cancel{4}}\times\overset{1}{\cancel{9}}\times\;5\times\overset{1}{\cancel{11}}}{\underset{1}{\underset{3}{\cancel{6}}}\times\underset{1}{\cancel{5}}\times\quad\underset{1}{\cancel{11}}\times\underset{\underset{2}{6}}{\cancel{12}}}$$

Multiply the numerators
Multiply the denominators:

$$\frac{1\times1\times1\times5\times1}{1\times1\times\quad1\times2}=\frac{5}{2}=2\frac{1}{2}\;\text{ or }\;2.5$$

PRACTICE PROBLEMS

Equations with Fractions in the Denominator

Show all your work. (Check your answers on page 316.)

11. $\dfrac{4 \times\ 1 \times 18 \times 9}{1/6 \times 24 \times 27 \times 8}$

14. $\dfrac{5 \times 9 \times 15 \times 2}{2/3 \times 4 \times 60 \times 1}$

12. $\dfrac{9 \times 1 \times 8 \times 1}{3/4 \times 8 \times 7 \times 3}$

15. $\dfrac{2 \times 3 \times 6 \times 3}{1\frac{1}{2} \times 6 \times 9 \times 8}$

13. $\dfrac{1 \times\ 4 \times\ 7 \times\ 5}{3 \times 21 \times 10 \times 1\frac{4}{7}}$

EQUATIONS WITH FRACTIONS AND/OR DECIMALS

Sometimes both common fractions and decimal fractions are in the numerators or the denominators of equations. Canceling decimals is sometimes tricky. When canceling decimals, make sure the decimal point is in the correct place. It is very easy to lose decimal points when canceling. One way to get rid of decimals is to multiply both the numerator and denominator by 10 or powers of 10. Unfortunately, this creates large numbers in either the numerator or denominator.

SAMPLE PROBLEM $\dfrac{11 \times\ 1 \times 1 \times 3}{1 \times 2.2 \times 6 \times 5}$

Cancel:

$$\dfrac{\overset{1}{\cancel{11}} \times\ 1 \times 1 \times \overset{1}{\cancel{3}}}{1 \times \underset{0.2}{\cancel{2.2}} \times \underset{2}{\cancel{6}} \times 5}$$

Multiply the numerator:
Multiply the denominator:

$$\dfrac{1 \times\ 1 \times 1 \times 1}{1 \times 0.2 \times 2 \times 5} = 1/2 = 0.5$$

The following sample problems include decimals and fractions in the same equation.

SAMPLE PROBLEM $\dfrac{3\frac{7}{16} \times\ 1 \times 12 \times 1}{1 \times 2.2 \times\ 5 \times 6}$

Convert the mixed number to an improper fraction:

$$\dfrac{(3 \times 16) + 7}{16} = \dfrac{55}{16}$$

$$\dfrac{55/16 \times\ 1 \times 12 \times 1}{1 \times 2.2 \times\ 5 \times 6}$$

Drop the fraction denominator into the equation denominator. Cancel.

$$\frac{1 \quad\quad\quad 1}{\cancel{5}\quad\quad\quad\cancel{3}}$$

$$\frac{\cancel{55} \times 1 \times \cancel{12} \times 1}{\cancel{16} \times 1 \times \cancel{2.2} \times \cancel{5} \times \cancel{6}}$$
$$\quad 4 \quad\quad 0.2 \quad 1 \quad 2$$

Multiply the numerator:
Multiply the denominator:

$$\frac{1 \times \quad\quad 1 \times 1 \times 1}{4 \times 1 \times 0.2 \times 1 \times 2} = \frac{1}{1.6}$$

$$\begin{array}{r} 0.625 \\ 1.6\overline{)1.0000} \\ \underline{9\ 6} \\ 40 \\ \underline{32} \\ 80 \\ \underline{80} \end{array}$$

SAMPLE PROBLEM $\dfrac{1/6 \times 0.4 \times 100 \times \quad 8}{4 \times \quad 1 \times \quad 2 \times 2/3}$

Drop the fraction denominator into the equation denominator. Invert the fraction in the equation denominator by placing the fraction denominator in the numerator of the equation. Cancel.

$$\begin{array}{cccc} 0.1 & & 1 \\ \cancel{0.2} & & \cancel{2} & 1 \\ \frac{1 \quad \times \cancel{0.4} \times 100 \times \cancel{8} \times \cancel{3}}{\cancel{6} \times \cancel{4} \times \quad 1 \times \quad \cancel{2} \times \quad \cancel{2}} \\ \cancel{2} \quad 1 \quad\quad\quad 1 \quad\quad 1 \\ 1 \end{array}$$

Multiply the numerator:
Multiply the denominator:

$$\frac{1 \quad \times 0.1 \times 100 \times 1 \times 1}{1 \times 1 \times \quad 1 \times \quad 1 \times \quad 1} = \frac{10}{1} = 10$$

Sometimes there is a portion of the numerator or denominator that must be solved first. This is indicated by putting that portion in parentheses. Portions within parentheses that are added, subtracted, or divided are solved before solving the remainder of the equation. Always solve parts of the problem within the parentheses first. Sometimes the solution to that portion of a problem is a fraction or may include decimals. The solution can still be treated like any other fraction within an equation.

SAMPLE PROBLEM $\dfrac{9 \times (1/4 + 2/3) \times \quad 6}{22 \times \quad\quad\quad 1 \times 18}$

Solve the portion in parentheses:

$$\begin{array}{rcl} \frac{1}{4} & = & \frac{3}{12} \\ + \quad \frac{2}{3} & = & \frac{8}{12} \\ \hline & & \frac{11}{12} \end{array}$$

$$\frac{9 \times 11/12 \times \quad 6}{22 \times \quad\quad\quad 1 \times 18}$$

Drop fraction denominator into denominator of equation. Cancel.

$$\begin{array}{ccc} 1 & 1 & 1 \\ \cancel{9} \times \cancel{11} \times & & \cancel{6} \\ \hline \cancel{22} \times \cancel{12} \times 1 \times \cancel{18} \\ 2 & 2 & 2 \end{array}$$

Multiply the numerator:
Multiply the denominator:

$$\frac{1 \times 1 \quad \times 1}{2 \times 2 \times 1 \times 2} = \frac{1}{8}$$

Sometimes the use of parentheses avoids confusion in setting up complex equations.   Portions in parentheses that are multiplied together can be treated like any other fraction within an equation.

SAMPLE PROBLEM
$$\frac{3 \times (\frac{100}{1} \times \frac{1}{2.2}) \times 55 \times 3}{2 \times \qquad 3 \times 60 \times 5}$$

Portion within parentheses involves multiplication and can be treated like any other fraction. Drop fraction denominators into the equation denominator. Cancel.

$$\frac{3 \times \cancel{100} \times 1 \quad \times \cancel{55} \times \cancel{3}}{2 \times \quad 1 \times \cancel{2.2} \times 3 \times \cancel{60} \times 5}$$

Multiply the numerator:
Multiply the denominator:

$$\frac{1 \times 1 \times \quad 1 \quad \times 5 \times 1}{2 \times 1 \times 0.2 \times 1 \times 1 \times 1} = \frac{5}{0.4}$$

$$
\begin{array}{r}
12.5 \\
0.4\overline{)5.00} \\
4 \\
\overline{1\,0} \\
8 \\
\overline{2\,0} \\
2\,0 \\
\end{array}
$$

PRACTICE PROBLEMS

Equations with Fractions and/or Decimals

Show all your work. (Check your answers on page 316.)

16. $\dfrac{0.5 \times 3 \times 1/6 \times 5}{4 \times 5 \times \quad 8 \times 3}$

19. $\dfrac{1 \times \quad 5 \times 7 \times 24}{4/7 \times 21 \times 4 \times \quad 1}$

17. $\dfrac{10 \times (\frac{110}{1} \times \frac{1}{2.2}) \times 33}{1 \times \qquad\qquad 1 \times 4}$

20. $\dfrac{2 \times \quad 5 \times (\frac{110}{1} \times \frac{1}{20}) \times 50}{1 \times 0.4 \times \qquad\qquad 1 \times 22}$

18. $\dfrac{2 \times (3\frac{1}{2} + \frac{1}{4}) \times \quad 4}{1 \times \qquad\qquad 9 \times 0.3}$

SELF-ASSESSMENT POSTTEST

Equations Written as Fractions

Show all your work. (Check your answers on page 351.)

1. $\dfrac{6 \times 12 \times 0.5 \times 3}{2 \times 15 \times \ 1 \times 1}$

6. $\dfrac{2 \times \ \ 3 \times \ 1 \times 9}{1 \times 1/6 \times 13 \times 5}$

2. $\dfrac{1/6 \times 50 \times 20 \times 3}{1 \times \ 8 \times \ 9 \times 5}$

7. $\dfrac{1/150 \times \ 1 \times 1000 \times 16}{1 \times 15 \times \ \ \ 2 \times \ 1}$

3. $\dfrac{30 \times \ \ 1 \times \ \ 1 \times 5/6}{1 \times 2.2 \times 20 \times \ 1}$

8. $\dfrac{15 \times (\frac{92}{1} \times \frac{1}{2.2}) \times 5.5 \times 3/10}{1 \times \ \ \ \ \ \ \ \ 1 \times \ 5 \times \ \ \ 2}$

4. $\dfrac{22 \times 5/6 \times 3 \times \ \ 1}{1 \times 2.2 \times 4 \times 0.5}$

9. $\dfrac{0.4 \times \ \ 1 \times 15}{1 \times 1.5 \times 1/6}$

5. $\dfrac{3/8 \times 5 \times 25 \times 15}{1 \times 6 \times 50 \times \ 1}$

10. $\dfrac{5 \times \ 1 \times \ 2 \times 16}{1 \times 15 \times 10 \times \ 1}$

Unit II

Introduction to Dimensional Analysis

OBJECTIVES *Upon completion of this unit, the student will have demonstrated the ability to correctly:*

• Relate the process involved in the dimensional analysis method of problem solving.

• Identify the factors necessary to solve various types of problems.

• Set up equations using the dimensional analysis method.

• Solve dimensional analysis equations.

• Check the accuracy of answers.

    All problems in this workbook are solved using the *dimensional analysis method,* which is sometimes called the *factor label* or *factor labeling method.* The dimensional analysis method is a systematic approach for problem solving that eliminates the need to remember formulas or to solve several parts of a problem prior to finding the answer. Based on the ratio and proportion method, this method uses a series of ratios with their unit of measurement labels, called *factors,* which are set up in one long equation. Once the equation is set up, most problems can be solved in three simple steps: (1) multiplying the numerator, (2) multiplying the denominator, and (3) dividing the numerator by the denominator.

Chapter 6

The Dimensional Analysis Method

The foundation of the dimensional analysis method is a series of ratios, called factors, that are carefully and systematically arranged in a long fractional equation. The fractional equation is treated as a large fraction. Any process that can be applied to a simple fraction can be applied to the fractional equation.

Factors are two quantities (numbers) with their units of measurement that are related to each other, that "go together," in a particular problem. Sometimes the factors are equivalents or two quantities and units of measurement that are always equal to each other; in this case they are called *conversion factors*. Usually, conversion factors are equivalents that must be memorized. Some problems can be solved using only factors contained within the problem. In other instances, conversion factors may be required. In this workbook, the factors given in the problem and the conversion factors necessary to solve the problem are called the "knowns" of the problem.

Factors are always written in fraction form in dimensional analysis. For instance, the conversion factor 1 foot = 12 inches can be written as follows:

$$\frac{1 \text{ foot}}{12 \text{ inches}} \qquad \frac{12 \text{ inches}}{1 \text{ foot}}$$

Because the two are equivalent, or have equal value, they can be written either way. The same applies to two quantities and their measurement units that are related to each other in a particular problem. If an item costs $0.90 per dozen, the $0.90 and one dozen are related to each other. They can be written as either of the following:

$$\frac{\$0.90}{1 \text{ dozen}} \qquad \frac{1 \text{ dozen}}{\$0.90}$$

In many of the problems in this workbook, there will be a quantity and unit of measurement that has no mate. It is related to nothing in the problem; nothing "goes with" it. Factors of this nature are always expressed as the quantity and unit of measure in the numerator while the denominator is 1. The 1 is implied. Remember, in a fraction, a number over 1 is equal to the number. It is written as follows:

$$\frac{\text{quantity and unit of measure}}{1} \qquad \text{such as} \qquad \frac{3 \text{ feet}}{1}$$

This factor would change in value if the 3 feet were written in the denominator and the 1 in the numerator. Therefore, it can only be written in one way.

Factors within the dimensional analysis equation are also related to each other. Each factor contains a unit of measurement that is the same as a unit of measurement in another factor in the problem or in a conversion factor. All dimensional analysis equations in this workbook are set up so that factors with the same units of measurement are adjacent to each other. Factors are separated from each other by a multiplication symbol. The multiplication symbol may be a centered period, parentheses, or an ×.

SETTING UP THE DIMENSIONAL ANALYSIS EQUATION

Problems can be set up in several ways using the dimensional analysis method. The easiest way, however, is to start with the unit of the answer and set up the problem backward to the "knowns."

It may be helpful to set up the *framework* of the equation first. The framework is the unit of measurement of the answer, followed by the equal symbol and the line separating the numerator and denominator of the equation.

$$\text{Unit of measurement of the answer} = \frac{\text{numerator}}{\text{denominator}}$$

The unit of measurement in the numerator of the first factor must be the same as that of the answer.

$$\text{Unit of measurement of the answer} = \frac{\text{Unit of measurement of answer}}{}$$

The next step is to search the problem for the factor containing the unit of measurement of the answer. This may be found within the problem or it may be a conversion factor. Record the quantity of that unit in the numerator and the related quantity and unit of measurement in the denominator. This is called the second unit of measurement in the example. This factor is separated from the next factor by the multiplication symbol.

$$\text{Unit of measurement of the answer} = \frac{\text{quantity and unit of measurement of answer} \times}{\text{quantity and second unit of measurement} \times}$$

The unit of measurement in the numerator of the second factor must be the same as in the denominator of the first factor.

$$\text{Unit of measurement of the answer} = \frac{\text{quantity and unit of measurement of answer} \times \text{second unit of measurement}}{\text{quantity and second unit of measurement} \times}$$

The next step is to search the problem for the factor containing the second unit of measurement. Each factor can be used only once. The factor containing the second unit of measurement can be found either in the problem or as a conversion factor. Record the quantity and second unit of measurement in the numerator and the related quantity and unit of measurement in the denominator. This is followed by the multiplication sign.

$$\text{Unit of measurement of the answer} = \frac{\text{quantity and unit of measurement of answer} \times \text{quantity and second unit of measurement} \times}{\text{quantity and second unit of measurement} \times \text{quantity and third unit of measurement} \times}$$

The unit of measurement in the numerator of the third factor and the denominator of the second factor must be the same.

$$\text{Unit of measurement of the answer} = \frac{\text{quantity and unit of measurement of answer} \times \text{quantity and second unit of measurement} \times \text{third unit of measurement}}{\text{quantity and second unit of measurement} \times \text{quantity and third unit of measurement} \times}$$

This sequence can be followed until the entire problem is set up. Once the equation is set up, it is treated as one large fraction. The units of measurement that appear in both the numerator and denominator are canceled by dividing the numerator and denominator by those units.

Cancellation is the process of dividing both the numerator and denominator by the same quantity or unit. The value of the fraction does not change if both the numerator and denominator are subjected to the same multiplication or division process.

After cancellation, the only units remaining are the units of the answer. Cancellation of the quantities may save some time and reduce the necessity of multiplying and dividing large numbers. Then complete the following steps:

(1) Multiply the numerator.

(2) Multiply the denominator.

(3) Divide the numerator by the denominator.

Some students prefer to set up the equation in a boxlike format in which the vertical lines indicate multiplication. The equation in this format is as follows:

$$\text{Unit of answer} = \frac{\begin{array}{c|c|c}\text{quantity and} & \text{quantity and} & \text{quantity and} \\ \text{unit of answer} & \text{second unit} & \text{third unit}\end{array}}{\begin{array}{c|c|c}\text{quantity and} & \text{quantity and} & \text{quantity and} \\ \text{second unit} & \text{third unit} & \text{fourth unit}\end{array}}$$

Use whichever format is most comfortable.

CONVERSIONS USING DIMENSIONAL ANALYSIS

Conversion problems are those in which a quantity and unit of measurement are changed to a different but equal quantity and unit of measurement.

SAMPLE PROBLEM   **15 kilometers (km) = _____ miles (mi)**

Often it helps set up the problems to find the knowns first. The first known is the unit of the answer, miles.

The second known is the unit from which the answer will be converted, kilometers. In this problem, 15 kilometers has no mate; it can be coupled with the implied 1 for the denominator. Therefore, the second known is 15 km/1.

Miles and kilometers are not related to each other within the problem. Therefore, a conversion factor is required. An equivalent chart shows that 1 kilometer is equal to 0.6 miles. The third known is the conversion factor of 1 km = 0.6 mi. The three knowns of the problem are as follows:

Unit of Answer: mi

Factor: 15 km/1

Conversion Factor: 1 km = 0.6 mi

Set up the framework for the equation, beginning with the unit of the answer, followed by the equal sign and the line separating the numerator from the denominator.

$$\text{mi} = \frac{}{}$$

The unit in the numerator of the first factor must be the same as the unit of the answer.

$$\text{mi} = \frac{\text{mi} \times}{}$$

Search the problem (knowns) for the factor containing mi. The factor is 1 km = 0.6 mi. Write 0.6 in front of mi in the numerator and 1 km in the denominator, followed by multiplication signs.

$$mi = \frac{0.6mi \times}{1km \times}$$

The numerator unit of the second factor must be the same as the denominator unit of the first factor. That unit is km.

$$mi = \frac{0.6mi \times km}{1km \times}$$

Search the knowns for the factor that contains km, 15 km/1. Write 15 in the numerator and 1 in the denominator.

$$mi = \frac{0.6mi \times 15km}{1km \times \ 1}$$

Cancel the units appearing in both the numerator and denominator.

$$mi = \frac{0.6mi \times 15}{1 \ \times \ 1}$$

The equation is set up correctly because the only unit remaining is the unit of the answer.

Multiply the numerator:
Multiply the denominator:

$$\frac{0.6mi \times 15}{1 \ \times \ 1} = \frac{9.0mi}{1}$$

Divide the numerator by the denominator:

$$= 9 \ mi$$

The last step, division of the numerator by the denominator, was unnecessary in the previous problem as any number over 1 is that number itself. Division of the numerator by the denominator is necessary when the denominator number is any number other than 1.

Some problems require several conversion factors. In the following problem, two conversions are necessary. In addition, one of the conversions involves a mixed number.

Mixed numbers cannot be multiplied or divided without conversion to improper fractions or decimals. To convert a mixed number to an improper fraction:

$$\frac{\left(\begin{matrix} whole \\ number \end{matrix} \times denominator\right) + \begin{matrix} existing \\ numerator \end{matrix}}{denominator} = \frac{new \ numerator}{denominator}$$

SAMPLE PROBLEM   **9 rods = _____ yards.**

Find the knowns. The unit of the answer is yards. The first factor is 9 rods with no mate or 9 rods/1. Yards and rods are not related to each other; therefore, conversion factors are required. An equivalents chart shows that 1 rod is equal to $16\frac{2}{3}$ feet and 1 yard is equal to 3 feet. The third known is 1 rod = $16\frac{2}{3}$ feet. The fourth known is 1 yard = 3 feet. The knowns are summarized as follows:

Knowns: Unit of Answer: yd
Factor: 9 rds/1
Conversion Factors: 1 yd = 3 ft
             1 rd = $16\frac{2}{3}$ ft

Set up the framework of the equation. Start with the unit of the answer. Write yd followed by the equal sign and the line separating the numerator and denominator.

$$yd = \frac{\qquad}{\qquad}$$

The numerator unit of the first factor must be the same as the unit of the answer. Write yd in the numerator.

$$\text{yd} = \frac{\text{yd}}{\qquad}$$

Search the knowns for the factor containing yards. The factor is 1 yd = 3 ft. Write 1 in the numerator and 3 ft in the denominator, followed by the multiplication signs.

$$\text{yd} = \frac{1 \ \text{yd} \ \times}{3 \ \text{ft} \ \times}$$

The numerator unit of the second factor must be the same as the denominator unit of the first factor. Write ft in the numerator.

$$\text{yd} = \frac{1 \ \text{yd} \ \times \qquad \text{ft}}{3 \ \text{ft} \ \times}$$

Search the knowns for the factor containing feet, 1 rd = $16\frac{2}{3}$ ft. Write $16\frac{2}{3}$ in the numerator and 1 rod in the denominator, followed by multiplication signs.

$$\text{yd} = \frac{1 \ \text{yd} \ \times \ 16\frac{2}{3} \ \text{ft} \ \times}{3 \ \text{ft} \ \times \qquad 1 \ \text{rd} \ \times}$$

The numerator unit of the third factor must be the same as the denominator unit of the second factor, rd. Write rod in the numerator.

$$\text{yd} = \frac{1 \ \text{yd} \ \times \ 16\frac{2}{3} \ \text{ft} \ \times \qquad \text{rd}}{3 \ \text{ft} \ \times \qquad 1 \ \text{rd} \ \times}$$

Search the knowns for the factor containing rd, 9 rd/1. Write 9 in the numerator and 1 in the denominator.

$$\text{yd} = \frac{1 \ \text{yd} \ \times \ 16\frac{2}{3} \ \text{ft} \ \times \ 9 \ \text{rd}}{3 \ \text{ft} \ \times \qquad 1 \ \text{rd} \ \times \ 1}$$

Cancel the units that appear in both the numerator and denominator.

$$\text{yd} = \frac{1 \ \text{yd} \ \times \ 16\frac{2}{3} \ \times \ 9}{3 \ \times \ 1 \ \times \ 1}$$

Convert the mixed number to an improper fraction.

$$\frac{(16 \times 3) + 2}{3} = \frac{50}{3}$$

$$\text{yd} = \frac{1 \ \text{yd} \ \times \ \frac{50}{3} \ \times \ 9}{3 \ \times \ 1 \ \times \ 1}$$

Drop the fraction denominator into the denominator of the equation. Cancel the evenly divisible quantities.

$$\text{yd} = \frac{1 \ \text{yd} \times 50 \qquad \times \overset{1}{\cancel{9}}}{\underset{1}{\cancel{3}} \ \times \ \underset{1}{\cancel{3}} \times 1 \times 1}$$

Multiply the numerator:
Multiply the denominator:

$$\frac{1 \ \text{yd} \ \times \ 50 \ \times \ 1}{1 \ \times \ 1 \ \times \ 1 \ \times \ 1} = \frac{50 \ \text{yd}}{1} = 50 \ \text{yd}$$

Occasionally, answers will have both a numerator and denominator unit of measurement. Examples are answers such as miles per hour or drops per minute. The symbol for per is /. Therefore, miles per hour may be written as miles/hour or miles per 1 hour.

SAMPLE PROBLEM   **60 miles per hour = ___ kilometers per hour**

The equivalent chart shows that 1 kilometer is equal to 0.6 mile.

Knowns: Unit of Answer: kilometers/hour (km/h)
Factor: 60 miles/hour (mi/1 h)
Conversion Factor: 1 kilometer (km) = 0.6 miles (mi)

Set up the framework of the equation. Begin with the unit of the answer, followed by the equal symbol and the line separating the numerator and the denominator.

$$\frac{km}{h} = \underline{\hspace{2cm}}$$

The numerator unit of the first factor must be the same as the numerator unit of the answer. Write km in the numerator.

$$\frac{km}{h} = \frac{km}{\underline{\hspace{1.5cm}}}$$

Find the factor containing km. Write 1 km in the numerator and 0.6 mi in the denominator, followed by multiplication signs.

$$\frac{km}{h} = \frac{1 \ km \ \times}{0.6 \ mi \ \times}$$

The numerator unit of the second factor must be the same as the denominator unit of the first factor. Write mi in the numerator.

$$\frac{km}{h} = \frac{1 \ km \ \times \quad mi}{0.6 \ mi \ \times}$$

Find the factor containing mi. Write 60 in the numerator and 1 h in the denominator.

$$\frac{km}{h} = \frac{1 \ km \ \times \ 60 \ mi}{0.6 \ mi \ \times \ 1 \ h}$$

Cancel the units appearing in both the numerator and denominator. The equation is set up correctly because the units remaining are the units of the answer, km and h. Cancel the evenly divisible quantities.

$$\frac{km}{h} = \frac{1 \ km \ \times \ \overset{10}{\cancel{60}}}{\underset{0.1}{\cancel{0.6}} \ \times \ 1 \ h}$$

Multiply the numerator:
Multiply the denominator:

$$\frac{1 \ km \ \times \ 10}{0.1 \quad \times \quad 1 \ h} = \frac{10 \ km}{0.1 \ h}$$

Divide the numerator by the denominator:

$$0.1.\overline{)10.0.} \overset{\textstyle 100 \ kilometers/hour}{}$$

PRACTICE PROBLEMS

Conversions Using Dimensional Analysis

(Answers on page 317)

Equivalents necessary to solve these problems
1 yard = 3 feet
1 foot = 12 inches
1 pound = 16 ounces
1 ounce = 2 tablespoons
1 cup = 8 ounces
1 pint = 2 cups

1. 16 tablespoons = _____cups

2. 28 inches = _____yards

3. 82 ounces = _____pounds

5. $8\frac{3}{4}$ pounds = _____ounces

4. 24 ounces = _____pints

WORD PROBLEMS

Word problems pose some difficulties because they often contain information that is not pertinent to the question being asked. The task, then, is to separate the relevant parts from the irrelevant parts. All of the information in the first problem is relevant. The second problem, however, contains some irrelevant information.

SAMPLE PROBLEM   **Three apples cost $1.11. How much will two apples cost?**

First, determine the unit of measurement of the answer, $. This is the first known of the problem.

Determine the factors in the problem. Which units are related to each other? There is a relationship between the three apples and $1.11. This is the second known of the problem. The third known is the two apples. It is not related to anything in the problem. Therefore, it is coupled with an implied 1 in the denominator. There are no conversion factors required in this problem. The knowns are summarized as follows:

Knowns: Unit of Answer: $
Factors: 3 apples = $1.11
          2 apples/1

Set up the framework for the equation. Start with the unit of the answer, followed by the equal sign and the line separating the numerator from the denominator.

$$\$ = \frac{\quad}{\quad}$$

The numerator unit of the first factor must be the same as the unit of the answer. Write $ in the numerator.

$$\$ = \frac{\$}{\quad}$$

Find the factor containing $, $1.11 = 3 apples. Write 1.11 with the $ in the numerator and 3 apples in the denominator, followed by multiplication signs.

$$\$ = \frac{\$1.11 \qquad \times}{3 \text{ apples} \ \times}$$

The numerator unit of the second factor must be the same as the denominator unit of the first factor, apples. Write apples in the numerator.

$$\$ = \frac{\$1.11 \qquad \times \qquad \text{apples}}{3 \text{ apples} \ \times}$$

Find the factor containing apples, 2 apples/1. Write 2 in the numerator and 1 in the denominator.

$$\$ = \frac{\$1.11 \qquad \times \ 2 \text{ apples}}{3 \text{ apples} \ \times \ 1}$$

Cancel the units that appear in both the numerator and denominator. Cancel the evenly divisible quantities.

$$\$ = \frac{\cancel{\$1.11}^{\$0.37} \times 2}{\cancel{3}_{1}}$$

Multiply the numerator:
Multiply the denominator:

$$\frac{\$0.37 \times 2}{1 \times 1} = \frac{\$0.74}{1 \times 1} = \$0.74$$

This problem could have been solved without cancellation as follows:

$$\$ = \frac{\$1.11 \times 2 \text{ apples}}{3 \text{ apples} \times 1} = \frac{\$1.11 \times 2}{3 \times 1} = \frac{\$2.22}{3} = \$0.74$$

SAMPLE PROBLEM   **Company A routinely produces 115 cogs per day. The company's largest competitor manufactures 130 cogs per day. Company A has instituted several processes intended to increase productivity. If company A's productivity were increased 20%, how many cogs would be produced each day?**

(This problem is also in Chapter 4.)

The irrelevant information in this problem is the number of cogs produced by company A's competitor. This has no bearing on this problem and is disregarded.

The first known is the unit of the answer. The problem asks for the number of cogs produced by company A with the 20% increase. Therefore, the unit of the answer is cogs.

The whole or the total amount is 115 cogs. The whole or total percentage is 100%. Therefore, 115 cogs are 100%, the second known of the problem.

The problem asks for a number of cogs that is 20% greater than the whole. Since 100% is the whole, an additional 20% would be 120%. This factor has no mate. Therefore, it is coupled with the implied 1 for the denominator.

Knowns: Unit of Answer: cogs
Factors: 115 cogs = 100%
       120%/1

Set up the framework of the equation. Start with the unit of the answer, cogs, followed by the equal sign and the line separating the numerator and the denominator.

$$\text{cogs} = \frac{\quad}{\quad}$$

The numerator unit of the first factor must be the same as the unit in the answer, cogs. Write cogs in the numerator.

$$\text{cogs} = \frac{\text{cogs}}{\quad}$$

Find the factor containing cogs, 115 cogs = 100%. Write 115 in the numerator and 100% in the denominator, followed by multiplication signs.

$$\text{cogs} = \frac{115 \text{ cogs} \times}{100\% \quad \times}$$

The numerator unit of the second factor must be the same as the denominator unit of the first factor, %. Write % in the numerator.

$$\text{cogs} = \frac{115 \text{ cogs} \times \quad \%}{100\% \quad \times}$$

Find the factor containing %, 120%/1. Write 120 in the numerator and 1 in the denominator.

$$\text{cogs} = \frac{115 \text{ cogs} \times 120\%}{100\% \quad \times \quad 1}$$

Cancel the units that appear in both the numerator and the denominator. Cancel the evenly divisible quantities in the numerator and denominator.

$$\text{cogs} = \frac{\overset{23}{\cancel{115}} \text{ cogs} \times \overset{6}{\cancel{120}}}{\underset{\underset{1}{20}}{\cancel{100}} \times 1}$$

Multiply the numerator:
Multiply the denominator:

$$\frac{23 \text{ cogs} \times 6}{1 \times 1} = \frac{138 \text{ cogs}}{1} = 138 \text{ cogs}$$

SAMPLE PROBLEM   **Mrs. Jones has a balance of $116.52 on her credit card. Interest on her credit card is 18% per year. If Mrs. Jones decides to pay the amount in full, how much money will she have to add to the balance for this month's interest?**

The problem asks for the interest for one month in dollars. Therefore, the unit of the answer is $. The second known is the 18% interest for one year.

The whole balance is $116.52. The whole of anything is 100%. Therefore, $116.52 is equal to 100%, the third known.

The interest of 18% is for one year. To find the interest for one month, the conversion factor to change years to months is 1 year equals 12 months, the fourth known.

The fifth known is the number of months of the interest, 1 month. It has no mate. Therefore, the factor is 1 month over the implied 1. The knowns are summarized as follows:

Knowns: Unit of Answer: $
Conversion Factor: 1 year = 12 months
Factors: 18% = 1 year
         $116.52 = 100%
         1 month/1

Some steps in this practice problem are consolidated because the combined processes go together. The steps of problems in later chapters are combined.

Set up the framework of the equation. Begin with the unit of the answer, followed by the equal sign and the line separating the numerator and denominator.

$$\$ = \underline{\qquad}$$

The unit in the numerator of the first factor must be the same as the unit of the answer, $. Find the factor containing $, $116.52 = 100%. Write $116.52 in the numerator and 100% in the denominator, followed by multiplication signs.

$$\$ = \frac{\$116.52 \quad \times}{100\% \quad \times}$$

The numerator unit of the second factor must be the same as the denominator unit of the first factor, %. Find the factor containing %, 18% = 1 year. Write 18% in the numerator and 1 year in the denominator, followed by multiplication signs.

$$\$ = \frac{\$116.52 \quad \times \quad 18\% \quad \times}{100\% \quad \times \quad 1 \text{ yr} \quad \times}$$

The numerator unit of the third factor must be the same as the denominator unit of the second factor, year. Find the factor containing year, 1 year = 12 months. Write 1 year in the numerator and 12 months in the denominator, followed by multiplication signs.

$$\$ = \frac{\$116.52 \times 18\% \times 1 \text{ yr} \times}{100\% \times 1 \text{ yr} \times 12 \text{ mo} \times}$$

The numerator unit of the fourth factor must be the same as the denominator unit of the third factor, months. Find the factor containing month, 1 month/1. Write 1 mo in the numerator and 1 in the denominator.

$$\$ = \frac{\$116.52 \times 18\% \times 1 \text{ yr} \times 1 \text{ mo}}{100\% \times 1 \text{ yr} \times 12 \text{ mo} \times 1}$$

Cancel the units that appear in both the numerator and denominator. Cancel evenly divisible quantities in the numerator and denominator.

$$\$ = \frac{\overset{58.26}{\cancel{\$116.62}} \times \overset{3}{\cancel{18}} \times 1 \times 1}{100 \times 1 \times \underset{\underset{1}{\cancel{2}}}{\cancel{12}} \times 1}$$

Multiply the numerator:
Multiply the denominator:

$$\frac{\$58.26 \times 3 \times 1 \times 1}{100 \times 1 \times 1 \times 1} = \frac{\$174.78}{100}$$

Divide the numerator by the denominator:

$$= \$1.7478 \text{ or } \$1.75$$

Cancellation in the previous problem could have included dividing $58.26 and 100 by 2. This was not done as it is easier to divide by 100 than by 50.

> To divide by powers of 10, move the decimal point one place to the left for each zero in the divisor.
> To multiply by powers of 10, move the decimal point one place to the right for each zero in the multiplier.

PRACTICE PROBLEMS

Word Problems

(Answers on page 317.)
Equivalents necessary to solve these problems
1 kilometer = 0.6 mi
1 square yard = 9 square feet

6. Bananas are on sale for 3 pounds for $1.04. A bunch of bananas weight $5\frac{5}{8}$ pounds. How much does the bunch cost?

7. What is the yearly interest on a $15,000 loan with an interest rate of 11% a year?

8. The speed limit is 80 kilometers per hour. The speedometer reads 55 miles per hour. Is the driver speeding?

10. How many square yards of carpet will be needed to cover 189 square feet?

9. The real estate tax on a property is $128.50. The tax has been increased 15%. What is the total dollar value of the new tax?

CHECKING THE ACCURACY OF ANSWERS

Students are expected to check their answers for accuracy. A mistake can happen anywhere in the problem, such as:
- Equation set up wrong
- Factors in problem not correctly related
- Conversion factor inaccurate
- Fractions inverted or dropped incorrectly
- Cancellation wrong
- Multiplication of numerator and/or denominator incorrect
- Division of numerator by denominator wrong
- Decimals incorrectly placed

If an answer looks wrong, it probably is. Always check the logic of the answer.

SAMPLE PROBLEM **Convert 22 pounds to kilograms.**

The incorrect solution is as follows:

Knowns: Unit of Answer: kg
Factor: 22 lb/1
Conversion Factor: 1 kg = 2.2 lb.

$$kg = \frac{1\ kg \times 22\ lb}{2.2\ lb \times 1} = \frac{1\ kg \times \overset{(10)}{\overset{1}{\cancel{22}}}}{\underset{1}{\cancel{2.2}} \times 1} = \frac{1\ kg}{1} = \overset{(10\ kg)}{1\ kg.}$$

The equation is set up correctly, but the answer to this problem cannot possibly be correct. Logically, if 1 kg = 2.2 lb, it cannot also equal 22 lb. A decimal error was made when canceling. The corrections are in parentheses above the mistakes.

The following is the same problem, but with a different mistake.

SAMPLE PROBLEM   **Convert 22 lb to kg.**

The incorrect solution is as follows:

$$kg = \frac{\overset{(1\ kg)}{2.2\ kg} \times 22\ lb}{\underset{(2.2\ lb)}{1\ lb} \times 1} = \frac{48.4\ kg}{1} \overset{(10\ kg)}{=} 48.4\ kg$$

The answer to this problem cannot be correct. A kilogram is larger than a pound. Therefore, the number of kilograms must be smaller than the number of pounds. The answer must be less than half the number of pounds. The conversion factor is written incorrectly. The correction is written in parentheses.

   Problems with percentages are frequently set up incorrectly.

SAMPLE PROBLEM   **Find the yearly interest in dollars of a loan of $500 at an interest rate of 16% a year.**

The incorrect solution is as follows:

Knowns: Unit of Answer: $
Factors: $500 = 16% ($500 = 100%)
      100%/1 (16%/1)

$$\$ = \frac{\$500 \times 100\ \%}{16\ \% \times 1} = \frac{\overset{125}{\cancel{\$500}} \times 100}{\underset{4}{\cancel{16}}} = \frac{\$12500}{4} = \$3125$$

$$\left(\$ = \frac{\$500 \times 16\ \%}{100\ \% \times 1} = \frac{\overset{5}{\cancel{\$500}} \times 16}{\underset{1}{\cancel{100}} \times 1} = \frac{\$80}{1} = \$80 \right)$$

Interest of less than 100% produces a number less than the whole. This answer is considerably greater than the whole, $500. The factors are wrong. The corrections are in parentheses.

   Students who set up dimensional analysis equations by beginning with the unit of the answer and working toward the knowns rarely make mistakes. Always check the relationship between the numerator unit of one factor and the denominator unit of the preceding factor.

TO CHECK THE ACCURACY OF THE EQUATION

If the factors are correct, the equation is correct if:
The numerator unit of the first factor is the same as that of the answer numerator.
The numerator unit of one factor is the same as the denominator unit of the preceding factor.
The units remaining after cancellation of units appearing in both the numerator and denominator are the units of the answer.

   The most common mistakes involve simple mathematical errors. Errors in division, especially of decimals, are very common.

CHECKING THE MATHEMATICS FOR ACCURACY

Division: Multiply the quotient by the divisor to find the dividend.

$$\begin{array}{r} \text{Quotient} \\ \times\ \text{Divisor} \\ \hline \text{Dividend} \end{array}$$

Multiplication: divide the product by the multiplier to find the multiplicand.

$$\text{Multiplier}\,\overline{)\,\text{Product}}^{\displaystyle \text{Multiplicand}}$$

Subtraction: Add the difference and the subtrahend to find the minuend.

$$\begin{array}{r} \text{Difference} \\ +\ \text{Subtrahend} \\ \hline \text{Minuend} \end{array}$$

Addition: In a column of numbers, add from the opposite direction.
    For two numbers, subtract one addend from the sum to find the other addend.

$$\begin{array}{r} \text{Sum} \\ -1\ \text{Addend} \\ \hline \text{Other Addend} \end{array}$$

SAMPLE PROBLEM   **The equation is set up correctly, but the answer is incorrect. Find the error and correct it.**

$$\$ = \frac{\$1.25 \times 1\ \text{dozen} \times 16\ \text{donuts}}{1\ \text{dozen} \times 12\ \text{donuts} \times 1} = \frac{\$1.25 \times 1 \times \overset{5}{\cancel{15}}}{1 \times \underset{4}{\cancel{12}} \times 1} = \frac{\$6.25}{4} = \overset{(\$1.5625)}{\$1.6525} = \$1.65$$

The mistake is the division of $6.25 by 4. The number should have been $1.5625.

SAMPLE PROBLEM   **The equation is set up correctly. Find the error.**

$$\frac{\$}{\text{mo}} = \frac{\$250 \times 20\ \% \times 1\ \text{yr}}{100\ \% \times 1\ \text{yr} \times 12\ \text{mo}} = \frac{\overset{1255}{\cancel{\$250}} \times \overset{1}{\cancel{20}} \times 1}{\underset{\underset{2}{4}}{\cancel{100}} \times 1 \times 12} = \frac{\$125}{4} = \$5.20$$

The error is cancellation of 100 (and 20) by 20. The corrected equation is

$$= \frac{\overset{(\$25)}{\overset{\cancel{(\$50)}}{\cancel{\$250}}} \times \overset{1}{\cancel{20}} \times 1}{\underset{\underset{(1)}{\cancel{(5)}}}{\cancel{100}} \times 1 \times \underset{6}{\cancel{12}}} = \frac{\$25}{6} = \$4.166 = \$4.17$$

SAMPLE PROBLEM   **The equation is set up correctly. Find the error and correct it.**

$$\text{mcg} = \frac{1000\ \text{mcg} \times 4\ \text{mg} \times 1\ \text{kg} \times 55\ \text{lb}}{1\ \text{mg} \times 1\ \text{kg} \times 2.2\ \text{lb} \times 1} = \frac{1000\ \text{mcg} \times \overset{2}{\cancel{4}} \times 1 \times \overset{5}{\cancel{55}}}{1 \times 1 \times \underset{\underset{0.1}{\cancel{1.1}}}{\cancel{2.2}} \times 1}$$

$$= \frac{\overset{(10000)}{10}}{\underset{(0.1)}{1}} = 10(100{,}000\,\text{mcg})$$

The error is multiplication of numerator (1000 forgotten) and denominator (decimal lost). The corrections are in parentheses.

PRACTICE PROBLEMS

Checking the Accuracy of Answers

(Answers on page 318)

The equations are set up correctly, but the solution is wrong. Find and correct the errors.

11. 36 mi = _____km

$$km = \frac{1km \times 36mi}{0.6mi \times 1} = \frac{1km \times \cancel{36}^{\,6}}{\cancel{0.6} \times 1} = \frac{6 \; km}{1}$$

$$= 6 \; km$$

12. 25 yd = _____rd

$$rd = \frac{1rd \times 3ft \times 25yd}{16\frac{2}{3}ft \times 1yd \times 1} = \frac{1rd \times 3 \times 25}{\frac{50}{3} \times 1 \times 1}$$

$$= \frac{50 \times 1rd \times \overset{1}{\cancel{3}} \times 25}{\underset{1}{\cancel{3}} \times 1 \times 1} = \frac{1250 \; rd}{1}$$

$$= 1250 \; rd$$

13. What is this month's interest on a loan of $300 with an interest rate of 20% per year?

$$\$ = \frac{\$300 \times 20\% \times 1yr \times 1mo}{100\% \times 1yr \times 12mo \times 1}$$

$$= \frac{\overset{3}{\cancel{\$300}} \times \overset{4}{\cancel{20}} \times 1 \times 1}{\underset{1}{\cancel{100}} \times 1 \times \underset{3}{\cancel{12}} \times 1} = \frac{\$12}{3} = \$4.00$$

14. 2 gal = _____oz

$$oz = \frac{8oz \times 2C \times 2pt \times 4qt}{1C \times 1pt \times 1qt \times 1gal}$$

$$= \frac{8oz \times 2 \times 2 \times 4}{1 \times 1 \times 1 \times 1}$$

$$= \frac{108 \; oz}{1} = 108 \; oz$$

15. Three dozen eggs cost $1.39. How much will 84 eggs cost?

$$\$ = \frac{\$1.39 \times 1dozen \times 84eggs}{3dozen \times 12eggs \times 1}$$

$$= \frac{\$1.39 \times 1 \times \overset{1}{\cancel{84}}}{3 \times \underset{1}{\cancel{12}} \times 1}$$

$$= \frac{\$9.73}{3} = \$3.333 = \$3.33$$

SELF-ASSESSMENT POSTTEST

Dimensional Analysis

(Answers on page 352)

Equivalents necessary to solve the problems

1 kilometer = 0.6 miles	1 cup = 8 ounces
1 pound = 16 ounces	1 pint = 2 cups
1 tablespoon = 3 teaspoons	1 quart = 2 pint
1 ounce = 2 tablespoons	Check all the answers for accuracy.

1. 90 kilometers/hour = ___miles/hour

2. $\frac{1}{4}$ quart = ___ounces

3. 18 teaspoons = ___tablespoons

4. $8\frac{1}{8}$ pounds = ___ounces

5. 6 tablespoons = ___ounces

6. What is the yearly interest on a $1200 savings account with an interest rate of 5.5% a year?

7. The balance of a charge account is $212.53. The interest rate is 16% per year. What is the dollar value of this month's interest?

8. The speed limit is 65 miles per hour. The speedometer reads 100 kilometers per hour. Is the driver speeding?

9. The marathon race course is 26 miles long. How many kilometers is the course?

10. Company B produces 28 handmade handbags each day. By adding three new people to their payroll, they have increased the daily production by 25%. How many handbags are they making each day now?

BASIC DOSAGE AND SOLUTIONS CALCULATIONS

Unit III

Systems of Measurement

OBJECTIVES *Upon completion of this unit, the student will have demonstrated the ability to correctly:*

- Name the units of measurement for the metric, apothecary, and household measurement systems.

- List the abbreviations and symbols used to indicate units within the metric, apothecary, and household measurement systems.

- Recall the equivalents (conversion factors) used to convert from one unit to another within the measurement systems.

- Write the approximate equivalents (conversion factors) used to convert from one system of measurement to another.

- Convert equivalent quantities within the metric, apothecary, and household measurement systems.

- Calculate equivalent quantities among the three measurement systems.

- Calculate fluid intake.

Three systems of measurement—household, apothecary and metric—are used by health care providers in the United States. Students entering health care professions must become familiar with all three systems. This involves the ability to convert measurements within and among the three systems.

Early in the history of man, the need for some way to measure mass, volume, and distance became apparent. Early methods seem crude by today's standards. A foot was the length of the foot; later, this unit was standardized to be the length of the foot of the ruling monarch. The yard was the distance from the nose to the end of one outstretched fingertip or the length of a man's stride. Weight or mass was measured using a stone as the measurement unit. This system developed into several distinct measurement systems that are still in existence today.

The mixture of these measurement systems was brought to America from England by the colonialists. Collectively, these systems are referred to as the English systems, which use pounds and ounces for mass, bushels and pecks for dry volume, gallons and quarts for liquid volume, and miles and yards for length. Conversion from one unit to another within the English systems is complex and requires rote memorization of many equivalents. Household measurements are part of the English system of measurement. They consist of such units as cups, teaspoons, and tablespoons, which are commonplace in American kitchens.

Although technically a part of the English system, the apothecary system is usually separated from the others since it is used almost exclusively by pharmacists, physicians, and nurses. This system is named for the apothecaries, the forerunner of today's pharmacists. When it was determined that a bit of a particular herb had medicinal properties but more than a bit could produce unwanted effects or even death, it became necessary to measure very small quantities. In the beginning, a grain of wheat was balanced with the amount of herb. Therefore, the measurement unit was labeled *grain*. Other measurements in this system include *scruples, drams,* and *minims.* This system of mismatched units is difficult to remember and to use for converting one unit of measurement to another.

The metric system was developed in 1790 in France and is based on the decimal system. The system has been improved and revised and is officially called the International Metric System. The metric system uses a base unit, such as the *gram*, and adds fixed prefixes to designate larger or smaller quantities.

Most countries use the metric system. In the 1970s, a plan was proposed to gradually convert the United States to the metric system, thus putting Americans in tune with the rest of the world. Proposals included changing road signs from miles to kilometers per hour and tools from inches to centimeters and millimeters. Household measurements were to be replaced by liters and milliliters, while pounds and ounces were to become kilograms, grams, and milligrams. The plan met with much public resistance and was largely abandoned, despite the simplicity of the metric system. However, some merchandise is labeled with both the metric and household or apothecary systems. Measuring cups are available with both ounces and milliliters listed on their sides. Soft drink containers and canned goods often have weight or liquid measures in both metric and household measurements.

Chapter 7

The English Measurement Systems

The English systems of measurement are each distinct. Each system has some common measurement units that may or may not be equivalent. Consider pounds and ounces. Three distinct systems use these units. In the troy and apothecary systems, there are 12 ounces in a pound, while in the avoirdupois system a pound is 16 ounces. In the United States, the standard pound is 16 ounces.

Some texts claim that only volume measures are true household measurements. Other sources claim that pints and quarts belong to the apothecary system. These measures are part of the English systems of measurement, however. For the purposes of this workbook, common linear and weight measurements used in the home are included in the household measurement portion of this section, although they may not be true household measurements. Only measurements units used by health care providers are included in this section.

HOUSEHOLD MEASUREMENT SYSTEM

The household measurement system is often used by health care providers when instructing clients on measuring liquid oral medications at home. Fluid intake is recorded in the metric system after being converted from household measurements. Infant weights are reported in the metric system but converted to pounds and ounces for parents.

Table 7-1 lists household abbreviations used by health care providers. This list contains both official and commonly used abbreviations.

The measurement equivalents of the household system are mismatched and require rote memorization to learn. Not all the equivalents listed in Table 7-2 are needed to solve problems in this book or in the clinical setting; therefore, there is no need to memorize them. The list of equivalents in Chapter 9 should be memorized, however.

As a general rule, conversion from one unit to a second unit can be done only within the type of measurement. For instance, only volume measurements can be converted to other volume measurements. Teaspoons cannot be converted to pounds.

TABLE 7-1 Household measurement abbreviations

Volume		Weight	Length
Drop(s)	= gtt(s)	Pound = lb	Foot = ft or '
Gallon	= gal	Ounce = oz	Inch = in or ''
Pint	= pt		
Ounce	= oz		
Quart	= qt		
Teaspoon	= tsp or t		
Tablespoon	= Tbsp, tbsp, or T		
Gallon	= Gal, gal		

TABLE 7-2 Common household measurement equivalents

Volume		Weight	Length
1 tablespoon	= 3 teaspoons	1 pound = 16 ounces	1 foot = 12 inches
1 ounce	= 2 tablespoons		
1 cup	= 8 ounces		
1 pint	= 2 cups		
1 quart	= 2 pints		
1 gallon	= 4 quarts		

Anyone who has ever tried to cut a recipe in half is familiar with the complexities of conversion within the household measurement system. A recipe, for instance, calls for $\frac{1}{3}$ cup of milk. If the recipe is cut in half, $\frac{1}{6}$ cup of milk is necessary. There is no $\frac{1}{6}$ cup on the standard household measuring cup, and most cooks aren't familiar enough with equivalents to be able to convert the calculation accurately. An accurate conversion of $\frac{1}{6}$ cup within the household measurement system would be 2 tablespoons plus 2 teaspoons. Instead, many cooks either make the entire recipe knowing there will be leftovers or estimate the $\frac{1}{6}$ cup.

Arabic numerals and common fractions are used to identify quantities within the household systems. The quantities precede the units of measurement.

Examples: 2 C   3 ft
         $1\frac{1}{2}$ tsp   3 qts

APOTHECARY MEASUREMENT SYSTEM

Although the metric measurement system is more commonly used for prescribing medication dosages, the apothecary system is still used for older drugs, such as aspirin, and by older physicians. The apothecary measurement system is a complex one of minims, fluid drams, fluid ounces, pints and gallons for volumes, and grains, drams, scruples, ounces, and pounds for weight units.

It is as cumbersome to convert within the apothecary system as within the household system. This does not really concern the health care professional because conversion within the system is not necessary. Therefore, no equivalents are listed in this section. Only commonly used apothecary unit abbreviations are listed in Table 7-3.

In common practice, the abbreviation indicating fluid is not used. The abbreviation and symbol for dram, dr and ʒ, are usually used to indicate liquid (volume) measurements only, while oz and ℥ indicate both volume and weight.

Roman numerals are commonly used to signify amounts in the apothecary system. Technically, lowercase roman numerals are to be used, but both uppercase and lowercase roman numerals are commonly used. The fraction $\frac{1}{2}$ is abbreviated as ss. Smaller fractions are written in arabic numerals.

The apothecary system unit is followed by the roman numeral and/or fraction.

Example: gr iv = 4 grains   gr $\frac{1}{150}$ = $\frac{1}{150}$ grain
        ʒ iss = $1\frac{1}{2}$ drams   ℥ iv = 4 ounces

TABLE 7-3 Apothecary measurement
abbreviations

Volume		Weight	
Minim	= M, mx, min, ℳ	grain	= gr
fluid dram	= fdr, fʒ	dram	= dr, ʒ
fluid ounce	= foz, f℥	ounce	= oz, ℥

CONVERSION BETWEEN THE ENGLISH MEASUREMENT SYSTEMS

Occasionally health care providers may need to convert measurements between the household and apothecary systems. Equivalents between the household and apothecary systems are only approximations. Table 7-4 shows these equivalents.

Some of the approximate equivalents are not used by health care providers. For instance, there is no need to know that a minim is the approximate equivalent of a standard drop. The size of a drop depends on the size of the opening through which the drop passes. It does, however, provide a frame of reference and helps visualize the relative size of a minim. The conversion of drops to teaspoons is not commonly used. Fractional parts of a teaspoon, such as $\frac{1}{4}$ or $\frac{1}{2}$ teaspoon, are easier to use and more accurate than counting 15 or 30 drops, respectively.

Health care professionals do not use the apothecary weight measurement of 1 oz = 60 grains because weights used in medication administration are smaller than an ounce. Neither do they use volumes larger than quarts.

Figures 7-1 and 7-2 show the relative sizes of some measurements in the household and apothecary systems. In reality, a dram is slightly smaller than a teaspoon. When considering one teaspoon and one dram, the amount is negligible. When comparing drams and teaspoons in an ounce, the difference is larger. There are 8 drams but only 6 teaspoons in an ounce.

To convert from one measurement unit to another:

$$\text{Unit of answer} = \frac{\text{conversion} \times \frac{\text{quantity and unit}}{\text{being converted}}}{\text{factor(s)} \quad \times 1}$$

TABLE 7-4   Approximate household and apothecary equivalents

	Household	*Apothecary*
Weight	1 oz (ʒ)	= 1 oz = 8 dr (ʒ) = 60 gr
	1 lb = 16 oz	
Volume	1 gtt	= 1 mx, M, (♏)
	1 tsp = 60 gtts	= 1 fdr = 60 mx
	1 tbsp = 3 tsp	= $\frac{1}{2}$ foz
	2 tbsp	= 1 foz = 8 fdr
	1 C	= 8 foz
	2 C = 1 pt	= 16 foz = 1 pt
	2 pt = 1 qt	= 32 foz
	4 qt = 1 gal	= 8 pt = 1 gal
Length	1 ft (′) = 12 in (″)	

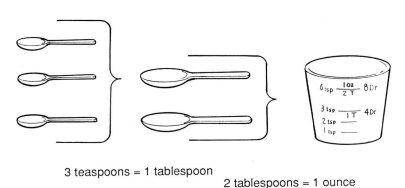

3 teaspoons = 1 tablespoon

2 tablespoons = 1 ounce

FIGURE 7-1 Comparison of household and apothecary volume measurements

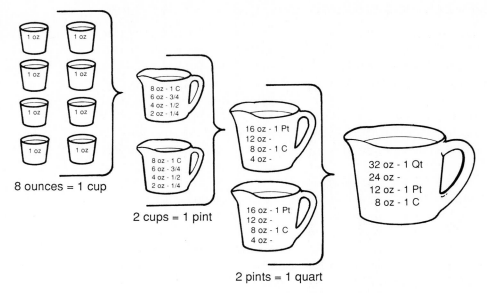

FIGURE 7.2 Comparison of household and apothecary volume measurements

The section introducing dimensional analysis utilized some conversion factors of the English measurement systems. Some of the problems will require the use of only one conversion factor and some will require several.

SAMPLE PROBLEM   **28 ounces (oz) = _____ cups (C)**

Knowns: Unit of Answer: C
Factor: 28 oz/1
Conversion Factor: 1 C = 8 oz
Set up the framework of the equation, beginning with the unit of the answer, followed by the equal sign and the line separating the numerator and denominator.

$$C = \underline{\hspace{3cm}}$$

The numerator unit of the first factor must be the same as the unit of the answer, C. Find the factor containing C, 1 C = 8 oz. Write 1 C in the numerator and 8 oz in the denominator, followed by multiplication signs.

$$C = \frac{1\,C\ \times}{8\,oz\ \times}$$

The numerator unit of the second factor must be the same as the denominator unit of the first factor, oz. Find the factor that contains oz, 28 oz/1. Write 28 oz in the numerator and 1 in the denominator.

$$C = \frac{1\,C\ \times 28\,oz}{8\,oz\ \times\ 1}$$

Cancel the units appearing in both the numerator and denominator by dividing both by oz. The problem is set up correctly because the unit remaining after cancellation is the unit of the answer. Then cancel the evenly divisible quantities by dividing both the numerator and denominator by 4.

$$C = \frac{1\,C \times \overset{7}{\cancel{28}}}{\underset{2}{\cancel{8}}\ \times\ 1}$$

Multiply the numerator;
Multiply the denominator:

$$\frac{1C \times 7}{2\ \times 1} = \frac{7C}{2}$$

Divide the numerator by the denominator:

$$\frac{7C}{2} = 3\tfrac{1}{2}\,C$$

SAMPLE PROBLEM   **How many cups are in 2 quarts?**

Knowns: Unit of Answer: Cups (C)
Factor: 2 Quarts (qt)/1
Conversion Factors: 1 Pint (pt) = 2 Cups (C)
              1 Quart (qt) = 2 Pints (pt)

Set up the framework of the equation, beginning with the unit of the answer, cups (C), followed by the equal sign and the line separating the numerator and the denominator.

$$C = \underline{\qquad}$$

The numerator unit of the first factor must be the same as the unit of the answer, C. Find the factor that contains C. Write 2 cups in the numerator and 1 pint in the denominator, followed by multiplication signs.

$$C = \frac{2\,C\,\times}{1\,pt\,\times}$$

The numerator unit of the second factor must be the same as the denominator unit of the first factor. Find the factor containing pt. Write 2 pt in the numerator and 1 quart in the denominator, followed by multiplication signs.

$$C = \frac{2\,C\,\times\,2\,pt\,\times}{1\,pt\,\times\,1\,qt\,\times}$$

The numerator unit of the third factor must be the same as the denominator unit of the second factor, qt. Find the factor containing qt. Write 2 qt in the numerator and 1 in the denominator.

$$C = \frac{2\,C\,\times\,2\,pt\,\times\,2\,qt}{1\,pt\,\times\,1\,qt\,\times\,1}$$

Cancel the units that appear in both the numerator and denominator.

$$C = \frac{2C\times2\times2}{1\times1\times1}$$

Multiply the numerator:
Multiply the denominator:

$$\frac{2C\times2\times2}{1\times1\times1} = \frac{8\,C}{1} = 8\,C$$

There was no need to divide the numerator with the denominator. The answer is 8 cups because any number over 1 is that number.

SAMPLE PROBLEM   **24 tsp = _____ oz**

Knowns: Unit of Answer: oz
Factor: 24 tsp/1
Conversion Factors: 1 T = 3 tsp
              1 oz = 2 tbsp

Set up the framework for the equation. Begin with the unit of the answer, followed by the equal sign and the line separating the numerator and the denominator.

$$oz = \underline{\qquad}$$

The numerator unit of the first factor must be the same as the unit of the answer. Find the factor containing oz. Write 1 oz in the numerator and 2 T in the denominator, followed by multiplication signs.

$$oz = \frac{1\,oz\,\times}{2\,T\,\times}$$

The numerator unit of the second factor must be the same as the denominator unit of the first factor. Find the factor containing T. Write 1 T in the numerator and 3 tsp in the denominator, followed by multiplication signs.

$$oz = \frac{1 \text{ oz} \times 1 \text{ T} \times}{2 \text{ T} \times 3 \text{ tsp} \times}$$

The numerator unit of the third factor must be the same as the denominator unit of the second factor. Find the factor containing tsp. Write 24 tsp in the numerator and 1 in the denominator.

$$oz = \frac{1 \text{ oz} \times 1 \text{ T} \times 24 \text{ tsp}}{2 \text{ T} \times 3 \text{ tsp} \times 1}$$

Cancel those units appearing in both the numerator and the denominator. Cancel the evenly divisible quantities.

$$oz = \frac{1oz \times 1 \times \overset{\overset{4}{\cancel{12}}}{\cancel{24}}}{\underset{1}{\cancel{2}} \times \underset{1}{\cancel{3}} \times 1}$$

Multiply the numerator: multiply the denominator:

$$\frac{1oz \times 1 \times 4}{1 \times 1 \times 1} = \frac{4 \text{ oz}}{1} = 4 \text{ oz}$$

PRACTICE PROBLEMS

Conversion between the English Measurement Systems

Use dimensional analysis to solve the practice problems. (Answers on page 312.)

Conversion factors: 1 qt = 2 pt
  1 pt = 2 C
  1 C = 8 oz
  1 oz = 2 tbsp

1 Tbsp, tbsp, T, tbs = 3 tsp
1 tsp = 1 dr. ӡ
1 lb = 16 oz
1 ft = 12 in

1. $\frac{1}{2}$ ӡ = _____ T

2. 2 qt = _____ oz

3. 4 tbs = _____ tsp

4. 12 ӡ = _____ tsp

5. 5 C = _____ ӡ

6. 6 pt = _____ qt

7. 7 ӡ = _____ ӡ

8. 30 oz = _____ qt

9. 18 ℥ = _____ lb

10. 7 oz = _____ C

11. 6 ℥ = _____ tbsp

12. 12 oz = _____ pt

13. 4 C = _____ tbsp

14. 12 ℥ = _____ tbsp

15. $1\frac{1}{2}$ qt = _____ C

16. 60 oz = _____ qt

17. 21" = _____ '

18. $6\frac{1}{2}$ lb = _____ oz

19. 24 ℥ = _____ lb

20. $3\frac{1}{6}$ ft = _____ in

SELF-ASSESSMENT POSTTEST

The English Measurement Systems

Show all your work. Check your answers (page   ).

Conversion factors: 1 dr = 1 tsp
       1 T = 3 tsp
       1 oz = 2 T
       1 C = 8 oz

1 pt = 2 C
1 qt = 2 pt
1 lb = 16 oz
1 ft = 12 in

1. 39 in = _____ ft

2. 45 oz = _____ lb

3. 3 pt = _____ oz

4. 24 T = _____ C

5. 5 qt = _____ oz

6. 30 oz = _____ lb

7. $2\frac{5}{8}$ ft = _____ in

8. 29 oz = _____ pt

9. $\frac{15}{16}$ lb = _____ oz

10. 24 tsp = _____ C

11. 64 oz = _____ pt

12. 26 oz = _____ lb

13. 14 C = _____ qt

14. 14 tsp = _____ oz

15. $3\frac{1}{2}$ C = _____ oz

16. $4\frac{1}{6}$ feet = _____ in

17. 27 T = _____ pt

18. 12 ʒ = _____ lb

19. 6 C = _____ ʒ

20. 20 ʒ = _____ tsp

Chapter 8

The Metric System

Metric is the preferred system of measurement for health care providers. American pharmaceutical companies have converted to the metric system or a combination of metric and apothecary systems for labeling medication dosages. Physicians educated in the last several decades prefer to use the metric system exclusively. Some physicians, however, tend to order medications, such as atropine or aspirin, using the apothecary system. Until clients become well-versed in the metric system, they should be taught to measure their medications using the household system.

The metric system is the simplest of all the measurement systems used today. It consists of three base units—grams, liters and meters—to signify weight, volume and distance. The base units are abbreviated as follows: gram = g, liter = L, and meter = m. To these base units are added fixed prefixes to signify larger or smaller sizes. Each prefix is 10 times larger or smaller than the prefix before or after it. Table 8-1 lists metric prefixes, their abbreviations, and the number by which the base unit is multiplied.

TABLE 8-1 Metric system prefixes

Prefix	Abbreviation	Base unit with prefix	Number by which base unit is multiplied
kilo	k	kg	1000.
centi	c	cm	0.01 or $\frac{1}{100}$
milli	m	mg, mL, mm	0.001 or $\frac{1}{1000}$
micro	μ or mc	μg or mcg	0.000001 or $\frac{1}{1,000,000}$

When handwritten, the symbol for micro, μ, is often confused with the abbreviation for milli, m, and should not be used. When writing microgram by hand, always use the abbreviation mcg. Even many drug companies use mcg to avoid confusion.

Only a few of the metric prefixes are used by health care providers. Table 8-2 shows the metric prefixes indicating 1000 to 0.000001 times the base unit. Only those prefixes that are combined with base units are used by health care providers.

TABLE 8-2 Metric measurements used by health care providers

Kilo (1000)	Hecto (100)	Deka (10)	Base Unit	Deci ($\frac{1}{10}$)	Centi ($\frac{1}{100}$)	Milli* ($\frac{1}{1000}$)	Micro ($\frac{1}{1,000,000}$)
kg			gram			mg	mcg, μg
			liter			mL, ml	
			meter		cm	mm	

* There are no terms for $\frac{1}{10,000}$ and $\frac{1}{100,000}$ of a base unit.

Table 8-3 shows the metric equivalents used by health care professionals. The first abbreviation listed after the unit of measure is the correct abbreviation while the others listed are abbreviations occasionally seen in practice.

TABLE 8-3   Equivalents within the metric system

Volume	1 liter (L)	= 1000 milliliter (mL or ml)
	1 liter (L)	= 1000 cubic centimeters (cc)
	1 milliliter (mL or ml)	= 1 cubic centimeter (cc)
Weight	1 kilogram (kg)	= 1000 grams (g, G, or gm)
	1 gram (g or gm)	= 1000 milligrams (mg or mgm)
	1 gram (g or gm)	= 1,000,000 micrograms (mcg or mcgm)
	1 milligram (mg or mgm)	= 1000 micrograms (mcg or mcgm)
Length	1 meter (m)	= 100 centimeters (cm)
	1 meter (m)	= 1000 millimeters (mm)
	1 centimeter (cm)	= 10 millimeters (mm)

Note that cubic centimeter is abbreviated cc. It is never abbreviated as ccm. A cubic centimeter occupies the same space as a milliliter and is used interchangeably with milliliter in practice. The current trend is to use ml, which is a more correct term for volume than cc. The nurse must know that 1 ml is equal to 1 cc, however. Syringes are calibrated in cc rather than ml to avoid confusion between ml and the apothecary unit, minims.

CONVERSION WITHIN THE METRIC SYSTEM

Converting from one unit of measurement to another is very simple within the metric system. Conversion involves multiplication or division by powers of 10.

Remember:
To multiply by powers of 10, move the decimal point one place to the right for each zero in the multiplier.
To divide by powers of 10, move the decimal point one place to the left for each zero in the divisor.

All fractional answers in the metric system are written as decimal fractions. Conversion from one measurement unit to another is as follows:

$$\text{Unit of answer} = \frac{\text{conversion} \times \text{quantity and unit being converted}}{\text{factor(s)} \times \quad 1}$$

CONVERSION OF METRIC WEIGHTS

SAMPLE PROBLEM   **1500 milligrams (mg) = _____ grams (g)**

Knowns: Unit of Answer: g
Factor: 1500 mg/1
Conversion Factor: 1 g = 1000 mg
Set up the framework of the equation. Start with the unit of the answer, g, followed by the equal symbol and the line separating the numerator and the denominator.

$$g = \underline{\qquad}$$

The numerator unit of the first factor must be the same unit as the answer. Find the factor containing g. Write 1 g in the numerator and 1000 mg in the denominator, followed by multiplication signs.

$$g = \frac{1\,g\ \times}{1000\,mg\ \times}$$

The numerator unit of the second factor must be the same as the denominator unit of the first factor. Find the factor containing mg. Write 1500 mg in the numerator and 1 in the denominator.

$$g = \frac{1\,g\ \times\ 1500\,mg}{1000\,mg\ \times\ \ \ 1}$$

Cancel the units appearing in both the numerator and denominator. Cancel the evenly divisible quantities.

$$g = \frac{1\,g \times \overset{1.5}{\cancel{1500}}}{\underset{1}{\cancel{1000}}\ \times\ \ \ 1}$$

Multiply the numerator:
Multiply the denominator:

$$\frac{1\,g \times 1.5}{1\ \times\ 1} = \frac{1.5\,g}{1} = 1.5\,g$$

There is no need to divide the numerator by the denominator because a number over 1 is that number. The cancellation in the previous problem could have been done as follows:

$$\frac{1\,g \times \overset{3}{\cancel{1500}}}{\underset{2}{\cancel{1000}}\ \times\ \ 1} = \frac{3\,g}{2} = 1.5\,g$$

SAMPLE PROBLEM   **0.4 g = _____ mcg**

Knowns: Unit of Answer: mcg
Factor: 0.4 g/1
Conversion Factors: 1 g = 1000 mg
                         1 mg = 1000 mcg
Set up the framework of the equation.

$$mcg = \underline{}$$

The numerator unit of the first factor must be the same as the unit of the answer. Find the factor containing mcg. Write 1000 mcg in the numerator and 1 mg in the denominator, followed by multiplication signs.

$$mcg = \frac{1000\,mcg\ \times}{1\,mg\ \times}$$

The numerator unit of the second factor must be the same as the denominator unit of the first factor containing 1000 mcg. Find the factor containing mg. Write 1000 mg in the numerator and 1 g in the denominator, followed by multiplication signs.

$$mcg = \frac{1000\,mcg\ \times\ 1000\,mg\ \times}{1\,mg\ \times\ \ \ \ 1\,g\ \ \ \ \times}$$

The numerator unit of the third factor must be the same as the denominator unit of the second factor. Find the factor containing g. Write 0.4 g in the numerator and 1 in the denominator.

$$mcg = \frac{1000\,mcg\ \times\ 1000\,mg\ \times 0.4\,g}{1\,mg\ \times\ \ \ \ 1\,g\ \ \ \ \times\ \ \ 1}$$

Cancel the units.

$$mcg = \frac{1000\,mcg\ \times\ 1000 \times 0.4}{1\ \times\ \ \ \ 1 \times\ \ \ 1}$$

Multiply the numerator:
Multiply the denominator:

$$\frac{1000 \text{ mcg} \times 1000 \times 0.4}{1 \quad \times \quad 1 \times \quad 1} = \frac{400,000 \text{ mcg}}{1}$$

$$= 400,000 \text{ mcg}$$

PRACTICE PROBLEMS

Conversion of Metric Weights

(Answers on page 319.)

Conversion factors: 1 kilogram (kg) = 1000 grams (g)
                   1 gram (g) = 1000 milligrams (mg)
                   1 milligram (mg) = 1000 micrograms

1. 4 g = ___ mg

6. 35 mcg = ___ mg

2. 2000 mcg = ___ g

7. 0.002 mg = ___ mcg

3. 250 g = ___ kg

8. 0.75 mg = ___ mcg

4. 0.04 g = ___ mg

9. 3050 g = ___ kg

5. 0.5 mg = ___ mcg

10. 6.3 kg = ___ g

CONVERSION OF METRIC LENGTHS

SAMPLE PROBLEM   **13 cm = ____ mm**

Knowns: Unit of Answer: mm
Factor: 13 cm/1
Conversion Factor: 1 cm = 10 mm
Set up the framework of the equation.

mm = ————

The numerator unit of the first factor must be the same as the unit of the answer. Find the factor containing mm. Write 10 mm in the numerator and 1 cm in the denominator, followed by multiplication signs.

$$mm = \frac{10\ mm\ \times}{1\ cm\ \ \times}$$

The numerator unit of the second factor must be the same as the denominator unit of the first factor. Find the factor containing cm. Write 13 cm in the numerator and 1 in the denominator.

$$mm = \frac{10\ mm\ \times\ 13\ cm}{1\ cm\ \ \times\ \ 1}$$

Cancel the units.

$$mm = \frac{10\ mm\ \times\ 13}{1\ \ \ \ \times\ \ 1}$$

Multiply the numerator:
Multiply the denominator:

$$\frac{10\ mm\ \times\ 13}{1\ \ \ \ \times\ \ 1} = \frac{130\ mm}{1} = 130\ mm$$

PRACTICE PROBLEMS

Conversion of Metric Lengths

(Answers on page 319.)
Conversion factors: 1 meter (m) = 100 centimeters (cm)
                   1 centimeter (cm) = 10 milliliters (mm)

11. 3 m = ___ cm

14. 22 mm = ___ cm

12. 15 mm = ___ cm

15. 0.1 cm = ___ mm

13. 6 cm = ___ mm

CONVERSION OF METRIC VOLUMES

SAMPLE PROBLEM   **0.75 L = _____ cc**

Knowns: Unit of Answer: cc
Factor: 0.75 L/1
Conversion Factors: 1 L = 1000 ml
                        ml = 1 cc
Set up the framework for the equation.

$$cc = \frac{}{}$$

The numerator unit of the first factor must be the same as the unit of the answer.
Find the factor containing cc. Write 1 cc in the numerator and 1 ml in the denominator, followed by multiplication signs.

$$cc = \frac{1 \text{ cc } \times}{1 \text{ ml } \times}$$

The numerator unit of the second factor must be the same as the denominator unit of the first factor. Find the factor containing ml.
Write 1000 ml in the numerator and 1 L in the denominator, followed by multiplication signs.

$$cc = \frac{1 \text{ cc } \times 1000 \text{ ml } \times}{1 \text{ ml } \times \quad 1 \text{ L } \times}$$

The numerator unit of the third factor must be the same as the denominator unit of the second factor. Find the factor containing L. Write 0.75 L in the numerator and 1 in the denominator.

$$cc = \frac{1 \text{ cc } \times 1000 \text{ ml } \times 0.75 \text{ L}}{1 \text{ ml } \times \quad 1 \text{ L } \times \quad 1}$$

Cancel the units.

$$cc = \frac{1 \text{ cc } \times 1000 \times 0.75}{1 \quad \times \quad 1 \times \quad 1}$$

Multiply the numerator:
Multiply the denominator:

$$\frac{1 \text{ cc } \times 1000 \times 0.75}{1 \quad \times \quad 1 \times \quad 1} = \frac{750 \text{ cc}}{1} = 750 \text{ cc}$$

PRACTICE PROBLEMS

Conversion of Metric Volumes

(Answers on page 320.)
Conversion factors: 1 milliliter (ml) = 1 cubic centimeter (cc)
                  1 liter (L) = 1000 milliliters

16. 0.5 L = ___ cc

19. 1.8 cc = ___ ml

17. 750 ml = ___ L

20. 1.5 L = ___ cc

18. 250 ml = ___ cc

SELF-ASSESSMENT POSTTEST

The Metric System

Show all your work. Check your answers (page 354).

Conversion factors: 1 kg = 1000 g   1 cm = 10 mm
                     1 g = 1000 mcg   1 L = 1000 ml
                     1 mg = 1000 mcg   1 cc = 1 ml

1. 44 mcg = ___ mg

2. 180 mm = ___ cm

3. 0.75 L = ___ cc

4. 26 mg = ___ g

5. 450 g = ___ kg

6. 1500 mcg = ___ g

7. 3 g = ___ mg

8. 0.51 kg = ___ g

9. 0.06 mg = ___ mcg

10. 5.5 kg = ___ g

11. 12 cc = ___ ml

12. 12 g = ___ mg

13. 2.5 kg = ___ g

14. 53 mcg = ___ mg

15. 8 cm = ___ mm

16. 225 ml = ___ L

17. 1200 mg = ___ mcg   19. 0.005 g = ___ mcg

18. 1500 ml = ___ L   20. 0.4 L = ___ ml

Chapter 9

Conversion Among the Measurement Systems

Conversions among the three systems of measurement are very difficult if the actual measurement equivalents are used. Consider the actual conversions between inches and centimeters. One centimeter is equal to 0.3937 inches; therefore, 2.5 centimeters equal 0.98425 inches. Memorizing the actual equivalents is a nearly impossible task. Multiplication and division of long decimals and fractions increase the possibility of error. Instead, approximate equivalents are used. Table 9-1 lists approximate equivalents that must be committed to memory. The abbreviations and symbols also must be memorized.

Because the equivalents are approximate, the resulting conversions will not be exact. Remember, conversions within a measurement system are exact; conversions among measurement systems are approximate. The more conversions among systems, the greater the variance from the actual measurement.

All problems in this workbook can be solved using the equivalents in Table 9-1. These equivalents are also used in clinical settings. This table does not include all conversions that health care professionals could use, but it is complete enough to solve any problem involving conversions in the clinical setting. An example is the equivalent weight of 1 milligram in grains. According to the equivalent table, there are 60 mg in 1 grain. There is no need to memorize the fact that 1 mg is equivalent to gr $\frac{1}{60}$. The conversion can be made by setting up the equation and solving the problem. Appendix A contains a complete list of approximate and actual equivalents.

TABLE 9-1 Metric, Apothecary, and Household Measurement Approximate Equivalents

	Metric	*Apothecary*	*Household*
WEIGHT	1 g = 1000 mg 60 mg 1 mg= 1000 mcg, mcgm, μg 1 Kg= 1000 Gm	= gr 15 = gr 1	 = 2.2 lb = 1 lb = 16oz,
VOLUME	1 ml = 1 cc 4 or 5 ml or cc 15 ml or cc 30 ml or cc 240 or 250 ml or cc 480 or 500 ml or cc 960 or 1000 ml or cc 1000 ml = 1 L	= 15-16 M, mx, ℥ = 1 dr, ℥ = 1/2 oz, ℥ = 1 oz = 8 oz = 16 oz = 32 oz = 32 oz	 = 1 tsp = 1 Tbsp = 2 Tbsp = 1 C = 1 pt = 1 qt = 1 qt
LENGTH	1 cm = 10 mm 2.5 cm 1 M		 = 1 inch, in, '' = 39 inches

Memorize the equivalents in this table. Some of them will be used each day in clinical practice; others will be used less frequently. Every nurse must know these conversions.

CONVERSION OF WEIGHTS

Sometimes it is difficult to understand and memorize equivalent measurements without frames of reference. Figure 9-1 shows some equivalents commonly used in medication administration. It is very difficult to perceive a weight measurement that is about the size of a pencil dot. Larger amounts are easier to conceptualize. Figure 9-2 shows the relationship between the larger measurements, kilograms and pounds. Figure 9-3 shows the corresponding weight and measurements of a woman in the metric and English systems.

Conversions among the three measurement systems are accomplished in the same manner as conversions within each system.

$$\text{Unit of answer} = \frac{\text{conversion} \times \begin{array}{c}\text{quantity and unit}\\ \text{being} \quad \text{converted}\end{array}}{\text{factor(s)} \times 1}$$

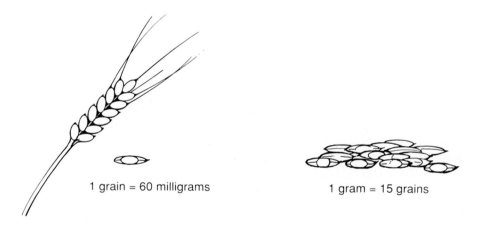

1 grain = 60 milligrams   1 gram = 15 grains

FIGURE 9-1 Comparison of apothecary and metric weights used in medication administration. A grain is about the size of a grain of wheat, about one-half inch long and less than an eighth of an inch in diameter. This grain of wheat contains 60 milligrams. Health care professionals use weights smaller than the mg. Each milligram contains 1000 micrograms. Therefore, 1 grain is equal to 60 milligrams or 60,000 micrograms.

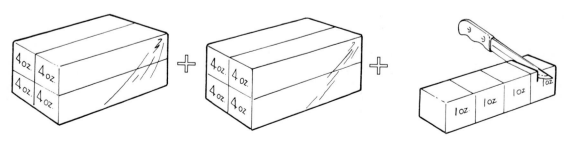

1 kilogram = 2.2 pounds or 2 pounds $3\frac{1}{5}$ ounce

FIGURE 9-2 Comparison between kilograms and pounds. One pound of butter contains four sticks, each of which weighs four ounces or approximately 113.6 grams. Two pounds plus almost a stick of butter is a kilogram.

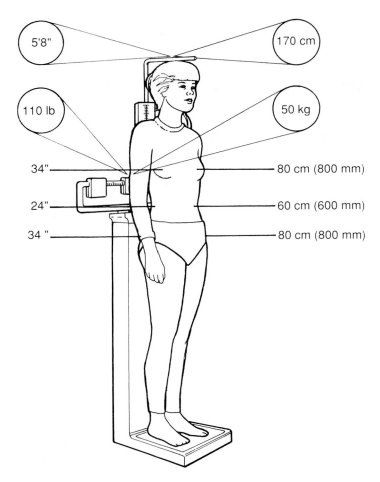

FIGURE 9-3 Comparison of household and metric length and weight measurements. A five feet eight inch young lady who weighs about 110 pounds has measurements of 34 inches, 24 inches, and 34 inches. This young lady does not mind weighing 50 kilograms or being 170 centimeters tall, but she is not enthusiastic about having measurements of 80, 60 and 80 centimeters. She would be appalled if those measurements were in millimeters.

SAMPLE PROBLEM   **1500 milligrams (mg) = _____ grains (gr)**

Knowns: Unit of Answer: gr
Factor: 1500 mg/1
Conversion Factor: 1 gr = 60 mg

Set up the framework of the equation, beginning with the unit of the answer, followed by the equal sign and the line separating the numerator and denominator.

$$gr = \underline{\qquad}$$

The numerator unit of the first factor must be the same as the unit of the answer. Find the factor containing gr. Write 1 gr in the numerator and 60 mg in the denominator, followed by multiplication signs.

$$gr = \frac{1\ gr\ \times}{60\ mg\ \times}$$

The numerator unit of the second factor must be the same as the denominator unit of the first factor. Find the factor containing mg. Write 1500 mg in the numerator and 1 in the denominator.

$$gr = \frac{1\ gr\ \times\ 1500\ mg}{60\ mg\ \times\quad 1}$$

Cancel the units appearing in both the numerator and denominator. Cancel the evenly divisible quantities.

$$gr = \frac{1 \text{ gr} \times \overset{25}{\cancel{1500}}}{\underset{1}{\cancel{60}} \times 1}$$

Multiply the numerator:
Multiply the denominator:

$$\frac{1 \text{ gr} \times 25 = 25 \text{ gr}}{1 \times 1 = 1} = 25\text{gr}$$

There was no need to divide the numerator by the denominator as any number over 1 is that number.

SAMPLE PROBLEM   **1.5 g = _____ gr**

Knowns: Unit of Answer: gr
Factor: 1.5 g/1
Conversion Factor: 1 g = 15 gr
Set up the equation framework.

$$gr = \text{————}$$

The numerator unit of the first factor must be the same as the unit of the answer. Find the factor containing gr. Write 15 gr in the numerator and 1 g in the denominator, followed by multiplication signs.

$$gr = \frac{15 \text{ gr} \times}{1 \text{ g} \times}$$

The numerator unit of the second factor must be the same as the denominator unit of the first factor. Find the factor containing g. Write 1.5 g in the numerator and 1 in the denominator.

$$gr = \frac{15 \text{ gr} \times 1.5 \text{ g}}{1 \text{ g} \times 1}$$

Cancel the units.

$$gr = \frac{15 \text{ gr} \times 1.5}{1 \times 1}$$

Multiply the numerator:
Multiply the denominator:

$$\frac{15 \text{ gr} \times 1.5 = 22.5 \text{ gr}}{1 \times 1 = 1} = 22.5 \text{ gr} = 22\tfrac{1}{2} \text{ gr}$$

Remember, fractional parts of an apothecary measurement are written in common fractions, while parts of a metric measurement are written in decimal fractions.

Consider the answers to these two problems. In problem 1, 1500 milligrams is equal to 25 grains, whereas in problem 2, 1.5 grams equals $22\tfrac{1}{2}$ grains. One gram is equal to 1000 milligrams; therefore, 1.5 grams is equal to 1500 milligrams. If 1.5 grams is equal to 1500 milligrams, why are the answers in grains different? The answers are not equivalent because the conversions used are approximate equivalents rather than actual. In general, it is probably more accurate to use the conversion factor 1 gr = 60 mg for amounts of less than 1 grain. For amounts greater than 1 grain, the conversion factors 1 g = 15 gr and 1000 mg = 15 gr are more accurate. Solutions using both conversion factors are shown in the answer section.

The more approximate equivalents that are used in a problem, the greater the discrepancy between the answer and the actual measurement. Therefore, it is much safer to remain within a measurement system whenever possible, since equivalents within a measurement system are actual measurements.

The following problem has a mixed number that must be converted to an improper fraction.

> To convert a mixed number to an improper fraction:
>
> $$\frac{(\text{whole number} \times \text{denominator}) + \text{existing numerator}}{\text{denominator}} = \frac{\text{new numerator}}{\text{denominator}}$$

SAMPLE PROBLEM   **2 lb 1 oz =** _____ **g**

Knowns: Unit of Answer: g
Factor: 2 lb 1 oz/1 = $2\frac{1}{16}$ lb
Conversion Factors: 1 kg = 1000 g
           1 kg = 2.2 lb
Set up the framework for the equation.

$$g = \frac{\rule{2cm}{0.4pt}}{}$$

The numerator unit of the first factor must be the same as the unit of the answer. Find the factor containing g. Write 1000 g in the numerator and 1 kg in the denominator, followed by multiplication signs.

$$g = \frac{1000\ g \ \times}{1\ kg \ \times}$$

The numerator unit of the second factor must be the same as the denominator unit of the first factor. Find the factor containing kg. Write 1 kg in the numerator and 2.2 lb in the denominator, followed by multiplication signs.

$$g = \frac{1000\ g \ \times \ 1\ kg \times}{1\ kg \times 2.2\ lb \ \times}$$

The numerator unit of the third factor must be the same as the denominator unit of the second factor. Find the factor containing lb. Write $2\frac{1}{16}$ lb in the numerator and 1 in the denominator.

$$g = \frac{100\ g \ \times \ 1\ kg \times 2\ 1/16\ lb}{1\ kg \times 2.2\ lb \ \times \qquad 1}$$

Cancel the units.

$$g = \frac{1000\ g \times \ 1 \times 2\ 1/16}{1 \ \times 2.2 \times \qquad 1}$$

Convert the mixed number to an improper fraction. $\frac{(2\times16)+1}{16} = \frac{32+1}{16} = \frac{33}{16}$

$$g = \frac{1000\ g \times \ 1 \times 33/16}{1 \ \times 2.2 \times \qquad 1}$$

Drop the fraction denominator into the equation denominator. Cancel.

$$g = \frac{\overset{125}{\cancel{1000}}\ g \times \ 1 \times \overset{3}{\cancel{33}}}{1 \ \times \underset{0.2}{\cancel{2.2}} \times \underset{2}{\cancel{16}}}$$

Multiply the numerator:
Multiply the denominator:

$$\frac{125\ g \times \ 1 \times 3}{1 \ \times 0.2 \times 2} = \frac{375\ g}{0.4} = 937.5\ g$$

SAMPLE PROBLEM   **gr $\frac{1}{150}$ =** _____ **mcg**

Knowns: Unit of Answer: mcg
Factor: gr $\frac{1}{150}$/1
Conversion Factors: 1 gr = 60 mg
           1 mg = 1000 mcg
Set up the framework for the equation.

$$mcg = \frac{\rule{2cm}{0.4pt}}{}$$

The numerator unit of the first factor must be the same as the answer unit. Find the factor containing mcg. Write 1000 mcg in the numerator and 1 mg in the denominator, followed by multiplication signs.

$$mcg = \frac{1000\ mcg \ \times}{1\ mg \ \times}$$

The numerator unit of the second factor must be the same as the denominator unit of the first factor. Find the factor containing mg. Write 60 mg in the numerator and 1 gr in the denominator, followed by multiplication signs.

$$\text{mcg} = \frac{1000 \text{ mcg} \times 60 \text{ mg} \times}{1 \text{ mg} \times 1 \text{ gr} \times}$$

The numerator unit of the third factor must be the same as the denominator unit of the second factor. Find the factor containing gr. Write gr $\frac{1}{150}$ in the numerator and 1 in the denominator.

$$\text{mcg} = \frac{1000 \text{ mcg} \times 60 \text{ mg} \times \text{gr} \quad 1/150}{1 \text{ mg} \times 1 \text{ gr} \times \quad\quad 1}$$

Cancel the units.

$$\text{mcg} = \frac{1000 \text{ mcg} \times 60 \times 1/150}{1 \times 1 \times 1}$$

Drop the fraction denominator into the denominator of the equation. Cancel the evenly divisible quantities.

$$\text{mcg} = \frac{\overset{200}{\cancel{1000}} \text{ mcg} \times \overset{2}{\cancel{60}} \times 1}{1 \times 1 \times \underset{\underset{1}{5}}{\cancel{150}} \times 1}$$

Multiply the numerator:
Multiply the denominator:

$$\frac{200 \text{ mcg} \times 2 \times 1}{1 \quad \times 1 \times 1 \times 1} = \frac{400 \text{ mcg}}{1} = 400 \text{ mcg}$$

PRACTICE PROBLEMS

Conversion of Weights

Conversion factors: 1 gram (g) = 1000 milligrams (mg)
1 gram (g) = 15 grains (gr)
1 grain (gr) = 60 milligrams (mg)
1 milligram = 1000 micrograms (mcg)
1 kilogram (kg) = 1000 grams (g)
1 kilogram (kg) = 2.2 pounds (lb)
1 pound (lb) = 16 ounces (oz,ʒ)

Writing the conversion factors for each problem will aid the process of memorization. Show all your work. Check your answers (page 320).

1. gr ii = _____ mg

2. 0.3 g = _____ gr

3. gr $\frac{1}{300}$ = _____ mcg

4. 45 kg = _____ lb

5. 200 mcg = gr _____

6. gr viiss = _____ g

7. 6 lb 6 oz = _____ g

14. 7 lb 14 oz = _____ kg

8. 0.04 g = _____ gr

15. 60 mcg = _____ gr

9. 154 lb = _____ kg

16. 250 g = _____ oz

10. gr XX = _____ mg

17. gr $\frac{1}{6}$ = _____ mg

11. 10 kg = _____ lb

18. 0.4 mg = _____ gr

12. 0.6 mg = _____ gr

19. 4.8 kg = _____ lb

13. gr $\frac{1}{150}$ = _____ mg

20. 0.8 g = _____ gr

CONVERSION OF LINEAR MEASUREMENTS

Conversion of measurements of length involves the memorization of several conversion factors. Rarely is the nurse expected to convert between meters and household lengths. Conversions between centimeters, millimeters, and inches are used with some regularity. Figure 9-3 shows equivalent metric and household measurements of a woman's figure. Other metric and English measurements of length are shown in Figure 9-4.

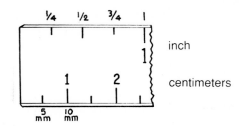

1 inch = 2.5 centimeters = 25 millimeters

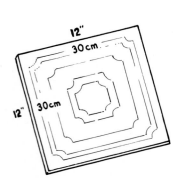

12 inches = 30 centimeters

FIGURE 9-4 Comparison of inches and centimeters. A standard floor tile is 12 inches square. In the metric system, the measurement is 30 centimeters square. An inch contains about 2.5 centimeters or 25 millimeters. Each short line on the centimeter rule is equal to 5 millimeters.

SAMPLE PROBLEM   **10 in = _____ mm**

Knowns: Unit of Answer: mm
Factor: 10 in/1
Conversion Factors: 1 in = 2.5 cm
                                    1 cm = 10 mm

Set up the framework for the equation.

$$mm = \frac{\rule{2cm}{0.4pt}}{}$$

The numerator unit of the first factor must be the same as the unit of the answer. Find the factor containing mm. Write 10 mm in the numerator and 1 cm in the denominator, followed by multiplication signs.

$$mm = \frac{10\ mm\ \times}{1\ cm\ \times}$$

The numerator unit of the second factor must be the same as the denominator unit of the first factor. Find the factor containing cm. Write 2.5 cm in the numerator and 1 in in the denominator, followed by multiplication signs.

$$mm = \frac{10\ mm \times 2.5\ cm\ \times}{1\ cm\ \times\ \ 1\ in\ \ \times}$$

The numerator unit of the third factor must be the same as the denominator unit of the second factor. Find the factor containing in. Write 10 in in the numerator and 1 in the denominator.

$$mm = \frac{10\ mm \times 2.5\ cm\ \times 10\ in}{1\ cm\ \times\ \ 1\ in\ \ \times\ \ 1}$$

Cancel the units.

$$mm = \frac{10\ mm \times 2.5 \times 10}{1\ \ \ \times\ \ 1 \times\ 1}$$

Multiply the numerator; multiply the denominator:

$$\frac{10\ mm \times 2.5 \times 10}{1\ \ \ \times\ \ 1 \times 1} = \frac{250\ mm}{1} = 250\ mm$$

PRACTICE PROBLEMS

Conversion of Linear Measurements

Conversion factors: 1 meter (m) = 39 inches (in)

1 inch (in) = 2.5 centimeters (cm)

1 centimeter (cm) = 10 millimeters (mm)

Writing the conversion factors for each problem will aid in memorization of equivalents. (Answers on page 321.)

21. 8 inches = _____ cm

22. 96 cm = _____ in

23. 28 cm = _____ in

24. 42 in = _____ m

25. 10 cm = _____ in

26. 16 in = _____ mm

27. 112 mm = _____ in

28. $1\frac{1}{2}$ in = _____ mm

29. 12.5 mm = _____ in

30. 3 in = _____ cm

CONVERSION OF VOLUMES

The bulk of the equivalents requiring memorization are volume measurements. Figure 9-5 compares volume measurements in apothecary, household, and metric systems. These measurements are used frequently in medication administration. Medicine cups traditionally are labeled in all three measurement systems. Note the discrepancy between drams and teaspoons on the cup. In the United States, the standard teaspoon is 5 ml.

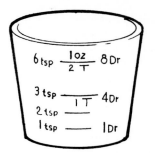
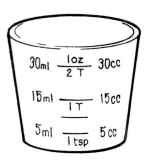

FIGURE 9-5 Comparison of volume measurements of the apothecary, household and metric systems. Notice that there are 8 drams but only 6 teaspoons in 30 milliliters. Remember that, although a dram and teaspoon are approximately equal, a dram is a little bit smaller. This difference is negligible with one or two teaspoons or drams but becomes apparent when three or four teaspoons or drams are considered. In the United States, the standard teaspoon is 5 milliliters.

Larger volume measurements are shown in Figure 9-6. These measurements most commonly are used for calculating fluid intake.

The syringe is the tool of choice for measuring small quantities accurately. Figure 9-7 shows a 1 milliliter tuberculin syringe and a 3 milliliter syringe. Notice that they are calibrated in minims on the left side and in cubic centimeters (milliliters) on the right side.

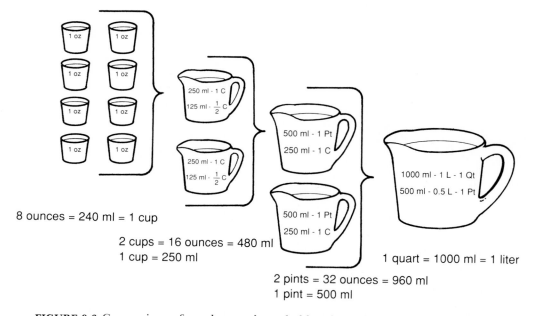

FIGURE 9-6 Comparison of apothecary, household and metric volume measurements.

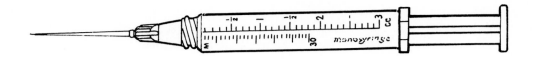

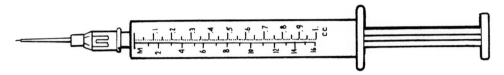

FIGURE 9-7 Relationship between minims and cubic centimeters (milliliters). Note that there are 8 minims in 0.5 cc and 16 minims in 1 cc. 3 cc = 48 minims; 2 cc = 32 minims. The conversion factor for minims to cc or ml, however, is 1 cc or ml = 15 to 16 minims.

SAMPLE PROBLEM   **3 pt =_____ ml**

Knowns: Unit of Answer: ml
Factor: 3 pt/1
Conversion Factor: 1 pt = 500 ml
Set up the framework for the equation.

$$ml = \underline{\hspace{3cm}}$$

The numerator unit of the first factor must be the same as the answer unit. Find the factor containing ml. Write 500 ml in the numerator and 1 pt in the denominator, followed by multiplication signs.

$$ml = \frac{500 \text{ ml} \times}{1 \text{ pt} \times}$$

The numerator unit of the second factor must be the same as the denominator unit of the first factor. Find the factor containing pt. Write 3 pt in the numerator and 1 in the denominator.

$$ml = \frac{500 \text{ ml} \times 3 \text{ pt}}{1 \text{ pt} \times 1}$$

Cancel the units.

$$ml = \frac{500 \text{ ml} \times 3}{1 \times 1}$$

Multiply the numerator:
Multiply the denominator:

$$\frac{500 \text{ ml} \times 3}{1 \times 1} = \frac{1500 \text{ ml}}{1} = 1500 ml$$

This problem could have been solved using the following conversion factors: 1 pt = 2 C, 1 C = 8 oz, and 1 oz = 30 ml. The equation using these conversion factors is:

$$ml = \frac{30 \text{ ml} \times 8 \text{ oz} \times 2 \text{ C} \times 3 \text{ pt}}{1 \text{ oz} \times 1 \text{ C} \times 1 \text{ pt} \times 1} = \frac{30 \text{ ml} \times 8 \times 2 \times 3}{1 \times 1 \times 1 \times 1} = \frac{1440 \text{ ml}}{1} = 1440 \text{ ml}$$

The discrepancy between 1440 and 1500 ml occurs as a result of the approximate equivalents used. One pint is actually 473.167 ml, so 3 pints equals 1419.501 or 1420 ml. Therefore, 1440 ml is actually more correct than 1500 ml. Throughout this workbook, either answer is considered correct.

PRACTICE PROBLEMS

Conversion of Volumes

Conversion factors: 1 ml = 1 cc
                         1 oz = 30 ml or cc
                         1 ml or cc = 15–16 minims
                         1 cup (C) = 8 oz or 250 ml or cc
                         1 tsp = 1 dr = 4–5 ml or cc
                         1 pint (pt) = 16 oz or 500 ml or cc
                         1 Tbsp = 15 ml or cc
                         1 quart (qt) = 32 oz or 1000 ml
                         1 oz = 2 tablespoons

Writing the conversion factors for each problem aids in the memorization of equivalents. (Answers on page 322.)

31. $7\frac{1}{2}$ minims = _____ cc

36. 6 drams = _____ ml

32. $1\frac{1}{2}$ oz = _____ cc

37. 12 Tbsp = _____ cc

33. 3 pt = _____ ml

38. 45 ml = _____ Tbsp

34. 6 ml = _____ minims

39. $\frac{1}{2}$ pt = _____ ml

35. 15 cc = _____ tsp

40. $\frac{1}{4}$ qt = _____ ml

CALCULATING FLUID INTAKE

One frequent clinical use of conversions among the measurement systems occurs with the calculation of intake and output. Frequently abbreviated I & O, intake and output is the monitoring of fluids entering and exiting the body. A variety of clients require I & O monitoring.

Intake and output is recorded using cubic centimeters or milliliters. Output is measured using metric calibrated containers, so conversions are not necessary. Oral intake, however, often must be converted from household measurements prior to recording.

Oral intake includes all fluids and solids that become liquid at body temperature, such as ice cream, popsicles, and jello. Cream soups and broths are included, as are the liquids in vegetable soups or milk in cereals. Intake does not include solids such as meat, bread, cereal, or vegetables.

To record individual fluids ingested, nonmetric measurements are converted to milliliters or cubic centimeters and recorded on the intake portion of the bedside record along with the appropriate time. Some agencies use metric calibrated cups or glasses to facilitate accurate I & O. Every time a client ingests oral fluids, including those taken with medications, the amount is recorded.

One point of confusion often occurs when recording cups of coffee or tea. Although a standard cup is 8 ounces, a coffee cup usually holds 5 or 6 ounces. Each agency has a standard measurement for the coffee cup used in its facility. Sometimes the bedside intake and output record contains a list of amounts specific to the agency, as shown in Figure 9-8. Note that the coffee cup holds 6 ounces or 180 cc. In the following problem, a cup of coffee will be considered to be 6 ounces and a glass of liquid will be recorded as a standard cup or 8 ounces.

Oral intake is calculated in the same manner as other conversion problems. The following problem has three separate problems that are set up in dimensional analysis equations. After each item is converted, the items are added together for the total intake.

SAMPLE PROBLEM **Calculate the following total breakfast intake in cubic centimeters:**

½ **glass juice**	½ **pint milk**
2 strips bacon	**1 C dry cereal**
1 poached egg	**1 cup coffee**

Knowns: Unit of Answer: cc
Conversion Factors: 1 oz = 30 cc
1 pt = 500 cc
1 coffee cup = 6 oz
1 glass = 1 C = 8 oz

The food ingested is:

½ glass juice

$$cc = \frac{30\,cc \times 8\,oz \times \frac{1}{2}\,C}{1\,oz \times 1\,C \times 1} = \frac{30\,cc \times \overset{4}{\cancel{8}} \times 1}{1 \times 1 \times \cancel{2}} = \frac{120\,cc}{1} = 120\,cc$$

2 strips bacon   not part of fluid intake

1 poached egg   not part of fluid intake

½ pint milk

$$cc = \frac{500\,cc \times \frac{1}{2}\,pt}{1\,pt \times 1} = \frac{\overset{250}{\cancel{500}}\,cc \times 1}{1 \times \cancel{2}} = \frac{250\,cc}{1} = 250\,cc$$

INTAKE AND OUTPUT
BEDSIDE RECORD

COFFEE CUP 180 CC	JUICE GLASS 120 CC
DESSERT BOWL 120 CC	SOUP BOWL 150 CC
GLASS 240 CC	TEAPOT 250 CC

INTAKE				OUTPUT			
TIME	PO	IV	OTHER	TIME	VOID	CATH	OTHER
9:00	Joe 120cc Milk 250cc Coffee 180cc						
TOTAL							
TOTAL							
TOTAL							
24 HOUR TOTAL							

FIGURE 9-8 Intake and output sheet

SAMPLE PROBLEM, continued

1 C dry cereal   not part of fluid intake

1 cup coffee

$$cc = \frac{30\,cc \times 6\,oz}{1\,oz \times 1} = \frac{30\,cc \times 6}{1\ \ \times 1} = \frac{180\,cc}{1} = 180\,cc$$

Total: 550cc

The conversions are recorded on the bedside I & O record as shown in Figure 9-8.
    The half-pint of milk could have been calculated by converting the half-pint to ounces prior to solving for cubic centimeters. That equation is written and solved as follows:

$$cc = \frac{30\,cc \times 16\,oz \times 1/2\,pt}{1\,oz \times 1\,pt \times 1\,oz} = \frac{30\,cc \times \overset{8}{\cancel{16}} \times 1}{1 \times 1 \times \underset{1}{\cancel{2}}} = \frac{240\,cc}{1} = 240\,cc$$

If this equation is used, the product differs from the previously calculated intake by 10 cc. Therefore, the total intake would be 540 instead of 550 cc. Both answers are correct. The discrepancy is due to the approximate equivalents used to convert from one measurement system to another.

The total intake includes intravenous fluids infused as well as those administered orally or by tube feeding. These are recorded separately on the bedside record. When the 24-hour intake is totaled, all fluids administered by any route are totaled. Figure 9-9 shows a completed, 24-hour bedside intake and output record that includes oral and intravenous fluids.

INTAKE AND OUTPUT
BEDSIDE RECORD

COFFEE CUP 180 CC   JUICE GLASS 120 CC
DESSERT BOWL 120 CC   SOUP BOWL 150 CC
GLASS 240 CC   TEAPOT 250 CC

INTAKE				OUTPUT			
TIME	PO	IV	OTHER	TIME	VOID	CATH	OTHER
0630 0700	H₂0 250cc	850 cc		0230 0640	200cc 350cc		NG 130cc
TOTAL	250cc	850cc			550 cc		130cc NG
0800 0900 1030 1200 1300 1430 1500	Juice 120cc Coffee 180cc Eggnog 250cc tea 250cc H₂0 120cc SHAKE 250cc	DSW 150cc DSW 850cc		1000 1230 1300 1430	325 cc 250 cc 300cc		80cc
TOTAL	1170 cc	1000 cc			875 cc		80cc NG
1530 1645 1800	H₂0 250cc H₂0 150cc tea 250cc Soup 150cc Ice cream 120cc	D5NS 150cc		1700 1830 2100 2230	425 cc 250 cc 350 cc 150 cc		
TOTAL	920 cc	150 cc			1175 cc		
24 HOUR TOTAL	2340 cc	2000 cc			2600		210 cc NG
	4340 cc				2810 cc		

FIGURE 9-9 Completed 24-hour intake and output sheet

PRACTICE PROBLEMS

Calculating Fluid Intake

(Answers on page 325.)

Assume that a coffee or tea cup holds 6 ounces and a glass holds 8 ounces for these problems.

41–44. Record Mrs. Jones's intake for each item and total intake in ml. She ate the following:

$\frac{1}{2}$ cup orange juice

$1\frac{1}{2}$ slices buttered wheat toast

1 cup coffee

1 cup raisin bran

$\frac{1}{2}$ of a half-pint container of milk

45–48. Record Mr. Brown's intake for each item and total in cc. He ate the following for lunch:

4 oz fresh fruit

$\frac{1}{2}$ C lettuce and tomato salad

5 Tbsp cream of chicken soup

3 oz roast beef

$\frac{1}{4}$ C broccoli

$\frac{1}{2}$ pt milk

1 cup coffee

49–57. Calculate Mrs. Rush's individual item and total day shift intake in ml. She drank the following:

$\frac{1}{2}$ C orange juice

$\frac{1}{2}$ pint container of milk

$\frac{1}{2}$ quart water

$\frac{1}{2}$ cup strawberry ice cream

7 Tbsp creamed soup

$\frac{1}{2}$ glass water

1 glass iced tea

12 oz Dr. Pepper

58–60. Calculate the following individual item and total intake in ml:

2 popsicles, 3 oz each

1 sliced apple

6 Tbsp jello

$\frac{1}{2}$ cup dry cereal

$\frac{1}{4}$ quart lemonade

CONVERSIONS AMONG MEASUREMENT SYSTEMS

Complete these problems without looking at the equivalent table. Remember that fractional parts of metric unit answers are written in decimals while household and apothecary unit answers are in common fractions. (Answers on page 355.)

1. gr $\frac{1}{300}$ = _____ mg

2. 200 mcg = _____ gr

3. 25 minims = _____ cc

4. gr viiss = _____ g

5. 7 lb 8 oz = _____ kg

6. 55 kg = _____ lb

7. 35 mm = _____ in

8. 0.4 mg = _____ gr

9. gr XXX = _____ mg

10. 0.75 ml = _____ minims

11. gr $\frac{1}{600}$ = _____ mcg

12. 2 g = _____ gr

13. 4 lb 5 oz = _____ g

14. 45 mg = _____ gr

15. gr iiss = _____ g

16. 6 mg = _____ gr

17–20. Calculate the individual item and total intake of the following in ml:

$\frac{1}{3}$ C creamed broccoli soup

1 C lettuce and tomato salad

2 slices roast beef

$\frac{1}{2}$ C oven-browned potatoes

$\frac{1}{2}$ pint milk

$\frac{1}{2}$ C sliced fresh fruit

2 glasses iced tea

UNIT III POSTTEST

Conversions Within and Among Measurement Systems
Test A

Complete these problems without looking at the equivalent table. (Answers on page 368.)

1. gr $\frac{1}{300}$ = _____ mcg

5. 12 mx = _____ ml

2. 200 mm = _____ ”

6. 4 mcg = _____ mg

3. 7 lb 12 oz = _____ kg

7. 15 mg = _____ gr

4. 0.03 g = _____ mg

8. 7 ʒ = _____ tsp

9. gr $\frac{1}{200}$ = _____ mg

16. 0.03 g = _____ mcg

10. 0.3 ml = _____ mx

17. 77 kg = _____ lb

11. ℥ iss = _____ Tbsp

18. 1 1/2 qt = _____ ml

12. 2.5 mcg = _____ mg

19. 600 mcg = _____ gr

13. 8 cc = _____ ml

20. 9 tsp = _____ ml

14. 6 lb 13 oz = _____ g

21. 750 cc = _____ qt

15. 12 cm = _____ in

22–25. Calculate the individual item and total intake in ml for the following:

$\frac{1}{2}$ C fresh fruit

10 Tbsp cream soup

$\frac{1}{2}$ tuna salad sandwich

$\frac{3}{4}$ C grapefruit juice

4 oz slice chocolate cake

10 oz Pepsi

UNIT III POSTTEST

Test B

(Answers on page 369.)

1. gr $\frac{1}{400}$ = _____ mcg

2. 100 mm = _____ ”

3. 9 lb 10 oz = _____ kg

4. 0.05 g = _____ mg

5. 20 mx = _____ ml

6. 12 mcg = _____ mg

7. 30 mg = _____ gr

8. 9 ℥ = _____ tsp

9. gr 1/150 = _____ mg

10. 0.6 ml = _____ mx

11. 5 oz = _____ Tbsp

17. 99 kg = _____ lb

12. 150 mcg = _____ mg

18. 1 3/4 qt = _____ ml

13. 10 cc = _____ ml

19. 200 mcg = _____ gr

14. 4 lb 2 oz = _____ g

20. 7 tsp = _____ ml

15. 6 cm = _____ in

21. 1250 cc = _____ qt

16. 0.007 g = _____ mcg

22–25. Calculate the individual item and total intake in ml for the following:

$\frac{1}{2}$ peach

8 Tbsp chicken broth

1 C tossed green salad

2 C Koolade

3 oz broiled chicken

$\frac{1}{2}$ C milk

UNIT III POSTTEST

Test C

(Answers on page 370.)

1. gr $\frac{1}{600}$ = _____ mcg

2. 50 mm = _____ ”

3. 8 lb 4 oz = _____ kg

4. 0.07 g = _____ mg

5. 4 mx = _____ ml

6. 8 mcg = _____ mg

7. 45 mg = _____ gr

8. 11 ʒ = _____ tsp

9. gr $\frac{1}{400}$ = _____ mg

10. 0.9 ml = _____ mx

11. ʒ viiss = _____ Tbsp

12. 25 mcg = _____ mg

13. 6 cc = _____ ml

14. 5 lb 8 oz = _____ g

15. 15 cm = _____ in

16. 0.06 g = _____ mcg

17. 110 kg = _____ lb

20. 5 tsp = _____ ml

18. $\frac{3}{4}$ qt = _____ ml

21. 400 cc = _____ qt

19. 300 mcg = _____ gr

22–25. Calculate the individual item and total intake in ml for the following:

1 orange

5 Tbsp tomato soup

1 C chicken salad

12 oz Coke

4 cookies

4 oz ice cream

Dosage Conversions and Calculations

OBJECTIVES *Upon completion of this unit, the student will have demonstrated the ability to correctly:*

- Utilize abbreviations and symbols used in medication administration to translate medication orders into lay terms.

- Calculate daily dosage.

- Read medication labels.

- Utilize unit of measurement equivalents to select appropriate medication strength.

- Calculate oral medication dosages in tablets, capsules, and liquid measurements.

- Calculate volumes for injectable medication dosages.

Prior to administering medications in the agency, nurses must have the ability to interpret medication orders and labels. This involves knowledge of medication terminology, abbreviations, and symbols as well as conversion equivalents.

Conversions are frequently used to determine which strengths or concentration of medication to use when there are several strengths from which to choose. Calculations of dosages are used each time medications are given and are the most common mathematical processes performed by nurses in the clinical setting. Most medication orders are written using weights, such as milligrams or grains. Units such as tablets, milliliters, or ounces are used to administer medications. Pharmaceutical companies prepare specific weights (dosages) of medication in solid or liquid form. The nurse is responsible for calculating the amounts of these pharmaceutical preparations that are equivalent to the dosage ordered. Some dosage calculations require only the recognition that an order and a label are the same quantity and unit of measurement. Other dosage calculations require more complicated computations.

Chapter 10

Interpretation of Medication Orders and Labels

Medication orders consist of four parts: (1) the medication name, either generic or trade (brand or proprietary); (2) the dosage; (3) the route; and (4) the frequency of administration. No order is complete without all four parts. The order will also include the date and the physician's signature. Some agencies also require the time the order was written.

Medication orders are written by physicians on the doctor's orders or physician's directions form. A doctor's order form is shown in Figure 10-1, complete with admission orders for the client. Note that the orders are written using abbreviations and symbols. The orders have been translated into lay terms in the box on the lower right side of the doctor's order sheet.

The original order is transcribed, or rewritten, on the record of medication administration by the unit secretary or nurse. Transcribed orders may be entered into a computerized medication administration record or handwritten on a medication administration record. Some facilities, especially those that provide extended care, also transcribe medications onto medication cards. Note that the orders from Figure 10-1 have been transcribed in Figure 10-2 onto a medication administration record. Figure 10-3 shows those same orders transcribed onto a computerized medication record.

Transcribed medication orders also may be recorded on a patient profile record, the form that is used for the client's nursing care plan. In Figure 10-4, those same orders were transcribed onto the patient profile and an inset medication card. Even though a medication administration record or card is used when medication is administered, that nurse is expected to verify the transcribed order with the original order.

Health care providers are expected to understand the abbreviations and symbols used on physician's orders. Table 10-1 lists common abbreviations and symbols used in medication and treatment orders. Learn these abbreviations. It is necessary to be able to recall the symbols and abbreviations used in conversion and calculation of dosage. Table 10-2 is a recapitulation of those symbols, abbreviations, measurement equivalents, and roman numerals.

Some medications are frequently abbreviated in medication orders. Abbreviation of medications on doctor's orders and medication administration records can be a hazardous practice unless all health care providers recognize the abbreviations. Some health care facilities have policies prohibiting the use of most abbreviations for medications. Some common medication abbreviations are shown in Table 10-3. Abbreviations of medications that are usually acceptable, such as ASA for aspirin, are marked with asterisks. Chemical symbols for elements, compounds, suffixes, and prefixes are usually acceptable also. A more complete list of chemical symbols is shown in Appendix C.

FORT WORTH OSTEOPATHIC MEDICAL CENTER FORT WORTH, TEXAS

ORDERS & DIRECTIONS	DOCTOR Indicate duration of medication in days or doses

DATE AND TIME: Jan 21 8:30 A

ALLERGIES:

NKA 1. Adm to 6T

2. BR c̄ BRP

3. Flds Ad lib

4. Reg diet NAS

5. Notify Dr. Coats of Adm ASAP

C Ngo DO

(right margin handwritten: 0900 Anderson LU / J. Bright Rn 0910)

02568   ROOM 603
DOE, MARY A
32429   DR G COATS

DATE AND TIME: Jan 21 10:30 A

1. ASA gr v PO qd

2. digoxin 0.125 mg. PO bid

3. aldomet 250 mg. PO tid

4. nitroglycerine gr. 1/150 SL PRN

5. Dalmane 30 mg. PO his prn

6. ECG stat

02568   ROOM 603
DOE, MARY A
32429   DR G COATS

DATE AND TIME:

7. Routine CBC, UA, lytes in AM

G Coats DO

(right margin handwritten: 1040 Anderson LU / J. Bright Rn 1100)

LAY TRANSLATION OF DOCTOR'S ORDERS

Jan 21, 8:30 AM
NO KNOWN ALLERGIES
1. Admit to 6 tower
2. Bedrest with bath room privileges
3. Fluids as desired
4. Regular diet, no added salt
5. Notify Dr. Coats of admission as soon as possible
Jan 21, 1030 AM
1. Aspirin grains 5 by mouth every day
2. Digoxin 0.125 milligrams by mouth twice a day
3. Aldomet 250 milligrams by mouth three times a day
4. Nitroglycerine grains 1/150 sublingually when necessary
5. Dalmane 30 milligrams by mouth at bedtime when necessary
6. Electrocardiogram immediately
7. Routine complete blood count, urinalysis and electrolytes in the morning
Jan 21, 1:00 PM
1. Morphine sulfate grains 1/6 intramuscularly immediately verbal order of Dr. Coats

DATE AND TIME: Jan 21 1300 MS gr 1/6 IM stat

VO Dr. Coats / L. Bright Rn

DOCTOR

(1) Your orders are being automatically copied. Please write or print legibly. Use a Ball Point Pen.
(2) *To comply with Medical Board action, for "Stop - orders on dangerous drugs.

PHYSICIANS DIRECTIONS
☐ GENERIC EQUIVALENTS ORDERED UNLESS MARKED HERE

(1) **ADDRESSOGRAPH IN ALL 4 SPACES BEFORE PUTTING THIS SHEET IN THE CHART.**
(2) If the doctor did not use all the lines in a segment, mark through these blank lines.
(3) Send carbon to Pharmacy **as soon as possible.**

CHART COPY   REV. 85-FS043
                                   4448

FIGURE 10-1 Physician's order sheet. (*Courtesy Fort Worth Osteopathic Medical Center, Fort Worth, Texas.*)

CURRENT DIAGNOSIS: __Hypertension, R/o CHF__   PAGE ___1___ OF ___1___ PAGES
ALLERGIES: __NKA__   RECOPIED BY: _____

Date Ordered / Start Date	MEDICATION Drug — Strength — Frequency	Route	Shift	DATE	Initials	DATE	Initials	DATE	Initials	DATE	Initials	DATE	Initials
1/21 1/22			11-7										
Reorder / Last Dose 1/27	Aspirin gr 5	PO	7-3										
Transcriber aa qd													
Times To Administer 8^A			3-11										
Date Ordered / Start Date	digoxin		11-7										
Reorder / Last Dose 1/26 0.125 mg		PO	7-3										
Transcriber aa bid													
Times To Administer 8^A - 8^A			3-11										
Date Ordered 1/21 / Start Date 1/21	Aldomet		11-7										
Reorder / Last Dose 1/26 250 mg		PO	7-3	2^P	JB								
Transcriber aa tid													
Times To Administer 8^A - 2^P - 8^P			3-11										
Date Ordered 1/21 / Start Date 1/21	Nitroglycerine		11-7										
Reorder / Last Dose 1/26 gr 1/150		SL	7-3										
Transcriber aa prn													
Times To Administer prn			3-11										
Date Ordered 1/21 / Start Date 1/21	Dalmane		11-7										
Reorder / Last Dose 1/26 30 mg		PO	7-3										
Transcriber aa HS PRN													
Times To Administer 10^P prn			3-11										
Date Ordered 1/21 / Start Date 1/21	MORPHINE SULFATE		11-7										
Reorder / Last Dose 1/21		IM	7-3	1^10	JB								
Transcriber gr 1/6 stat													
Times To Administer Stat			3-11										
Date Ordered / Start Date			11-7										
Reorder / Last Dose			7-3										
Transcriber													
Times To Administer			3-11										
Date Ordered / Start Date			11-7										
Reorder / Last Dose			7-3										
Transcriber													
Times To Administer			3-11										

PATIENT IDENTIFICATION

02568   ROOM 603
DOE, MARY A
32429   DR G COATS

	SIGNATURE & TITLE	I	SIGNATURE & TITLE	I	SIGNATURE & TITLE	I	SIGNATURE & TITLE	I	SIGNATURE & TITLE	I
11-7	Jill Bright	JB								
7-3										
3-11										

I = Initials   **MEDICATION ADMINISTRATION RECORD —**
FSO30W REV. 9/84

FIGURE 10-2 Medication administration record (*Courtesy Fort Worth Osteopathic Medical Center, Fort Worth, Texas.*)

DAILY MEDICATION RECORD FOR 01/21/89
PAGE 1 OF 1
02568   DOE, MARY A
                                                     ROOM 603

MEDICATION 1	ASPIRIN 325 MG (GR 5) PO QD		
DATE ORDERED 1/21/89	NIGHT SHIFT	DAY SHIFT	EVENING SHIFT
DR G COATS	0	0	2100
LAST DOSE 1/27/89:0900			

MEDICATION 2	DIGOXIN 0.125 MG PO BID		
DATE ORDERED 1/21/89	NIGHT SHIFT	DAY SHIFT	EVENING SHIFT
DR G COATS	0	0	2100
LAST DOSE 1/26/89:2100			

MEDICATION 3	ALDOMET 250 MG PO TID		
DATE ORDERED 1/21/89	NIGHT SHIFT	DAY SHIFT	EVENING SHIFT
DR G COATS		0900	1700
LAST DOSE 1/26/89:1700		1300	

MEDICATION 4	NITROGLYCERIN 0.4 MG (GR 1/150) SL PRN		
DATE ORDERED 1/21/89	NIGHT SHIFT	DAY SHIFT	EVENING SHIFT
DR G COATS			
LAST DOSE 1/26/89:2359			

MEDICATION 5	DALMANE 30 MG PO HS PRN		
DATE ORDERED 1/21/89	NIGHT SHIFT	DAY SHIFT	EVENING SHIFT
DR G COATS	0	0	2100 PRN
LAST DOSE 1/26/89:2100			

FIGURE 10-3 Computerized medication administration record

ROUTINE MEDICATIONS

Date Ordered	Start Date	Stop Date	Medication and Frequency		Route	7-3	3-11	11-7
1/21	1/22	1/27	ASA qd	gr 5	PO	9		
1/21	1/21	1/26	Digoxin bid	0.125mg	PO	9	9	
1/21	1/21	1/26	Aldomet tid	250 mg	PO	9-1	5	

PRN MEDICATIONS

Date Ordered	Start Date	Stop Date	Medication	Dose	Route	Frequency
1/21	1/21	1/26	NTG	gr 1/150	SL	PRN
1/21	1/21	1/26	Dalmane	30 mg	PO	HS PRN

ONE TIME MEDICATIONS

Date Ordered	Date to Be Given	Time to Be Given	Medication and Dosage	Route	Date Ordered	Date to Be Given	Time to Be Given	Medication and Dosage	Route
			1.					4.	
			2.					5.	
			3.					6.	

I.V. THERAPY

Start Date	I.V. #	Solution	Volume	Additives	Rate

HYPERALIMENTATION I.V. THERAPY

Start Date	I.V. #	Solution	Volume	Additive

```
MEDICATION CARD

Name  DOE, MARY A
Room  603
Medication
  digoxin
Dosage  0.125 mg
Route  PO
Frequency  bid
Times  9 A - 9 P
```

Admission Date	Age	Sex	Religion	Attending Physician	Surgery Date:_____
1/21	60	F	Prot	G. Coats	Type:

Room	Name		Admitting Diagnosis	Current Diagnosis
603	DOE, MARY A		Hypertension R/o CHF	
FS 024 Rev. 9/84				

FIGURE 10-4 Patient profile with medication card (*Courtesy Fort Worth Osteopathic Medical Center, Fort Worth, Texas.*)

TABLE 10-1 Common abbreviations and symbols used in medication and treatment orders

a, $\bar{a}$	before	post-op, PO	postoperatively
aa	of each	preop	preoperatively
a.c., ac	before meals	p.r.n., PRN	when required, as needed
ad	up to	q	every
ad lib	as freely as desired	q.d., qd	every day
aq	water, aqueous	q.h., qh	every hour
ASAP	as soon as possible	q.2h., q2h	every two hours
b.i.d., bid	two times a day	q.3h., q3h	every three hours
c or $\bar{c}$	with	q.4h., q4h	every four hours
cap(s)	capsule(s)	q.6h., q6h	every six hours
D5W, 5%DW	5% dextrose in water	q.8h., q8h	every eight hours
D5NS, 5%DNS	5% dextrose in normal saline	q.i.d., qid	four times a day
elix	elixir	q.o.d., qod	every other day
fld, Fl	fluid	q.s., qs	quantity sufficient
H	hypodermic	R	right
h	hour	RL	Ringer's lactate, lactated
h.s., hs	at bedtime		Ringer's
IM	intramuscularly	Rx	take, take thou[*]
IV	intravenously	s or $\bar{s}$	without
KVO	keep vein open, pertains	S or Sig	write, label[*]
	to intravenous fluids	s.c., subq, sc	subcutaneously
L	left (liter)	S L	sublingually, under tongue
mEq	milliequivalent	SOS	if necessary, once only
min	minutes	stat.	immediately
Noct, noc	night	supp	suppository
NS	normal saline	Syr	syrup
	0.9% sodium chloride	t.i.d., tid	three times a day
1/2 NS	one-half normal saline	tab(s)	tablet(s)
	0.45% sodium chloride	TKO	to keep open; same as KVO
O.D., OD	right eye	tr or tinct	tincture
O.S., OS	left eye	ung	ointment
os	mouth	X	times
O.U., OU	both eyes	VO	verbal order
p, $\bar{p}$	after	w.a., wa	while awake (as q.4h.wa)
PB	piggyback	>	greater than, more than
p.c., pc	after meals	<	less than
per	by, through	=	equal to
PO	by mouth	≠	not equal to
PO, TO	phone (telephone) order		
	per order		

[*]Used almost exclusively for writing prescriptions

TABLE 10-2   Conversion equivalents, symbols, abbreviations, and roman numerals

Measurement Symbols and Abbreviations

C	= cup	mg	= milligram
cc	= cubic centimeter	ml	= milliliter
cm	= centimeter	mx, M, min	= minim
G, g, gm	= gram	m	= meter
gr	= grain	pt	= pint
gtt, gtts	= drop/drops	qt	= quart
kg	= kilogram	Tbsp, T, tbsp	= tablespoon
L,l	= liter	tsp, t	= teaspoon
lb	= pound	U	= unit
mcgm, mcg, μg	= microgram		
ʒ/dr	= dram	ʒ/oz	= ounce

Measurement Conversion Equivalents
(Approximate only)

		Metric	Apothecary	Household
WEIGHT	✓	1 g = 1000 mg	= gr 15	
	✓	60 mg	= gr 1	
		1 mg = 1000 mcgm, mcg, μg		
		1 kg = 1000 g		= 2.2 lb
				= 1 lb = 16oz
VOLUME	✓	1 ml = 1 cc	= 15-16 mx, M, ℳ	
	✓	4 or 5 ml or cc	= 1 dr, ʒ	= 1 tsp
	✓	15 ml or cc	= 1/2 oz, ʒ	= 1 Tbsp, T, tbsp
	✓	30 ml or cc	= 1 oz	= 2 Tbsp
		240 or 250 ml or cc	= 8 oz	= 1 C
		480 or 500 ml or cc	= 16 oz	= 1 pt
		960 or 1000 ml or cc	= 32 oz	= 1 qt
		1000 ml = 1 L	= 32 oz	= 1 qt
LENGTH		1 cm = 10 mm		
		2.5 cm		= 1 inch
		1 m		= 39 inches

Roman Numerals
(used only in apothecary system)

ss	= 1/2	viiss	= 7 1/2
I or i	= 1	XV	= 15
V or v	= 5	IV	= 4
X or x	= 10	XI	= 11

TABLE 10-3   Common abbreviations for medications

ASA*	aspirin, acetylsalicylic acid	NaCl	sodium chloride, salt
FeSO$_4$	ferrous sulfate	NTG*	nitroglycerine
HCl	hydrochloride	O$_2$	oxygen
HCTZ	hydrochlorothiazide	PCN	penicillin
KCl*	potassium chloride	PO$_4$	phosphate
MgSO$_4$	magnesium sulfate	SO$_4$	sulfate
MO*	mineral oil	SSKI*	saturated solution of
MOM*	milk of magnesia		potassium iodide
m s, M S*	morphine sulfate	TCN	tetracycline

*These medication abbreviations usually acceptable in health care agencies.

PRACTICE PROBLEMS

Interpretation of Medication and Treatment Orders

Show all your work. Check your answers (page 324). Translate the following medication and treatment orders into lay terms:

1. Ampicillin 250 mg PO q.i.d.

   miligrams
   250 mg of Ampacillin by mouth
   4 x's day

2. Garamycin 80 mg IV PB q.8h.

   80 mg Gara intravenous
   every 8 hours Piggy Back

3. Demerol and phenergan 50 mg aa IM stat.

   50 mg of each Dem & Phenergan Intramuscular
   Immediatly

4. Nitroglycerine ung 1 inch to chest q.d.

   Nitro ointment 1" to chest every day

5. 1000 ml D5W c KCl 20 mEq IV to run 8 h; then KVO with D5NS.

   1000 mililiter 5% Dextros with water with 20 mili equivilant Potassium
   Chloride intravenous to run 8 hours. Than keep vein open with 5% Dextros
   with Normal Saline

6. MOM 30 ml c cascara 5 ml PO q.o.d. SOS

   30 mililiters Milk of Magnesia with 5 mililiters cascara by mouth
   every other day if necessary

7. Pantapon gr 1/3 s.c. preop on call

   1/3 grains Pantapon subcutaneous injection preoperation

8. Mylanta ʒ I PO t.i.d. p.c.

   1 oz Mylanta by mouth three times a day after meals

9. Donnatal tab I PO q.i.d. a.c. & h.s.

   1 Tablet of Donnatal by mouth four times a day
   before meals and at bedtime

10. SSKI gtt. 10 in orange juice q.s. to 60 ml PO q.6h.

    10 drops of Saturated solution of
    potassium iodine in O.J. in quantity sufficiant to make 60 mililiters
    By mouth every 6 hours

11. Neodecadron gtt. i OS q.h. w a & q.2h. at noc

    one drop of Neodecadron Right eye every hour while awake at every
    two hours at night

12. Calomine lotion to rash L leg ad lib

    Calomine lotion to Rash on left leg as frequently as desired

13. Lasix 20 mg IV b.i.d.

    20 miligrams of Lasix intraveinouse twice a day

14. ephinephrine 1:1000 0.3 ml s.c. stat.

    1:1000 .3 mililiter ephinephrine   Subcutaneous Immediatly

15. Dyazide cap i PO b.i.d.

    1 capsuale Dyazide By mouth twice daily

16. boric acid 5% gtt. i OU t.i.d.

    one 5% drop boric acid Both eyes three times day

17. Irrigate O.D. c 50 ml NS ASAP

    Irrigate Right eye with 50 mililiter Normal saline as soon as possible

18. nitroglycerine 0.4 mg SL PRN

    .04 miligram Nitroglycerine Sublingually as needed

19. Procaine penicillin 300,000 U IM q.d.

    300,000 units Procaine penicillin intramuscular every day

20. ASA gr V PO q.d.

    5 grain aspirin by mouth every day

CALCULATION OF DAILY DOSAGE

Nurses frequently have to calculate the total daily dosages of medication orders. The most common reason is to compare the medication the patient receives with the normal dosage.

Calculation of daily dosage requires two knowns: the dosage the patient receives at each dose and the number of doses per day. The equation is as follows:

$$\frac{\text{dosage}}{\text{day}} = \frac{\text{dosage} \quad \times \text{number doses}}{\text{(per) dose} \times \quad \text{(per) day}}$$

SAMPLE PROBLEM **Calculate the daily dosage of the order "ampicillin 500 mg q.i.d. PO."**

500 Miligrams ampicillin by mouth four times per day

Knowns: Unit of Answer: mg/d

Factors: 500 mg = 1 Dose

4 Doses per Day

Set up the framework of the equation.

$$\text{mg/d} = \underline{\hspace{2cm}}$$

The numerator unit of the first factor must be the same as the numerator unit of the answer, mg. Find the factor containing mg. Write 500 mg in the numerator and 1 dose in the denominator, followed by multiplication signs.

$$\frac{\text{mg}}{\text{d}} = \frac{500 \text{ mg} \times}{1 \text{ dose} \times}$$

The numerator unit of the second factor must be the same as the denominator unit of the first factor. Find the factor containing dose. Write 4 doses in the numerator and 1 d in the denominator.

$$\frac{\text{mg}}{\text{d}} = \frac{500 \text{ mg} \times 4 \text{ doses}}{1 \text{ dose} \times 1 \text{ d}}$$

Cancel the units that appear in both the numerator and denominator.

$$\frac{\text{mg}}{\text{d}} = \frac{500 \text{ mg} \times 4}{1 \quad \times 1 \text{ d}}$$

Multiply the numerator:
Multiply the denominator:

$$\frac{500 \text{ mg} \times 4}{1 \quad \times 1 \text{ d}} = \frac{2000 \text{ mg}}{1 \text{ d}} = 2000 \text{ mg/d}$$

Dosages orders written as frequencies of a specific number of hours rather than times per day can cause confusion. For instance, dosages ordered q.8h. are really three times a day. The frequencies that cause the most confusion are q.4h. and q.6h. Instead of converting the dosage from the frequency of a specific number of hours into times per day, these problems can be solved by using the frequency and the number of hours per day, 24 hours. Thus the problem can be solved as follows:

$$\frac{\text{dosage}}{\text{day}} = \frac{\text{dosage} \quad \times 24 \text{ hours}}{\text{(q) number hours} \times \quad 1 \text{ day}}$$

SAMPLE PROBLEM   **Calculate the daily dosage of the order, "Garamycin 80 mg IV PB q.4h."**

Knowns: Unit of Answer: mg/d
Factors: 80 mg/4h
1 Day = 24 Hours

Set up the framework of the equation.

$$\frac{mg}{d} = \underline{\hspace{2cm}}$$

The numerator unit of the first factor must be the same as the numerator unit of the answer. Find the factor containing mg. Write 80 mg in the numerator and 4 h in denominator, followed by multiplication signs.

$$\frac{mg}{d} = \frac{80\ mg\ \times}{4\ h\ \ \times}$$

The numerator unit of the second factor must be the same as the denominator unit of the first factor. Find the factor containing h. Write 24 h in the numerator and 1 d in the denominator.

$$\frac{mg}{d} = \frac{80\ mg \times 24\ h}{4\ h\ \times\ 1\ d}$$

Cancel the units. Cancel the evenly divisible quantities.

$$\frac{mg}{d} = \frac{80\ mg \times \overset{6}{\cancel{24}}}{\underset{1}{\cancel{4}}\ \times\ 1\ d}$$

Multiply the numerator:
Multiply the denominator:

$$\frac{80\ mg \times 6}{1\ \ \ \times 1\ d} = \frac{480\ mg}{1\ d} = 480\ mg/d$$

PRACTICE PROBLEMS

Calculating Daily Dosages

(Answers on page 325.)

21. Dalmane 30 mg PO h.s.

$$\frac{mg}{d} = \frac{30mg \times 1\,dose}{1\,dose \times 1\,d} = 30\,mg/d$$

22. Robinul 2 mg PO q.i.d. a.c. & h.s.

$$\frac{mg}{d} = \frac{2mg \times 4\,dose}{1\,dose \times 1\,d} = 8\,mg/d$$

23. Pen Vee K 400,000 U q.6h. PO

$$\frac{U}{D} = \frac{400,000 \times \overset{4h}{\cancel{24h}}}{\underset{1\,h}{\cancel{6h}} \times 1\,d} = 1,600,000\,u/d$$

24. Phenergan 50 mg IM q.8h.

$$\frac{mg}{D} = \frac{50mg \times \overset{3}{\cancel{24h}}}{\cancel{q8h} \times 1d} = \frac{50mg \times 3}{1 \times 1d} = 150mg/d$$

25. Solu-cortef 100 mg IV q.3h

$$\frac{Mg}{D} = \frac{100mg \times \overset{8}{\cancel{24h}}}{\underset{1}{\cancel{q3h}} \times 1d} = \frac{100mg \times 8}{1 \times 1d}$$

$$800mg/d$$

MEDICATION DELIVERY SYSTEMS

Several systems of medication delivery are available for use in health care facilities. The oldest system is the time-consuming stock supply system, in which each nursing unit has stock bottles of commonly used medication tablets in various strengths. A second system is the individual client supply, where each client has a labeled section, such as a drawer or bin, which contains bottles containing several days' supply of medications in an appropriate strength. With either of these systems, the nurse removes the correct amount of medication from the stock or client's bottle, places it in a medication cup, and administers it to the patient. Figure 10-5 shows the same medication in both stock supply and individual client supply delivery systems.

Most acute care facilities have adopted a form of the unit dose medication system which has simplified dosage calculation in many instances. In this system, the medications are supplied in labeled single dosage units which are usually stored in drawers

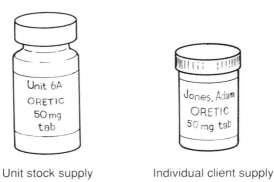

Unit stock supply   Individual client supply

FIGURE 10-5 Unit stock and individual client medication supplies

in a portable cart, shown in Figure 10-6, that the pharmacy restocks daily. Many pharmaceutical companies package medications in single units, called *unit dose*. The daily supply of the medication in unit dose packaging is placed in the client's drawer by the pharmacy. The nurse takes the appropriate amount of unit doses from the drawer for each medication administration. The amount may be one or more unit doses, or a part of the unit dose, such as one half. The unit dose system has a special safety feature: the medication is labeled until it is removed from the packaging at the client's bedside. Some pharmacies also prepare injectable medications in single client doses in premixed syringes. Others stock the client's drawer with the appropriate ampules or vials and the nurse prepares the injection. Figure 10-7 shows a variety of oral medication unit dose labels.

Regardless of the medication delivery system used, the nurse is responsible for the correct administration of medications. This includes administering the accurate amount of the correct medication by the ordered route at the appropriate time to the correct patient. This is called the FIVE RIGHTS of medication administration.

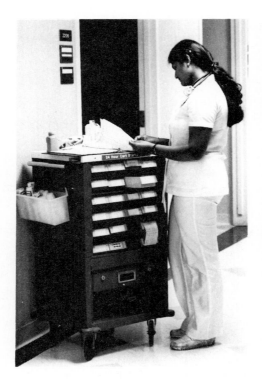

FIGURE 10-6 Medication cart for unit dose medication administration system. (From Potter, P.A., and Perry, A.G.: Fundamentals of nursing: concepts, process and practice, St. Louis, 1985, The C.V. Mosby Co.)

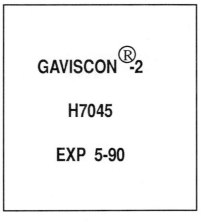

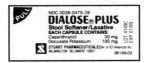

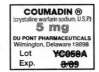

FIGURE 10-7 Examples of unit dose labels

THE FIVE RIGHTS OF MEDICATION ADMINISTRATION

Right CLIENT
Right MEDICATION
Right DOSAGE
Right ROUTE
Right TIME

Since charting the medication after administration is very important, some authors add a sixth right.

Right DOCUMENTATION

When medications are prepared in the agency by the pharmacist, the nurse is still responsible for ensuring that the patient receives the correct dosage. *Never administer any medication without checking the dosage.* Pharmacists are very conscious of their responsibility to assure the correct dosage of medications and rarely make mistakes. Both the nurse and the pharmacist are legally liable if a mistake occurs; therefore, the nurse must check all dosages prior to administration.

TIME SCHEDULES

The time schedules of medications vary with the health care agency. Medications administered four times a day might be on a 9 AM, 1 PM, 5 PM and 9 PM in one agency and 6 AM, 12 noon, 6 PM and 10 PM at another facility. A third agency may have an entirely different time schedule. The policy for medication administration time schedules can be found in the agency procedure or policy book. Note the differences in the time schedules in Figures 10-2, 10-3, and 10-4. The time schedule in the computerized medication record in Figure 10-3 utilizes the 24-hour clock, commonly called *military time*. Conversion from standard to military time is shown in Appendix D.

READING MEDICATION LABELS

Medication orders are written in weights: grains, grams, milligrams, and micrograms. Medications are administered in units other than weights, such as tablets, capsules, or volumes such as milliliters.

Oral medications are available in tablets, capsules, powders, and liquids. Parenteral medications, those which are injected, are available as liquids or powders reconstituted as liquids. Ampules, single or multiple dose vials, and prefilled syringe cartridges are the most common containers for injectable medications.

Administration of medications requires the ability to correctly read the medication labels. Medication labels always contain the following information: the generic name, the dosage per unit (tablet, milliliter, etc.), the lot number, the expiration date, and the manufacturer. The label also may contain a trade or brand name. Figure 10-8 shows a medication label with the information identified.

SELECTION OF APPROPRIATE MEDICATION STRENGTH

Many medications are available in several strengths or concentrations. Concentration is the amount of medication dissolved in a particular unit of solution. Figure 10-9 shows labels and amounts for three containers of atropine for injection. To compare the concentrations, convert the weights to the same unit of measurement and the volumes to the same amount. Note the conversions in Figure 10-9. The largest volume, vial A, has the lowest concentration.

It is very easy to select the appropriate strength when the units of measurement are the same in the doctor's order and on the label. For instance, if the order reads digoxin 0.125 mg PO q.d. and digoxin is available in tablets of 0.125 mg, 0.25 mg, and 0.5 mg, the obvious selection is the 0.125 mg tablet. Figure 10-10 depicts labels that are in the same unit of measurement as the medication order and labels that differ from the ordered unit of measurement.

Conversions are needed to choose the appropriate strength of medication when the order and the labels use different units of measurement. When the units of measurement are different, convert the unit of the medication order to the unit on the labels and compare the amount of the converted medication order to the amounts on the labels.

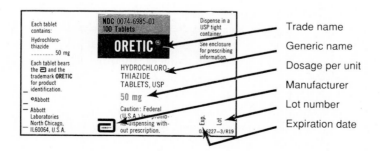

FIGURE 10-8 Drug label information

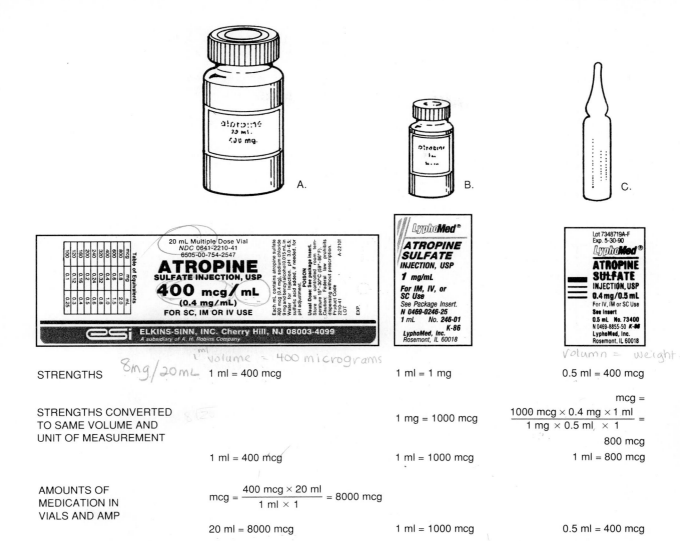

FIGURE 10-9 Comparison of strengths and total amounts of medication in certain atropine containers

To select the appropriate strength of medication from several strengths:

(1) Convert dosage ordered measurement unit to label measurement unit, if necessary.

(2) Compare converted ordered dosage to the dosages on medication labels.

(3) Select the label dosage closest to the ordered dosage.

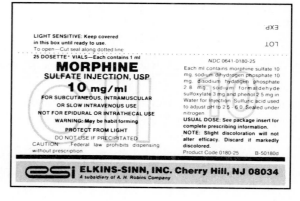

MEDICATION: Drug – Strength – Frequency	Route	Shift	DATE
Lanoxin *0.125 mg* *qd.*	*PO*	11-7	
		7-3	
9 Am		3-11	

A

MEDICATION: Drug – Strength – Frequency	Route	Shift	DATE
Morphine *Sulfate* *gr 1/6*	*IM*	11-7	
		7-3	
Stat		3-11	

B

FIGURE 10-10 Labels with the same and different units of measurement as medication orders. Note that the units of measurement of order A are the same as the units on the label. It is obvious that the medication to choose is 0.125 mg. Order B must be converted to the same unit of measurement as the label prior to selection. Grains 1/6 is 10 mg.

SAMPLE PROBLEM   **Select the ordered strength aspirin tablet from the two labels representing two strengths of aspirin.**

1 gr = 60 mg   *5×*

Date Ordered	Start Date	MEDICATION: Drug – Strength – Frequency	Route	Shift	DATE
3|10	3|10				
Reorder	Last Dose	Aspirin	PO	11-7	
	3|17	gr 5 qd		7-3	
Transcriber as					
Times To Administer		10ᴬ		3-11	

```
┌─────────────────┐     ┌─────────────────┐
│     Aspirin     │     │     Aspirin     │
│   325 MG TAB    │     │   500 MG TAB    │
└─────────────────┘     └─────────────────┘
        A                       B
```

(1) Convert ordered dosage measurement unit to label dosage unit.

Knowns: Unit of Answer: mg
Factor: gr 5/1
Conversion Factor: 1 gr = 60 mg
Set up the framework of the equation.

$$mg = \frac{\quad\quad}{\quad\quad}$$

The numerator unit of the first factor must be the same as the answer unit. Find the factor containing mg. Write 60 mg in the numerator and 1 gr in the denominator, followed by multiplication signs.

$$mg = \frac{60\ mg\ \times}{1\ gr\ \times}$$

The numerator unit of the second factor must be the same as the denominator unit of the first factor. Find the factor containing gr. Write 5 gr in the numerator and 1 in the denominator.

$$mg = \frac{60\ mg \times 5\ gr}{1\ gr\ \times 1}$$

Cancel the units.

$$mg = \frac{60\ mg \times 5}{1\quad \times 1}$$

Multiply the numerator:
Multiply the denominator:

$$\frac{60\ mg \times 5}{1\quad \times 1} = \frac{300\ mg}{1} = 300mg$$

If the conversion factor 1000 mg = 15 gr is used, the equation is as follows:

$$mg = \frac{1000\ mg \times 5\ gr}{15\ gr\ \times 1} = \frac{1000\ mg \times \overset{1}{\cancel{5}}}{\underset{3}{\cancel{15}}\ \times 1} = \frac{1000\ mg}{3} = 333.3\ mg$$

(2) Compare the converted ordered dosage to label dosages.

Ordered dosage: 300 mg or 333 mg
Label dosages: Label A- 325 mg
Label B- 500 mg

(3) Select the label dosage closest to the ordered dosage. Because 300 mg or 333 mg is closest to 325 mg, tablet A is the one to choose. Five grains of aspirin is actually equivalent to 325 mg. The discrepancy between either 300 or 333 mg and 325 mg is due to the approximate equivalents used when converting from one measurement system to another.

SAMPLE PROBLEM **The physician's order reads "Ampicillin 0.5 g PO qid." Select the correct ampicillin strength from the two labels representing ampicillin strengths.**

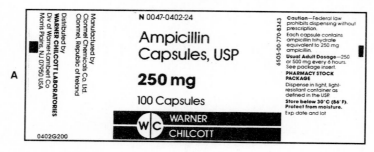

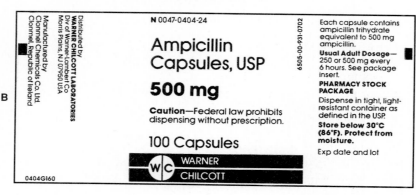

(1) Convert the measurement unit of the medication order to the unit on the medication label.

Knowns: Unit of answer: mg
Factor: 0.5 g/1
Conversion Factor: 1 g = 1000 mg
Set up the framework of the equation.

$$mg = \underline{\qquad}$$

The numerator unit of the first factor must be the same as the answer unit. Find the factor containing mg. Write 1000 mg in the numerator and 1 g in the denominator, followed by multiplication signs.

$$mg = \frac{1000 \text{ mg} \times}{1 \text{ g} \times}$$

The numerator unit of the second factor must be the same as the denominator unit of the first factor. Find the factor containing g. Write 0.5 g in the numerator and 1 in the denominator.

$$mg = \frac{1000 \text{ mg} \times 0.5 \text{ g}}{1 \text{ g} \times 1}$$

Cancel the units.

$$mg = \frac{1000 \text{ mg} \times 0.5}{1 \quad \times \quad 1}$$

Multiply the numerator:
Multiply the denominator:

$$\frac{1000 \text{ mg} \times 0.5}{1 \quad \times \quad 1} = \frac{500 \text{ mg}}{1} = 500 \text{ mg}$$

(2) Compare the converted ordered dosage to the label dosages.

Ordered dosage: 500 mg
Label dosages: Label A- 250 mg
Label B- 500 mg

(3) Select the label dosage closest to the ordered dosage. The ordered dosage is the same as the 500 mg label dosage. The conversion from grams to milligrams is exact because measurement equivalents within a measurement system are exact.

Injectable medications are selected the same way as oral medications. When there are several strengths from which to choose, always select the strength that requires opening only one ampule or single dose vial, whenever possible, to avoid wasting copious amounts. The rubber stoppers on multidose vials reseal themselves and can be used several times. Once ampules have been opened, they cannot be resealed and used again.

SAMPLE PROBLEM   **From the labels representing two strengths of morphine sulfate, select the appropriate ampule to use for the following medication order:**

ONE TIME MEDICATIONS

Date Ordered	Date to Be Given	Time to Be Given	Medication and Dosage	Route
6/1	6/1	1300	1. Morphine gr 1/6	IM
			2.	
			3.	

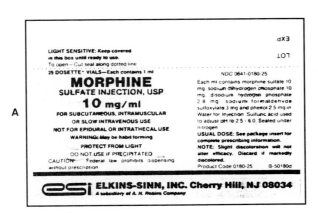

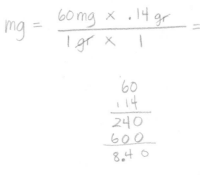

$$mg = \frac{60 mg \times .14 gr}{1 gr \times 1} =$$

$$\begin{array}{r} 60 \\ .14 \\ \hline 240 \\ 600 \\ \hline 8.4\,0 \end{array}$$

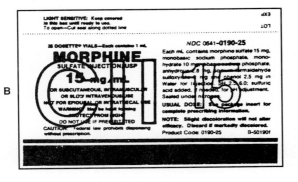

(1) Convert the ordered dosage unit to the ampule label unit.

Knowns: Unit of Answer: mg
Factor: 1/6 gr/1
Conversion Factor: 1 gr = 60 mg
Set up the framework for the equation.

$$mg = \underline{}$$

The numerator unit of the first factor must be the same as the answer unit. Find the factor containing mg. Write 60 mg in the numerator and 1 gr in the denominator, followed by multiplication signs.

$$mg = \frac{60 \text{ mg} \times}{1 \text{ gr} \times}$$

The numerator unit of the first factor must be the same as the denominator unit of the first factor. Find the factor containing gr. Write gr $\frac{1}{6}$ in the numerator and 1 in the denominator.

$$mg = \frac{60 \text{ mg} \times \text{gr } 1/6}{1 \text{ gr} \times 1}$$

Cancel the units.

$$mg = \frac{60 \text{ mg} \times 1/6}{1 \times 1}$$

Drop the denominator of the fraction into the denominator of the equation. Cancel the evenly divisible numbers.

$$mg = \frac{\overset{10}{\cancel{60}} \text{ mg} \times 1}{1 \times \cancel{6}}{}_{1}$$

Multiply the numerator; multiply the denominator

$$\frac{10 \text{ mg} \times 1}{1 \times 1} = \frac{10 \text{ mg}}{1} = 10 \text{ mg}$$

(2) Compare the converted ordered dosage to the morphine ampule labels.

Ordered dosage: 10 mg
Label dosages: Label A- 10 mg
Label B- 15 mg

(3) Select the label dosage closest to the ordered dosage. The ordered dosage is the same as the 10 mg label. Therefore, the correct ampule to choose is A.

Not all injectable medications ordered convert to the dosage on the medication label. When this occurs, select the nearest dosage higher than the ordered dosage.

SAMPLE PROBLEM   **From the two labels representing two strengths of morphine sulfate, select the appropriate ampule for the following medication order:**

ONE TIME MEDICATIONS

Date Ordered	Date to Be Given	Time to Be Given	Medication and Dosage	Route
6|1	6|1	1300	1. Morphine gr $\frac{1}{5}$	IM
			2.	
			3.	

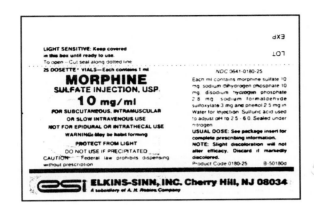

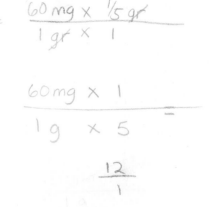

Convert the measurement unit of the medication order to the unit on the medication label.

Knowns: Unit of Answer: mg.

Factor: 1/5 gr/1

Conversion Factor: 1 gr = 60 mg

Set up the framework of the equation.

The numerator unit of the first factor must be the same as the answer unit. Find the factor containing mg. Write 60 mg in the numerator and 1 gr in the denominator, followed by multiplication signs.

The numerator unit of the second factor must be the same as the denominator unit of the first factor. Find the factor containing gr. Write gr $\frac{1}{5}$ in the numerator and 1 in the denominator.

Cancel the units.

$$mg = \underline{\quad\quad\quad}$$

$$mg = \frac{60 \text{ mg} \times}{1 \text{ gr} \times}$$

$$mg = \frac{60 \text{ mg} \times \text{gr } 1/5}{1 \text{ gr} \times 1}$$

$$mg = \frac{60 \text{ mg} \times 1/5}{1 \times 1}$$

Drop the denominator of the fraction in
the numerator into the equation denominator.
Cancel evenly divisible numbers.

$$mg = \frac{\overset{12}{\cancel{60}} \, mg \times 1}{1 \quad \times \cancel{5}}$$
$$\frac{1}{1}$$

Multiply the numerator:
Multiply the denominator:

$$\frac{12 \, mg \times 1}{1 \quad \times 1} = \frac{12 \, mg}{1} = 12 \, mg$$

(2) Compare the converted ordered dosage to the medication label dosages.

Ordered dosage: 12 mg
Label dosages: Label A— 10 mg
**   Label B— 15 mg**

(3) Select the medication label that is closest to the ordered dosage. The closest label dosage is 10 mg. This choice requires opening two ampules. Since the ordered dosage is more than 10 mg, the label selected must be higher than the ordered dosage. Therefore, the label to choose is B, 15 mg. Only a portion (0.8 ml) of this ampule will be administered. Calculation of administration volumes is covered in Chapters 11 and 12.

PRACTICE PROBLEMS

Selection of Appropriate Medication Strength

For the following medication orders, select the appropriate labels. (Answers on page 326.)

26. Aspirin gr viiss PO q.4h. p.r.n.

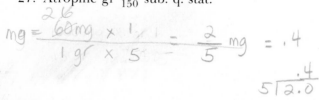

Aspirin 325 MG TAB	Aspirin 500 MG TAB

27. Atropine gr $\frac{1}{150}$ sub. q. stat.

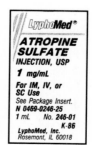
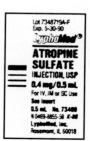

28. NTG gr $\frac{1}{100}$ SL p.r.n. chest pain

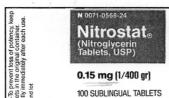

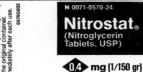

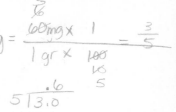

$$mg = \frac{60mg \times 1}{1\ gr \times 100} = \frac{3}{5}$$

$$5\overline{)3.0} = .6$$

29. morphine sulfate gr $\frac{1}{5}$ s.c. stat.

$$mg = \frac{60mg \times gr\ \frac{1}{5}}{1\ gr \times 1} = \frac{60mg \times 1}{1 \times 1 \times 5} = 12$$

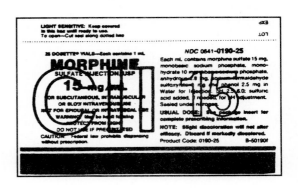

30. Aspirin 0.5 g t.i.d. PO

$$mg = \frac{1000\,mg \times .5\,g}{1\,g \times 1} = 500\,mg$$

Aspirin 325 MG TAB	Aspirin 500 MG TAB

31. Atropine 0.4 mg IM ASAP

$$mg = $$

LyphoMed®
ATROPINE SULFATE
INJECTION, USP
1 mg/mL
For IM, IV, or SC Use
See Package Insert.
N 0469-0246-25
1 mL   No. **246-01**
K-86
LyphoMed, Inc.
Rosemont, IL 60018

LyphoMed®
ATROPINE SULFATE
INJECTION, USP
0.5 mg/mL
For IM, IV, or SC Use
See Package Insert.
N 0469-0243-25
1 mL   No. **243-01**
LyphoMed, Inc. K-86
Rosemont, IL 60018

LyphoMed®
ATROPINE SULFATE
INJECTION, USP
0.4 mg/mL
For IM, IV, or SC Use
See Package Insert.
N 0469-1234-25
1 mL   No. **234-01**
K-86
LyphoMed, Inc.
Rosemont, IL 60018

32. Pyridium 0.1 g PO t.i.d.

$$mg = \frac{1000\,mg}{1\,g} \times \frac{.1\,g}{1} = \frac{100\,mg}{1}$$

Adult Dosage—One tablet 3 times a day after meals.
See package insert for complete prescribing information.
Keep this and all drugs out of the reach of children.
Store at controlled room temperature 15° to 30° C (59° to 86° F).
0181G014

N 0071-0181-24
Pyridium®
(Phenazopyridine HCl Tablets, USP)
200 mg
Caution—Federal law prohibits dispensing without prescription.
100 TABLETS
PARKE-DAVIS
Div of Warner-Lambert Co
Morris Plains, NJ 07950 USA

Dispense in tight container as defined in the USP.
Exp date and lot

Adult Dosage—Two tablets 3 times a day after meals.
See package insert for complete prescribing information.
Keep this and all drugs out of the reach of children.
Store at controlled room temperature 15°-30° C (59°-86° F).
0180G054

N 0071-0180-24
Pyridium®
(Phenazopyridine HCl Tablets, USP)
100 mg
Caution—Federal law prohibits dispensing without prescription
100 TABLETS
PARKE-DAVIS
Div of Warner-Lambert Co
Morris Plains, NJ 07950 USA

Dispense in tight container as defined in the USP.
Exp date and lot
6505-00-138-8461

33. Atropine gr $\frac{1}{100}$ s.c. stat.

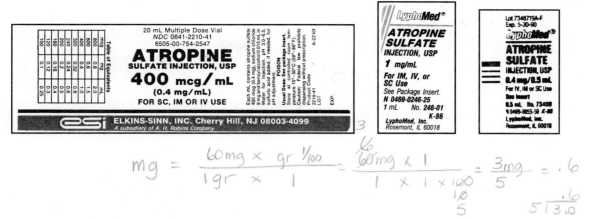

$$mg = \frac{60mg \times gr \frac{1}{100}}{1 gr \times 1} = \frac{60mg \times 1}{1 \times 1 \times 100} = \frac{3mg}{5} = .6$$

$$\frac{\quad}{10}\quad\quad\quad 5\overline{)3.0}$$

34. Dynapen 0.250 g PO q.i.d.

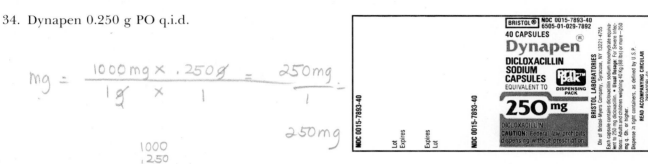

$$mg = \frac{1000mg \times .250g}{1g \times 1} = \frac{250mg}{1} = 250mg$$

$$\begin{array}{r} 1000 \\ .250 \\ \hline 50,000 \\ 200000 \\ \hline 250.000 \end{array}$$

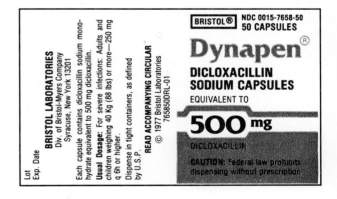

35. Lanoxin 125 mcg PO q.d.

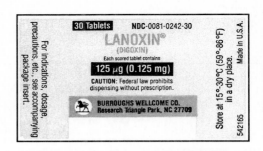

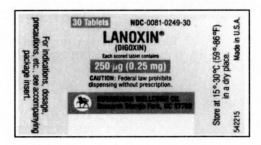

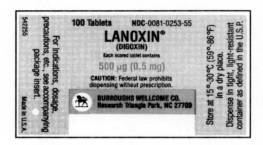

SELF-ASSESSMENT POSTTEST

INTERPRETATION OF MEDICATION ORDERS AND LABELS

Translate the following orders into lay terms. (Answers on page 357.)

1. Esidrex 50 mg PO b.i.d.

2. 1000 cc D5NS IV q.8h.

3. Pyridium 200 mg PO t.i.d.

4. Morphine sulfate gr $\frac{1}{8}$ sub. q. q.4h. p.r.n.

5. Phenobarbital gr $\frac{1}{2}$ PO q.i.d.

6. Demerol 75 mg c̄ Vistaril 25 mg IM q.4h. PRN

7. Digoxin 0.25 mg q.d. PO

8. Bicillin 1,200,000 U IM stat

9. Amphogel 30 cc PO q.2h.

10. 1000 ml D5W c̄ KCl 20 mEq IV q.8h.

Calculate the daily dosages of the following:

11. Keflex 500 mg q.4h. PO

12. Dynapen 250 mg q.i.d. PO

13. Hydrochlorothiazide 50 mg PO b.i.d.

14. Aspirin gr X q.3h. PO

Select the appropriate medication for the doctor's order from the two labels representing different strengths of medication.

15. Medication order: Atropine 0.2 mg sc noc

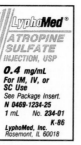 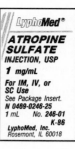

16. Medication order: nitroglycerine gr $\frac{1}{200}$ SL p.r.n.

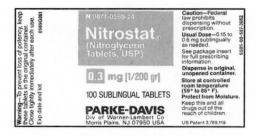

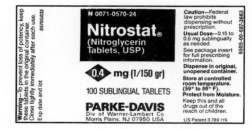

17. Medication order: morphine sulfate gr $\frac{1}{4}$ s.c. stat.

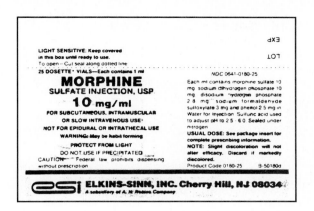

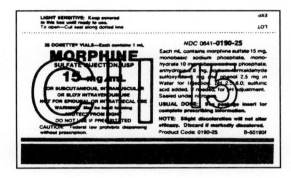

18. Medication order: acetaminophen gr V PO q.4h. p.r.n.

ACETAMINOPHEN
325 MG TAB

ACETAMINOPHEN
500 MG TAB

19. Medication order: morphine sulfate gr $\frac{1}{7}$ IM
q.4h. p.r.n.

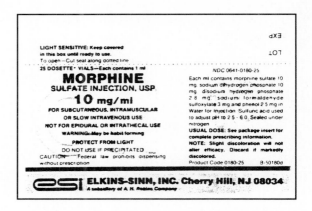

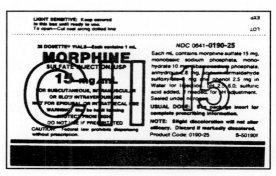

20. Medication order: amoxicillin 0.5 g q.6h. PO

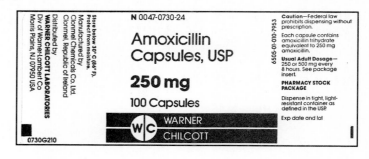

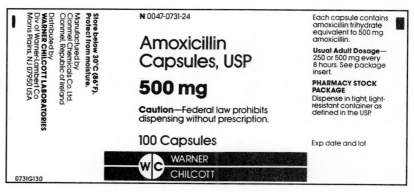

Chapter 11

Calculation of Oral Medication Dosages

Most medications are administered orally. Oral medications are easier to administer and easier for most patients to take. Medications administered orally are cheaper and more comfortable than their injectable counterparts.

Oral medications are available in solid and liquid form. Tablets, capsules, and powders are examples of solid oral medications. In response to a growing population of persons who have difficulty swallowing tablets and capsules, some pharmaceutical companies now package sprinkles, which are designed to be mixed with soft food. Liquid medications are in the form of solutions or suspensions that must be agitated prior to each administration.

DOSAGE CALCULATION OF MEDICATIONS AVAILABLE IN SOLID FORMS

The majority of oral medications are available in tablets and capsules. Tablets are manufactured in a variety of shapes and sizes. They may be scored, or indented, for breaking into two or four equal parts. Only scored tablets can be broken into evenly divided doses. Tablets may have a smooth surface for ease in swallowing. Enteric-coated tablets are covered with a material designed to dissolve in the intestines rather than the stomach and protect the stomach from irritating medications. Some tablets may be crushed and administered in liquids or soft foods. Enteric-coated tablets are never crushed, for to do so would defeat the purpose of the enteric coating. A *caplet* is a tablet in the shape of a capsule. Figure 11-1 shows various types of tablets and capsules.

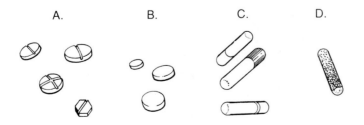

FIGURE 11-1 Various tablets and capsules. A, scored tablets. B, unscored tablets. C, capsules. D, spansules.

Capsules are cylindrical gelatin shells into which powders or liquids are packed. Capsules containing time-released pellets are often called *spansules.* Liquid medications encapsulated in firm gelatin coatings are sometimes called *perles.* Many capsules may be opened for administering in liquid. Others should never be opened. The nurse is responsible for knowing which capsules may be dissolved or suspended in liquid. Capsules should never be opened to administer less than the entire capsule as the amount cannot be assured.

Powders are always administered in liquid. Many powders are stable for only a short time when mixed in liquid. Some powders, such as Metamucil, solidify if allowed to remain in liquid more than several minutes. Therefore, powders are mixed immediately prior to administration.

Calculation of dosage requires the ordered dosage and the dosage and amount available. Conversion factors are used as needed. The dimensional analysis equation for dosage calculation is as follows:

$$
\begin{array}{c}
\text{Unit and} \\
\text{amount to} \\
\text{administer}
\end{array}
=
\frac{
\begin{array}{c}
\text{conversion} \\
\text{factor if} \\
\text{necessary}
\end{array}
\times
\begin{array}{c}
\text{amount} \\
\text{available}
\end{array}
\times
\begin{array}{c}
\text{conversion} \\
\text{factor if} \\
\text{necessary}
\end{array}
\times
\begin{array}{c}
\text{dosage} \\
\text{ordered}
\end{array}
}{
\begin{array}{c}
\text{dosage} \\
\text{available}
\end{array}
\times \quad\quad \times \quad\quad 1
}
$$

The dosage and amount available, also called *on hand* in this workbook, is written on the medication label.

Dosage calculation involving the same quantity and unit of measurement requires only the recognition that the order and medication label are exactly the same.

SAMPLE PROBLEM **Physician's order: Acetaminophen 325 mg PO q4h PRN. How many Acetaminophen tablets are to be administered?**

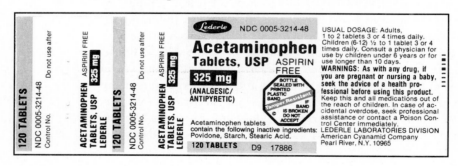

Knowns: Dosage ordered: 325 mg
Label dosage and amount: 325 mg per tablet.
(*Every four hours as needed* is extraneous information in this problem, since only one dose is given at a time.)
If the dosage ordered is 325 mg and there are 325 mg in one tablet, it is obvious that one tablet is to be administered.

Many medications are ordered in different units of measurement or in dosage amounts that are different from that on the label. Then recognition alone is not adequate to solve the problem.

SAMPLE PROBLEM **Dosage ordered: aspirin gr XV PO q.i.d.**
Dosage available: aspirin 500 mg per tab. How many tabs are to be administered?

Knowns: Unit of answer: tab
Factors: 500 mg = 1 tab
      15 gr/1
Conversion factor: 15 gr = 1000 mg

$$
\text{Tab} = \frac{1 \text{ Tab} \times 1000 \text{ mg} \times 15 \text{ gr}}{500 \text{ mg} \times 15 \text{ gr} \times 1} = 2 \text{ Tab}
$$

Set up the framework for the equation.

$$\text{tab} = \underline{\hspace{3cm}}$$

The numerator unit of the first factor must be the same as the unit of the answer. Find the factor containing tab. Write 1 tab in the numerator and 500 mg in the denominator, followed by multiplication signs.

$$\text{tab} = \frac{1 \ \text{tab} \ \times}{500 \ \text{mg} \ \times}$$

The numerator unit of the second factor must be the same as the denominator unit of the first factor. Find the factor containing mg. Write 1000 mg in the numerator and 15 gr in the denominator, followed by multiplication signs.

$$\text{tab} = \frac{1 \ \text{tab} \times 1000 \ \text{mg} \times}{500 \ \text{mg} \times \quad 15 \ \text{gr} \quad \times}$$

The numerator unit of the third factor must be the same as the denominator unit of the second factor. Find the factor containing gr. Write 15 gr in the numerator and 1 in the denominator.

$$\text{tab} = \frac{1 \ \text{tab} \times 1000 \ \text{mg} \times 15 \ \text{gr}}{500 \ \text{mg} \times \quad 15 \ \text{gr} \quad \times \quad 1}$$

Cancel the units. Cancel the evenly divisible quantities.

$$\text{tab} = \frac{1 \ \text{tab} \times \overset{2}{\cancel{1000}} \times \overset{1}{\cancel{15}}}{\underset{1}{\cancel{500}} \quad \times \quad \underset{1}{\cancel{15}} \times \quad 1}$$

Multiply the numerator:
Multiply the denominator:

$$\frac{1 \ \text{tab} \times 2 \times 1}{1 \quad \times 1 \times 1} = \frac{2 \ \text{tab}}{1} = 2 \ \text{tab}$$

If the conversion factor 1 gr = 60 mg is used, the equation would be as follows:

$$\text{tab} = \frac{1 \ \text{tab} \times 60 \ \text{mg} \times 15 \ \text{gr}}{500 \ \text{mg} \times 1 \ \text{gr} \quad \times \quad 1} = \frac{1 \ \text{tab} \times \overset{3}{\cancel{60}} \times \overset{3}{\cancel{15}}}{\underset{\underset{5}{25}}{\cancel{500}} \quad \times \quad 1 \times \quad 1} = \frac{1 \ \text{tab} \times 3 \times 3}{5 \quad \times 1 \times 1} = \frac{9 \ \text{tab}}{5} = 1\frac{4}{5} \ \text{tab}$$

Since there is no way to give 1 4/5 tabs, 2 tabs will be given. The conversion factor 1000 mg = 15 gr is more accurate than 1 gr = 60 mg for amounts greater than 1 grain. Some problems require several conversion factors.

SAMPLE PROBLEM   **Dosage ordered: gr 1/150 PO b.i.d.**
Dosage on hand (available): 200 mcg per capsule. How many capsules should be administered?

Knowns: Unit of answer: cap
Factors: 200 mcg = 1 cap
    1/150 gr/1
Conversion factors: 1 gr = 60 mg
        1 mg = 1000 mcg

Set up the framework for the equation.

$$\text{cap} = \underline{\hspace{3cm}}$$

The numerator unit of the first factor must be the same as the unit of the answer. Find the factor containing cap. Write 1 cap in the numerator and 200 mcg in the denominator, followed by multiplication signs.

$$\text{cap} = \frac{1 \ \text{cap} \ \times}{200 \ \text{mcg} \ \times}$$

[handwritten] $Cap = \dfrac{1\ cap \times \overset{5}{\cancel{1000\,mcg}} \times \overset{2}{\cancel{60\,mg}} \times \frac{1}{\cancel{150}}}{\underset{\underset{1}{2}}{\cancel{200}}\,mcg \times 1\,mg \times 1\,gr \times \underset{\cancel{5}}{150} \times 1}$

$\dfrac{2}{1} = 2$

The numerator unit of the second factor must be the same as the denominator unit of the first factor. Find the factor containing mcg. Write 1000 mcg in the numerator and 1 mg in the denominator, followed by multiplication signs.

$$\text{cap} = \frac{1 \text{ cap} \times 1000 \text{ mcg} \times}{200 \text{ mcg} \times 1}$$

The numerator unit of the third factor must be the same as the denominator unit of the second factor. Find the factor containing mg. Write 60 mg in the numerator and 1 gr in the denominator, followed by multiplication signs.

$$\text{cap} = \frac{1 \text{ cap} \times 1000 \text{ mcg} \times 60 \text{ mg} \times}{200 \text{ mcg} \times \quad 1 \text{ mg} \times 1 \text{ gr} \times}$$

The numerator unit of the fourth factor must be the same as the denominator unit of the third factor. Find the factor containing gr. Write gr 1/150 in the numerator and 1 in the denominator.

$$\text{cap} = \frac{1 \text{ cap} \times 1000 \text{ mcg} \times 60 \text{ mg} \times \text{gr } 1/150}{200 \text{ mcg} \times \quad 1 \text{ mg} \times 1 \text{ gr} \times \quad 1}$$

Cancel the units.

$$\text{cap} = \frac{1 \text{ cap} \times 1000 \times 60 \times 1/150}{200 \quad \times \quad 1 \times 1 \times \quad 1}$$

Drop the denominator of the fraction into the denominator of the equation. Cancel the evenly divisible numbers.

$$\text{cap} = \frac{1 \text{ cap} \times \overset{5}{\cancel{1000}} \times \overset{2}{\cancel{60}} \times \quad 1}{\underset{1}{\cancel{200}} \quad \times \quad 1 \times 1 \times 1 \times \underset{\underset{1}{\cancel{5}}}{\cancel{150}}}$$

Multiply the numerator:
Multiply the denominator:

$$\frac{1 \text{ cap} \times 1 \times 2 \times 1}{1 \quad \times 1 \times 1 \times 1} = \frac{2 \text{ cap}}{1} = 2 \text{ cap}$$

Sometimes the answers to problems will be in half tablets. Remember, only scored tablets can be divided into two equal amounts. Tablets that are scored in fourths can be divided into four equal amounts. Capsules cannot be divided into equal parts.

PRACTICE PROBLEMS

Dosage Calculation of Oral Medications Available in Solid Forms

Show all your work. Check your answers (page 326).

1. Dosage ordered: 16 mg PO q.i.d. Dosage on hand: 4 mg scored tablets. How many tablets should be administered?

$$\text{Tab} = \frac{1 \text{ Tab} \times \overset{4}{\cancel{16}}\text{mg}}{\underset{1}{\cancel{4}}\text{mg} \times \quad 1} = 4 \text{ Tab}$$

2. Dosage ordered: gr iii PO ASAP. Dosage on hand: 0.1 g capsule. How many caps will you administer?

15 gr 1000 mg
15 gr 1 g

$$\text{caps} = \frac{1 \text{ cap} \times 1 \text{ g} \times 3 \text{ gr}}{0.1 \text{ g} \times 15 \text{ gr} \times 1} = \frac{1}{.5} =$$

5

2 cap

$$\begin{array}{r} 2 \\ 5 \overline{)1.0} \end{array}$$

3. Dosage ordered: 200 U q.i.d. PO. Dosage available: 400 U per scored tablet. How many tabs will be administered?

$$Tab = \frac{1\ Tab \times 200U}{\underset{2}{\cancel{400}}\ U \times 1} = \frac{1}{2}\ Tab$$

4. Dosage ordered: 250 mg PO q.i.d. Dosage on hand: 0.5 g scored tablets. How many tablets will be administered?

$$Tab = \frac{1\ Tab \times 1g \times \overset{25}{\cancel{250}}mg}{0.5g \times \cancel{1000}mg \times 1} = \frac{1}{2}\ \frac{1}{2}\ Tab$$

5. Dosage ordered: 1 g PO b.i.d. Dosage on hand: 250 mg unscored tablets. How many tablets will be given?

$$Tab = \frac{1\ Tab \times \overset{4}{\cancel{1000}}mg \times 1g}{\cancel{250}mg \times 1g \times 1} = 4\ Tab$$

6. Dosage ordered: gr 1/8 PO q.6h. Dosage on hand: 4 mg scored tablets. How many tabs will be given.

$$Tab = \frac{1\ Tab \times \overset{15}{\cancel{60}}mg \times 1/8\ gr}{\cancel{4}mg \times 1\ gr \times 1 \times 8} = \frac{15}{8}\ or\ 1\tfrac{7}{8}\ or\ 2\ Tab$$

7. Dosage ordered: 0.25 mg PO q.8h. Dosage on hand: 100 mcg per scored tablet. How many tablets will be administered?

$$Tab = \frac{1\ Tab \times \overset{10}{\cancel{1000}}mcg \times .25mg}{\cancel{100}mcg \times 1\ mg \times 1} = 2.5 = 2\tfrac{1}{2}\ Tab$$

8. Dosage ordered: gr iss PO b.i.d. Dosage available: 0.1 g scored tab. How many tabs will be administered?

$$Tab = \frac{1\ Tab \times 1g \times 1.5\ gr}{.1g \times 15\ gr \times 1} = \frac{.1}{.1}\ or\ 1$$

9. Dosage ordered: gr 1/500 PO q.4h. Dosage on hand: 120 mcg cap. How many caps will be administered?

$$cap = \frac{1\ cap \times 1000\ mg \times 60mg \times 1/500}{120\ mcg \times 1\ mg \times 1\ gr \times 1 \times 500} = \frac{1}{1}\ or\ 1$$

10. Dosage ordered: 25 mg PO b.i.d. Dosage on hand: 0.05 g scored tablets. How many tabs should be given?

$$Tab = \frac{1\ Tab \times 1g \times 25mg}{.05g \times 1000\ mg \times 1} = \frac{1}{2}\ Tab$$

Solve the following problems using the medication labels that appear to the right of the medication order.

11. Dosage ordered: Decadron 0.75 mg PO q AM. How many tabs will be given?

$$Tab = \frac{1\ Tab \times .75mg}{.5mg \times 1} = \frac{1.5}{1} = 1\tfrac{1}{2}\ Tab$$

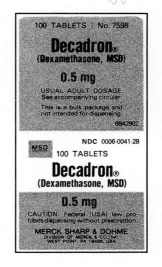

12. Dosage ordered: Ampicillin 500 mg PO q.4h.
    How many tabs will be administered?

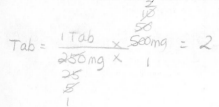

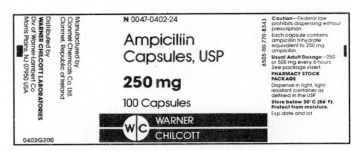

13. Dosage ordered: Acetaminophen gr X q4h
    prn. How many caps will be given?

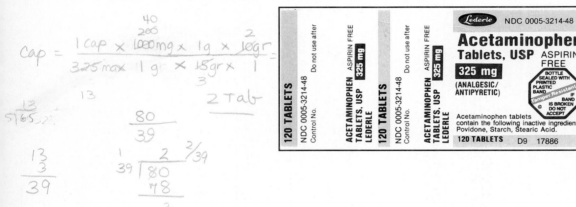

14. Dosage ordered: Aldomet 250 mg PO t.i.d.
    How many tabs will be given?

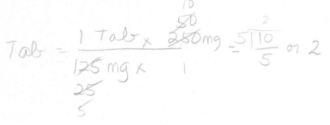

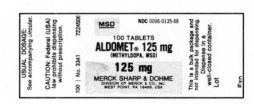

15. Dosage on hand: Decadron 750 mcg PO
    ASAP How many tabs will be administered?

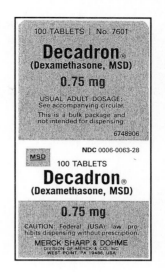

$$Tab = \frac{1\,Tab}{.75\,mg} \times \frac{1\,mg}{1000\,mg} \times \frac{750\,mg}{1} = \frac{1}{1} \quad or \quad 1$$

.125

20

4

$$\frac{20}{50\overline{)1000}} \qquad 50\overline{)750}^{\,15} \qquad 3\overline{)0.75}^{\,.25} \qquad \frac{.25}{100}^{\,2}$$

16. Dosage ordered: Dilantin 60 mg t.i.d. PO.
    How many caps will be given?

$$cap = \frac{1\,cap}{30\,mg} \times \frac{60\,mg}{1} = 2$$

17. Dosage ordered: Myambutal 1 g PO q.d.
    How many tabs will be administered?

$$Tab = \frac{1\,Tab}{400\,mg} \times \frac{1000\,mg}{1\,g} \times \frac{1\,g}{1}$$

$$\frac{5}{2} \quad or$$

$$2\frac{1}{2} \quad Tab$$

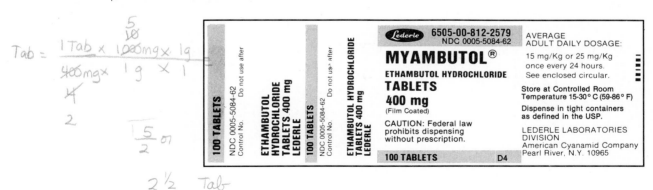

18. Dosage ordered: Ferrous sulfate gr V PO t.i.d. How many tabs will be administered?

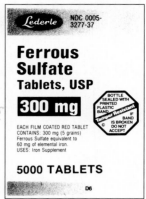

$$Tab = \frac{1\,Tab \times \overset{10}{\cancel{1000}}\,mg \times 1\,g}{\underset{3}{\cancel{300}}\,mg \times 1\,g \times \underset{3}{\cancel{15}}\,gr} \times \frac{\overset{1}{\cancel{5}}\,gr}{1} = \frac{10}{9} \text{ or } 1\tfrac{1}{9} \text{ or } 1\,Tab$$

19. Dosage ordered: Benadryl 50 mg PO h.s. How many caps will be given?

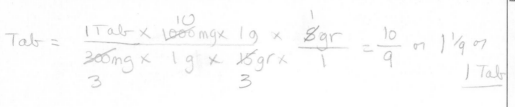

$$Cap = \frac{1\,cap}{\underset{5}{\underset{1}{\cancel{25}}}\,mg} \times \frac{\overset{2}{\overset{10}{\cancel{50}}}\,mg}{1} = 2 \ cap$$

20. Dosage ordered: Restoril 15mg hs prn. How many caps will be given?

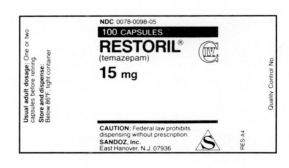

$$Cap = \frac{1\,cap}{\cancel{15}\,mg} \times \frac{\cancel{15}\,mg}{1} = 1$$

order + dosage same
order is 1 cap.

CALCULATION OF ORAL MEDICATIONS
UTILIZING DRUGS OF SEVERAL STRENGTHS

Some medications are ordered in dosages that can be obtained only by combining tablets or capsules of several strengths. Such a medication is Coumadin, which is available in 2 mg, 2.5 mg, 5 mg, 7.5 mg and 10 mg scored tablets. To determine which tablets to give, select a combination that provides the correct dosage using the fewest tablets or capsules. Sometimes, several combinations work equally well.

SAMPLE PROBLEM   **Dosage ordered: Coumadin 17 mg PO qd.**
Select the correct dosage using the fewest tablets possible from the following labels:

COUMADIN ®	COUMADIN ®	COUMADIN ®	COUMADIN ®	COUMADIN ®
(crystalline warfarin sodium, U.S.P.)	(crystalline warfarin sodium, U.S.P.)	(crystalline warfarin sodium, U.S.P.)	(crystalline warfarin sodium, U.S.P.)	(crystalline warfarin sodium, U.S.P.)
2 mg	**2½ mg**	**5 mg**	**7½ mg**	**10 mg**
DU PONT PHARMACEUTICALS	DU PONT PHARMACEUTICALS	DU PONT PHARMACEUTICALS	DU PONT PHARMACEUTICALS	DU PONT PHARMACEUTICALS
Wilmington, Delaware 19898	Wilmington, Delaware 19898	Wilmington, Delaware 19898	Wilmington, Delaware 19898	Wilmington, Delaware 19898
Lot YA007A	Lot YA021A	Lot YC058A	Lot XC009A	Lot XL077A
Exp. 1/89	Exp. 1/89	Exp. 8/89	Exp. 3/88	Exp. 10/88

Three combinations equal 17 mg: (1) three 5 mg tab + one 2 mg tab = 17 mg
(2) one 10 mg tab + one 5 mg tab + one 2 mg tab = 17
(3) two 7.5 mg tab + one 2 mg tab = 17 mg

Thus combinations (2) or (3) = 17 mg uses the least number of tablets.

The least number of tablets is used whenever possible. The more capsules or tablets the client is required to take, the less likely the client is to follow the medication regime. However, the more complicated the regime, the less likely they are to follow the regime. The client would tend to follow regime 3 better than regime 2. Two strengths are easier to handle than three strengths.

PRACTICE PROBLEMS

Calculation of Oral Medication Using Drugs of Several Strengths

Utilizing the labels to the right of the medication order, select the combination of medication strengths that provides the correct dosage while using the fewest tabs or caps possible. (Answers on page 327.)

21. Dosage ordered: Coumadin 13 mg PO q.d.

COUMADIN ®	COUMADIN ®	COUMADIN ®
(crystalline warfarin sodium, U.S.P.)	(crystalline warfarin sodium, U.S.P.)	(crystalline warfarin sodium, U.S.P.)
2 mg	**2½ mg**	**5 mg**
DU PONT PHARMACEUTICALS	DU PONT PHARMACEUTICALS	DU PONT PHARMACEUTICALS
Wilmington, Delaware 19898	Wilmington, Delaware 19898	Wilmington, Delaware 19898
Lot YA007A	Lot YA021A	Lot YC058A
Exp. 1/89	Exp. 1/89	Exp. 8/89

2 - 5 mg
1½ - 2½ mg

22. Dosage ordered: Thorazine 35 mg PO q.i.d.

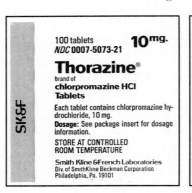
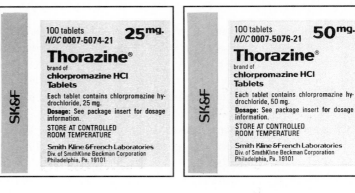

1 — 10 mg

1 — 25 mg

23. Dosage ordered: Coumadin 3.5 mg h.s. PO

1 — 2 1/2

1/2 — 2

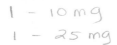

24. Dosage ordered: Decadron 1.25 mg bid PO
    X 2 d

.75   .75

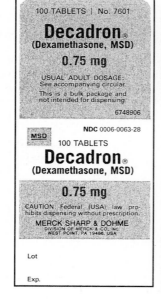
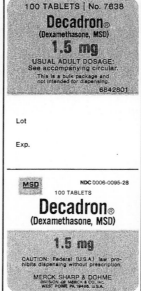
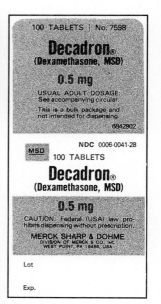

25. Dosage ordered: Synthroid 0.125 mg PO q
    AM

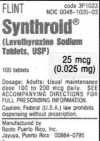

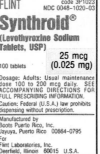

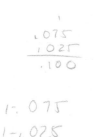

.075
.025
───
.100

1. 075
1-.025

1- .075
1- .05

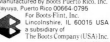

CALCULATION OF ORAL MEDICATIONS IN LIQUID FORM

Oral pediatric medications have been available in liquid form for many years. Many medications primarily given to adults are now available in liquid form as a response to the growing number of older adults who have difficulty swallowing pills.

Some liquid medications are available in unit dose form. Others must be carefully measured in a medication cup held at eye level. Syringes provide the most accurate measurement of small quantities.

Calculation of dosages for oral liquid medications is the same as for solid medications. The equation is as follows:

$$\text{Unit and amount to administer} = \frac{\text{conversion factor if necessary}}{} \times \frac{\text{amount available}}{\text{dosage available}} \times \frac{\text{conversion factor if necessary}}{} \times \frac{\text{dosage ordered}}{1}$$

SAMPLE PROBLEM **Dosage ordered: 500 mg b.i.d. PO.**
Dosage on hand: 500 mg per 5 ml. How many teaspoons will be administered?

Knowns: Unit of answer: tsp
Factors: 500 mg = 5 ml
         500 mg/1

$$\text{Tsp} = \frac{1\,\text{Tsp} \times 5\,\text{ml} \times 500\,\text{mg}}{5\,\text{ml} \times 500\,\text{mg} \times 1} = 1\,\text{tsp.}$$

Conversion factor: 1 tsp = 5 ml
Since 500 mg are ordered and there are 500 mg per 5 ml, it is obvious that 5 ml will be given: 5 ml = 1 tsp; therefore, 1 tsp will be given. The equation for this problem is as follows:

$$\text{tsp} = \frac{1\,\text{tsp} \times 5\,\text{ml} \times 500\,\text{mg}}{5\,\text{ml} \times 500\,\text{mg} \times 1} = \frac{1\,\text{tsp} \times \frac{1}{5} \times \frac{1}{500}}{\frac{5}{1} \times \frac{500}{1} \times 1} = \frac{1\,\text{tsp} \times 1 \times 1}{1 \times 1 \times 1} = \frac{1\,\text{tsp}}{1} = 1\,\text{tsp}$$

Many liquid medications are ordered in units of measurement or quantities differing from those on the medication label. Recognition alone is not adequate to solve the problem.

[handwritten: gR ½]

SAMPLE PROBLEM   **Dosage ordered: gr ss PO t.i.d.**
Dosage on hand: 50 mg/5 ml. How many ml will be given?

[handwritten calculation:
$$ml = \frac{5\,ml \times 60\,mg \times \frac{1}{2}\,gr}{\frac{50\,mg}{5} \times 1\,gR \times 1 \times 2} = \frac{15}{5}\,ml$$
3 ml]

Knowns: Unit of answer: ml
Factors: 50 mg = 5 ml
          1/2 gr/1
Conversion factor: 1 gr = 60 mg
Set up the framework of the equation.

ml = _____

The numerator unit of the first factor must be the same as the answer unit. Find the factor containing ml. Write 5 ml in the numerator and 50 mg in the denominator, followed by multiplication signs.

$$ml = \frac{5\ ml \times}{50\ mg \times}$$

The numerator unit of the second factor must be the same as the denominator unit of the first factor. Find the factor containing mg. Write 60 mg in the numerator and 1 gr in the denominator, followed by multiplication signs.

$$ml = \frac{5\ ml \times 60\ mg \times}{50\ mg \times \ 1\ gr\ \times}$$

The numerator unit of the third factor must be the same as the denominator unit of the second factor. Find the factor containing gr. Write gr 1/2 in the numerator and 1 in the denominator.

$$ml = \frac{5\ ml \ \times 60\ mg \times gr\ 1/2}{50\ mg \times \ 1\ gr\ \times \qquad 1}$$

Cancel the units.

$$ml = \frac{5\ ml \times 60 \times 1/2}{50 \quad \times \ 1 \times \ 1}$$

Drop the denominator of the fraction into the denominator of the equation. Cancel evenly divisible quantities.

$$ml = \frac{\overset{1}{\cancel{5}}\ ml \times \overset{\overset{3}{\cancel{30}}}{\cancel{60}} \times 1}{\underset{\underset{1}{\cancel{10}}}{\cancel{50}} \quad \times \ 1 \times \underset{1}{\cancel{2}}}$$

Multiply the numerator:
Multiply the denominator:

$$\frac{1\ ml \times 3 \times 1}{1 \quad \times 1 \times 1} = \frac{3\ ml}{1} = 3\ ml$$

Some answers are fractional parts of a measurement unit. This is no problem with liquid medications; quantities can be measured very precisely with a syringe. Remember, fractional parts of metric measurements are always written as decimals and those in apothecary and household measurements are written as fractions.

The following problem has a mixed number that must be converted to an improper fraction. The conversion is as follows:

$$\frac{(\text{whole number} \times \text{denominator}) + \text{existing numerator}}{\text{denominator}} = \frac{\text{new numerator}}{\text{denominator}}$$

SAMPLE PROBLEM   **Dosage ordered: gr 1 1/2 PO q.i.d.**
Dosage available: 50 mg/ml. How many ml will be given?

Knowns: Unit of answer: ml
Factors: 50 mg = 1 ml
     1 1/2 gr/1
Conversion factor: 1 gr = 60 mg
Set up the framework of the equation.

$$ml = \underline{\hspace{3cm}}$$

The numerator unit of the first factor must be the same as the answer unit. Find the factor containing ml. Write 1 ml in the numerator and 50 mg in the denominator, followed by multiplication signs.

$$ml = \frac{1\ ml\ \times}{50\ mg\ \times}$$

The numerator unit of the second factor must be the same as the denominator unit of the first factor. Find the factor containing mg. Write 60 mg in the numerator and 1 gr in the denominator, followed by multiplication signs.

$$ml = \frac{1\ ml\ \times\ 60\ mg\ \times}{50\ mg\ \times\ 1\ gr\ \times}$$

The numerator unit of the third factor must be the same as the denominator unit of the second factor. Find the factor containing gr. Write gr 1 1/2 in the numerator and 1 in the denominator.

$$ml = \frac{1\ mg\ \times\ 60\ mg\ \times\ gr\ 1\ 1/2}{50\ mg\ \times\ 1\ gr\ \times\ \quad 1}$$

Cancel the units.

$$ml = \frac{1\ mg\ \times\ 60\ \times\ 1\ 1/2}{50\ \times\ 1\ \times\ \quad 1}$$

Convert the mixed number to an improper fraction. $\frac{(1\times2)+1}{2} = \frac{3}{2}$

$$ml = \frac{1\ mg\ \times\ 60\ \times\ 3}{50\ \times\ 1\ \times\ 2}$$

Drop the fraction denominator into the denominator of the equation. Cancel the evenly divisible quantities.

$$ml = \frac{1\ mg\ \times\ \overset{3}{\cancel{60}}\ \times\ 3}{\underset{5}{\cancel{50}}\ \times\ 1\ \times\ \cancel{2}\underset{1}{}}$$

Multiply the numerator:
Multiply the denominator:

$$\frac{1\ ml\ \times\ 3\ \times\ 3}{5\ \times\ 1\ \times\ 1} = \frac{9\ ml}{5} = 1.8\ ml$$

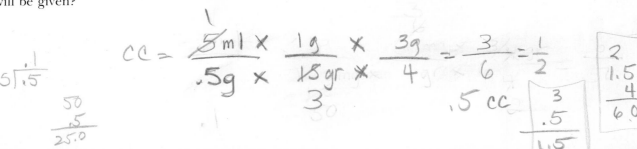

PRACTICE PROBLEMS

Calculation of Oral Medications Available in Liquid Forms

Show all your work. Check your answers (page 328).

26. Dosage ordered: gr 3/4 PO q.d. Dosage on hand: 0.5 g per 5 ml. How many cc
    will be given?

27. Dosage ordered: 75 mg t.i.d. PO. Dosage on hand: 300 mg per ml. How many ml will be given?

$$ml = \frac{1\ ml}{\underset{4}{300}mg} \times \frac{\overset{1}{75}mg}{1} = \frac{1}{4} \quad .25\ ml$$

28. Dosage ordered: gr 1/300 b.i.d. PO. Dosage available: 50 mcg per 5 ml How many teaspoons will be administered?

1 g = 15 g
60 mg =
1000 mg = 15 g00
1 mg = 1000 mg
1000 mcg =

$$Tsp = \frac{1\ Tsp}{\underset{1}{5\ ml}} \times \frac{\overset{1}{5}ml}{50mcg} \times \frac{\overset{20}{1000}mcg}{1\ mg} \times \frac{60mg}{1\ gr} \times \frac{1}{\underset{5}{300}} = 4\ Tsp$$

29. Dosage ordered: 1.5 g PO q.4h. Dosage on hand: 150 mg/ml. How many drams will be given?

$$DRS = \frac{1\ dR}{5\ ml} \times \frac{1\ ml}{\underset{15}{150}mg} \times \frac{1000mg}{1\ g} \times \frac{1.5\ g}{1} = \quad 2$$

30. Dosage ordered: 0.4 mg b.i.d. PO. Dosage available: 200 mcg/ml. How many ml will be administered?

$$ml = \frac{1\ ml}{200mcg} \times \frac{\overset{5}{1000}mg}{1\ mg} \times \frac{.4\ mg}{1} = \quad 2$$

31. Dosage ordered: gr 1/100 PO q.8h. Dosage on hand: 300 mcg/ml. How many ml will be administered?

$$ml = \frac{1\ ml}{\underset{5}{300}mcg} \times \frac{1000\ mcg}{1\ mg} \times \frac{60\ mg}{1\ gr} \times \frac{1\ g}{100} = \quad 2$$

32. Dosage ordered: gr 1/8 PO b.i.d. Dosage available: 100 mg per 5 ml. How many ml will be given?

$$ml = \frac{5\ ml}{\underset{5}{100}mg} \times \frac{60\ mg}{1\ g} \times \frac{1}{8} = \frac{3}{8}$$

.375

$$8\overline{)3.10}$$

33. Dosage ordered: 0.25 g PO q.d. Dosage available: 1 g per ml. How many cc will be administered?

$$cc = \frac{1\ mg}{1\ g} \times \frac{.25\ g}{1} = .25\ cc$$

34. Dosage ordered: gr iii h.s. p.r.n. PO. Dosage available: 0.5 g per 5 ml. How many ml will be given?

$$ml = \frac{5\ ml}{.5\ g} \times \frac{1\ g}{15\ gr} \times \frac{3\ gr}{1} = \frac{1}{.5} = 2\ ml$$

35. Dosage ordered: 600 mcg PO b.i.d. Dosage available: 1 mg per 5 ml. How many cc will be administered?

$$cc = \frac{5\ ml}{1\ mg} \times \frac{1\ mg}{1000\ mcg} \times \frac{600\ mcg}{1} = 3\ cc$$

Solve the following problems using the dosages on the medication labels.

36. Dosage ordered: Erythromycin 400 mg q.i.d. PO. How many ml will be given?

$$ml = \frac{5\ ml}{200\ mg} \times \frac{400\ mg}{1} = 10\ ml$$

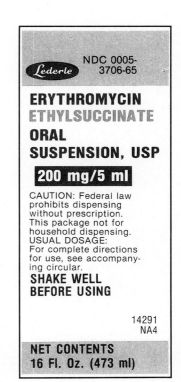

NDC 0005-3706-65

Lederle

ERYTHROMYCIN ETHYLSUCCINATE ORAL SUSPENSION, USP

200 mg/5 ml

CAUTION: Federal law prohibits dispensing without prescription. This package not for household dispensing. USUAL DOSAGE: For complete directions for use, see accompanying circular.

SHAKE WELL BEFORE USING

14291
NA4

NET CONTENTS 16 Fl. Oz. (473 ml)

37. Dosage ordered: V-Cillin K suspension 250 mg PO q.i.d. How many ml will be administered?

$$ml = \frac{5\ ml}{125\ mg} \times \frac{250\ mg}{1} = \frac{5\ ml}{125} \times \frac{250}{1} = 10\ ml$$

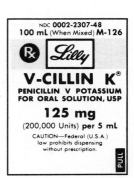

NDC 0002-2307-48
100 mL (When Mixed) M-126

Rx *Lilly*

V-CILLIN K®
PENICILLIN V POTASSIUM
FOR ORAL SOLUTION, USP

125 mg
(200,000 Units) per 5 mL

CAUTION—Federal (U.S.A.) law prohibits dispensing without prescription.

38. Dosage ordered: Dilantin 100 mg t.i.d. PO.
    How many cc will be given?

$$cc = \frac{5\ ml}{125\ mg} \times \frac{100\ mg}{1} = \frac{5\ ml}{\overset{125}{\underset{5}{\cancel{125}}}} \times \frac{\overset{4}{\cancel{100}}}{1} = 4\ cc$$

N 0071-2214-20   *Shake Well*

Dilantin-125®
(Phenytoin Oral Suspension, USP)

125 mg per 5 mL potency

Important—Another strength available; verify unspecified prescriptions.

Caution—Federal law prohibits dispensing without prescription.

8 fl oz (237 mL)

PARKE-DAVIS
Div of Warner-Lambert Co/ Morris Plains, NJ 07950 USA

39. Dosage ordered: Benadryl 50 mg PO h.s.
    p.r.n. How many tsp will be administered?

N 0071-2220-17

ELIXIR

Benadryl®
(Diphenhydramine Hydrochloride Elixir, USP)

Caution—Federal law prohibits dispensing without prescription.

4 FLUIDOUNCES

PARKE-DAVIS
Div of Warner-Lambert Co
Morris Plains, NJ 07950 USA

Elixir P-D 2220 for prescription dispensing only.

Contains—12.5 mg diphenhydramine hydrochloride in each 5 mL. Alcohol, 14%.

Dose—Adults, 2 to 4 teaspoonfuls; children over 20 lb, 1 to 2 teaspoonfuls; three or four times daily.

See package insert.

Keep this and all drugs out of the reach of children.

Store below 30°C (86°F). Protect from freezing and light.

Exp date and lot

2220G10 2

$$tsp = \frac{1\ tsp \times 5\ ml \times 50\ mg}{5\ ml \times 12.5\ mg \times 1} =$$

$$\frac{1\ tsp \times \cancel{5} \times \overset{2}{\cancel{50}}}{\underset{\underset{.5}{\cancel{2.5}}}{\cancel{5} \times \cancel{12.5} \times 1}} = \frac{2}{.5} = 4\ tsp$$

40. Dosage ordered: Pen-Vee K 400,000 U PO t.i.d. How many tsp will be given?

$$tsp = \frac{1\,tsp}{5\,ml} \times \frac{5\,ml}{250\,mg} \times \frac{250\,mg}{400,000\,U} \times \frac{400,000\,U}{1}$$

$$\frac{1\,tsp \times 5 \times 250 \times 400,000}{5 \times 250 \times 400,000} \qquad 1\,tsp$$

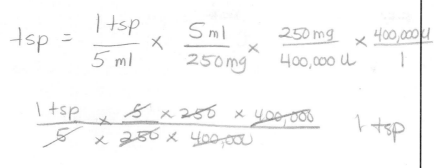

Wyeth®
Pen·Vee® K
(penicillin V potassium for oral solution)

250 mg **(400,000 units)**
penicillin V per 5 ml
1 bottle powder
to make **200 ml** liquid

PHARMACIST:
Note larger bottle and
new mixing instructions.

®

41. Dosage ordered: Kaon Chloride 20 mEq PO q.d. How many ml will be administered?

$$ml = \frac{15\,ml}{40\,mEq} \times \frac{20\,mEq}{1} =$$

$$\frac{15\,ml \times \overset{1}{\cancel{20}}}{\underset{2}{\cancel{40}} \times 1} = \frac{15\,ml}{2} = 7.5\,ml$$

NDC 0013-3113-51

KAON-CL
20%®
(POTASSIUM CHLORIDE)

40 mEq/15 ml

CHERRY

Sugar-Free

Each 15 ml (tablespoonful) supplies 40 mEq each of potassium and chloride (as potassium chloride, 3 g), with saccharin and alcohol 5%.

CAUTION: Federal law prohibits dispensing without prescription.

ONE PINT

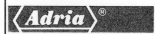

Adria ®

42. Dosage ordered: Mycostatin suspension 100,000 U PO q.i.d. How many ml will be administered?

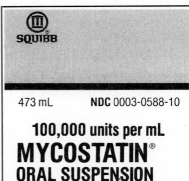

1 ml

43. Dosage ordered: amoxicillin 250 mg PO q4h. How many cc will be administered?

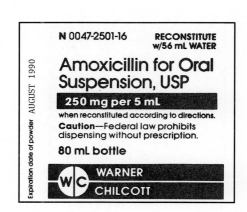

$$CC = \frac{5\,ml}{250\,mg} \times \frac{250\,mg}{1} = 5\ CC$$

44. Dosage ordered: morphine sulfate gr 1/4 PO q.4h. p.r.n. How many ml will be given?

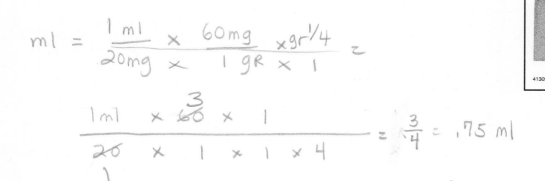

$$ml = \frac{1\,ml}{20\,mg} \times \frac{60\,mg}{1\,gR} \times \frac{gr^{1/4}}{1} =$$

$$\frac{1\,ml \times \overset{3}{\cancel{60}} \times 1}{\underset{1}{20} \times 1 \times 1 \times 4} = \frac{3}{4} = .75\ ml$$

45. Dosage ordered: Lithium citrate 600 mg t.i.d. PO. 8 mEq lithium is equal to 300 mg. How many ml will be given?

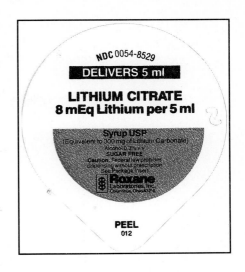

$$ml = \frac{5\,ml}{8\,mEq} \times \frac{8\,mEq}{300\,mg} \times \frac{600\,mg}{1} =$$

$$\frac{5\,ml \times 8 \times 600}{8 \times 300 \times 1} = 10\,ml$$

SELF-ASSESSMENT POSTTEST

Calculation of Oral Dosages

Show all your work. Check your answers (page 358).

1. Dosage ordered: 200,000 U q.i.d. PO. Dosage on hand: 400,000 U scored tabs. How many tablets will be administered?

$$Tab = \frac{1\,Tab}{400,000\,U} \times \frac{200,000\,U}{1} = \frac{1}{2}\,Tab$$

2. Dosage ordered: 0.25 mg q.4h. PO. Dosage on hand: 100 mcg per 5 ml. How many cc will be administered?

$$CC = \frac{5\,ml}{100\,mcg} \times \frac{1000\,mcg}{1\,mg} \times \frac{0.25\,mg}{1} = \frac{12.5}{1} \quad 12.5\,cc$$

3. Dosage ordered: 100 mg PO q.6h. Dosage available: 0.25 g per 5 ml. How many ml will be given?

$$ml = \frac{5\,ml}{0.25\,g} \times \frac{1\,g}{1000\,mg} \times \frac{100\,mg}{1} = \frac{5}{2.5} \quad 2\,ml$$

4. Select the correct dosage using the smallest number of tablets from the labels to the right of the ordered dosage.
   Dosage ordered: Coumadin 12 mg PO q.d.

2 – 5 mg Tab

1 – 2 mg Tab

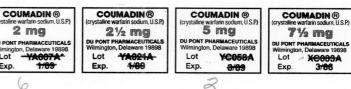

6   2

5. Dosage ordered: gr 1/60 PO t.i.d. Dosage available: 2 mg scored tabs. How many tabs will be given?

$$Tab = \frac{1\ Tab}{2\ mg} \times \frac{60\ mg}{1\ gr} \times \frac{1/60\ gr}{1 \times 60} = \frac{1}{2}\ Tab$$

6. Dosage ordered: 0.6 mg PO stat. Dosage on hand: 400 mcg scored tabs. How many tabs will be given?

$$Tab = \frac{1\ Tab}{400\ mcg} \times \frac{1000\ mcg}{1\ mg} \times \frac{0.6\ mg}{1} = \frac{600}{400} \quad 1.5\ Tab$$

7. Dosage ordered: gr 1/3 PO t.i.d. Dosage available: 10 mg/ml. How many ml will be given?

$$ml = \frac{1\ ml}{10\ mg} \times \frac{60\ mg}{1\ gr} \times \frac{1/3\ gr}{1 \times 3} = \frac{60}{30} = 2\ ml$$

8. Dosage ordered: gr 1/300 q.4h. PO. Dosage on hand: 400 mcg scored tabs. How many tabs will be administered?

$$Tab = \frac{1\ Tab}{400\ mcg} \times \frac{1000\ mcg}{1\ mg} \times \frac{60\ mg}{1\ gr} \times \frac{1/300\ gr}{1 \times 300} = \frac{60,000}{120,000} =$$

0.5 Tab   1/2 Tab

9. Dosage ordered: 0.2 mg q.12h. PO. Dosage on hand: 25 mcg/ml. How many ml will be given?

10. Dosage ordered: gr 1/30 PO q.i.d. Dosage available: 4 mg scored tabs. How many tabs will be given?

11. Dosage ordered: 0.05 mg PO t.i.d. Dosage on hand: 25 mcg scored tabs. How many tabs will be administered?

12. Dosage ordered: gr III PO q.d. Dosage on hand: 0.1 g scored tabs. How many tabs will be given?

$$Tab = \frac{1\ Tab}{0.1g} \times \frac{1g}{1000mg} \times \frac{1000mg}{15gr} \times \frac{3gr}{1} = \frac{3}{1.5} = 2\ Tab$$

13. Dosage ordered: 30 mcg q.d. PO. Dosage on hand: 0.25 mg per 5 ml. How many cc will be given?

14. Dosage ordered: gr viiss PO h.s. p.r.n. Dosage available: 0.5 g per 5 ml. How many teaspoons will be administered?

$$Tsp = \frac{1\ tsp}{5\ ml} \times \frac{5ml}{0.5g} \times \frac{1g}{1000mg} \times \frac{1000mg}{15gr} \times \frac{7.5g}{1} = \frac{7.5}{12.5} =$$

$$Tsp = \frac{1\ tsp}{5\ ml} \times \frac{5ml}{0.5g} \times \frac{1g}{1000mg} \times \frac{1000mg}{15gr} \times \frac{7.5g}{1} = \quad 0.6\ Tsp \quad n\ 1\ tsp$$

$$\frac{37500}{37500}$$

15. Dosage ordered: gr 1/3 PO t.i.d.   Dosage available: 40 mg scored tabs.   How many tabs will be given?

16. Dosage ordered: 50 mg PO q.i.d.   Dosage available: 20 mg scored tabs.   How many tabs will be given?

17. Dosage ordered: 400 mg b.i.d. PO. Dosage on hand: 0.1 g caps. How many caps will be administered?

18. Dosage ordered: 250 mg PO q.6h.   Dosage on hand: 500 mg per 5 ml.   How many tsp will be given?

19. Dosage ordered: 1.25 g a.c. t.i.d. PO. Dosage available: 500 mg scored tabs. How many tabs will be administered?

20. Dosage ordered: gr 1/30 PO t.i.d. Dosage on hand: 2 mg/ml. How many ml will be given?

Chapter 12

Calculation of Parenteral Medication Dosages

Parenteral medications are injectable medications administered subcutaneously, intramuscularly, intradermally, and intravenously. Only subcutaneous, intradermal, and intramuscular medications are included in this chapter. Intravenous solutions and medications are covered in Unit VIII.

Parenteral medication preparations are available as liquids or as powders to be reconstituted into liquids. Injectable medications are often available in several strengths. Parenteral medications are packaged in single and multiple dose vials, ampules, prefilled syringes, and syringe cartridges used with cartridge holders as shown in Figure 12-1.

Intradermal injections are administered almost exclusively for skin testing for allergies or disease. Very minute amounts of allergen are deposited just below the skin. Figure 12-2 shows a tuberculin syringe with an average amount of solution for skin testing.

Only small amounts of solution can be administered by subcutaneous and intramuscular routes. Large volumes of medication are painful for the client. Additionally, absorption is much slower and tissue damage is more likely to occur when large amounts of medication are administered. Table 12-1 shows the amount of medication that may be administered safely into a single injection site.

The amount of solution that can be administered safely into an injection site is dependent upon the size of the client. The maximum amount of medication injected into the deltoid muscle of a large adult might be 2 ml, whereas the maximum amount for a 10-year-old child might be only 0.5 ml. Injections of volumes greater than the maximum must be divided and given in two sites. The acceptable amounts to administer must be kept in mind when determining the strength of medication to use when there are several concentrations from which to choose.

Health care professionals are expected to know the conversion from ml to minims. Therefore, minims are frequently included in dosage calculation workbooks. Remember, there is a discrepancy when converting from one measurement system to another due to the use of approximate equivalents. The more conversions among the measurement systems, the greater the discrepancy. In the clinical setting, therefore,

TABLE 12-1 Volumes per Injection Site

Injection Route	Solution Volumes	
	Usual Range	*Maximum*
Intramuscular	0.5 - 3 ml	5 ml
Subcutaneous	0.1 - 1 ml	2 ml
Intradermal	0.01 - 0.1 ml	0.2 ml

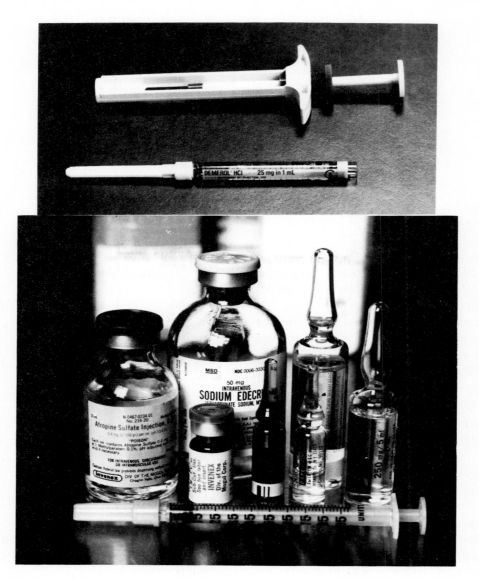

FIGURE 12-1 Parenteral medication packaging. A, syringe cartridge and holder (Tubex by Wyeth). B, variety of vials, ampules and pre-filled syringe. (From Potter, P.A. & Perry, A.G., Fundamentals of nursing: concepts, process and practice, St. Louis, 1985, The C.V. Mosby Co.)

conversions to minims are rarely done. Minims can be used as measurement aids, however. Figure 12-3 shows two syringes used to administer 0.25 ml of medication. Note that 4 minims is equal to 0.25 ml on the tuberculin syringe. There is no 0.25 measurement on the 2.5 ml syringe, but 4 minims is marked. Therefore, it is easier to withdraw the medication to the 4 minim mark than to approximate 0.25 ml.

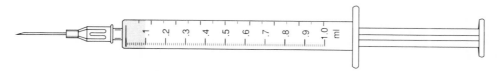

FIGURE 12-2 Tuberculine syringe for skin testing

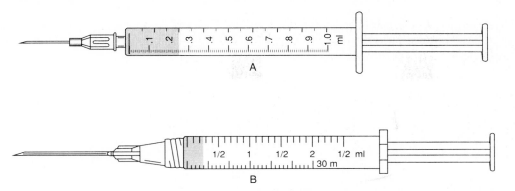

FIGURE 12-3 Comparison of the same amount of medication in two syringes. The upper tuberculin syringe and the lower 2.5 ml syringe both have 0.25 ml (4 minims) of medication.

Calculations of parenteral medication dosages are accomplished in exactly the same way as oral liquids. The equation is as follows:

$$\text{Unit and amount to administer} = \frac{\text{conversion factor if necessary} \times \text{amount available} \times \text{conversion factor if necessary} \times \text{dosage ordered}}{\text{necessary} \times \text{dosage available} \times \text{necessary} \times 1}$$

SAMPLE PROBLEM   **Dosage ordered: meperdine 37.5 mg IM stat.**
How many ml will be administered?

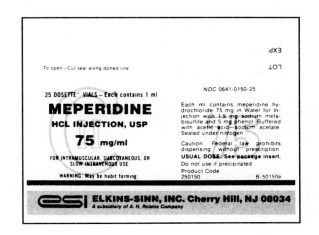

Knowns: Unit of Answer: ml
Factors: 75   mg = 1 ml
          37.5 mg/1
Set up the equation framework.   ml = _____

The first factor numerator unit must be the same
as the answer unit. Find the factor containing ml.
Write 1 ml in the numerator and 75 mg in the
denominator, followed by multiplication signs.

$$ml = \frac{1 \ ml \ \times}{75 \ mg \ \times}$$

$$ml = \frac{1 \ ml}{75 \ mg} \times \frac{37.5 \ mg}{1} =$$

$$\frac{1 \ ml \times 37.5}{75 \times 1} = .5 \ ml$$

The second factor numerator unit must be the same as the first factor denominator unit. Find the factor containing mg. Write 37.5 mg in the numerator and 1 in the denominator.

$$ml = \frac{1 \ ml \ \times \ 37.5 \ mg}{75 \ mg \ \times \ 1}$$

Cancel the units and evenly divisible quantities.

$$ml = \frac{1 \ ml \ \times \ \overset{1}{\cancel{37.5}}}{\underset{2}{\cancel{75}} \ \times \ 1}$$

Multiply the numerator:
Multiply the denominator:

$$\frac{1 \ ml \times 1}{2 \ \times 1} = \frac{1 \ ml}{2} = 0.5 \ ml$$

Figure 12-4 shows the syringe with the appropriate amount of meperidine.

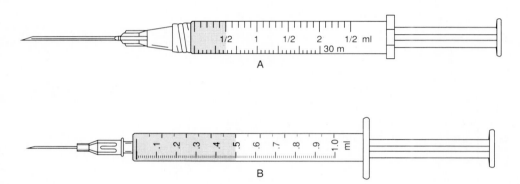

FIGURE 12-4 Two syringes with 0.5ml solution. Note that 0.5 ml is equal to 8 minims. It is much easier to measure small amounts using the tuberculin syringe (B) than the 2.5 ml syringe (A).

The instructions accompanying the following problems are shortened versions of previous instructions. Refer to previous instructions if you have difficulty in setting up the equation.

SAMPLE PROBLEM   **Dosage ordered: scopolamine gr 1/300**
How many minims will be given?

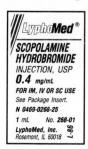

Knowns: Unit of Answer: mx
Factors: 0.4 mg = 1 ml
      $\frac{1}{300}$ **gr/1**
Conversion factors: 1 gr = 60 mg
                1 ml = 16 mx

$$mx = \frac{\overset{4}{\cancel{16} \ mx}}{1 \ ml} \times \frac{1 \ ml}{\underset{.1}{\cancel{.4 \ mg}}} \times \frac{\overset{\overset{1}{\cancel{6}}}{\cancel{60} \ mg}}{1 \ gr} \times \frac{g \ 1/300}{} = \frac{4}{.5}$$

$$\frac{300}{30}$$

$$= 8 \ mx$$

$$= 8 \ mx$$

Set up the equation framework.

$$mx = \underline{\hspace{2cm}}$$

The first factor numerator unit is the same as the answer unit.

$$mx = \frac{16 \text{ mx} \times}{1 \text{ ml} \times}$$

The second factor numerator unit is the same as the first factor denominator unit.

$$mx = \frac{16 \text{ mx} \times 1 \text{ ml} \times}{1 \text{ ml} \times 0.4 \text{ mg} \times}$$

The third factor numerator unit is the same as the second factor denominator unit.

$$mx = \frac{16 \text{ mx} \times 1 \text{ ml} \times 60 \text{ mg} \times}{1 \text{ ml} \times 0.4 \text{ mg} \times 1 \text{ gr} \times}$$

The fourth factor numerator unit is the same as the third factor denominator unit.

$$mx = \frac{16 \text{ mx} \times 1 \text{ ml} \times 60 \text{ mg} \times \text{gr}\frac{1}{300}}{1 \text{ ml} \times 0.4 \text{ mg} \times 1 \text{ gr} \times 1}$$

Drop the fraction denominator in the numerator into the equation denominator. Cancel the units and evenly divisible quantities.

$$mx = \frac{\overset{4}{\cancel{16}} \text{ mx} \times 1 \times \overset{1}{\cancel{60}} \times 1}{\underset{0.1}{1 \times \cancel{0.4}} \times 1 \times \underset{5}{\cancel{300}}}$$

Multiply the numerator:
Multiply the denominator:

$$\frac{4 \text{ mx} \times 1 \times 1 \times 1}{1 \times 0.1 \times 1 \times 5} = mx$$

$$= \frac{4 \text{ mx}}{0.5} = 8 \text{ mx}$$

Figure 12-5 shows the syringe with 8 minims of scopolamine. Note that this is 0.5 ml. (The answer would have been 7.5 mx if the conversion 1 ml = 15 mx had been used.)

Narcotics and other controlled substances are frequently available on nursing units in several strengths. Other medications in several strengths may be available as well. It is necessary to choose the appropriate strength from the several strengths. Remember to consider the volume of medication to be administered. The number of ampules or vials necessary to supply that volume is another important factor when using unit dose ampules or vials. It is not a consideration when using multiple dose vials.

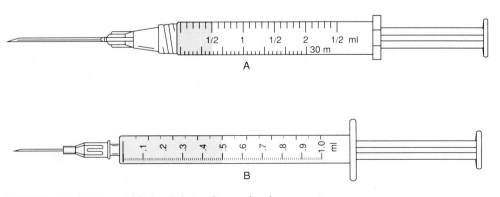

FIGURE 12-5 Syringe with 8 minims of scopolamine.

SAMPLE PROBLEM   **Dosage ordered: atropine gr 1/100**
Which vial would be most appropriate?
How many ml will be administered?

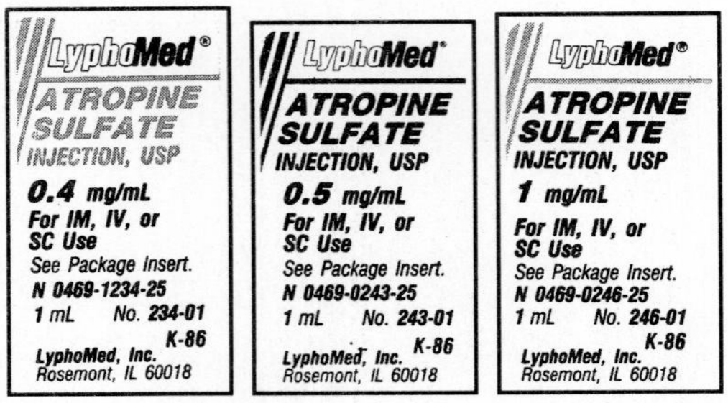

Handwritten notes in left margin:

$$3$$
$$6$$
$$mg = \frac{60mg}{1gr} \times \frac{1/100\,gr}{1 \times 100} = =$$

$$10$$
$$\frac{3\,mg}{5} = .6\,mg \qquad 5$$

$$5\overline{)3.0}^{.6}$$

Three vial labels:

A — LyphoMed® ATROPINE SULFATE INJECTION, USP **0.4** mg/mL For IM, IV, or SC Use See Package Insert. N 0469-1234-25 1 mL No. 234-01 K-86 LyphoMed, Inc. Rosemont, IL 60018

B — LyphoMed® ATROPINE SULFATE INJECTION, USP **0.5** mg/mL For IM, IV, or SC Use See Package Insert. N 0469-0243-25 1 mL No. 243-01 K-86 LyphoMed, Inc. Rosemont, IL 60018

C — LyphoMed® ATROPINE SULFATE INJECTION, USP **1** mg/mL For IM, IV, or SC Use See Package Insert. N 0469-0246-25 1 mL No. 246-01 K-86 LyphoMed, Inc. Rosemont, IL 60018

Begin by selecting the appropriate vial to use. To do this, convert the ordered apothecary dosage to metric.

Knowns: Unit of Answer: mg.

Factor: $\frac{1}{100}$ gr/1

Conversion Factor: 1 gr = 60 mg

Set up the equation framework.

$$mg = \underline{\qquad\qquad}$$

The first factor numerator unit is the same as the answer unit.

$$mg = \frac{60\ mg\ \times}{1\ gr\ \times}$$

The second factor numerator unit is the same as the first factor denominator unit.

$$mg = \frac{60\ mg\ \times\ gr\ \frac{1}{100}}{1\ gr\ \times\ 1}$$

Drop the fraction denominator in the numerator into the equation denominator. Cancel the units and evenly divisible quantities.

$$mg = \frac{\overset{3}{\cancel{60}}\ mg\ \times\ 1}{1\ gr\ \times\ \underset{5}{\cancel{100}}}$$

Multiply the numerator:
Multiply the denominator:

$$\frac{3\ mg \times 1}{1\ \times 5} = \frac{3\ mg}{5} = 0.6\ mg$$

Compare the converted dosage to the dosage on the vial labels. Because 0.6 mg is greater than 0.4 or 0.5 mg, it would take two vials of vials A or B to obtain 0.6 mg. 0.6 mg is less than the 1 mg vial. Therefore, vial C, 1 mg/ml, would be the most appropriate vial to choose.

Now find the volume of medication to administer. The dosage ordered was gr 1/100, which has already been converted to 0.6 mg. The dosage available is 1 mg/ml.

Knowns: Unit of Answer: ml

Factors: 1 mg = 1 ml
0.6 mg/1

Set up the equation framework.

$$ml = \underline{\qquad\qquad}$$

The first factor numerator unit is the same as the answer unit.

$$ml = \frac{1\ ml\ \times}{1\ mg \times}$$

The second factor numerator unit is the same as the first factor denominator unit.

$$ml = \frac{1\ ml\ \times\ 0.6\ mg}{1\ mg\ \times\ 1}$$

Cancel the units.

$$ml = \frac{1\ ml \times 0.6}{1\ \times\ 1}$$

Multiply the numerator:
Multiply the denominator:

$$\frac{1\ ml \times 0.6}{1\ \times\ 1} = \frac{0.6\ ml}{1} = 0.6\ ml$$

Figure 12-6 shows 0.6 ml of atropine in a syringe. Note that 0.6 ml = 9 mx.

15 mx = 1 ml

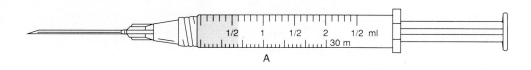

A

B

FIGURE 12-6 Syringes with 0.6 ml solution

Dosage Calculation of Parenteral Medications

Show all your work. Check your answers (page 329).

1. Dosage ordered: 35 mg IM q.4h.   p.r.n. Dosage on hand: 50 mg per ml. How many ml will be administered?

$$ml = \frac{1\ ml}{\underset{5}{50}mg} \times \frac{\overset{3}{30mg}}{1} = \frac{3}{5} = 0.6\ ml$$

2. Dosage ordered: gr ii IM h.s. p.r.n. Dosage on hand: 75 mg per ml. How many ml will be administered?

$$ml = \frac{1\ ml}{75mg} \times \frac{1000mg}{15gr} \times \frac{2gr}{1} = \frac{2000}{1125}$$

2
75
15
375
150
1125   15
        5⟌75

3. Dosage ordered: 100 mg s.c. stat. Dosage on hand: 250 mg per 1 ml. How many ml will be given?

$$ml = \frac{1\ ml}{250mg} \times \frac{100mg}{1} = \frac{2}{5} = 0.4\ ml$$

$$5\overline{)2.0}\ ^4$$

4. Dosage ordered: 200 mcg IM q.4h. Dosage on hand: 1.5 mg/1 ml. How many mx will be administered?

$$mx = \frac{\overset{2}{15}mx}{1\ ml} \times \frac{1\ ml}{1.5mg} \times \frac{1mg}{1000mcg} \times \frac{200mcg}{1} =$$

1.5⟌30.0 ^2

5. Dosage ordered: 250 mg IM t.i.d. Dosage on hand: 0.1 g per ml. How many ml will be given?

6. Dosage ordered: gr 1/150 s.c. b.i.d. Dosage on hand: 500 mcg per ml. How many ml will be given?

1.8 ml

7. Dosage ordered: gr i IM q.4h. Dosage available: 1 g per 10 ml. How many mx will be given?

8. Dosage ordered: 400,000 U IM b.i.d. Dosage available: 1,000,000 U/ml. How many ml will be administered?

2 mx

9. Dosage ordered: gr 1/300 s.c. q.8h. Dosage on hand: 0.6 mg per 2 ml. How many ml will you give?

10. Dosage ordered: 0.25 g q.12h. Dosage on hand: 500 mg/ml. How many ml will be administered?

Select the appropriate ampule, vial, or prefilled cartridge labels and solve the calculations.

11. Dosage ordered: heparin 3000 U s.c. q.6h. Which tubex is most appropriate? How many ml will be administered?

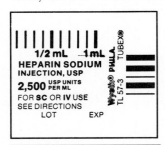

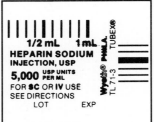

12. Dosage ordered: Dilaudid gr 1/16 s.c. stat. Which ampule is most appropriate? How many ml will be administered?

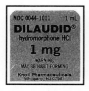 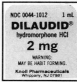 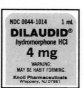

Find the volume to adminster in the following problems:

13. Dosage ordered: phenobarbital gr 1/2 IM t.i.d. How many ml will be administered?

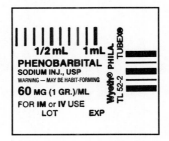

14. Dosage ordered: codeine gr 3/4 IM q.4h. p.r.n. How many ml will be given?

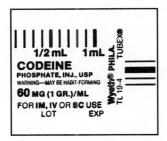

15. Dosage ordered: Vistaril 35 mg IM preop on call. How many ml will be given?

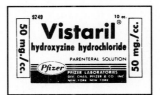

16. Dosage ordered: meperidine 25 mg IM stat. How many ml will be given?

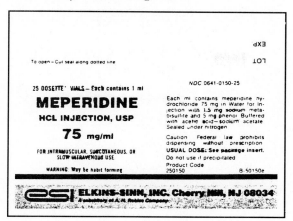

17. Dosage ordered: Cyanocobalamin 1000 mcg IM q month. How many ml will be given?

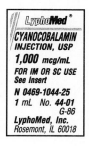

$$ml = \frac{1\,ml}{1000\,mcg} \times \frac{1000\,mcg}{1} = 1\,ml$$

18. Dosage ordered: procaine penicillin 900,000 U IM stat. How much of this 1 ml tubex will be administered?

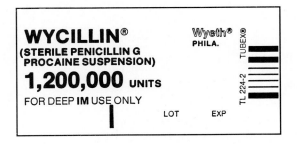

19. Dosage ordered: stadol 0.5 mg IM stat. How many mx will be given?

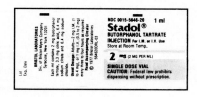

20. Dosage ordered: scopolamine gr 1/300 s.c. stat. How many ml will be given?

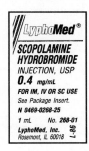

21. Dosage ordered: Bicillin CR 600,000 U IM stat. How many ml will be given?

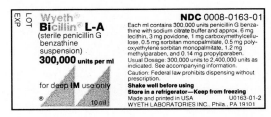

22. Dosage ordered: haloperidol 2 mg IM q.8h. p.r.n. How many ml will be given?

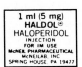

23. Dosage ordered: Ativan 3 mg IM stat. How many ml will be administered?

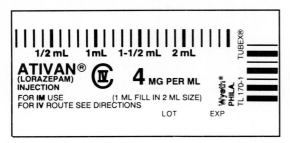

24. Dosage ordered: Kantrex 250 mg IM q.4h. How many ml will be administered?

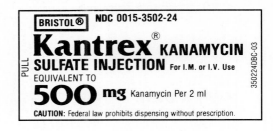

25. Dosage ordered: Robinul 300 mcg IM preop on call. How many ml will be administered?

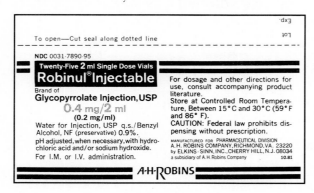

RECONSTITUTION OF PARENTERAL MEDICATIONS

Parenteral medications are reconstituted by adding sterile liquid, usually water or normal saline, to a powder to obtain a specific concentration of solution per unit. Powders are reconstituted by the pharmacist, especially in agencies employing the unit dose system, or by the person administering the medication. Most medications requiring reconstitution are not stable for long periods of time in liquid form. Because they deteriorate, it is important to know when the solution was reconstituted. After reconstitution, the vial must be labeled with the date and time of reconstitution and the initials of the person who reconstituted the medication.

Medication labels give directions for the reconstitution of powders. Figure 12-7 shows a medication label of an Ancef vial with those instructions. Note that the directions for reconstitution state that 2.5 ml of sterile water will provide 3 ml of solution per gram or 333 mg per ml. The powder in the vial occupies 0.5 ml space. To prove this, subtract the amount of sterile solution added from the total amount: 3 ml − 2.5 ml = 0.5 ml.

Practice reading the label directions in the following problems. Answer the questions asked. Cover the answers that follow the questions.

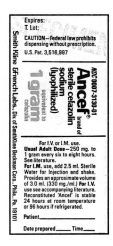

FIGURE 12-7 Medication label with directions for reconstitution.

Label 1:

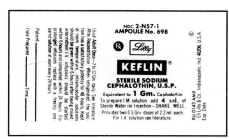

4.4 ml − 4 = .4

a. How many total grams of Keflin are in the vial?___1 g___
b. Which solution is to be used to reconstitute the medication?_Sterile water_
c. How much sterile solution is to be added?__4 ml__
d. What is the dosage per unit given on the vial?_2.2 ml_ .05g
e. What is the total amount of the solution in the vial after reconstitution?__4.4 ml__
f. How much space does the dry powder occupy?__0.4 cc__

Answers:

a. 1 g
b. sterile water
c. 4 cc
d. 0.5 g per 2.2 ml
e. 4.4 cc; two 0.5 g doses of 2.2 cc each
f. 0.4 cc; 4.4 cc − 4 cc = 0.4 cc

Label 2:

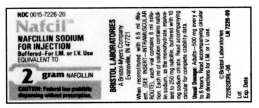

a. How many total grams of nafcillin are in the vial?___2 g___ Sterile water
b. Which solution is to be used to reconstitute the medication?___Sterile water___
c. How much sterile solution is to be added?___6.6 ml___
d. What is the dosage per unit given on the vial?___250 mg___
e. What is the total amount of the solution in the vial after reconstitution?__8 ml__
f. How much space does the dry powder occupy?_____

Answers:

a. 2 g
b. sterile water

8 ml − 6.6 = 1.4 ml

7.10
8.10
6.6
_____
14

c. 6.6 ml.

d. 250 mg per ml

e. $ml = \dfrac{1\ ml \times 1000\ mg \times 2\ g}{250\ mg \times\ 1\ g\ \times 1} = \dfrac{1\ ml \times \cancel{1000}^{\,4} \times 2}{\cancel{250}_{\,1}\ \times\ 1 \times 1} = \dfrac{1\ ml \times 4 \times 2}{1\ \times 1 \times 1} = \dfrac{8\ ml}{1} = 8\ ml$

f. 8 ml − 6.6 ml = 1.4 ml

Label 3:

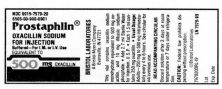

[handwritten: $9\frac{1}{1000\text{ml}}\frac{1}{2}$ $\frac{560\text{mg}}{1} = 5$]

a. How many grams of Prostaphlin are in the vial? *.5 g*

b. Which solution is to be used to reconstitute the medication? *Sterile water*

c. How much solution is to be added? *2.7 ml*

d. What is the dosage per unit given on the vial? *250 mg*

e. What is the total amount of the solution in the vial after reconstitution? *3 ml*

f. How much space does the dry powder occupy? *.3 ml*

[handwritten: $\frac{2}{3.00}$ $\frac{2.7}{}$ 3]

Answers:

a. 0.5 g (500 mg)

b. sterile water

c. 2.7 ml

d. 250 mg/1.5 ml

e. $ml = \dfrac{1.5\ ml\ \times 500}{250\ mg \times\ 1} = \dfrac{1.5\ ml\ \times \cancel{500}^{\,2}}{\cancel{250}_{\,1}\ \times\ 1} = \dfrac{1.5\ ml \times 2}{1\ \times 1} = \dfrac{3\ ml}{1} = 3\ ml$

f. 3 ml − 2.7 ml = 0.3 ml

Label 4:

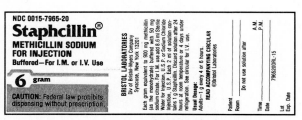

a. How many total grams of Staphcillin are in the vial?_____

b. Which solution is to be used to reconstitute the medication?_____

c. How much sterile solution is to be added?_____

d. What is the dosage per unit given on the vial?_____

e. What is the total amount of solution in the vial after reconstitution?_____

f. How much space does the dry powder occupy?_____

Answers:

a. 6 g

b. sterile water

c. 8.6 ml

d. 1 ml = 500 mg

e. $ml = \dfrac{1\ ml\ \times 1000\ mg \times 6\ g}{500\ mg \times\ 1\ g\ \times 1} = \dfrac{1\ ml \times \cancel{1000}^{\,2} \times 6}{\cancel{500}_{\,1}\ \times\ 1 \times 1} = \dfrac{12\ ml}{1} = 12\ ml$

f. 12 ml − 8.6 ml = 3.4 ml

   Some medications have directions for reconstitution into several strengths. Read the following drug label for reconstitution of intramuscular injection. Answer the following questions. Be careful to answer only the question asked.

Label 5:

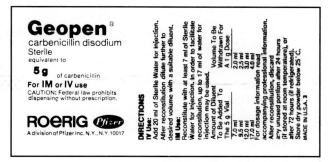

a. How many total grams of carbenicillin are in the vial?_____

b. Which solution is to be used to reconstitute the medication?_____

c. How much sterile solution is to be added to provide 1 g per 2.5 ml?_____

d. What is the dosage per unit if 17 ml solution are added?_____

e. What is the total amount of solution in the vial after reconstitution with 7 ml solution?_____

f. How much space does the dry powder occupy?_____

Answers:

a. 5 g

b. sterile water

c. 9.5 ml

d. 1 g = 4 ml

e. $\text{ml} = \dfrac{2\text{ ml} \times 5\text{ g}}{1\text{ g} \times 1} = \dfrac{2\text{ ml} \times 5}{1 \times 1} = \dfrac{10\text{ ml}}{1} = 10\text{ ml}$

f. 10 ml − 7 ml = 3 ml

Most medications have directions for reconstitution. An occasional medication, however, may not have directions. When reconstituting medications without instructions, the space occupied by the dry powder must always be taken into consideration. To reconstitute these medications, determine the total amount of solution desired. Mix the dry powder with about half of the desired amount of solvent. Then add solvent in the quantity sufficient to obtain the desired amount of solution.

ADMINISTRATION OF INSULIN

Insulin, used in the treatment of diabetes, is available in three major types: rapid, intermediate, and long acting insulins. The rapid acting insulin may be administered subcutaneously or intravenously; intermediate and long acting insulins, which are in suspension, are only administered subcutaneously. Most insulin is produced from beef, although pork (porcine) or human sources are also used. Insulin labels contain all this information and may be confusing, as shown in Figure 12-8. Always read insulin labels with special care.

Insulin is given in units. Two strengths of insulin are produced; U-100 is more commonly used. The other strength of insulin is gradually being phased out in this country and is not discussed here. U-100 insulin has 100 units per ml. Nearly all health care agencies use U-100 insulin exclusively, as recommended by The American Diabetic Association, to avoid confusion for clients and lessen the chances of errors in medication administration. Errors of three or four units can cause a well-controlled diabetic to become uncontrolled. For this reason, many agencies require that two nurses check insulin dosages prior to administration.

Insulin is administered using insulin syringes with the units marked. Figure 12-9 shows two U-100 syringes in 0.5 and 1 ml sizes. Note the scales for the units on each syringe. Figure 12-10 shows some syringes with varying dosages of insulin.

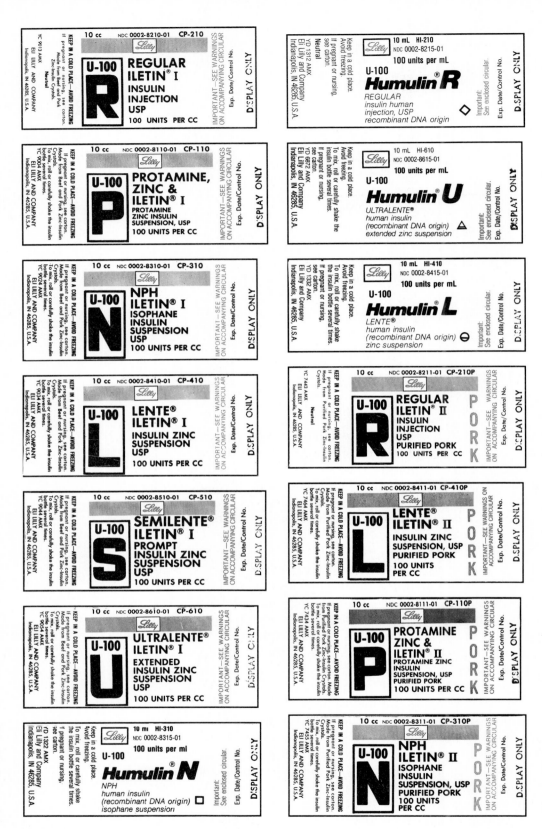

FIGURE 12-8 Insulin labels. Note that all the labels have the same dosage, 100 U per ml. The large R, P, N, L, S, and U help identify regular, protamine zinc, NPH, lente, semilente and ultralente respectively.

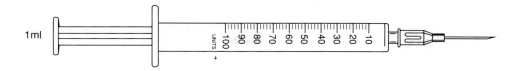

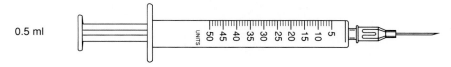

FIGURE 12-9 U-100 insulin syringes

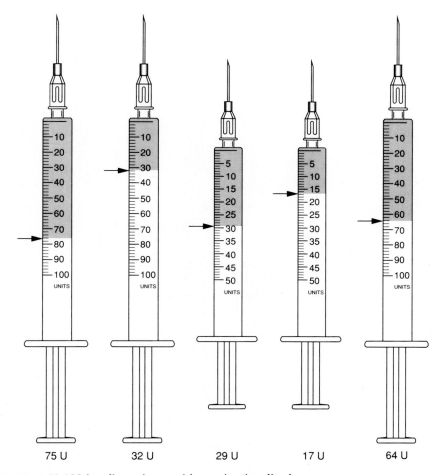

FIGURE 12-10 U-100 insulin syringes with varying insulin dosages

Calculation of volume is not necessary when using insulin syringes, since the units are calibrated on the syringes. The major concern in insulin administration is assuring correct measurement. Practice reading the amounts and types of insulin on the following syringes.

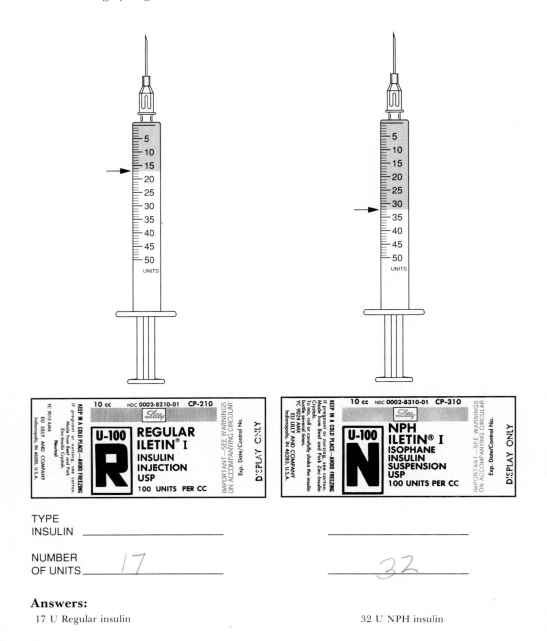

TYPE
INSULIN _____   _____

NUMBER
OF UNITS _____*17*_____   _____*32*_____

Answers:

17 U Regular insulin   32 U NPH insulin

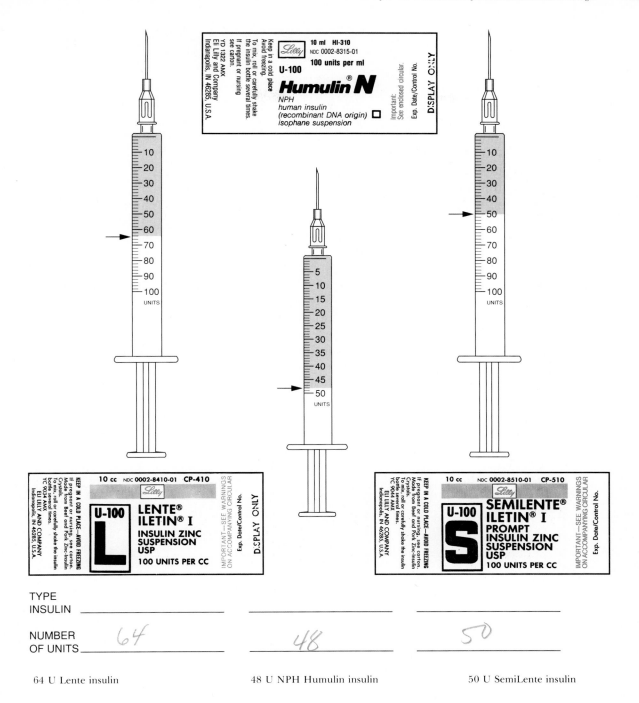

TYPE
INSULIN _____   _____   _____

NUMBER
OF UNITS _____64_____   _____48_____   _____50_____

64 U Lente insulin   48 U NPH Humulin insulin   50 U SemiLente insulin

Regular insulin, which is clear, is often mixed with an intermediate or long acting insulin, which is in suspension and cloudy, in one syringe for administration. Practice reading the amounts on each type of insulin on the syringes.

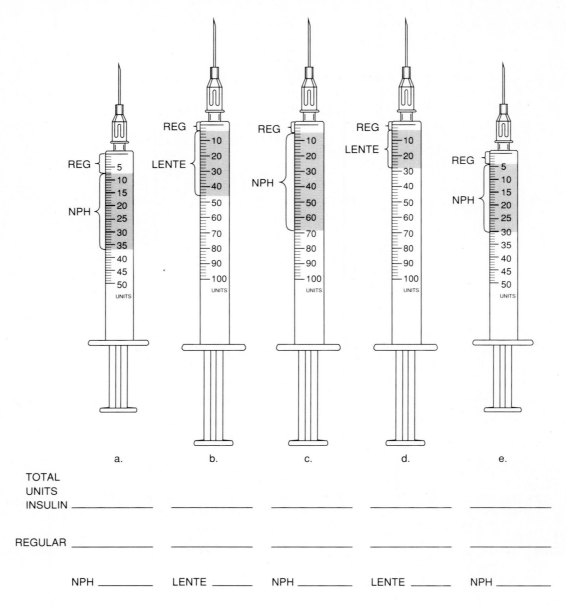

TOTAL
UNITS
INSULIN _____   _____   _____   _____   _____

REGULAR _____   _____   _____   _____   _____

NPH _____   LENTE _____   NPH _____   LENTE _____   NPH _____

Answers:

a. Total insulin 37 U; NPH insulin 29 or 30 U; Regular insulin 7 or 8 U.
b. Total insulin 45 U; Lente insulin 40 U; Regular insulin 5 U.
c. Total insulin 68 U; NPH insulin 62 U; Regular insulin 6 U.
d. Total insulin 28 U; Lente insulin 24 U; Regular insulin 4 U.
e. Total insulin 30 U; NPH insulin 25 U; Regular insulin 5 U.

    Insulin can be administered using a tuberculin syringe when insulin syringes are not available. Keep this in mind: if 100 U are equal to 1 ml, then 1 unit is 0.01 of a ml. Calculate the insulin dosages in the same manner as other parenteral dosages. The administration volume must be carried out to two decimal places (hundredths) when calculating insulin to be administered with a tuberculin syringe.

SAMPLE PROBLEM   **Medication order: NPH insulin 33 U s.c. a.c. breakfast q.d. NPH insulin available: 100 U/ml**

Knowns: Unit of answer: ml
Factors: 100 U = 1 ml
      33 U/1

$$ml = \frac{1\ ml}{100\ U} \times \frac{33}{1} = \frac{33}{100} = .33\ ml$$

The equation is as follows:

$$ml = \frac{1 \text{ ml} \times 33 \text{ U}}{100 \text{ U} \times 1} = \frac{1 \text{ ml} \times 33}{100 \times 1} = \frac{33}{100} = 0.33 \text{ ml}$$

Calculate the amont of insulin to administer in a tuberculin syringe using the following dosages of U-100 insulin (100 U per ml). Mark the volume on the tuberculin syringe beside the order. Regardless of the type of insulin ordered, the dosage on the label is 100 units per milliliter.

a. Dosage ordered: Regular insulin 28 U

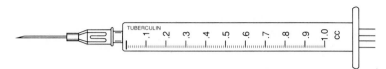

b. Dosage ordered: NPH insulin 40 U

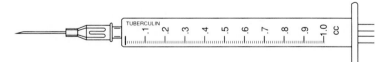

c. Dosage ordered: Lente insulin 75 U

d. Dosage ordered: Regular insulin 12 U

e. Dosage ordered: NPH insulin 38 U

Answers:

a. 28 U = 0.28 ml

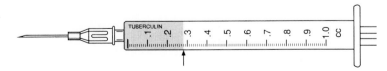

b. 40 U = 0.4 ml

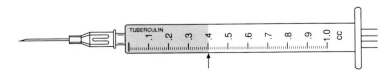

c. 75 U = 0.75 ml

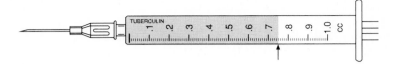

d. 12 U = 0.12 ml

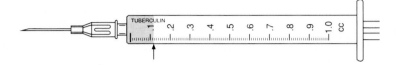

e. 38 U = 0.38 ml

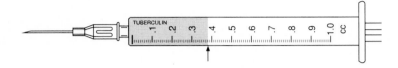

SELF-ASSESSMENT POSTTEST

CALCULATION OF PARENTERAL MEDICATION DOSAGES

Show all your work. Check your answers (page 359).

1. Dosage ordered: 35 mg IM. Dosage on hand: 12.5 mg per ml. How many ml will be administered?

2. Dosage ordered: 200 mg s.c. stat. Dosage on hand: 300 mg/ml. How many minims will be administered?

3. Dosage ordered: 250 mg IM noc. Dosage on hand: 6 g per 4 ml. How many ml will be given?

4. Dosage ordered: 900,000 U IM stat. Dosage on hand: 600,000 U per 2 ml. How many ml will be administered?

5. Dosage ordered: 36 U q AM s.c. Dosage on hand: 100 U per ml. How many ml will be administered?

6. Dosage ordered: 0.6 mg s.c. q.4h. Three strengths of the medication are available:
   Amp A: 6 mcg/ml in a 1 ml amp
   Amp B: 60 mcg/ml in a 1 ml amp
   Amp C: 600 mcg/ml in a 1 ml amp
   Which is the appropriate amp?

7. Dosage ordered: NPH porcine insulin 68 U s.c. a.c. breakfast. Dosage available: 100 U per ml. How many ml will be administered in a tuberculin syringe?

8. Dosage ordered: 7500 U s.c. q.6h. Dosage available: 10,000 U per ml. How many ml will be administered?

9. Dosage ordered: gr 1/200 IM preop. Dosage on hand: 400 mcg/ml. How many ml will be administered?

10. Dosage ordered: gr iss h.s. p.r.n. IM. Dosage available: 100 mg/ml. How many ml will be given?

$$ml = \frac{1\,ml}{100mg} \times \frac{\overset{10}{1000mg}}{15gr} \times \frac{1.5\,gr}{1} = \frac{15}{15} =$$
$$1\ ml$$

11. Dosage ordered: gr 1/4 IM stat. Dosage on hand: 130 mg/2 ml. How many ml will be administered?

$$ml = \frac{2ml}{130mg} \times \frac{60mg}{1gr} \times \frac{1}{4} = \frac{120}{520} = \frac{12}{52} =$$
$$\frac{6}{26} = \frac{3}{13} = .23\,ml$$

12. Dosage ordered: 0.5 g IM t.i.d. Dosage on hand: 500 mg/ml. How many ml will be administered?

13. Dosage ordered: 0.125 mg IM q.d. Dosage available: 250 mcg per ml. How many ml will be administered?

14. Dosage ordered: 600 mg s.c. t.i.d. Dosage available: 1 g per ml. How many ml will be administered?

15. Dosage ordered: 0.05 mg t.i.d. IM. Dosage available: 25 mcg per ml. How many ml will be given?

16. Dosage ordered: gr iii IM h.s. Dosage available: 1 g per 5 ml. How many ml will be administered?

$$ml = \frac{5ml}{1g} \times \frac{1g}{1000mg} \times \frac{1000mg}{15gr} \times \frac{3gr}{1} = \frac{\cancel{15}}{5}\frac{5}{5}$$
$$0.6\,ml = 1$$

17. Dosage ordered: 30 mg IM q.4h. p.r.n. Dosage on hand: 60 mg per ml. How many ml will be administered?

18. Dosage ordered: 10,000 U stat. Dosage on hand: 20,000 U per ml. How many ml will be administered?

19. Dosage ordered: 125 mg IM q.8h. Dosage on hand: 1 g per 2 ml. How many ml will be given?

20. Dosage ordered: 800 mg q.12h. Dosage available: 1 g per ml. How many ml will be given?

UNIT IV POSTTEST

DOSAGE CONVERSIONS AND CALCULATIONS TEST A

Show all your work. Check your answers (page 372).
Translate the following medication orders into lay terms:

1. Bicillin CR 1,200,000 U IM stat.

2. Oretic 50 mg PO b.i.d.

3. Lanoxin 0.5 mg PO stat., then 0.125 mg q.d.

Calculate the following:

4. Dosage ordered: NPH Humulin insulin 45 U. Dosage available: 100 U/ml. How many ml will be given in a tuberculin syringe?

5. Dosage ordered: gr 1/60 IM q.4h. p.r.n. Dosage available: 3 mg/ml. How many ml will be administered?

6. Dosage ordered: 0.2 mg s.c. t.i.d. Dosage on hand: 500 mcg/5 ml. How many ml will be administered?

7. Dosage ordered: 200 mg PO t.i.d. Dosage on hand: 0.5 g/5 ml. How many ml will be given?

8. Dosage ordered: gr X PO t.i.d. Dosage on hand: 300 mg per 5 ml. How many tsp will be administered?

9. Dosage ordered: 0.5 g t.i.d. IM. Dosage on hand: 250 mg per ml. How many ml will be administered?

10. Dosage ordered: gr ss IM t.i.d. Dosage available: 0.1 g/ml. How many ml will be administered?

11. Dosage ordered: gr 1/200 PO stat. Dosage on hand: 600 mcg scored tab. How many tabs will be administered?

12. A 20 ml vial contains 500 mg of medication. Directions state to add 2.8 ml normal saline to obtain a solution of 250 mg/2.5 ml. How many total ml of medication solution are in the vial after dilution?
How much space did the dry powder occupy?

13. Dosage ordered: 250 mg IM q.i.d. Dosage on hand: 2.5 g per 5 ml. How many ml will be administered?

14. Dosage ordered: 100 mcg s.c. b.i.d. Dosage available: 20 ml vial with 10 mg dry powder with directions to add 18.2 ml of sterile water to obtain concentration of 1 mg/2 ml. How many ml of reconstituted solution will be given?

15. Dosage ordered: gr XV PO t.i.d. Dosage available: 0.325 g tab. How many tabs will be administered?

16. Dosage ordered: 0.2 mg t.i.d PO. Dosage available: 50 mcg scored tab. How many tabs will be administered?

17. Dosage ordered: atropine 200 mcg s.c. stat. Dosage available: atropine 0.4 mg/ml. How many minims will be administered?

18. Dosage ordered: 0.6 mg PO b.i.d. Dosage available: 200 mcg scored tab. How many tablets will be given?

19. Dosage ordered: gr 1/30 PO t.i.d. Dosage available: 5 mg per 5 ml. How many ml will be administered?

20. Dosage ordered: 250 mg PO q.6h. Dosage available: 500 mg per 5 ml. How many tsp would be administered?

21. Dosage ordered: gr 1/60 PO t.i.d. The medication is available in three strengths:
Tab A: 1 mg scored tab
Tab B: 5 mg scored tab
Tab C: 20 mg scored tab.
Select the appropriate tablet.

22. Dosage ordered: 0.5 g PO q.i.d. Dosage available: 250 mg scored tablet. How many tablets will be administered?

23. Dosage ordered: 20 mcg IM stat. The medication is available in three strengths:
Amp A: 0.01 mg/ml in a 1 ml amp
Amp B: 0.2 mg/ml in a 1 ml amp
Amp C: 0.02 mg/ml in a 1 ml amp
Select the appropriate ampule.

24. Dosage ordered: 1.5 g PO ASAP. Dosage on hand: 500 mg scored tablet. How many tablets will be administered?

25. Dosage ordered: 75 mg s.c. stat. Dosage on hand: 100 mg/ml. How many ml will be given?

UNIT IV POSTTEST

DOSAGE CONVERSIONS AND CALCULATIONS TEST B

(Answers on page 374).

Translate the following medication orders into lay terms:

1. epinephrine 0.3 mg s.c. stat.

2. Seconal gr iss PO h.s. PRN

3. Lanoxin 0.125 mg PO q.o.d.

Calculate the following:

4. Dosage ordered: NPH Humulin insulin 35 U. Dosage available: 100 U/ml. How many ml will be given in a tuberculin syringe?

$$ml = \frac{1\,ml}{100\,u} \times \frac{35\,u}{1} = \frac{35}{100} \cdot .35\,ml$$

5. Dosage ordered: gr 1/100 IM q.4h. p.r.n. Dosage available: 3 mg/ml. How many ml will be administered?

6. Dosage ordered: 0.3 mg IM t.i.d. Dosage on hand: 200 mcg/1 ml. How many ml will be administered?

7. Dosage ordered: 150 mg PO t.i.d. Dosage on hand: 0.5 g/5 ml. How many ml will be given?

8. Dosage ordered: gr XV PO t.i.d. Dosage on hand: 500 mg per 5 ml. How many tsp will be administered?

$$tsp = \frac{1\,tsp}{5\,ml} \times \frac{5\,ml}{500\,mg} \times \frac{1000\,mg}{15\,gr}^{2} \times \frac{15\,gr}{1} = \frac{10}{5}\ or\ 2$$

9. Dosage ordered: 0.25 g t.i.d. IM. Dosage on hand: 500 mg per ml. How many ml will be administered?

10. Dosage ordered: gr iss IM t.i.d. Dosage available: 0.1 g/ml. How many ml will be administered?

11. Dosage ordered: gr 1/300 PO stat. Dosage on hand: 100 mcg scored tab. How many tabs will be administered?

12. A 20 ml vial contains 2 g of medication. Directions state to add 4.8 ml normal saline to obtain a solution of 250 mg/1 ml. How many ml of medication solution are in the vial after dilution?

How much space did the dry powder occupy?

13. Dosage ordered: 300 mg IM q.i.d. Dosage on hand: 2 g per 5 ml. How many ml will be administered?

14. Dosage ordered: 300 mcg s.c. b.i.d. Dosage available: 20 ml vial with 10 mg dry powder with directions to add 18.2 ml of sterile water to obtain concentration of 1 mg/2 ml. How many ml of reconstituted solution will be given?

15. Dosage ordered: gr XX PO t.i.d. Dosage available: 0.325 g tab. How many tabs will be administered?

16. Dosage ordered: 0.1 mg t.i.d. PO. Dosage available: 25 mcg scored tab. How many tabs will be administered?

17. Dosage ordered: atropine 400 mcg s.c. stat. Dosage available: atropin 0.4 mg/ml. How many minims will be administered?

18. Dosage ordered: 0.5 mg PO b.i.d. Dosage available: 200 mcg scored tab. How many tablets will be given?

19. Dosage ordered: gr 1/3 PO t.i.d. Dosage available: 5 ml. How many ml will be administered?

20. Dosage ordered: 750 mg PO q.6h. Dosage available: 500 mg per 5 ml. How many tsp would be administered?

21. Dosage ordered: gr 1/2 PO t.i.d. The medication is available in three strengths:
Tab A: 20 mg scored tab
Tab B: 30 mg scored tab
Tab C: 60 mg scored tab.
Select the appropriate tablet.

22. Dosage ordered: 0.25 g PO q.i.d. Dosage available: 500 mg scored tablet. How many tablets will be administered?

23. Dosage ordered: 400 mcg IM stat. The medication is available in three strengths:
Amp A: 0.01 mg/ml in a 1 ml amp
Amp B: 0.4 mg/ml in a 1 ml amp
Amp C: 0.04 mg/ml in a 1 ml amp
Select the appropriate ampule.

24. Dosage ordered: 0.5 g PO ASAP. Dosage on hand: 250 mg scored tablet. How many tablets will be administered?

25. Dosage ordered: 60 mg s.c. stat. Dosage on hand: 100 mg/ ml. How many ml will be given?

DOSAGE CONVERSIONS AND CALCULATIONS TEST C

(Answers on page 376). Translate the following medication orders into lay terms:

1. Keflin 1 g IV PB stat., then 500 mg IV PB q.6h.

2. Dilantin 100 mg PO t.i.d.

3. Benadryl elix 12.5 mg PO q.4h. PRN

Calculate the following:

4. Dosage ordered: NPH Humulin insulin 28 U. Dosage available: 100 U/ml. How many ml will be given in a tuberculin syringe?

5. Dosage ordered: gr 1/30 IM q.4.h p.r.n. Dosage available: 3 mg/2 ml. How many ml will be administered?

6. Dosage ordered: 0.4 mg s.c. t.i.d. Dosage on hand: 500 mcg/ml. How many ml will be administered?

7. Dosage ordered: 300 mg PO t.i.d. Dosage on hand: 0.5 g/5 ml. How many ml will be given?

8. Dosage ordered: gr viiss PO t.i.d. Dosage on hand: 500 mg per 5 ml. How many tsp will be administered?

9. Dosage ordered: 0.25 g t.i.d IM. Dosage on hand: 500 mg per ml. How many ml will be administered?

10. Dosage ordered: gr iss IM t.i.d. Dosage available: 0.5 g/5 ml. How many ml will be administered?

11. Dosage ordered: gr 1/150 PO stat. Dosage on hand: 200 mcg scored tab. How many tabs will be administered?

12. A 20 ml vial contains 1 g of medication. Directions state to add 7.3 ml normal saline to obtain a solution of 250 mg/2.5 ml. How many total ml of medication solution are in the vial after dilution?

How much space did the dry powder occupy?

13. Dosage ordered: 400 mg IM q.i.d. Dosage on hand: 2 g per 5 ml. How many ml will be administered?

14. Dosage ordered: 200 mcg s.c. b.i.d. Dosage available: 20 ml vial with 10 mg dry powder with directions to add 18.2 ml of sterile water to obtain concentration of 1 mg/2 ml. How many ml of reconstituted solution will be given?

15. Dosage ordered: gr XV PO t.i.d. Dosage available: 0.5 g tab. How many tabs will be administered?

16. Dosage ordered: 0.15 mg t.i.d PO. Dosage available: 50 mcg scored tab. How many tabs will be administered?

17. Dosage ordered: atropine 300 mcg s.c. stat. Dosage available: atropine 0.4 mg/ml. How many minims will be administered?

18. Dosage ordered: 0.5 mg PO b.i.d. Dosage available: 200 mcg scored tab. How many tablets will be given?

19. Dosage ordered: gr 1/4 PO t.i.d. Dosage available: 5 mg per 5 ml. How many ml will be administered?

20. Dosage ordered: 250 mg PO q.6.h. Dosage available: 100 mg per 5 ml. How many tsp would be administered?

21. Dosage ordered: gr 1/3 PO t.i.d. The medication is available in three strengths:
Tab A: 20 mg scored tab
Tab B: 30 mg scored tab
Tab C: 60 mg scored tab.
Select the appropriate tablet.

22. Dosage ordered: 0.125 g PO q.i.d. Dosage available: 250 mg scored tablet. How many tablets will be administered?

23. Dosage ordered: 30 mcg IM stat. The medication is available in 3 strengths:
Amp A: 0.01 mg/ml in a 1 ml amp
Amp B: 0.3 mg/ml in a 1 ml amp
Amp C: 0.03 mg/ml in a 1 ml amp
Select the appropriate ampule.

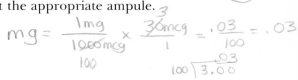

24. Dosage ordered: 0.25 g PO ASAP. Dosage on hand: 500 mg scored tablet. How many tablets will be administered?

25. Dosage ordered: 40 mg s.c. stat. Dosage on hand: 100 mg/ml. How many ml will be given?

CALCULATIONS BASED ON BODY WEIGHT

OBJECTIVES: *Upon completion of this unit, the student will have demonstrated the ability to correctly:*

- Calculate dosages based on body weight.

- Compute administration amounts according to body weight.

- Calculate recommended daily dosages.

- Compare ordered daily dosage with recommended daily dosage.

Some medications are ordered according to the weight of the client. Pediatric dosages are often calculated for the individual's body weight. Dosages based on body weight are used frequently by oncology and critical care nurses. Calories or fluid volumes ordered according to body weight are covered in Unit X.

Drug reference books report the recommended dosages for some drugs based on client weight. Nurses are expected to know the usual or recommended dosage for each drug administered. Comparison of the client's dosage with the recommended dosage often requires calculations based on weight.

Chapter 13

Dosages Based on Client Weight

Dosages based on body weight may be ordered as dosage per kilogram or pound. The equation for calculation of dosages based on weight is as follows:

$$\text{dosage} = \frac{\substack{\text{conversion} \\ \text{factor if} \\ \text{necessary}} \times \text{dosage} \times \substack{\text{conversion} \\ \text{factor if} \\ \text{necessary}} \times \substack{\text{client's} \\ \text{weight} \\ \times 1}}{\times \text{weight unit}}$$

Dosages per pounds of body weight are very easy as most facilities weigh clients in pounds.

SAMPLE PROBLEM   **Dosage ordered: 3 mg per lb. Client weight: 81 lb. What is the client's dosage?**

Knowns: Unit of answer: mg
Factors: 3 mg = 1 lb
       81 lb/1

Set up the equation framework.

$$mg = \underline{\qquad}$$

The first factor numerator unit is the same as the answer unit.

$$mg = \frac{3 \text{ mg} \times}{1 \text{ lb} \times}$$

The second factor numerator unit is the same as the first factor denominator unit.

$$mg = \frac{3 \text{ mg} \times 81 \text{ lb}}{1 \text{ lb} \times 1}$$

Cancel the units.

$$mg = \frac{3 \text{ mg} \times 81}{1 \times 1}$$

Multiply the numerator:
Multiply the denominator:

$$\frac{3 \text{ mg} \times 81}{1 \times 1} = \frac{243 \text{ mg}}{1} = 243 \text{ mg}$$

Health care facilities weigh pediatric clients in either pounds or kilograms, while most adults are weighed in pounds. Most dosages based on body weight are calculated per kilogram; therefore, a conversion factor must be used. The dosage may be desired in units other than the unit ordered. If so, a conversion factor from one dosage unit to another is necessary.

SAMPLE PROBLEM   **Dosage ordered: 0.5 mg/kg. Patient weight: 154 lb. What is the dosage for the client?**

Knowns: Unit of answer: mg.
Factors: 0.5 mg = 1 kg
       154 lb/1
Conversion factor: 1 kg = 2.2 lb

Set up the equation framework.

$$mg = \underline{\qquad}$$

The first factor numerator unit is the same as the answer unit.

$$mg = \frac{0.5 \text{ mg} \times}{1 \text{ kg} \times}$$

The second factor numerator unit is the same as the first factor denominator unit.

$$mg = \frac{0.5 \text{ mg} \times 1 \text{ kg} \times}{1 \text{ kg} \times 2.2 \text{ lb} \times}$$

The third factor numerator unit is the same as the second factor denominator unit.

$$mg = \frac{0.5\,mg \times 1\,kg \times 154\,lb}{1\,kg \times 2.2\,lb \times 1}$$

Cancel the units.

$$mg = \frac{0.5\,mg \times 1 \times 154}{1 \times 2.2 \times 1}$$

Cancel the evenly divisible quantities.

$$mg = \frac{0.5\,mg \times 1 \times \overset{70}{\cancel{154}}}{1 \times \cancel{2.2} \times 1}$$
$$1$$

Multiply the numerator:
Multiply the denominator:

$$\frac{0.5\,mg \times 1 \times 70}{1 \times 1 \times 1} = \frac{35.0\,mg}{1} = 35\,mg$$

SAMPLE PROBLEM   **Dosage ordered: 50 mcg/kg. Client weight: 170 lb. What is the client's dosage in mg?**

Knowns: Unit of answer: mg.
Factors: 50 mcg = 1 kg
          170 lb/1
Conversion factors: 1 kg = 2.2 lb
                  1 mg = 1000 mcg

Set up the equation framework.

$$mg = \underline{\hspace{3cm}}$$

The first factor numerator unit is the same as the answer unit.

$$mg = \frac{1\,mg \times}{1000\,mcg \times}$$

The second factor numerator unit is the same as the first factor denominator unit.

$$mg = \frac{1\,mg \times 50\,mcg \times}{1000\,mcg \times 1\,kg \times}$$

The third factor numerator unit is the same as the second factor denominator unit.

$$mg = \frac{1\,mg \times 50\,mcg \times 1\,kg \times}{1000\,mcg \times 1\,kg \times 2.2\,lb \times}$$

The fourth factor numerator unit is the same as the third factor denominator unit.

$$mg = \frac{1\,mg \times 50\,mcg \times 1\,kg \times 170\,lb}{1000\,mcg \times 1\,kg \times 2.2\,lb \times 1}$$

Cancel the units.

$$mg = \frac{1\,mg \times 50 \times 1 \times 170}{1000 \times 1 \times 2.2 \times 1}$$

Cancel the evenly divisible quantities.

$$mg = \frac{1\,mg \times \overset{5}{\cancel{50}} \times 1 \times \overset{17}{\cancel{170}}}{\underset{\underset{10}{\cancel{100}}}{\cancel{1000}} \times 1 \times 2.2 \times 1}$$

Multiply the numerator:
Multiply the denominator:

$$\frac{1\,mg \times 5 \times 1 \times 17}{10 \times 1 \times 2.2 \times 1} = \frac{85\,mg}{22} = 3.86\,mg$$

*Note that cancellation could have been continued by dividing the 5 and 10 by 5. This was not done because it is easy to multiply by 10 and, in doing so, the decimal point is removed. It is easier to divide by 22 than by 4.4.

PRACTICE PROBLEMS

Dosages Based on Body Weight

Show all your work. Check your answers (page 331).

1. Dosage ordered: 5 mcg per pound. Client weight: 100 lb. How many mg is the client to receive?

2. Dosage ordered: 20 mcg per kg. Client weight: 50 kg. What is the dosage for this client in mg?

3. Dosage ordered: 4 mcg/kg. Patient weight: 176 lb. How many mcg should the patient receive?

4. Dosage ordered: 0.5 mg per kg. Patient weight: 12 kg. What is the dosage in mg?

5. Dosage ordered: 25 mg/lb. Client weight: 85 kg. What is the dosage for this client?

6. Dosage ordered: 30 mcg/kg. Client weight: 88 lb. What is the dosage for this client in mg?

7. Dosage ordered: 0.3 mg/kg. Client weight: 231 lb. How many grams will this client receive?

8. Dosage ordered: 10 mcg per kg. Client weight: 24 kg. What is the dosage for this client?

9. Dosage ordered: 0.15 mcg per kg. Client weight: 198 lb. How many mcg will the client receive?

10. Dosage ordered: 0.03 mg per kg. Client weight: 121 lb. How many mcg should the client receive?

CALCULATION OF DOSAGE BASED ON BODY WEIGHT

Administration of medications ordered as dosages per body weight involves the calculation of dosages as in Chapters 11 and 12. The equation for calculating dosages based on body weight is as follows:

$$\text{Amount and unit to administer} = \frac{\text{conversion factor if necessary} \times \text{amount available} \times \text{conversion factor if necessary} \times \text{dosage available} \times \text{conversion factor if necessary} \times \text{dosage} \times \text{weight unit} \times \text{conversion factor if necessary} \times \text{client's weight}}{1}$$

SAMPLE PROBLEM   **Dosage ordered: 30 mg/kg. Dosage available: 500 mg scored tablets. Client weight: 165 lb. How many tablets will be administered?**

Knowns: Unit of answer: tab
Conversion factor: 1 kg = 2.2 lb
Factors: 30 mg = 1 kg
       500 mg = 1 tab
       165 lb/1

Set up the equation framework.

$$\text{tab} = \underline{\qquad\qquad}$$

The first factor numerator unit is the same as the answer unit.

$$\text{tab} = \frac{1\ \text{tab} \times}{500\ \text{mg} \times}$$

The second factor numerator unit is the same as the first factor denominator unit.

$$\text{tab} = \frac{1\ \text{tab} \times 30\ \text{mg} \times}{500\ \text{mg} \times \ 1\ \text{kg} \ \times}$$

The third factor numerator unit is the same as the second factor denominator unit.

$$\text{tab} = \frac{1\ \text{tab} \times 30\ \text{mg} \times \ 1\ \text{kg} \ \times}{500\ \text{mg} \times 1\ \text{kg} \ \times 2.2\ \text{lb} \ \times}$$

The fourth factor numerator unit is the same as the third factor denominator unit.

$$\text{tab} = \frac{1\ \text{tab} \ \times \ 30\ \text{mg} \times 1\ \text{kg} \ \times \ 165\ \text{lb}}{500\ \text{mg} \ \times 1\ \text{kg} \ \ \times \ 2.2\ \text{lb} \times \ \ \ 1}$$

Cancel the units and evenly divisible quantities.

$$\text{tab} = \frac{1\ \text{tab} \times \overset{3}{\cancel{30}} \times \ 1 \ \times \overset{\overset{3}{\cancel{75}}}{\cancel{165}}}{\underset{2}{\underset{\cancel{50}}{\cancel{500}}}\ \text{mg} \ \times \ 1 \ \times \underset{1}{2.2} \times \ \ \ 1}$$

Multiply the numerators:
Multiply the denominators:

$$\frac{1\ \text{tab} \times 3 \times 1 \times 3}{2 \ \ \ \times 1 \times 1 \times 1} = \frac{9\ \text{tab}}{2} = 4\tfrac{1}{2}\ \text{tab}$$

SAMPLE PROBLEM   **Dosage ordered: 2 mg/kg. Patient weight: 132 lb. Dosage on hand: 0.15 g per ml. How many ml will you administer?**

Knowns: Unit of answer: ml
Factors: 2 mg = 1 kg
       0.15 g = 1 ml
       132 lb/1
Conversion factor: 1 kg = 2.2 lb
                     1 g = 1000 mg

Set up the equation framework.

$$\text{ml} = \underline{\qquad\qquad}$$

The first factor numerator unit is the same as the unit of the answer.

$$\text{ml} = \frac{1\ \text{ml} \ \times}{0.15\ \text{g} \ \ \times}$$

The second factor numerator unit is the same as the first factor denominator unit.

$$\text{ml} = \frac{1\ \text{ml} \times \ \ \ 1\ \text{g} \ \ \times}{0.15\ \text{g} \ \times 1000\ \text{mg} \times}$$

The third factor numerator unit is the same as the second factor denominator unit.

$$\text{ml} = \frac{1\ \text{ml} \times \ \ \ 1\ \text{g} \ \ \times 2\ \text{mg} \times}{0.15\ \text{g} \ \times 1000\ \text{mg} \times 1\ \text{kg} \ \times}$$

The fourth factor numerator unit is the same as the third factor denominator unit.

$$\text{ml} = \frac{1\ \text{ml} \times \ \ \ 1\ \text{g} \ \ \times 2\ \text{mg} \times \ \ \ 1\ \text{kg} \times}{0.15\ \text{g} \ \times 1000\ \text{mg} \times 1\ \text{kg} \ \times 2.2\ \text{lb} \ \times}$$

The fifth factor numerator unit is the same as the fourth factor denominator unit.

$$\text{ml} = \frac{1\ \text{ml} \times \ \ \ 1\ \text{g} \ \ \times 2\ \text{mg} \times 1\ \text{kg} \ \times 132\ \text{lb}}{0.15\ \text{g} \ \times 1000\ \text{mg} \times 1\ \text{kg} \ \times 2.2\ \text{lb} \times \ \ \ 1}$$

Cancel the units and evenly divisible quantities.

$$ml = \frac{1\ ml\ \times \quad 1 \times \cancel{2}^{1} \times \quad 1 \times \cancel{132}^{4}}{\cancel{0.15}_{0.01} \quad \times \cancel{1000}_{500} \times 1 \times \cancel{2.2}_{1} \times \quad 1}$$

Multiply the numerator:
Multiply the denominator:

$$\frac{1\ ml\ \times \quad 1 \times 1 \times 1 \times 4}{0.01 \quad \times 500 \times 1 \times 1 \times 1} = \frac{4\ ml}{5}$$

$$= 0.8\ ml$$

Sometimes the dosage ordered is a total dosage per day that is divided into several doses during that day. Reference books often report recommended dosages for medications in this manner. Then it is necessary to divide the total dosage per day by the number of doses given per day. This can be accomplished in several ways. Calculation of the quantity to administer per dose can be done in one long equation. The equation is as follows:

$$\text{Unit and amount to give per dose} = \frac{\text{conversion factor if necessary}}{} \times \frac{\text{amount available}}{\text{dosage available}} \times \frac{\text{conversion factor if necessary}}{} \times \left(\frac{\text{dosage} \times \text{conversion factor if necessary} \times \text{client weight}}{\text{weight unit} \times \quad \times 1}\right) \times \frac{\text{day}}{\text{number doses}}$$

This equation can be simplified by dropping the fraction denominators in the numerator into the equation denominator. The portion of the equation enclosed in parentheses is usually solved first. Because the factors in the equation are multiplied, each factor in parentheses can be treated like a separate fraction. The simplified equation is as follows:

$$\text{Unit and amount to give per dose} = \frac{\text{conversion factor if necessary} \times \text{amount available} \times \text{conversion factor if necessary} \times \text{dosage} \times \text{conversion factor if necessary} \times \text{client's weight} \times \text{day}}{\text{necessary} \times \text{dosage available} \times \text{necessary} \times \text{weight unit} \times \text{necessary} \times 1 (X\ day) \times \text{number doses}}$$

It may be easier to solve the problem in two steps as follows:
1. Solve for dosage in one day.
2. Solve for amount per dose, using the answer from the first step for the dosage ordered.

SAMPLE PROBLEM   **Dosage ordered: 10 mcg/kg/day in four divided doses. Client weight: 176 lb. Dosage available: 0.2 mg tab. How many tabs will be given with each dose?**

Knowns: Unit of final answer: tab/dose
           Unit of dosage/day answer: mg
Factors: 10 mcg/1 kg/day
          0.2 mg = 1 tab
          4 doses = 1 day
          176 lb/1
Conversion factor: 1 kg = 2.2 lb
1 mg = 1000 mcg

(1) Solve for dosage per day.
Set up the equation framework.

$$mg = \underline{\qquad\qquad}$$

The first factor numerator unit is the same as the answer unit.

$$mg = \frac{1\ mg\ \times}{1000\ mcg\ \times}$$

The second factor numerator unit is the same as the first factor denominator unit.

$$mg = \frac{1\ mg\ \times 10\ mcg\ \times}{1000\ mcg\ \times\ 1\ kg\ \times}$$

The third factor numerator unit is the same as the second factor denominator unit.

$$mg = \frac{1\ mg \times 10\ mcg \times 1\ kg \times}{1000\ mcg \times 1\ kg \times 2.2\ lb \times}$$

The fourth factor numerator unit is the same as the third factor denominator unit.

$$mg = \frac{1\ mg \times 10\ mcg \times 1\ kg \times 176\ lb}{1000\ mcg \times 1\ kg \times 2.2\ lb \times 1}$$

Cancel the units and evenly divisible quantities.

$$mg = \frac{1\ mg \times \cancel{10} \times 1 \times \overset{\overset{8}{\cancel{80}}}{\cancel{176}}}{\underset{\underset{10}{\cancel{100}}}{\cancel{1000}} \times 1 \times \overset{1}{\cancel{2.2}} \times 1}$$

Multiply the numerator:
Multiply the denominator:

$$\frac{1\ mg \times 1 \times 1 \times 8}{10 \times 1 \times 1 \times 1} = \frac{8\ mg}{10}$$

$$= 0.8\ mg\ daily\ dosage$$

(2) Solve for administration amount per dose using dosage per day from answer in part 1.

Set up the equation framework.

$$\frac{tab}{dose} = \underline{\hspace{2cm}}$$

The first factor numerator unit is the same as the numerator unit of the answer.

$$\frac{tab}{dose} = \frac{1\ tab \times}{0.2\ mg \times}$$

The second factor numerator unit is the same as the first factor denominator unit.

$$\frac{tab}{dose} = \frac{1\ tab \times 0.8\ mg \times}{0.2\ mg \times 1\ d \times}$$

The third factor numerator unit is the same as the second factor denominator unit.

$$\frac{tab}{dose} = \frac{1\ tab \times 0.8\ mg \times 1\ d}{0.2\ mg \times 1\ d \times 4\ doses}$$

Cancel the units and evenly divisible quantities.

$$\frac{tab}{dose} = \frac{1\ tab \times \overset{1}{\cancel{0.8}} \times 1}{\underset{1}{\cancel{0.2}} \times 1 \times \underset{1}{\cancel{4}}\ doses}$$

Multiply the numerator:
Multiply the denominator:

$$\frac{1\ tab \times 1 \times 1}{1 \times 1 \times 1\ dose} = \frac{1\ tab}{1\ dose}$$

$$= 1\ tab/dose$$

The equation set up in one long equation, using the simplified equation, is as follows:

$$\frac{tab}{dose} = \frac{1\ tab \times (\ 1\ mg \times 10\ mcg \times 1\ kg \times 176\ lb\ ) \times 1\ d}{0.2\ mg \times (\ 1000\ mcg \times 1\ kg \times 2.2\ lb \times 1\ ) \times 1\ d \times 4\ doses}$$

Note that the portion enclosed in parentheses is the same equation as the daily dosage equation with the addition of 1 d in the denominator. The problem is then solved as follows:

$$\frac{tab}{dose} = \frac{1\ tab \times 1 \times \cancel{10} \times 1 \times \overset{\overset{1}{\overset{\cancel{4}}{\cancel{80}}}}{\cancel{176}} \times 1}{0.2 \times \underset{\underset{5}{\underset{\cancel{100}}{}}}{\cancel{1000}} \times 1 \times \overset{1}{\cancel{2.2}} \times 1 \times 1 \times \underset{1}{\cancel{4}}\ doses}$$

$$\frac{1\ tab \times 1 \times 1 \times 1 \times 1 \times 1}{0.2 \times 5 \times 1 \times 1 \times 1 \times 1 \times 1\ dose} = \frac{1\ tab}{1\ dose} = 1\ tab/dose$$

Medication such as immune globulin may be ordered as a volume per body weight. These problems are solved in the same manner as dosage per body weight.

SAMPLE PROBLEM   **Dosage ordered: 0.02 ml per kg. Client weight: 127 1/2 lb. How many ml will be administered?**

Knowns: Unit of answer: ml
Factors: 0.02 mg = 1 kg
       127 1/2 lb/1
Conversion factor: 1 kg = 2.2 lb
Set up the equation framework.

$$ml = \frac{}{}$$

The first factor numerator unit is the same as the answer unit.

$$ml = \frac{0.02\ ml \times}{1\ kg \times}$$

The second factor numerator unit is the same as the first factor denominator unit.

$$ml = \frac{0.02\ ml \times\quad 1\ kg \times}{1\ kg \times 2.2\ lb \times}$$

The third factor numerator unit is the same as the second factor denominator unit.

$$ml = \frac{0.02\ ml \times\quad 1\ kg \times\ 127.5\ lb}{1\ kg \times\ 2.2\ lb \times\quad 1}$$

Cancel the units and evenly divisible quantities.

$$ml = \frac{\overset{0.01}{\cancel{0.02}} \times\quad 1 \times\ 127.5}{1 \times \underset{1.1}{\cancel{2.2}} \times\quad 1}$$

Multiply the numerator:
Multiply the denominator:

$$\frac{0.01\ ml \times\quad 1 \times\ 127.5}{1\quad \times\ 1.1 \times\quad 1} = \frac{1.275\ ml}{1.1}$$

$$= 1.159\ ml = 1.2\ ml$$

PRACTICE PROBLEMS

Calculation of Dosages Based on Body Weight

Show all your work. Check your answers (page 332).

11. Dosage ordered: 1 mg per kg. Patient weight: 110 lb. Dosage on hand: 50 mg tablets. How many tablets will be administered?

12. Dosage ordered: 6 mcg/kg. Patient weight: 121 lb. Dosage on hand: 0.5 mg/ml. How many minims will be administered?

13. Dosage ordered: 0.01 ml/kg. Patient weight: 180 lb. How many ml will be administered?

14. Dosage ordered: 10 mcg/kg/24 hours in three divided doses. Patient weight: 66 lb. Dosage on hand: 0.1 mg tablets. What is the daily dosage in mg?

How many tablets will be given at each dose?

15. Dosage ordered: 20 mg/kg. Patient weight: 19 lb 4 oz. (Suggestion: 19 lb 4 oz = 19 4/16 lb or 19 1/4 lb or 19.25 lb). Dosage on hand: 250 mg/ml. How many minims will you administer?

16. Mr. Jones, who weighs 198 lb, is to receive 3 mcg/kg in three divided doses per day. How many mcg will he receive in each dose?

17. Bobby Jordan weighs 8 lb 15 oz. He is to receive an injection of 10 units per kg. Dosage on hand: 50 U/ml. How many minims will you administer?

18. Mrs. Halen has medication orders for 25 mg/kg/day in four divided doses. She weighs 141 lb. The medication is available in 200 mg scored tablets. How many tablets will be administered at each dose?

19. Dosage ordered: 50 mcg/kg. Client weight: 220 lb. Dosage available: 2.5 mg tablets. How many tablets will the client receive?

20. Mrs. Price is to receive 15 mg per pound per day. She weighs 134 lb. The medication is available in 1 g per 5 ml. How many tsp will she receive?

Calculate the administration amount for the dosages ordered using the following labels.

21. Dosage ordered: chlorambucil 0.03 mg per kg q.d. PO. Client weight: 149 1/2 lb. How many tablets will the client receive?

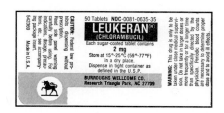

22. Dosage ordered: Imuran 2.5 mg/kg PO q.d. Client weight: 154 lb. How many tabs will the client receive?

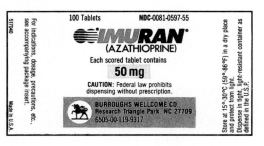

23. Dosage ordered: Furadantin oral suspension 5 mg/kg/d PO in four divided doses. Client weight: 57 1/2 lb. What is the daily dosage of the Furadantin?

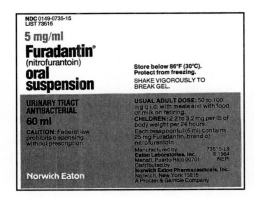

How many ml will be given at each dose?

24. Mr. Perout has an order for Hydrea 25 mg/kg PO q.d. Client weight: 132 lb. How many capsules will Mr. Perout receive each day?

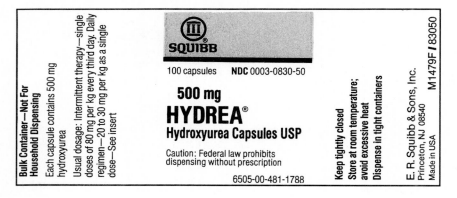

25. Mrs. Lawrence is to receive asparaginase 200 IU/kg IM q.d. Client weight: 110 lb. How many IU will be administered to Mrs. Lawrence each day?

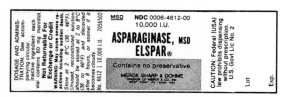

RECOMMENDED DOSAGES

Physicians rarely write orders in which the dosages are based on body weight. Instead, the physician determines the dosage based on the recommended dosage of the manufacturer. For instance, the pharmaceutical manufacturer recommends that Alkeran 0.2 milligrams per kilogram per day be administered for five days. For the client who weighs 50 kilograms, the daily dosage would be 10 milligrams. The physician writes the order "Alkeran 10 mg q.d. PO × 5 days."

The nurse administering the medication is expected to know the recommended dosage for each drug administered. If the recommended dosage differs from the dosage ordered, the nurse is responsible for notifying the physician. The nurse charts that notification and the physician's response on the nursing or progress notes. It is obvious that the nurse should check the nursing and progress notes prior to notifying the physician. The notification may already have been made and recorded by another nurse, or there may be a notation in the physician's notes explaining the dosage ordered.

There are occasions when the physician wishes to give a higher or lower dosage than the recommended dosage. Clients with renal disease are unable to eliminate drugs readily; therefore, dosages for these clients are smaller than the recommended dosages. Certain conditions warrant use of higher than recommended dosages.

Comparison of the ordered dosage with the recommended dosage requires calculation of the daily dosage ordered, as shown in Chapter 10. When the ordered dosage measurement unit differs from the unit of the recommended dosage, convert the ordered dosage unit to that of the recommended dosage. The equations for calculation of daily dosage are as follows:

$$\frac{dosage}{day} = \frac{conversion\ factor}{if\ necessary} \times \frac{dosage}{dose} \times \frac{number\ doses}{day} \quad or$$

$$\frac{dosage}{day} = \frac{conversion\ factor}{if\ necessary} \times \frac{dosage}{(q)\ number\ hours} \times \frac{24\ hours}{1\ day}$$

The ordered daily dosage is compared to the recommended daily dosage. Some recommended dosages require no calculations for adults but require calculations for pediatric clients. These problems are solved in two steps: (1) calculate ordered daily dosage and (2) compare ordered daily dosage with recommended daily dosage.

SAMPLE PROBLEM   **Dosage ordered: NegGram 500 mg PO q.i.d. × 10 d. Recommended dosage: 4 grams per day for one to two weeks. Compare the ordered dosage with the recommended dosage.**

Calculate the daily ordered dosage.
Knowns: Unit of answer: g/day
Factors: 500 mg = 1 dose
          4 doses = 1 day
Conversion factor: 1 g = 1000 mg
Set up the equation framework.

$$\frac{g}{d} = \underline{\hspace{3cm}}$$

The first factor numerator unit is the same as the answer numerator unit.

$$\frac{g}{d} = \frac{1\ g \quad \times}{1000\ mg \quad \times}$$

The second factor numerator unit is the same as the first factor denominator unit.

$$\frac{g}{d} = \frac{1\ g \quad \times \quad 500\ mg \quad \times}{1000\ mg \quad \times \quad 1\ dose \quad \times}$$

The third factor numerator unit is the same as the second factor denominator unit.

$$\frac{g}{d} = \frac{1\ g \quad \times \quad 500\ mg \quad \times \quad 4\ doses}{1000\ mg \quad \times \quad 1\ dose \quad \times \quad 1\ d}$$

Cancel the units and evenly divisible quantities

$$\frac{g}{d} = \frac{1 \text{ g} \times \overset{1}{\cancel{500}} \times \overset{2}{\cancel{4}}}{\underset{\underset{1}{\cancel{2}}}{\cancel{1000}} \times 1 \times 1 \text{ d}}$$

Multiply the numerator:
Multiply the denominator:

$$\frac{1 \text{ g} \times 1 \times 2}{1 \times 1 \times 1 \text{ d}} = \frac{2 \text{ g}}{1 \text{ d}} = 2 \text{ g/d}$$

Compare ordered daily dosage, 2 g/d, with recommended daily dosage, 4 g/d. The ordered dosage is only half of the recommended dosage. Therefore, prior to administration of the medication, the nurse would check with the physician if no notation had been made on the nursing or progress notes.

When the ordered dosage is half the recommended dosage, there is no problem determining whether the difference is significant enough to notify the physician. There is no rule for determining when the difference between ordered and recommended dosage is sufficient to notify the physician. In general, the smaller the dosage, the closer the ordered dosage should be to the recommended dosage. For instance, a difference of 100 milligrams per day means very little for dosages of 4 or 5 grams a day. On the other hand, differences of 5 to 10 micrograms per day may be critical when dealing with small microgram dosages. Most of these dosage differences involve nursing rather than mathematical judgments.

Recommended daily dosages based on body weight must be calculated prior to comparison with ordered dosage. This requires two separate equations that must be compared to each other. These problems are solved in three steps: (1) calculate ordered daily dosages, (2) calculate recommended daily dosage, and (3) compare ordered daily dosage to recommended daily dosage.

Dosages based on weight are rarely the exact recommended dosages. The dosages are adjusted to coincide with the dosages in which the medication is available. For instance, there is no way to give a sixth of a tablet; therefore, the dosage is adjusted to the nearest attainable tablet dosage.

SAMPLE PROBLEM   **Dosage ordered: NegGram suspension 400 mg q.i.d. Client weight: 66 lb. Recommended dosage: 55 mg/kg/d. The dosage on hand is 250 mg per 5 ml. Is the ordered dosage the same as, larger than, or smaller than the recommended dosage? If larger or smaller, what is the difference?**

Calculate the daily dosage ordered.
Knowns: Unit of measure: mg/d
Factors: 400 mg = 1 dose
            4 doses = 1 day
The equation is as follows:

$$\frac{\text{mg}}{\text{d}} = \frac{400 \text{ mg} \times 4 \text{ doses}}{1 \text{ dose} \times 1 \text{ d}}$$

Solve the equation.

$$\frac{\text{mg}}{\text{d}} = \frac{400 \text{mg} \times 4}{1 \times 1\text{d}} = \frac{1600 \text{mg}}{1\text{d}} = 1600 \text{ mg/d}$$

Calculate the recommended daily dosage.
Knowns: Unit of measure: mg (/d)
Factors: 55 mg/kg (/d)
          66 lb/1
Conversion factor: 1 kg = 2.2 lb
The equation is as follows:

$$\text{mg (/d)} = \frac{55 \text{mg} \times 1 \text{kg} \times 66 \text{lb}}{1 \text{kg} \times 2.2 \text{lb} \times 1}$$

Solve the equation.

$$mg \, (/d) = \frac{55mg \times \overset{30}{\underset{1}{\frac{1}{}}} \times \cancel{66}}{1 \quad \times \cancel{2.2} \times \; 1} = \frac{1650mg}{1} = 1650 \, mg \, (/d)$$

Compare the ordered dosage, 1600 mg/d, with the recommended dosage, 1650 mg/d. The ordered dosage is smaller than the recommended dosage by 50 mg.

PRACTICE PROBLEMS

Comparison of Recommended and Ordered Dosages

For the following problems, identify the ordered dosage as the same as, larger than, or smaller than the recommended dosage. If the dosage is not the same, what is the difference between the two? (Answers on page 334.)

26. Ordered dosage: 300 mg q.4h. PO. Client weight: 176 lb. Recommended dosage: 30 mg/kg/d. Dosage available: 150 mg tab.

27. Dosage ordered: 500 mg t.i.d. PO. Recommended dosage: 1.5 g/d. Client weight: 134 lb. Dosage on hand: 250 mg tab.

28. Digoxin 0.125 mg PO q.d. Recommended dosage: 2 mcg/kg/d. Client weight: 136 lb. Dosage on hand: 62.5 mcg/ml.

29. Dosage ordered: 50 mg q.8h. PO. Recommended dosage: 2 mg/kg/d in divided doses. Client weight: 165 lb. Dosage available: 100 mg scored tab.

30. Dosage ordered: 1 g q.i.d. PO. Recommended dosage: 5 g/d. Client weight: 204 lb. Dosage available: 500 mg tab.

RECOMMENDED DOSAGE RANGES

Many medications have a safe therapeutic dosage range. Too little of the medication will not produce the desired results, whereas too large an amount of the medication could be toxic. The safe therapeutic dosage range in medication reference books provides a range from the minimum dosage to achieve the desired effect of the drug to the maximum dosage that is not expected to produce toxic symptoms. Recommended dosage ranges may be minimum and maximum dosages per day, minimum to maximum dosages per body weight, or up to a specific amount per day.

Comparison of ordered dosage with a recommended dosage of a minimum and maximum per day requires calculation of the ordered dosage per day and determining whether that dosage is between the minimum and maximum dosage recommended. These problems are solved in two steps: (1) calculate ordered daily dosage and (2) compare ordered daily dosage with the minimum and maximum daily dosage range.

SAMPLE PROBLEM   **Mr. Harris has the following ordered dosage: 500 mg q.i.d. PO. The *Physician's Desk Reference* (PDR) reports the range of this medication is 1.5 to 3 g/day in four to six divided doses. Is Mr. Harris' medication order within the recommended dosage range?**

Calculate the ordered dosage per day.
Knowns: Unit of answer: g/d
Factors: 500 mg = 1 dose
         4 doses = 1 d
Conversion factor: 1 g = 1000 mg
The equation is as follows:

$$\frac{g}{d} = \frac{1\ g \quad \times \quad 500\ mg \quad \times \quad 4\ doses}{1000\ mg \quad \times \quad 1\ dose \quad \times \quad 1\ d}$$

Solve the equation.

$$\frac{g}{d} = \frac{1\ g \times \overset{1}{\cancel{500}} \times \overset{2}{\cancel{4}}}{\underset{\underset{1}{\cancel{2}}}{\cancel{1000}} \times 1 \times 1\ d} = \frac{2\ g}{1\ d} = 2\ g/d$$

    Mr. Harris' daily dosage is 2 grams. Compare his dosage with the recommended dosage of 1.5 to 3 grams/day. Since 2 grams is within the 1.5 to 3 g range, the ordered dosage is within the recommended range.

    Comparison of ordered dosages with recommended dosage ranges based on body weight usually requires three calculation equations. Four steps are required for these problems: (1) calculate the ordered daily dosage, (2) calculate the minimum recommended dosage, (3) calculate the maximum recommended dosage, and (4) compare the ordered daily dosage with the calculated dosage range.

SAMPLE PROBLEM   **Dosage ordered: 2 mcg IM q.8h. Recommended dosage range: 0.06 to 0.07 mcg/kg/d. Client weight: 187 lb. Is the ordered dosage within the recommended range?**

Calculate the ordered dosage per day.
Knowns: Unit of answer: mcg/d
Factors: 2 mcg = 8 h (or 2 mcg = 1 dose)
        24 h = 1 d (or 3 doses = 1 day)
The equation is as follows:

$$\frac{mcg}{d} = \frac{2\ mcg \times 24\ h}{8\ h \times 1\ d}$$

Solve the equation.

$$\frac{mcg}{d} = \frac{2\,mcg \times \overset{3}{\cancel{24}}}{\underset{1}{\cancel{8}}\,h \times 1d} = \frac{6\,mcg}{1d} = 6\ mcg/d$$

Calculate the minimum recommended dosage.
Knowns: Unit of answer: mcg (/d)
Factors: 0.06 mcg = 1 kg
        187 lb/1
Conversion factor: 1 kg = 2.2 lb
The equation is as follows:

$$mcg = \frac{0.06\ mcg \times 1\ kg \times 187\ lb}{1\ kg \times 2.2\ lb \times 1}$$

Solve the equation:

$$\text{mcg} = \frac{0.06\text{mcg} \times\ \ 1 \times \overset{85}{\cancel{187}}}{1\ \ \ \times \cancel{2.2} \times\ \ 1} = \frac{5.1\text{mcg}}{1} = 5.1\ \text{mcg(/d)}$$

Calculate the maximum recommended dosage.

Knowns: Unit of answer: mcg (/d)

Factors: 0.07 mcg = 1 kg

   187 lb/1

Conversion factor: 1 kg = 2.2 lb

The equation is as follows:

$$\text{mcg} = \frac{0.07\text{mcg} \times\ \ 1\text{kg}\ \ \times 187\text{lb}}{1\text{kg}\ \ \times 2.2\text{lb}\ \ \times\ \ 1}$$

Solve the equation.

$$\text{mcg} = \frac{0.07\text{mcg} \times\ \ 1 \times \overset{85}{\cancel{187}}}{1\ \ \ \times \cancel{2.2} \times\ \ 1} = \frac{5.95\text{mcg}}{1} = 5.95\ \text{mcg (/d)}$$

Note that the ordered daily dosage, 6 mcg, is not within the recommended range of 5.1 to 5.95 mcg. If 5.95 was rounded off to 6 mcg, it would be within the dosage range. With minute dosages, however, the 5.95 would probably not be rounded off to 6 mcg. For problems in this book, the answer will be no.

Dosage ranges up to a maximum dosage per day require two calculations, the ordered daily dosage and the maximum daily dosage. The three steps of these problems are: (1) calculate ordered daily dosage, (2) calculate maximum daily dosage, and (3) compare the ordered daily dosage with the maximum dosage.

SAMPLE PROBLEM   **Dosage ordered: 0.3 mg q.2h. PO. Recommended dosage range: up to 50 mcg/kg/d. Client weight is 84 kg. Is the dosage ordered within the recommended range?**

Calculate the ordered daily dosage.

The unit of the answer may be either mcg or mg/d. Since mg/d produces smaller numbers, it was chosen for this problem.

Knowns: Unit of answer: mg/d

Factors: 0.03 mg = (q)2 h

   24 h = 1 d

The equation is as follows:

$$\frac{\text{mg}}{\text{d}} = \frac{0.3\text{mg} \times 24\text{h}}{(q)2\text{h}\ \times\ 1\text{d}}$$

Solve the equation.

$$\frac{\text{mg}}{\text{d}} = \frac{0.3\text{mg} \times \overset{12}{\cancel{24}}}{\underset{1}{\cancel{2}}\ \times\ 1\text{d}} = \frac{3.6\text{mg}}{1\text{d}} = 3.6\ \text{mg/d}$$

Calculate the maximum dosage. The answer unit is mg since mg were used in the ordered dosage equation.

Knowns: Unit of answer: mg (/d)

Factors: 50 mcg = 1 kg

   84 kg/1

Conversion factor: 1 mg = 1000 mcg

The equation is as follows:

$$\text{mg} = \frac{1\text{mg}\ \ \times 50\text{mcg} \times 84\text{kg}}{1000\text{mcg} \times\ \ 1\text{kg}\ \ \times\ \ 1}$$

Solve the equation.

$$mg = \frac{1mg}{1000} \times \frac{\overset{1}{\cancel{50}} \times \overset{42}{\cancel{84}}}{\times 1 \times 1} = \frac{42mg}{10} = 4.2 \text{ mg(/d)}$$

$$\frac{\overset{2}{\cancel{20}}}{10}$$

Note the ordered daily dosage, 3.6 mg, is less than the maximum recommended daily dosage, 4.2 mg. Therefore, the ordered dosage is within the dosage range.

PRACTICE PROBLEMS

Recommended Dosage Ranges

Show all your work. Check your answers (page 334).

31. Dosage ordered: 25 mg q.4h. PO. Recommended daily dosage range: 100 to 150 mg/day. Client weight: 159 lb. Is this medication order within the recommended dosage range?

32. Dosage ordered: 250 mg q.6h. IM. Recommended daily dosage range: 10 to 15 mg/kg per day. Client weight: 98 kg. Is this medication order within the recommended dosage range?

33. Dosage ordered: 750 mcg q.3h. PO. Recommended dosage range: 2 to 5 mg/day. Client weight: 98 lb. Is this medication within the recommended dosage range?

34. Dosage ordered: gr 1/300 q.i.d. s.c. Recommended daily dosage range: 10 to 15 mcg/kg per 24 hours. Client weight: 176 lb. Is this medication order within the recommended dosage range?

35. Dosage ordered: 400 mg t.i.d. Recommended dosage range: 20 to 30 mg/kg/day. Patient weight: 110 lb. Is this medication order within the recommended dosage range?

36. Dosage ordered: 500 mg q.4h. Recommended dosage range: up to 3 g/day. Patient weight: 192 lb. Is this medication order within the recommended dosage range?

37. Dosage ordered: 0.5 g b.i.d. IM. Recommended dosage range: . up to 1 mg/lb/d. Client weight: 70 kg. Is this medication order within the recommended dosage range?

38. Dosage ordered: 0.15 mg PO b.i.d. Recommended dosage range: 2 to 5 mcg per kg per day. Patient weight: 165 lb. Dosage on hand: 0.05 mg tablets. Is this medication order within the recommended dosage range?

39. Dosage ordered: gr XXX PO q.i.d. Recommended dosage range: 5 to 10 g/day. Is this medication order within the recommended dosage range?

40. Dosage range: 1.2 mg t.i.d. a.c. PO. Patient weight: 132 lb. Recommended dosage range: 50 to 60 mcg/kg/day. Is the prescribed dosage within the recommended dosage range?

Dosages Based on Client Weight

Show all your work. Check your answers (page 361).

1. Dosage ordered: 0.7 mcg/lb. Client weight: 45 kg. What is the client's dosage?

2. Dosage ordered: 30 mcg/kg/d in two divided doses. Client weight: 132 lb. What is the daily dosage?

   What is the dosage per dose?

3. Dosage ordered: 400 mg q.4h. PO. Client weight: 209 lb. Recommended daily dosage range: up to 30 mg/kg/d. Is the prescribed dosage within the recommended dosage range?

4. Dosage ordered: 25 mg/kg/day. Client weight 110 lb. Dosage available: 250 mg scored tabs. How many tabs will be administered?

5. Dosage ordered: 0.5 mg per pound in 3 divided doses. Client weight: 150 lb. Dosage on hand: 25 mg tabs. How many tabs will be given at each dose?

6. Dosage ordered: 20 U/kg/d. Client weight: 189 lb. Dosage on hand: 1000 U/ml. How many ml will be administered?

7. Dosage ordered: 1.5 mcg/kg/d in six divided doses. Client weight: 220 lb. Dosage on hand: 25 mcg/ml. What is the daily dosage?

8. Dosage ordered: 500 mg t.i.d. PO. Client weight: 132 lb. Recommended dosage range: 20 to 30 mg/kg/d. Is the dosage within the dosage range?

9. Dosage ordered: 0.004 ml per pound. Client weight: 185 lb. How many ml will be given?

10. Dosage ordered: 1 mg/kg/d. Client weight: 71 kg. Dosage available: 50 mg/ml. What is the daily dosage?

UNIT V POSTTEST

Calculations Based on Body Weight

Test A

Show all your work. Check your answers (page 378).

1. Dosage ordered: 1 mg/lb. Client weight: 50 kg. What is the client's dosage?

2. Dosage ordered: 50 mcg/kg/d in two divided doses. Client weight: 176 lb. What is the daily dosage?

   What is the dosage per dose?

3. Dosage ordered: 500 mg q.4h. PO. Client weight: 198 lb. Recommended daily dosage range: up to 35 mg/kg/d. Is the prescribed dosage within the recommended dosage range?

4. Dosage ordered: 30 mg/kg/day. Client weight 110 lb. Dosage available: 500 mg scored tabs. How many tabs will be administered?

5. Dosage ordered: 0.5 mg/lb q.d. PO. Client weight: 120 lb. What is the daily dosage in mg?

6. Dosage ordered: 20 U/kg/d. Client weight: 189 lb. How many U will be administered each day?

7. Dosage ordered: 1.5 mcg/kg/d. Client weight: 88 lb. What is the daily dosage?

8. Dosage ordered: 500 mg q.4h. PO. Client weight: 132 lb. Recommended dosage range: 20 to 50 mg/kg/d. Is the dosage within the dosage range?

9. Dosage ordered: 0.01 ml per kg. Client weight: 121 lb. How many ml will be given?

10. Dosage ordered: 10 mcg/kg/d. Client weight: 68 kg. Dosage available: 5 mg/ml. What is the daily dosage?

Calculations Based on Body Weight
Test B

Show all your work. Check your answers (page 379).

1. Dosage ordered: 2 mg/lb. Client weight: 50 kg. What is the client's dosage?

2. Dosage ordered: 100 mcg/kg/d in two divided doses. Client weight: 176 lb. What is the daily dosage?

   What is the dosage per dose?

3. Dosage ordered: 750 mg q.4h. PO. Client weight: 198 lb. Recommended daily dosage range: up to 50 mg/kg/d. Is the prescribed dosage within the recommended dosage range?

4. Dosage ordered: 40 mg/kg/day. Client weight: 110 lb. Dosage available: 500 mg scored tabs. How many tabs will be administered?

5. Dosage ordered: 0.05 mg/lb q.d. PO. Client weight: 120 lb. What is the daily dosage in mg?

6. Dosage ordered: 30 U/kg/d. Client weight: 189 lb. How many U will be administered each day?

7. Dosage ordered: 1.8 mcg/kg/d. Client weight: 88 lb. What is the daily dosage?

8. Dosage ordered: 250 mg q.4h. PO. Client weight: 132 lb. Recommended dosage range: 20 to 50 mg/kg/d. Is the dosage within the dosage range?

9. Dosage ordered: 0.05 ml per kg. Client weight: 121 lb. How many ml will be given?

10. Dosage ordered: 10 mcg/kg/d. Client weight: 78 kg. Dosage available: 5 mg/ml. What is the daily dosage?

UNIT V

Posttest Calculations Based on Body Weight
Test C

Show all your work. Check your answers (page 380).

1. Dosage ordered: 8 mg/lb. Client weight: 50 kg. What is the client's dosage?

2. Dosage ordered: 25 mcg/kg/d in two divided doses. Client weight: 176 lb. What is the daily dosage?

   What is the dosage per dose?

3. Dosage ordered: 250 mg q.4h. PO. Client weight: 198 lb. Recommended daily dosage range: up to 25 mg/kg/d. Is the prescribed dosage within the recommended dosage range?

4. Dosage ordered: 35 mg/kg/day. Client weight 110 lb. Dosage available: 500 mg scored tabs. How many tabs will be administered?

5. Dosage ordered: 0.005 mg/lb q.d. PO. Client weight: 120 lb. What is the daily dosage in mg?

6. Dosage ordered: 15 U/kg/d. Client weight: 189 lb. How many U will be administered each day?

7. Dosage ordered: 2.5 mcg/kg/d. Client weight: 88 lb. What is the daily dosage?

8. Dosage ordered: 1 g q.4h. PO. Client weight: 198 lb. Recommended dosage range: 20 to 50 mg/kg/d. Is the dosage within the dosage range?

9. Dosage ordered: 0.02 ml per kg. Client weight: 121 lb. How many ml will be given?

10. Dosage ordered: 10 mcg/kg/d. Client weight: 98 kg. Dosage available: 5 mg/ml. What is the daily dosage?

Unit VI

Solutions

OBJECTIVES *Upon completion of this unit, the student will have demonstrated the ability to correctly:*

- Calculate quantities of solid or stock solutes required for specific percentage solution preparation.

- Calculate quantities of solid or stock solutions required for preparation of solutions ordered or supplied as ratios.

- Calculate amount of solutes present in prepared solutions.

- Calculate kilocalories of solutions with specific percentage of carbohydrate.

- Compute dosage per volume for medication solutions ordered as ratios.

The solutions most commonly used by health care providers are medication solutions and intravenous fluids. Nurses also use solutions for enemas, irrigations, soaks, and gargles. Nurses in the community or in home health care frequently teach clients to make solutions.

Most solutions are premixed by the manufacturer. Occasionally, however, nurses have to make specified solutions from either solids or stock solutions. The nurse may have to make a normal saline solution from plain table salt for mouth care, gargles, or enemas. It is too costly to use premixed solutions for these purposes. Nurses may make soak solutions from stock solutions. When the strength of a stock solution is greater than ordered, the nurse must be able to dilute the solution to the proper strength.

Sometimes nurses need to know how much solute is found in a particular prepared solution. Some medications, such as epinephrine, may be ordered in milligrams, whereas medication solutions may be labeled as ratios. Finding the amount of solutes in intravenous infusions is sometimes necessary.

Chapter 14

Calculation of Solutes and Solvents

Solutions are made by combining solutes with solvents. A *solute* is a substance to be dissolved. The *solvent* is the liquid in which the solute is dissolved. In a normal saline solution, which contains 0.9% sodium chloride in water, the sodium chloride is the solute, while the water is the solvent.

Sometimes several solutes are dissolved in a solvent. An example of this is the 5% dextrose in normal saline intravenous solution. In this case, the solvent is water to which the solutes, both dextrose and sodium chloride, have been added.

SOLUTIONS FROM SOLIDS

Solutes in solutions made by manufacturers are weighed rather than measured by volume. Manufactured solutions, such as medications and intravenous fluids, must contain precise quantities of solutes, which can be obtained only by weight. When nurses make solutions from solids, the solutions are only approximately the percentage ordered, because nurses do not have access to precision scales on which to weigh the small quantities of solutes. Instead, nurses rely on the chemical principle that 1 gram of water is equal to 1 milliliter which occupies the same space as 1 cubic centimeter. Therefore, 1 gram of water = 1 milliliter of water = 1 cubic centimeter of water. Since this principle applies only to water, it is not true to say that 1 milliliter of water weighs the same as 1 milliliter of a solid. However, it is close enough for producing normal saline solutions for enemas, soaks, and gargles.

Calculation of quantities of solutes required for solutions requires the percentage of solute required in the solution, the percentage of the solute available, and the total amount of solution to be made. Consider normal saline, the most common solution that nurses prepare. The percentage of solute required for the solution is 0.9%. By definition, normal saline is 0.9% sodium chloride (table salt). A quantity of salt, by itself, is wholly salt. The whole of anything is 100%. Therefore, the percentage of the salt is 100%.

One factor that is present in solution problems involving percentages is the ratio of the total quantity of solution and the total percentage of the solute. All solution equations involving percentages contain the following:

$$\text{quantity solute} = \frac{\text{total quantity of solution} \times \% \text{ of solute needed}}{\text{total } \% \text{ of solute available} \times 1}$$

SAMPLE PROBLEM   **How many ml of salt are needed to make 1000 ml of normal saline solution?**

Knowns: Unit of answer: ml salt.
Factors: 1000 ml = 100%
          0.9%/1

The equation is as follows:

$$\text{ml salt} = \frac{1000 \text{ ml} \times 0.9\%}{100\% \times 1}$$

Solve the equation.

$$\text{ml salt} = \frac{\overset{10}{\cancel{1000}} \text{ ml} \times 0.9}{\underset{1}{\cancel{100}} \times 1} = \frac{10 \text{ ml} \times 0.9}{1 \times 1} = \frac{9.0 \text{ ml}}{1} = 9 \text{ ml salt}$$

To prepare the solution, add solvent to the solute in a quantity sufficient (q.s.) to make the desired amount of solution. To get a rough estimate of the amount of water to be used, subtract the amount of solute from the total volume of solution.

SAMPLE PROBLEM   **How much water is needed to prepare the solution in previous sample problem?**

Total amount of solution − amount of solute = approximate amount of solvent

ml water = 1000 ml solution − 9 ml solute = 991 ml

SAMPLE PROBLEM   **Mary Jones is to have normal saline gargles q.4h. Her mother must be shown how to prepare the gargle. How many tsp salt are required to make 8 ounces of normal saline for a gargle?**

Known: Unit of answer: tsp salt
Factors: 8 oz = 100%
     0.9%/1
Conversion factor: 1 tsp = 5 ml
       1 oz = 30 ml
The equation is as follows:

$$\text{tsp} = \frac{1 \text{ tsp} \times 30 \text{ ml} \times 8 \text{ oz} \times 0.9\%}{5 \text{ ml} \times 1 \text{ oz} \times 100\% \times 1}$$

Solve the equation.

$$\text{tsp} = \frac{1 \text{ tsp} \times \overset{6}{\cancel{30}} \times \overset{2}{\cancel{8}} \times 0.9}{\underset{1}{\cancel{5}} \times 1 \times \underset{25}{\cancel{100}} \times 1} = \frac{10.8 \text{ tsp}}{25} = 0.432 \text{ tsp} = 0.4 \text{ tsp} = 4/10 \text{ or } 2/5$$

Teaspoon, a household measurement, is not expressed as a decimal but can be expressed as $\frac{4}{10}$ or $\frac{2}{5}$ tsp. Mrs. Jones does not have a measuring spoon for $\frac{4}{10}$ tsp. Compare $\frac{4}{10}$ tsp with a measuring spoon that is available, $\frac{1}{2}$ tsp. You know that $\frac{1}{2} = \frac{5}{10}$, which is slightly larger than $\frac{4}{10}$. Therefore, Mrs. Jones should use a scant $\frac{1}{2}$ tsp. (Refer to Chapter 2 for help in comparing fractions, if necessary.)

SAMPLE PROBLEM   **How many ml salt are required to make 1000 ml of 1/2 normal saline solution?**

Half-strength normal saline is half of 0.9%, or 0.45%. This problem can be solved by using the 0.45% or by multiplying the equation by $\frac{1}{2}$, as in this sample problem.

Knowns: Unit of answer: ml salt
Factors: 1000 ml = 100%
      0.9%/1
      1/2
The equation is as follows:

$$\text{ml} = \frac{1000 \text{ ml} \times 0.9\% \times 1}{100\% \times 1 \times 2}$$

Solve the equation.

$$\text{ml salt} = \frac{\overset{5}{\cancel{10}}}{\underset{1}{\cancel{100}}} \frac{ml \times 0.9 \times 1}{\times 1 \times \cancel{2}} = \frac{5 \text{ ml} \times 0.9 \times 1}{1 \times 1 \times 1} = \frac{4.5 \text{ ml}}{1} = 4.5 \text{ ml salt}$$

The equation using 0.45% for $\frac{1}{2}$ normal saline produces the same answer and is as follows:

$$\text{ml} = \frac{1000 \text{ ml} \times 0.45\%}{100\% \times 1}$$

Solutions other than normal saline are made from solid solutes. These problems are solved in the same manner as the normal saline problems.

SAMPLE PROBLEM   **How many ml of boric acid crystals are needed to make 500 ml of 5% solution?**

Knowns: Unit of answer: ml boric acid
Factors: 500 ml = 100%
        5%/1
The equation is as follows: $$\text{ml boric acid} = \frac{500 \text{ ml} \times 5\%}{100\% \times 1}$$

Solve the equation.

$$\text{ml boric acid} = \frac{\overset{5}{\cancel{500}} \text{ ml} \times 5}{\underset{1}{\cancel{100}} \times 1} = \frac{5 \text{ ml} \times 5}{1 \times 1} = \frac{25 \text{ ml}}{1} = 25 \text{ ml boric acid}$$

It is easy to put the percentages in the wrong place when setting up the equation. This will yield an answer that is larger than the total amount of solution. If the answer is larger than the total amount of solution, check the placement of percentages.

PRACTICE PROBLEMS

Solutions from Solids

Show all your work. Check your answers (page 336).

1. How many ml salt will you use to make 500 ml of normal saline?

2. How many ml of boric acid crystals are needed to make 100 ml of a 5% solution?

Approximately how many ml of water will be required?

3. How many ml of a solid solute will be required to make 800 ml of a 20% solution?

4. How many tsp of salt will be used to make 1500 ml of normal saline?

5. How many ml of salt are necessary to make 1.5 L of half-strength normal saline?

Solutes and Calories in Prepared Solutions

Sometimes it is necessary to know the amount of solute in a particular strength prepared solution. This problem is solved in exactly the same manner as the solution preparation problems. Prepared solutions are weighed rather than measured by volume. Remember, when solving solution problems, 1 g = 1 ml = 1 cc.

SAMPLE PROBLEM   **How many grams of dextrose are in an intravenous solution of 1000 ml of 5% dextrose in normal saline? How many grams of sodium chloride (salt) are in this IV?**

Solve for grams of dextrose first.
Knowns: Unit of answer: g dextrose
Factors: 1000 ml = 100%
    5%/1
Conversion factor: 1 g = 1 ml
The equation is as follows:

$$\text{g dextrose} = \frac{1\ \text{g} \times 1000\ \text{ml} \times 5\%}{1\ \text{ml} \times 100\% \times 1}$$

Solve the equation.

$$\text{g dextrose} = \frac{1\ \text{g} \times \overset{10}{\cancel{1000}} \times 5}{1 \times \underset{1}{\cancel{100}} \times 1} = \frac{1\ \text{g} \times 10 \times 5}{1 \times 1 \times 1} = \frac{50\ \text{g}}{1} = 50\ \text{g dextrose}$$

Solve for grams of sodium chloride.
Knowns: Unit of answer: g sodium chloride (NaCl)
Factors: 1000 ml = 100%
    0.9%/1
Conversion factor: 1 g = 1 ml
The equation is as follows:

$$\text{g NaCl} = \frac{1\ \text{g} \times 1000\ \text{ml} \times 0.9\%}{1\ \text{ml} \times 100\% \times 1}$$

Solve the equation.

$$\text{g NaCl} = \frac{1\ \text{g} \times \overset{10}{\cancel{1000}} \times 0.9}{1 \times \underset{1}{\cancel{100}} \times 1} = \frac{1\ \text{g} \times 10 \times 0.9}{1 \times 1 \times 1} = \frac{9.0\ \text{g}}{1} = 9\ \text{g NaCl}$$

The 1000 milliliters of 5% dextrose in normal saline contain both 50 grams of dextrose and 9 grams of sodium chloride.

Calories can be calculated for solutions in which the percentage of the carbohydrate dextrose and the total amount of solution are known. There are 4 Calories (kilocalories) per gram of carbohydrate. Calculation of Calories is covered in Appendix F.

SAMPLE PROBLEM   **Calculate the Calories for an intravenous infusion of 1000 ml of 10% dextrose in normal saline.**

Knowns: Unit of answer: Cal
Factors: 4 Cal = 1 g
       1000 ml = 100%
       10%/1

Conversion factor: 1 g = 1 ml
The equation is as follows:

Solve the equation.

$$Cal = \frac{4\ Cal \times 1\ g \times 1000\ ml \times 10\%}{1\ g \times 1\ ml \times 100\% \times 1}$$

$$Cal = \frac{4\ Cal \times 1 \times \overset{10}{\cancel{1000}} \times 10}{1 \times 1 \times \underset{1}{\cancel{100}} \times 1} = \frac{4\ Cal \times 1 \times 10 \times 10}{1 \times 1 \times 1 \times 1} = \frac{400\ Cal}{1} = 400\ \text{Calories}$$

PRACTICE PROBLEMS

Solutes and Calories in Solution

Show all your work. Check your answers (page 337).

6. How many Calories are in 1000 ml of 10% dextrose in water?

7. How many grams of dextrose are in a 500 ml IV of 5% dextrose in normal saline?

   How many grams of sodium chloride are in this IV?

   How many Calories are in this IV?

8. How many Calories are in 100 ml of 50% dextrose in water?

9. Mrs. Brown is receiving 1000 ml of 5% dextrose in water IV every 12 hours. How many Calories is Mrs. Brown receiving in her IVs each day (24 hours)?

10. How many grams of dextrose are in 1500 ml of 2.5% dextrose in 0.45% normal saline?

    How many grams of sodium chloride are in this IV?

Solutions from Stock Solutions

Stock solutions are prepared solutions used to prepare lesser strength solutions. The percentage of the stock solution may vary from very mild to nearly 100%.

Calculations involving stock solution use the factor of the total amount of solution and the percentage of the stock solution. The total percentage of the solute is the stock solution percentage.

SAMPLE PROBLEM   **How much 50% stock solution will be needed to make 100 ml of 10% solution?**

Knowns: Unit of answer: ml
Factors: 100 ml = 50%
          10%/1
The equation is as follows:

$$ml = \frac{100 \ ml \ \times \ 10\%}{50\% \ \times \ 1}$$

Solve the equation.

$$ml = \frac{\overset{2}{\cancel{100}} \ ml \times 10}{\underset{1}{\cancel{50}} \times 1} = \frac{2 \ ml \times 10}{1 \times 1} = \frac{20 \ ml}{1} = 20 \ ml$$

PRACTICE PROBLEMS

Solutions from Stock Solutions

Show all your work. Check your answers (page 337).

11. How many ml of 20% stock solution will be needed to make 400 ml of 10% solution?

12. Make 300 ml of 20% solution from a 30% stock solution. How many ml of stock solution will be used?

13. How many ounces of 50% stock solution will be needed to make 900 ml of 10% solution?

14. How many ounces of 50% stock solution will you need to make 1500 ml of 10% solution?

15. How many ml of 60% stock solution will be needed to make 300 ml of 5% solution?

Solutions Expressed as Ratios

Some solutions are ordered or available as ratios rather than percentages. Remember, a ratio is nothing more than a fraction. The ratio 1:1000 could be written as $\frac{1}{1000}$. A 1:1000 solution consists of 1 part solute to 1000 parts of total solution. This means that 1 part solute plus 999 parts solvent equal 1000 parts solution. Therefore, for 1000 ml of solution, there is 1 ml of solute.

Because a ratio is a fraction, it can be changed to a percentage by dividing the numerator, the first number of the ratio, by the denominator, the second number, and multiplying the quotient by 100%. This could be written in equation form as follows:

$$\frac{Numerator \ \times \ 100\%}{Denominator \ \times \ 1}$$

Therefore, changing the ratio 1:1000 to a percentage is as follows:

$$\frac{\overset{1}{\cancel{1}} \times \cancel{100\%}}{\underset{10}{\cancel{1000}} \times 1} = \frac{1\%}{10} = 0.1\%$$

Changing a ratio to a percentage can be done within the framework of the problem equation as shown in the following sample problem.

SAMPLE PROBLEM   **Make 1000 ml of a 1:1000 solution from a 5% stock solution. How much stock solution will you use?**

Knowns: Unit of answer: ml
Factors: 1000 ml = 5%
            1/1000
Conversion factor: 1 = 100%
The equation is as follows:

$$ml = \frac{1000 \text{ ml} \times 100\% \times 1}{5\% \times 1 \times 1000}$$

Solve the equation.

$$ml = \frac{\overset{1}{\cancel{1000}} \text{ ml} \times \overset{20}{\cancel{100}} \times 1}{\underset{1}{\cancel{5}} \times 1 \times \underset{1}{\cancel{1000}}} = \frac{1 \text{ ml} \times 20 \times 1}{1 \times 1 \times 1} = \frac{20 \text{ ml}}{1} = 20 \text{ ml}$$

When stock solutions are expressed as ratios, the conversion of ratios to percentages also can be done within the equation. To do so, however, involves the use of complex fractions. Usually it is easier to convert the ratio to a percentage prior to setting up the equation.

SAMPLE PROBLEM   **How much 1:20 solution will be needed to make 500 ml of 2% solution?**

Convert 1:20 solution to a percentage. This can be done by dividing the numerator by the denominator and multiplying by 100 or by the following equation. Remember, 1 is equal to 100%.

$$\% = \frac{\overset{5}{\cancel{100\%}} \times 1}{1 \times \underset{1}{\cancel{20}}} = \frac{5\%}{1} = 5\%$$

Solve the problem.
Knowns: Unit of answer: ml
Factors: 500 ml = 5%
            2%/1
The equation is as follows:

$$ml = \frac{500 \text{ ml} \times 2\%}{5\% \times 1}$$

Solve the equation.

$$ml = \frac{\overset{100}{\cancel{500}} \text{ ml} \times 2}{\underset{1}{\cancel{5}} \times 1} = \frac{100 \text{ ml} \times 2}{1 \times 1} = \frac{200 \text{ ml}}{1} = 200 \text{ ml}$$

The equation set up without converting the ratio to a percentage first is as follows:

$$ml = \frac{500 \text{ ml} \times 1 \times 2\%}{\frac{1}{20} \times 100\% \times 1}$$

Solve the equation.

$$ml = \frac{500 \text{ ml} \times 1 \times 2}{\frac{1}{20} \times 100 \times 1} = \frac{\overset{5}{\cancel{500}} \text{ ml} \times 20 \times 1 \times 2}{1 \times \underset{1}{\cancel{100}} \times 1} = \frac{5 \text{ ml} \times 20 \times 1 \times 2}{1 \times 1 \times 1} = \frac{200 \text{ ml}}{1} = 200\text{ml}$$

PRACTICE PROBLEMS

Solution Expressed as Ratios

Show all your work. Check your answers (page 338).

16. How much 20% stock solution will be needed to make 2000 ml of a 1:1000 solution?

19. How much 10% stock solution will be needed to make 200 ml of a 1:10 solution?

17. How much 50% stock solution will be needed to make 500 ml of a 1:10 solution?

20. How many ml of 1:100 stock solution will be required to make 50 ml of a 0.05% solution?

18. How much 1:100 stock solution will be needed to make 1000 ml of a 0.5% solution?

Medications Labeled as Ratios

Some medication solutions, such as epinephrine, are labeled as ratios. The medication may be ordered as a specific amount of the ratio solution or as a specific dosage. When the dosage is ordered, it is necessary to determine the dosage of the medication on hand.

For a medication labeled 1:100, there is 1 part solute (medication) in the 100 parts of solution. This means that for every 100 milliliters of solution, there is 1 milliliter of medication. One milliliter of solution is equal to 1 gram of solution. Therefore, for every 100 ml of solution, there is 1 gram of medication. One point to remember is that 1 gram = 1 milliliter only when dealing with solutions. This conversion does not apply at any other time.

SAMPLE PROBLEM   **What is the dosage in mg of 1 ml of 1:1000 solution?**

This means that 1000 ml of solution contains 1 ml of medication; 1 ml = 1 g, therefore, 1000 ml = 1 g.

Knowns: Unit of answer: mg/ml

Factors: 1 g = 1000 ml

Conversion factor: 1 g = 1000 mg

The equation is as follows:

$$\frac{mg}{ml} = \frac{1000\ mg \times\ 1\ g}{1\ g\ \times\ 1000\ ml}$$

Solve the equation.

$$\frac{mg}{ml} = \frac{\overset{1}{\cancel{1000}}\ mg\ \times\ 1}{1\ \ \times\ \underset{1}{\cancel{1000}}\ ml} = \frac{1\ mg\ \times\ 1}{1\ \ \times\ 1\ ml} = \frac{1\ mg}{1\ ml} = 1\ mg/ml$$

PRACTICE PROBLEMS

Medications Labeled as Ratios

Show all your work. Check your answers (page 338).

21. What is the dosage in mg per ml of a 1:100 solution?

22. What is the dosage in mg per ml of a 1:40 solution?

23. What is the dosage in mg per ml of a 1:50 solution?

24. What is the dosage in mg per ml of a 1:500 solution?

25. What is the dosage in mg per ml of a 1:10 solution?

SELF-ASSESSMENT POSTTEST

Solutions

Show all your work. Check your answers (page 362).

1. How many tsp of salt will be used to make 500 ml of normal saline?

2. How many Calories are in an intravenous infusion of 1000 ml 10% dextrose in normal saline?

3. How many ml of boric acid crystals will be required to make 200 ml of 5% solution?

4. How many teaspoons of salt will be used to make 1000 ml of half-strength normal saline?

   How many ml of water will be used?

5. What is the dosage in mg per ml of a 1:1000 solution?

6. How many ml of salt will be needed to make 500 ml of 1/2 normal saline?

7. Make 500 ml of 15% solution from a 60% stock solution. How much stock solution will be used?

8. Make 1 L of 1% solution from a 1:50 stock solution. How much stock solution will be required?

9. How many grams of dextrose are in 500 ml of 2.5% dextrose in normal saline?

   How many grams of sodium chloride are in this solution?

10. Make 250 ml of 1:1000 solution from a 10% stock solution. How much stock solution must be used?

UNIT VI POSTTEST

Solutions

Test A

Show all your work. Check your answers (page 381).

1. What is the dosage in mg per ml of a 1:500 solution?

2. How much sodium chloride must be used to make 2 L of normal saline solution?

3. How many ounces of 50% stock solution are required to make 150 ml of 20% solution?

4. How many ml of 1:10 stock solution are required to make 200 ml of 5% solution?

5. How many calories are in 50 ml of 50% dextrose solution?

6. How many ml of boric acid crystals are required to make 50 ml of 5% solution?

7. How many tsp of salt are required to make 2 L of 1/2 normal saline solution?

8. How much 30% stock solution will be used to make 250 ml of 15% solution?

9. How many grams of dextrose are in 1 L of 5% dextrose in normal saline?

10. How many ml of 5% acetic acid solution will be used to make 1 L of 1:1000 solution?

UNIT VI POSTTEST

Solutions

Test B

Show all your work. Check your answers (page 382).

1. What is the dosage in mg per ml of a 1:40 solution?

2. How much sodium chloride must be used to make 1.5 L or normal saline solution?

3. How many ounces of 40% stock solution are required to make 100 ml of 20% solution?

4. How many ml of 1:10 stock solution are required to make 100 ml of 2.5% solution?

5. How many calories are in 100 ml of 50% dextrose solution?

6. How many ml of boric acid crystals are required to make 500 ml of 5% solution?

7. How many tsp of salt are required to make 1 L of 1/2 normal saline solution?

8. How much 30% stock solution will be used to make 250 ml of 10% solution?

9. How many grams of dextrose are in 0.5 L of 5% dextrose in normal saline?

10. How many ml of 5% acetic acid solution will be used to make 500 ml of 1:1000 solution?

UNIT VI POSTTEST

Solutions

Test C

Show all your work. Check your answers (page 383).

1. What is the dosage in mg per ml of a 1:100 solution?

2. How much sodium chloride must be used to make 1 L of normal saline solution?

3. How many ounces of 50% stock solution are required to make 200 ml of 25% solution?

4. How many ml of 1:5 stock solution are required to make 200 ml of 10% solution?

5. How many calories are in 250 ml of 10% dextrose solution?

6. How many ml of boric acid crystals are required to make 150 ml of 5% solution?

7. How many tsp of salt are required to make 1.5 L of 1/2 normal saline solution?

8. How much 50% stock solution will be used to make 500 ml of 15% solution?

9. How many grams of sodium chloride are in 0.5 L of 5% dextrose in normal saline?

10. How many ml of 10% acetic acid solution will be used to make a liter of 1:1000 solution?

Unit VII

Intravenous Fluid Administration

OBJECTIVES: *Upon completion of this unit, the student will have demonstrated the ability to correctly:*

- Calculate fluid volumes per hour.
- Calculate drip (flow) rates.
- Compare actual infused volumes with expected volumes.
- Recalculate drip rates.

Intravenous fluids are solutions administered directly into a vein. Nurses are responsible for assuring that intravenous fluids infuse as ordered by the physician. This involves the regulation of the rate of flow of the intravenous solution and the monitoring of volume infused.

Chapter 15

Calculations Associated with Intravenous Fluid Administration

Physician's orders for intravenous fluids may be written for single or continuous infusions. Examples of IV orders are as follows:

1. Single IV orders
    a. 1000 cc D5NS IV to run 8 hours.
    b. 500 cc 10% glucose in water IV to run 6 hours.
2. Continuous IV orders:
    a. 1000 cc 5% dextrose in lactated Ringer's IV q.10h.
    b. 1000 ml D5W with 40 mEq KCl alternating c 1000 ml D5NS IV q.12h.
    c. D5NS IV 125 ml/h
    d. 1000 ml D5W IV TKO (to keep open) or KVO (keep vein open)

A single IV order means that the IV is discontinued after the infusion is completed. Continuous IV orders mean that another infusion is started as soon as one is completed.

Most intravenous infusion orders have time frames for completion. This means that a specific amount of fluid is to infuse in a given amount of time. The first five IV order examples have a specific amount and time frame. The last order, however, does not. The purpose of the last intravenous order is to ensure a patent or open intravenous line for medications or in emergency situations rather than to supply a specific amount of fluid within a time frame.

Intravenous infusions consist of the intravenous solutions in plastic bags or glass bottles and the infusion set as shown in Figure 15-1. All intravenous fluids must be monitored frequently to ensure that the fluids are infusing as ordered. Intravenous infusion pumps are sometimes used to make monitoring easier. Infusion pumps are usually very accurate in administering precise amounts of solutions. The use of infusion pumps does not negate the need for frequent monitoring, however.

HOURLY VOLUMES

The basic calculation necessary to monitor intravenous fluids is *volume per hour*. Volume per hour is the amount of fluid that is to infuse in 1 hour. Some infusion pumps are set to deliver specific quantities of fluid per hour.

Calculation of volumes per hour requires the total amount of fluid and the total number of hours. Infusions ordered as ml per hour, such as 125 ml/hour in order 2c, do not have to be calculated. The equation for hourly volumes is as follows:

$$\text{ml/hr} = \frac{\text{total amount of IV fluid}}{\text{number of hours IV to infuse}}$$

SAMPLE PROBLEM   **IV order: 1000 ml D5NS to run 8 hours. What is the volume per hour to be administered?**

Knowns: Unit of answer: ml/h
Factor: 1000 ml = 8 h

$$\text{ml/h} = \frac{1000 \text{ml}}{8 \text{ hr}} = 125 \text{ ml/hr}$$

236

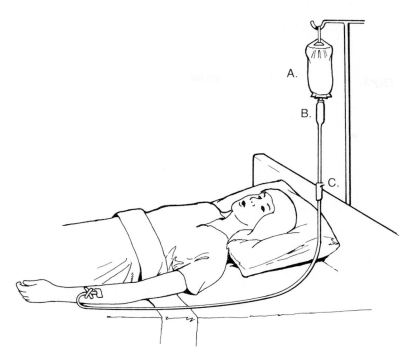

FIGURE 15-1 Intravenous solution bag and infusion set. A, intravenous solution bag. B, drip chamber. C, regulating clamp.

The equation is as follows:

$$\frac{ml}{h} = \frac{1000\ ml}{8\ h}$$

Solve the Equation.

$$\frac{ml}{h} = \frac{125\ ml}{1\ h} = 125\ ml/h$$

A quick reference for monitoring intravenous solution is a label indicating the expected fluid levels at hourly intervals. This label, shown in Figure 15-2, is placed on the inverted solution container. Note that each 125 ml is marked with an hour. Each time the IV is monitored, the fluid level of the solution is checked with the hour mark. If the fluid level is not at the expected level, the infusion is not on time.

A second way to monitor the infusion is to multiply the hourly volume by the number of hours the solution has been infusing. Logically, when half the time has passed, half the solution should have infused. The equation for finding expected infused volumes is as follows:

$$ml = \frac{hourly\ \times\ number\ of\ hours}{volume\ \times\ \ \ \ IV\ has\ infused}$$

SAMPLE PROBLEM   **IV order: 500 cc 10% Glucose in water to run 6 hours. How much solution should infuse in 4 hours?**

Knowns: Unit of answer: ml

Factors: 500 ml = 6 h

        4 h/1

The equation for this problem is as follows:

$$ml = \frac{500\ ml\ \times\ 4\ h}{6\ h\ \times\ 1}$$

Solve the equation.

$$ml = \frac{500\ ml\ \times\ \overset{2}{\cancel{4}}}{\underset{3}{\cancel{6}}\ \times\ 1} = \frac{500\ ml\ \times\ 2}{3\ \times\ 1} = \frac{1000\ ml}{3} = 333.3\ ml\,(in\ 4\ hours)$$

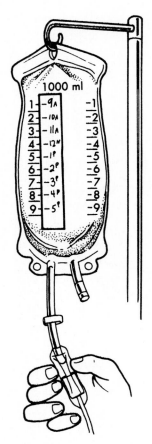

FIGURE 15-2 Intravenous bag with monitoring label. (From Dison, N.: Simplified drugs and solutions for nurses, ed. 9, St. Louis, The C.V. Mosby Co.)

PRACTICE PROBLEMS

Hourly Volumes

Show all your work. Check your answers (page 338.)

1. What is the hourly volume for 1000 ml D5W IV to run 10 hours?

$$ml/hr = \frac{1000\ ml}{10\ hrs} = 100\ ml/hr$$

2. What is the hourly volume for 250 ml D5NS IV to run 4 hours?

$$ml/hr = \frac{250\ ml}{4\ hrs} = 62.5\ ml/hr$$

$$\begin{array}{r}63.5\\4\overline{)250.}\\\underline{24}\\10\\\underline{8}\\20\end{array}$$

3. IV order: 1000 ml of 10% dextrose in water IV q.12h. How much solution should infuse in 6 hours?

$$ml/hr = \frac{1000\ ml}{\underset{2}{12\ hr}} \times \frac{6\ hr}{1} = 500\ ml\ in\ 6\ hr$$

4. IV order: 500 ml lactated Ringer's IV q.8h. What is the hourly volume?

$$ml/hr = \frac{500\ ml}{8\ hr} = 62.5\ ml/hr.$$

How much should infuse in 4 hours?

$$ml/hr = \frac{500\ ml}{4} = 250\ ml/hr$$

5. IV order: 1000 ml D5NS IV q.6h. What is the   How much should infuse in 3 hours?
   hourly volume?

CALCULATION OF DRIP (FLOW) RATES

The most commonly used intravenous fluid calculation is the *drip* or *flow* rate. Calculations of drip rates are essential to regulating intravenous infusions using some pumps that have sensors to count the drips. Drip rates are always used when infusion pumps are not used.

Infusion sets are the tubings that deliver the fluids from the intravenous solution containers to the patients. Manufacturers label the infusion sets with approximate drops per milliliter, as shown in Figure 15-3. The common infusion sets are labeled 10, 15, 20, or 60 drops per milliliter. The size of the drop depends on the size of the lumen through which it passes. Infusion sets that deliver large drops, 10, 15 or 20 drops per milliliter, are called *macrodrip infusion sets*. The larger the drop, the fewer the drops required per milliliter. *Microdrip infusion sets*, sometimes called *minidrip*, deliver very small drops, 60 drops per milliliter. Most infusion sets used in pediatrics are *microdrip sets*. The number of drops per milliliter of an infusion set is sometimes called a *drop factor*.

Drip (flow) rates are calculated as drops per minute. To calculate a drip rate, the following information is necessary:
1. the total amount of fluid to be administered in ml or cc.
2. the total time the IV fluid is to be administered.
3. the drop factor of the infusion set.
4. The conversion factor 1 hour = 60 minutes when necessary.

The equation for drip rates is as follows:

$$\frac{gtt}{min} = \frac{drop}{factor} \times \frac{total\ amount\ of\ IV\ fluid}{total\ time\ IV\ is\ to\ infuse} \times \frac{Conversion\ hours\ to\ minutes\ if\ necessary}{}$$

Note that part of the information necessary to solve drip rate problems is the hourly volume.

SAMPLE PROBLEM   **An IV of 1000 ml of 5% dextrose in water is to run 8 hours. The infusion set delivers 60 gtt/ml. What is the drip rate?**

Knowns: Unit of answer: gtt/min
Factors: 60 gtt = 1 ml
        1000 ml = 8 h
Conversion factor: 1 h = 60 min
The equation is as follows:

$$\frac{gtt}{min} = \frac{60\ gtt \times 1000\ ml \times 1\ h}{1\ ml \times 8\ h \times 60\ min}$$

Solve the equation.

$$\frac{gtt}{min} = \frac{\overset{1}{\cancel{60}}\ gtt \times \overset{125}{\cancel{1000}} \times 1}{1 \times \cancel{8} \times \cancel{60}\ min} = \frac{1\ gtt \times 125 \times 1}{1 \times 1 \times 1\ min} = \frac{125\ gtt}{1\ min} = 125gtt/min$$

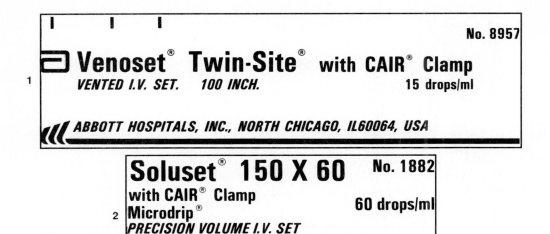

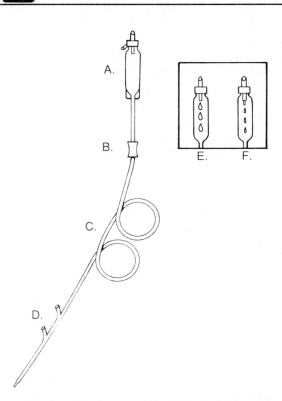

FIGURE 15-3 Infusion set labels and infusion tubing. The infusion set labels indicate the drop factor, the number of drops delivered per milliliter. Infusion set label 1 is a macrodrip set while label 2 is a microdrip set. The infusion set shows the drip chamber (A), the regulating clamp (B), the tubing (C) and the ports for piggyback administration (D). The inset shows the drip chambers of macrodrip (E) and microdrip (F) infusion sets.

The drip rate is used to adjust the infusion flow. Drops are counted as they enter the drip chamber of the infusion set, as shown in Figure 15-4, while the number of drops per minute is regulated by adjusting the screw clamp.

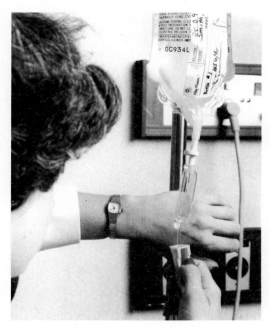

FIGURE 15-4 Regulation of the drip rate. (*From Potter, P.A. & Perry, A.G., Fundamentals of nursing: concepts, process and practice, St. Louis, ed. 2, 1989, The C.V. Mosby Co.*)

SAMPLE PROBLEM   **IV order: 1000 ml D5NS q.10h. IV. The infusion set delivers 15 gtt/ml. What is the drip rate of this IV?**

Knowns: Unit of answer: gtt/min
Factors: 1000 ml = 10 h
**   15 gtt = 1 ml**
Conversion factor: 1 h = 60 min
The equation is as follows:

$$\frac{gtt}{min} = \frac{15 \; gtt \times 1000 \; ml \times 1 \; h}{1 \; ml \times 10 \; h \times 60 \; min}$$

Solve the equation.

$$\frac{gtt}{min} = \frac{15 \; gtt \times 1000 \times 1}{1 \times 10 \times 60 \; min} = \frac{1 \; gtt \times 25 \times 1}{1 \times 1 \times 1 \; min} = \frac{25 \; gtt}{1 \; min} = 25 \; gtt/min$$

Calculations for administration of whole blood and packed cells are the same as those for other intravenous fluids. Blood is ordered as units rather than ml. A unit of whole blood is 500 ml, while a unit of packed cells is about half that amount. Blood is administered using an infusion set with a filter and a drop factor of 10 drops per milliliter. The infusion set for blood is shown in Figure 15-5.

SAMPLE PROBLEM   **Mr. Jones has 1 unit of whole blood ordered to run 4 hours. The infusion set delivers 10 gtt/ml. What is the drip rate for the blood?**

Knowns: Unit of answer: gtt/min
Factors: 500 ml = 4 h
**   10 gtt = 1 ml**
Conversion factor: 1 h = 60 min

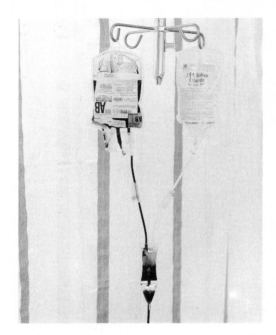

FIGURE 15-5 Blood administration set with blood and normal saline solution. (*From Potter, P.A. & Perry, A.G., Fundamentals of nursing: concepts, process and practice, St. Louis, ed. 2, 1989, The C.V. Mosby Co.*)

The equation is as follows:

$$\frac{gtt}{min} = \frac{10\ gtt \times 500\ ml \times 1\ h}{1\ ml \times 4\ h \times 60\ min}$$

Solve the equation.

$$\frac{gtt}{min} = \frac{\overset{1}{\cancel{10}}\ gtt \times \overset{125}{\cancel{500}} \times 1}{1 \times \underset{1}{\cancel{4}} \times \underset{6}{\cancel{60}}\ min} = \frac{1\ gtt \times 125 \times 1}{1 \times 1 \times 6\ min} = \frac{125\ gtt}{6\ min} = 20.8 gtt/min$$

Drops are rounded off to the nearest whole number as there is no way to measure a fraction of a drop. Therefore, the drip rate for the unit of blood is 21 gtt/min.

Sometimes the intravenous solutions are small amounts intended to infuse in less than an hour. In these problems, conversion from hours to minutes may not be necessary.

SAMPLE PROBLEM **What is the drip rate of 50 ml NS c ampicillin 125 mg to infuse in 30 minutes using an infusion set that delivers 20 gtt/ml?**

Knowns: Unit of answer: gtt/min
Factors: 50 ml = 30 min
  20 gtt = 1 ml

$$gtt/min = \frac{\overset{2}{\cancel{20}gtt}}{1ml} \times \frac{50ml}{\underset{3}{30min}} = \frac{100}{3} = 33,3$$

$$33\ gtt/min$$

(Ampicillin 125 mg is extraneous information for solving this problem.)

The equation is as follows:

$$\frac{gtt}{min} = \frac{20\ gtt \times 50\ ml}{1\ ml \times 30\ min}$$

Solve the equation.

$$\frac{gtt}{min} = \frac{20\ gtt \times \overset{5}{\cancel{50}}}{1 \times \underset{3}{\cancel{30}}\ min} = \frac{20\ gtt \times 5}{1 \times 3\ min} = \frac{100\ gtt}{3\ min} = 33.3\ gtt/min$$

This problem could have used the time frame of 1/2 hour instead of 30 minutes. The conversion from hours to minutes is required for that problem. Problems involving the delivery of small infusion amounts within time frames of less than an hour are usually for piggyback intravenous medication infusions. Piggyback infusions are covered more thoroughly in Chapter 16.

Infusion pumps are programmed with either the drip rate or the hourly volume. Therefore, use of the infusion pump does not eliminate the calculations associated with intravenous fluid administration.

PRACTICE PROBLEMS

Calculation of Drip Rates

Show all your work. Check your answers (page 339).

6. IV order: 1000 ml of 5% dextrose in lactated Ringer's in 12 hours. The infusion set delivers 20 gtt/ml. What is the drip rate?

$$\frac{gtt}{min} = \frac{20\,gtt}{1\,ml} \times \frac{1000\,ml}{12\,h} \times \frac{1\,h}{60\,min} = \frac{20,000}{}$$

$$27\ gtt/min$$

7. Calculate the drip rate for 1000 ml of 5% dextrose in normal saline to infuse in 6 hours using an infusion set that delivers 15 gtt/ml.

$$\frac{gtt}{min} = \frac{15\,gtt}{1\,ml} \times \frac{1000\,ml}{6\,h} \times \frac{1\,h}{60\,m} = \frac{15,000}{360}$$

$$42\ gtt/min$$

8. An IV of 500 ml of normal saline is to infuse in 6 hours. Calculate the drip rate using an infusion set with a drop factor of 10 gtt/ml.

$$36\overline{)500}\ \frac{13}{340}$$

$$\frac{gtt}{min} = \frac{10\,gtt}{1\,ml} \times \frac{500}{6h} \times \frac{1\,h}{60} = \frac{500}{36}$$

$$14\ gtt/min$$

9. Calculate the drip rate of the following IV order using an infusion set that delivers 15 gtt/ml: 100 ml D5W c̄ garamycin 80 mg to infuse in 30 minutes.

10. An IV of 500 ml of normal saline with 40 mEq KCl is to run 10 hours. The drop factor of the infusion set is 60 gtt/ml. What is the drip rate?

11. Calculate the drip rate of a unit of blood that is to run 5 hours. The drop factor of the infusion set is 10 gtt/ml.

12. IV order: 500 cc D5W to run 12 hours. The infusion set delivers 60 gtt/ml. What is the flow rate?

13. Calculate the drip rate of an IV of 1000 ml of 5% dextrose in normal saline q.8h. using an infusion set that delivers 15 gtt/ml.

14. Calculate the drip rate of an IV of 1000 ml of 1/2 NS q.12h. using an infusion set that delivers 10 gtt/ml.

$$gtt/min = \frac{10\,gtt}{1\,ml} \times \frac{1000\,ml}{12\,h} \times \frac{1\,h}{60\,min} =$$

15. Calculate the drip rate of the following IV order using an infusion set with a drop factor of 15 gtt/ml: 50 ml NS with Keflin 1 gram to run 1/2 hour.

RECALCULATION OF DRIP RATES

Intravenous fluids must be monitored closely to assure that the correct amount of fluid is infusing within the proper time frame. Although the drip rate may have been correctly established initially, any number of factors can increase or decrease that flow. The patient's arm may move slightly, causing the lumen of the intravenous needle to rest against the wall of the vein, or the patient may be compressing the infusion tubing. Raising or lowering the height of the intravenous fluid container will increase or decrease the rate of flow, respectively.

The nurse assesses whether the IV is on time by comparing the amount of fluid expected to be infused at any given time with the actual amount infused. An IV for an adult usually is considered to be on time if the actual infused volume is within 25 ml of the expected infused volume. This is because the markings on intravenous bags and bottles is approximate only.

Comparing of actual infused volumes is easy when labels marking the expected level each hour have been attached to the solution container. If the actual infused volume is 25 ml more or less than the expected infused volume, the drip rate must be changed. The following problems have no labels on the solution container. Therefore, the expected infused volume must be calculated for comparison.

SAMPLE PROBLEM   **IV order: 1000 ml D5W q.8h. The IV was started at 8 AM using an infusion set that delivers 15 gtt/ml. It is now 10 AM, and 400 ml have infused. Is the IV on time, infusing too rapidly, or infusing too slowly?**

Calculate the expected infused volume. The IV has been infusing for 2 hours.
Knowns: Unit of answer: ml
Factors: 1000 ml = 8 h
        2 h/1
The equation is as follows:

$$ml = \frac{1000 \ ml \ \times \ 2 \ h}{8 \ h \ \times \ 1}$$

Solve the equation.

$$ml = \frac{\overset{125}{\cancel{1000}} \ ml \ \times \ 2}{\underset{1}{\cancel{8}} \ \times \ 1} = \frac{250 \ ml}{1} = 250 \ ml \ (in \ 2 \ h)$$

Compare the expected infused volume with the actual infused volume.
Expected volume: 250 ml ± 25 = 225 to 275 ml.
Actual volume: 400 ml.
400 ml > 225 to 275 ml. Therefore, the IV is running too rapidly. The drip rate must be recalculated.

Drip rates are recalculated in the same manner as the original drip rate. The time is decreased by the number of hours the IV has infused. The volume is reduced by the amount that has already infused. The new equation is as follows:

$$\text{Recalculated gtt/min} = \frac{\text{drop} \ \times \ \left(\begin{array}{c} \text{total} \\ \text{volume} \end{array} - \begin{array}{c} \text{infused} \\ \text{volume} \end{array} \right) \ \times \ \text{conversion hours}}{\text{factor} \ \times \ \left(\begin{array}{c} \text{total} \\ \text{hours} \end{array} - \begin{array}{c} \text{hours} \\ \text{infused} \end{array} \right) \ \times \ \text{to minutes}}$$

Consider the previous sample problem. The infusion is not on time; it is infusing too rapidly. Therefore, the IV drip rate must be recalculated. The equation can be set up as shown or the infused volumes and hours can be subtracted first as shown in this sample problem.

SAMPLE PROBLEM   **Recalculate the drip rate using the information in the previous problem.**

The original volume − the amount already infused = amount of fluid remaining

$$1000 \text{ ml} - 400 \text{ ml} = 600 \text{ml}$$

The original time frame − the hours the infusion has been running = time remaining

$$8 \text{ h} - 2 \text{ h} = 6 \text{ h}$$

The new knowns are as follows:
Knowns: Unit of answer: gtt/min
Factors: 600 ml = 6 h
$$15 \text{ gtt} = 1 \text{ ml}$$
Conversion factor: 1 h = 60 min
The equation is as follows:

$$\frac{\text{gtt}}{\text{min}} = \frac{15 \text{ gtt} \times 600 \text{ ml} \times 1 \text{ h}}{1 \text{ ml} \times 6 \text{ h} \times 60 \text{ min}}$$

Solve the equation.

$$\frac{\text{gtt}}{\text{min}} = \frac{\overset{1}{\cancel{15}} \text{ gtt} \times \overset{\overset{25}{\cancel{100}}}{\cancel{600}} \times 1}{1 \times \underset{\underset{1}{1}}{\cancel{6}} \times \underset{\underset{1}{\cancel{4}}}{\cancel{60}} \text{ min}} = \frac{1 \text{ gtt} \times 25 \times 1}{1 \times 1 \times 1 \text{ min}} = \frac{25 \text{ gtt}}{1 \text{ min}} = 25 \text{ gtt/min}$$

The recalculated drip rate of an IV that infused too rapidly must be less than the original drip rate. Conversely, the drip rate of an IV running too slowly will be greater than the original drip rate.

PUTTING IT ALL TOGETHER

SAMPLE PROBLEM   **IV order: 1000 ml D5W q.10h. IV. The drop factor of the infusion set is 20 gtt/ml. What is the drip rate for the IV?**

Knowns: Unit of answer: gtt/min
Factors: 1000 ml = 10 h
$$20 \text{ gtt} = 1 \text{ ml}$$
Conversion factor: 1 h = 60 min
The equation is as follows:

$$\frac{\text{gtt}}{\text{min}} = \frac{20 \text{ gtt} \times 1000 \text{ ml} \times 1 \text{ h}}{1 \text{ ml} \times 10 \text{ h} \times 60 \text{ min}}$$

Solve the equation.

$$\frac{\text{gtt}}{\text{min}} = \frac{\overset{1}{\cancel{20}} \text{ gtt} \times \overset{100}{\cancel{1000}} \times 1}{1 \times \underset{1}{\cancel{10}} \times \underset{3}{\cancel{60}} \text{ min}} = \frac{100 \text{ gtt}}{3 \text{ min}} = 33.3 \text{ gtt/min}$$

The original drip rate is 33 gtt/min.

The IV was started at 0600 hours. It is now 1200 hours and 550 ml remain in the bottle. Is the IV on time, infusing too rapidly, or infusing too slowly?

If 550 ml remain in the bottle, 450 ml have infused. The IV has been infusing for 6 hours.

The equation for expected infused volumes is as follows:

$$\text{ml} = \frac{1000 \text{ ml} \times 6 \text{ h}}{10 \text{ h} \times 1}$$

Solve the equation.

$$ml = \frac{\overset{100}{\cancel{1000}} \text{ ml} \times 6}{\underset{1}{\cancel{10}} \times 1} = \frac{600 \text{ ml}}{1} = 600 \text{ ml (expected in 6 h)}$$

Compare the expected infused volume with the infused volume.

450 ml infused < 600 ml expected volume. The IV is infusing too slowly.

Recalculate the drip rate.

There are 550 ml remaining in the bottle. There is no need to calculate this as it is given in the problem. If the IV has infused for 6 hours, 4 hours remain. 10 hours − 6 hours = 4 hours. The new knowns are as follows:

Knowns: Unit of answer: gtt/ml

Factors: 550 ml = 4 h

20 gtt = 1 ml

Conversion factor: 1 h = 60 min

The equation is as follows:

$$\frac{gtt}{min} = \frac{20 \text{ gtt} \times 550 \text{ ml} \times 1 \text{ h}}{1 \text{ ml} \times 4 \text{ h} \times 60 \text{ min}}$$

Solve the equation.

$$\frac{gtt}{min} = \frac{\overset{5}{\cancel{20}} \text{ gtt} \times \overset{55}{\cancel{550}} \times 1}{\underset{1}{1} \times \cancel{4} \times \underset{6}{\cancel{60}} \text{ min}} = \frac{5 \text{ gtt} \times 55 \times 1}{1 \times 1 \times 6 \text{ min}} = \frac{275 \text{ gtt}}{6 \text{ min}} = 45.8 \text{ gtt/min}$$

The recalculated drip rate is 46 gtt/min.

Increasing the drip rate from 34 to 46 gtt/min at one time may harm the client. Therefore, the rate should be increased by small increments, perhaps 5 drops. The client should be observed closely for circulatory overload for 15 to 30 minutes. If no deleterious effects are noted, the rate is increased again and the client observed once more. It may be necessary to recalculate the drip rate several times before the IV is on time. Careful monitoring of the IV is easier than trying to "catch up."

Always check with the physician before increasing an IV rate above that ordered. An IV more than 25 ml off schedule is as much of a nursing error as giving the wrong medication. Nurses are legally responsible for following IV orders just as they are for following medication orders.

PRACTICE PROBLEMS

Recalculation of drip rates

Show all your work. Check your answers (page 340).

16. Mrs. Roberts has the following order: 1000 ml D5NS with 1 amp Multivits alternating with 1000 ml D5W with 20 mEq KCl IV q.10h. The first IV was started at 6:00 AM using an infusion set with the drop factor of 20 gtt/ml. What was the drip rate for Mrs. Roberts's IV?

What is the volume per hour that her IV should infuse?

How much solution should have infused by 11 AM?

It is now 11 AM and 650 ml remain in the IV bottle. Is the IV on time, infusing too rapidly, or infusing too slowly?

If the IV is not on time, recalculate the drip rate so that it will be completed on time.

17. An IV is ordered as follows: 500 ml normal saline to run for 6 hours. This IV was started at 0700 using an infusion set that delivers 10 gtt/ml. It is now 0800 and 250 ml have infused. Is the IV on time, infusing too slowly, or infusing too rapidly?

$$g tt/m in = \frac{100 gtts}{1 ml} \times \frac{500 ml}{6 h} \times \frac{1 h}{60 min} = 9\overline{)1250}$$

$$ml = \frac{500 ml}{6 hrs} \times \frac{1 h}{1} = 83 ml$$

If the IV is not on time, recalculate the drip rate.

To Fast.

$$gtt/min = \frac{10 gtt}{1 ml} \times \frac{250 ml}{5 h} \times \frac{1 h}{60 min} = \frac{25}{3} = 8 gtt/min$$

18. Calculate the drip rate of 1000 cc D5W to infuse in 10 hours using an infusion set that delivers 15 gtt/ml.

This IV was started at 4 AM. At 10 AM 600 ml remain in the bottle. Is the IV on time?

If the IV is not on time, recalculate the drip rate.

19. An IV of 1000 cc 5% dextrose in normal saline was started at 9 AM using an infusion set that delivers 60 gtt/ml. It should run 12 hours. What is the initial drip rate?

What is the expected hourly volume?

It is now 3 PM and 500 ml remain in the bottle. Is the IV on time?

If the IV is not on time, recalculate the drip rate so that the IV will finish in 12 hours.

20. IV order: 1000 ml D5W c̄ 500 mg aminoplylline q.8h. The drop factor of the infusion set is 20 gtt/ml. The IV was started at 2 PM. What is the drip rate?

What is the expected infused volume at 6 PM?

At 6 PM, 400 ml remain in the IV bag. Is the IV on time, infusing too rapidly, or infusing too slowly?

If the IV is not on time, recalculate the drip rate.

Intravenous Fluid Administration

Show all your work. Check your answers (page 363).

1. IV order: 1000 ml D5 1/2 NS c̄ 20 mEq KCl to run 10 hours. The infusion set has a drop factor of 15 gtt/ml. What is the drip rate?

If the IV is not on time, recalculate the drip rate.

2. IV order: 500 ml 5% glucose in water q.6h. The drop factor of the infusion set is 20 gtt/ml. What is the hourly volume of the IV?

4. IV order: 2 units whole blood (500 ml each) to run 3 hours each. The infusion set delivers 10 gtt/ml. What is the drip rate?

How much fluid should infuse in 3 hours?

5. IV order: 3 L D5NS q.24h. The infusion set delivers 20 gtt/ml. What is the drip rate?

3. An IV of 1000 ml D5NS was started at 10 AM using an infusion set delivering 60 gtt/ml. The IV is to run 12 hours. What is the drip rate?

6. 250 ml 2.5% dextrose in water is to run 8 hours. The infusion set drop factor is 60 gtt/ml. What is the drip rate?

7. IV order: 1 unit packed cells (250 ml) to run 4 hours. The drop factor of the infusion set is 10 gtt/ml. What is the drip rate?

At 3 PM, 500 ml remain in the IV bag. Is the IV on time, infusing too rapidly, or infusing too slowly?

8. IV order: 500 ml 10% dextrose in normal saline to run 8 hours. The drop factor of the infusion set is 15 gtt/ml. What is the hourly volume?

If the IV is not on time, recalculate the drip rate.

9. 50 ml D5NS with ampicillin 250 mg to infuse in 30 min. The infusion set delivers 20 gtt/ml. What is the drip rate?

What is the drip rate?

The IV was started at 3 AM. It is now 7 AM and 250 ml remain in the IV bottle. Is the IV on time, infusing too rapidly, or infusing too slowly?

10. IV order: 1000 ml 5% dextrose in Ringer's lactate q.8h. The drop factor is 15 gtt/ml. What is the drip rate?

UNIT VII POSTTEST

Intravenous Fluid Administration

Test A

Show all your work. Check your answers (page 383).

1. IV order: 1000 ml 5% glucose in water q.6h. The drop factor of the infusion set is 20 gtt/ml. What is the hourly volume of the IV?

$$ml/m = \frac{1000 ml}{6 h} \times \frac{1 h}{1} = 166.6 m/m$$

How much fluid should infuse in 3 hours?

$$166.6 \times 3 = 499.8 \, ml$$

$$ml/3h = \frac{1000 ml}{6 h} \times \frac{3 h}{1} = \quad or \; 500 ml$$

2. IV order: 1000 ml D5 1/2 NS c̄ 20 mEq KCl to run 12 hours. The infusion set has a drop factor of 15 gtt/ml. What is the drip rate?

3. An IV of 1000 ml D5NS was started at 4 AM using an infusion set delivering 60 gtt/ml. The IV is to run 24 hours. What is the drip rate?

$$41 \, gtt/min$$

At 2 PM, 500 ml remain in the IV bag. Is the IV on time, infusing too rapidly, or infusing too slowly?

To Fast

If the IV is not on time, recalculate the drip rate.

4. IV order: 1 unit whole blood (500 ml) to run 6 hours. The infusion set delivers 10 gtt/ml. What is the drip rate?

$$\text{gtt/min} = \frac{10\,\text{gtt}}{1\,\text{ml}} \times \frac{500\,\text{ml}}{6\,\text{h}} \times \frac{1\,\text{h}}{60\,\text{min}} = \frac{125}{9} = 15\,\text{gtt/min}$$

5. IV order: 100 ml D5W c̄ Keflin 1 g to run 1/2 hour. The infusion set delivers 20 gtt/ml. What is the drip rate?

$$\text{gtt/min} = \frac{20\,\text{gtt}}{1\,\text{ml}} \times \frac{100\,\text{ml}}{\tfrac12\,\text{h}} \times \frac{1\,\text{h}}{60\,\text{min}}$$

6. 1 L of 5% dextrose in water is to run 50 ml/h. The infusion set drop factor is 60 gtt/ml. What is the drip rate?

7. IV order: 1 unit packed cells (250 ml) to run 2 hours. The drop factor of the infusion set is 10 gtt/ml. What is the drip rate?

8. IV order: 1000 ml normal saline to run 4 hours. The drop factor of the infusion set is 10 gtt/ml. What is the hourly volume?

250 ml/h

What is the drip rate?

41 gtt/min

The IV was started at 6 AM. It is now 7:30 AM and 350 ml remain in the IV bottle. Is the IV on time, infusing too rapidly, or infusing too slowly?

Too rapidly.

If the IV is not on time, recalculate the drip rate.

17 gtt/min

9. 1000 ml lactated Ringer's is to run 6 hours. The infusion set delivers 15 gtt/ml. What is the drip rate?

10. IV order: 500 ml 5% dextrose in Ringer's lactate q.8h. The drop factor is 15 gtt/ml. What is the drip rate?

UNIT VII POSTTEST

Intravenous Fluid Administration
Test B
Show all your work. Check your answers (page 385).

1. IV order: 1000 ml 5% glucose in water q.8h. The drop factor of the infusion set is 15 gtt/ml. What is the hourly volume of the IV?

$$\text{ml/h} = \frac{1000\,\text{ml}}{8\,\text{h}} \times \frac{1\,\text{h}}{} = 125\,\text{ml/h}$$

How much fluid should infuse in 3 hours?

$$\text{ml/h} = \frac{1000\,\text{ml}}{8\,\text{h}} \times \frac{3\,\text{h}}{1} = 375\,\text{ml}$$

2. IV order: 1000 ml D5 1/2 NS c̄ 20 mEq KCl to run 10 hours. The infusion set has a drop factor of 20 gtt/ml. What is the drip rate?

3. An IV of 1000 ml D5NS was started at 6 AM using an infusion set delivering 60 gtt/ml. The IV is to run 12 hours. What is the drip rate?

$$gtt/min = \frac{60\,gtt}{1\,ml} \times \frac{1000\,ml}{12\,hr} \times \frac{1\,hr}{60\,min} = $$

83 gtt/min

At 2 PM, 500 ml remain in the IV bag. Is the IV on time, infusing too rapidly, or infusing too slowly?

$$ml = \frac{1000\,ml}{12\,hr} \times \frac{8\,hr}{1} = 667\,ml$$

to slowly

If the IV is not on time, recalculate the drip rate.

$$gtt/min = \frac{60\,gtt}{1\,ml} \times \frac{500\,ml}{4\,hr} \times \frac{1\,hr}{60\,min} = 125\,gtt/min$$

4. IV order: 1 unit whole blood (500 ml) to run 4 hours. The infusion set delivers 10 gtt/ml. What is the drip rate?

5. IV order: 100 ml D5W c̄ Keflin 1 g to run 1/3 hour. The infusion set delivers 15 gtt/ml. What is the drip rate?

$$gtt/min = \frac{15\,gtt}{1\,ml} \times \frac{100\,ml}{.33\,hr} \times \frac{1\,hr}{60\,min} = \frac{1500}{19.8}$$

75.7 gtt/min

$$\begin{array}{r} .33 \\ 3\ )\overline{1.0} \\ 9 \end{array}$$

6. 1 L of 5% dextrose in water is to run 80 ml/h. The infusion set drop factor is 60 gtt/ml. What is the drip rate?

7. IV order: 1 unit packed cells (250 ml) to run 3 hours. The drop factor of the infusion set is 10 gtt/ml. What is the drip rate?

8. IV order: 1000 ml normal saline to run 2 hours. The drop factor of the infusion set is 10 gtt/ml. What is the hourly volume?

$$ml/hr = \frac{1000\,ml}{2\,hr} \times \frac{1\,hr}{} = 500\,ml/hr$$

What is the drip rate?

$$gtt/min = \frac{10\,gtt}{1\,ml} \times \frac{500\,ml}{1\,hr} \times \frac{1\,hr}{60\,min} = \frac{5000}{60} =$$

83.3 gtt/min

The IV was started at 5 AM. It is now 6:30 AM and 350 ml remain in the IV bottle. Is the IV on time, infusing too rapidly, or infusing too slowly?

$$ml = \frac{1000\,ml}{2\,hr} \times \frac{1.5\,hr}{} = \frac{1500}{2} = 750$$

$$\begin{array}{r} 1000 \\ -350 \\ \hline 650 \end{array}$$

650 has infused

650 < 750   to slowly

If the IV is not on time, recalculate the drip rate.

$$gtt/min = \frac{10\,gtt}{1\,ml} \times \frac{350\,ml}{.5\,hr} \times \frac{1\,hr}{60} = \frac{3500}{30}$$

116.6 gtt/min

9. 1000 ml lactated Ringer's is to run 6 hours. The infusion set delivers 20 gtt/ml. What is the drip rate?

10. IV order: 500 ml 5% dextrose in Ringer's lactate q.10h. The drop factor is 20 gtt/ml. What is the drip rate?

UNIT VII POSTTEST

Intravenous Fluid Administration
Test C

Show all your work. Check your answers (page 386).

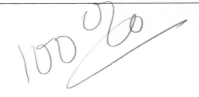

1. IV order: 1000 ml 5% glucose in water q.10h. The drop factor of the infusion set is 20 gtt/ml. What is the hourly volume of the IV?

$$ml/h = \frac{1000\,ml}{10\,hr} \times \frac{1\,hr}{1} = \frac{1000\,ml}{10} = 100\,ml$$

How much fluid should infuse in 3 hours?

$$ml = \frac{1000\,ml}{10\,hr} \times \frac{3\,hr}{1} = \frac{3000\,ml}{10} = 300\,ml$$

2. IV order: 1000 ml D5 1/2 NS c 20 mEq KCl to run 8 hours. The infusion set has a drop factor of 15 gtt/ml. What is the drip rate?

$$gtt/min = \frac{15\,gtt}{1\,ml} \times \frac{1000\,ml}{8\,hr} \times \frac{1\,hr}{60\,min} = \frac{15,000\,gtt}{480\,min} =$$
$$31.25\,gtt/min \quad 32\,gtt/min$$

3. An IV of 1000 ml D5NS was started at 7 AM using an infusion set delivering 60 gtt/ml. The IV is to run 10 hours. What is the drip rate?

$$gtt/min = \frac{60\,gtt}{1\,ml} \times \frac{\overset{100}{1000\,ml}}{10\,hr} \times \frac{1\,hr}{60\,min} = 100\,gtt/min$$

At 2 PM, 500 ml remain in the IV bag. Is the IV on time, infusing too rapidly, or infusing too slowly?

$$\frac{10}{\frac{7}{3}}$$

$$ml = \frac{1000\,ml}{10\,hr} \times \frac{7\,hr}{1} = \frac{7000\,ml}{10} = 700\,ml$$

$$\begin{array}{r}1000\\-\;500\\\hline 500\end{array} \qquad 500 < 700\,ml \qquad \text{to slowly}$$

If the IV is not on time, recalculate the drip rate.

$$gtt/min = \frac{60\,gtt}{1\,ml} \times \frac{500\,ml}{3\,hr} \times \frac{1\,hr}{60\,min} = \frac{500\,gtt}{3\,min} =$$
$$166.6\,gtt/min$$
$$167\,gtt/min$$

4. IV order: 1 unit whole blood (500 ml) to run 3 hours. The infusion set delivers 10 gtt/ml. What is the drip rate?

$$gtt/min = \frac{10\,gtt}{1\,ml} \times \frac{500\,ml}{3\,hr} \times \frac{1\,hr}{60\,min} = \frac{500\,gtt}{18\,min} =$$
$$27.7\,gtt/min \text{ or}$$
$$28\,gtt/min$$

5. IV order: 100 ml D5W c Keflin 1 g to run 30 minutes. The infusion set delivers 20 gtt/ml. What is the drip rate?

$$gtt/min = \frac{20\,gtt}{1\,ml} \times \frac{100\,ml}{.5\,hr} \times \frac{1\,hr}{60\,min} = \frac{2000}{30}$$
$$66.6\,gtt/min \text{ or}$$
$$67\,gtt/min$$

6. 1 L of 5% dextrose in water to run 100 ml/h. The infusion set drop factor is 60 gtt/ml. What is the drip rate?

$$gtt/min = \frac{60\,gtt}{1\,ml} \times \frac{100\,ml}{1\,hr} \times \frac{1\,hr}{60\,min} = 100\,gtt/min$$

7. IV order: 1 unit packed cells (250 ml) to run 4 hours. The drop factor of the infusion set is 10 gtt/ml. What is the drip rate?

$$gtt/min = \frac{10\,gtt}{1\,ml} \times \frac{250\,ml}{4\,hr} \times \frac{1\,hr}{60\,min} = \frac{250}{24} =$$
$$10\,gtt/min.$$

8. IV order: 1000 ml normal saline to run 5 hours. The drop factor of the infusion set is 20 gtt/ml. What is the hourly volume?

$$ml/hr = \frac{1000\,ml}{5\,hr} \times \frac{1\,hr}{1} = 200\,ml$$

What is the drip rate?

$$gtt/min = \frac{\overset{2}{20\,gtt}}{1\,ml} \times \frac{1000\,ml}{5\,hr} \times \frac{1\,hr}{60\,min} = \frac{1000}{15}$$
$$66.6\,gtt/min \quad 3$$
$$\text{or}\ 67\,gtt/min.$$

The IV was started at 5 AM. It is now 7:30 AM and 350 ml remain in the IV bottle. Is the IV on time, infusing too rapidly, or infusing too slowly?

$$ml = \frac{1000ml}{5hr} \times \frac{2.5hr}{1} = \frac{2500}{5} = 500ml$$

$$\begin{array}{r} 1000 \\ -350 \\ \hline 650 \end{array}$$

$650 > 500\ ml$ to fast

If the IV is not on time, recalculate the drip rate.

$$gtt/min = \frac{20\ gtt}{1ml} \times \frac{350ml}{2.5hr} \times \frac{1hr}{60min} =$$

$$\frac{7000}{150} =$$

$$46.6 \quad \text{or } 47\ gtt/min$$

9. 1000 ml lactated Ringer's is to run 8 hours. The infusion set delivers 15 gtt/ml. What is the drip rate?

$$gtt/min = \frac{15\ gtt}{1ml} \times \frac{1000\ ml}{8hr} \times \frac{1hr}{60min} = \frac{125}{4} =$$

$$\begin{array}{c} 31.25 \\ 31\ gtt/min \end{array}$$

10. IV order: 500 ml 5% dextrose in Ringer's lactate q.12h. The drop factor is 15 gtt/ml. What is the drip rate?

$$gtt/min = \frac{15\ gtt}{1ml} \times \frac{500ml}{12hr} \times \frac{1hr}{60min} = \frac{7500}{720}$$

$$10\ gtt/min$$

DOSAGE AND SOLUTION CALCULATIONS IN CLINICAL SPECIALITY SITUATIONS

Unit VIII

INTRAVENOUS MEDICATIONS

OBJECTIVES *Upon completion of this unit, the student will have demonstrated the ability to correctly:*

- Calculate the drip rate of piggyback medications.
- Dilute medications for bolus medication administration.
- Find the dosage per ml for titrated medications.
- Calculate the dosage per minute received by the client on titrated medications.
- Calculate the dosage per kilogram per minute received by the client on titrated medications.
- Compute the drip rate of titrated medications.
- Calculate the maximum safe dosage for the client receiving titrated medications.

Intravenous medications, once used only for critically ill clients, are becoming as common as any other form of medication administration except oral administration. Some intravenous medications are administered by continuous drip. A specific dosage of medication is added to the intravenous fluid and administered for the duration of the infusion. Potassium chloride, added to some of the infusions in Chapter 17, is one example of medication administered by continuous drip.

Calculations for three types of intravenous medication administration are covered in this unit, bolus, piggyback and titrations. Drip rates are the calculations used for piggyback medications. Many bolus medications are diluted for administration. Several calculations are used for titrated intravenous medications.

Chapter 16

Piggyback, Bolus and Titrated Medications

Piggyback medications are added to small volumes of fluid, usually 50 to 200 ml, which infuse over a short period of time. The problems in Chapter 15 that infused in less than an hour were actually piggyback problems. Piggyback medications are given through a port of an existing intravenous site. This port may be in an infusion set line or a heparin lock. Figure 16-1 shows both methods for administering piggyback medications.

Antibiotics are the most common medications administered intravenous piggyback, although bronchodilators, antihypertensives, and other medications may be administered in this manner. Piggybacks almost always infuse in less than an hour. Calculation of the drip rate for piggybacks is the same as any other drip rate. Therefore, the information necessary is the drop factor, volume of fluid, and the time frame. When the time frame is in minutes, the conversion of hour to minutes is not necessary. The equation is as follows:

$$\text{gtt/min} = \frac{\text{drop} \times \text{total amount of piggyback fluid} \times \text{conversion factor}}{\text{factor} \times \text{total time piggyback is to infuse} \times \quad \text{if necessary}}$$

SAMPLE PROBLEM **Mrs. Henderson has the following order: 1 g Keflin q6h. IV PB. Keflin 1 g is prepared by the pharmacy in 100 ml normal saline. The piggyback is to infuse in 30 minutes. The drop factor of the infusion set selected is 20 gtt/ml. What is the drip (flow) rate?**

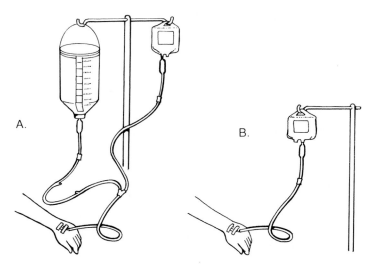

FIGURE 16-1 Piggyback medication administration. The piggyback on the left is administered through an existing infusion line port. The piggyback on the right is administered through a heparin lock.

The IV order means that this piggyback is administered every six hours rather than infusing for six hours.

Knowns: Unit of answer: gtt/min

Factors: 100 ml = 30 min

20 gtts = 1 ml

(The Keflin dosage is extraneous information when solving for drip rate.)

The equation is as follows:

Solve the equation.

$$\frac{gtt}{min} = \frac{20\ gtt \times 100\ ml}{1\ ml \times 30\ min}$$

$$\frac{gtt}{min} = \frac{\overset{2}{\cancel{20}}\ gtt \times 100}{1 \times \underset{3}{\cancel{30}}\ min} = \frac{2\ gtts \times 100}{1 \times 3\ min} = \frac{200\ gtts}{3\ min} = 66.6\ gtt/min$$

The drip rate is 67 gtt/min.

SAMPLE PROBLEM   **Mrs Bronson's IV medication order is methicillin 500 mg IV PB q.4h. Dosage available: methicillin 500 mg in 50 ml solution. The drop factor of the infusion set in 15 gtt/ml. The methicillin is to infuse in 1/3 hour. What is the drip rate?**

The time frame, 1/3 hour, may be converted to 20 minutes prior to setting up the equation or converted within the equation as in this sample.

Knowns: Unit of answer: gtt/min

Factors: 50 ml = 1/3 h

15 gtt = 1 ml

Conversion factor: 1 h = 60 min

The equation is as follows:

Solve the equation.

$$\frac{gtt}{min} = \frac{15\ gtt \times 50\ ml \times 1\ h}{1\ ml \times {}^{1}/_{3}\ h \times 60\ min}$$

$$\frac{gtt}{min} = \frac{15\ gtt \times 50 \times 3 \times 1}{1 \times 1 \times 60\ min} = \frac{15\ gtt \times \overset{5}{\cancel{50}} \times \overset{1}{\cancel{3}} \times 1}{1 \times 1 \times \underset{\underset{2}{\cancel{6}}}{\cancel{60}}\ min}$$

$$= \frac{15\ gtt \times 5 \times 1 \times 1}{1 \times 1 \times 2\ min} = \frac{75\ gtt}{2\ min} = 37.5\ gtt/min$$

The drip rate is 38 gtt/min.

PRACTICE PROBLEMS

Piggyback Medications

Show all your work. Check your answers (page 341).

1. Medication ordered: 200 mg q.i.d. IV PB. Medication available: 200 mg in 50 ml solution. Drop factor: 60 gtt/ml. Infusion time: 30 min. What is the drip rate?

2. Dosage ordered: 0.5 g q.4h. IV PB. Pharmacy supplies 0.5 g in 100 ml solution. Drop factor of the infusion set: 15 gtt/ml. Infusion time: 40 min. What is the drip rate?

3. Ordered: 400 mg b.i.d. IV PB. Medication available: 400 mg in 50 ml normal saline. Infusion set drop factor: 20 gtt/ml. Infusion time: 20 min. What is the drip rate?

4. Dosage ordered: 0.5 g IV piggyback t.i.d. On hand: 0.5 g in 150 ml normal saline. Drop factor: 15 gtt/ml. Infusion time: 40 min. What is the drip rate?

5. Dosage ordered: 250 mg IV PB q.4h. Available: 250 mg/100 ml. Drop factor: 20 gtt/ml. Infusion time: 1/2 hour. What is the drip rate?

6. Ordered: Ampicillin 500 mg IV PB q.4h. On hand: Ampicillin 500 mg in 100 ml solution. Infusion set drop factor: 20 gtt/ml. Ampicillin should infuse within 30 minutes. What is the drip rate?

7. Dosage ordered: gentamycin 80 mg IV PB q.8h. Dosage available: 80 mg in 50 ml NS. Infusion set drop factor: 15 gtt/ml. Gentamycin is to infuse in 20 min. What is the drip rate?

8. Dosage ordered: Keflin 1 g q.4h. IV PB. The pharmacy recommends that the Keflin 1 g in 100 ml solution infuse over 30 min. The drop factor of the infusion set is 15 gtt/ml. What is the drip rate?

9. Medication order: Nafcillin 500 mg q.6h. IV PB. Dosage available: Nafcillin 500 mg in 100 ml solution. The piggyback is to infuse in 15 min. The infusion set delivers 15 gtt/ml. What is the drip rate?

10. Mandol 750 mg IV PB q.6h. Dosage available: Mandol 750 mg in 100 ml solution to infuse in 30 min. Drop factor: 20 gtt/ml. What is the drip rate?

BOLUS MEDICATIONS

A bolus is a specific dosage of medication which is slowly injected directly into an intravenous site. The order for a bolus is sometimes written as "IV push." Many classifications of drugs may be given by bolus. The patient-controlled analgesia (PCA) pump is a form of bolus that allows clients to regulate the amount of pain medication received.

Bolus medications usually are given over a period of several minutes. Some bolus dosages are very small. It is very difficult to administer small volumes over several minutes. Therefore, small volumes of medications are diluted so that the slow intravenous administration can be controlled easily.

Two methods can be used to dilute the medication to the desired dosage per unit: (1) remove the ordered dosage from the vial and add the solvent (usually normal saline or water) in a sufficient quantity (qs) to make the desired total amount or (2) the entire vial or ampule can be diluted so that each volume unit will be the desired dosage.

Three things must be considered when diluting entire vials or ampules of medications: (1) the volume of solution prior to dilution, (2) the dosage per volume unit desired, and (3) the total volume after dilution. To find the amount of solvent to add, subtract the volume available from the total volume of the contents of the vial after dilution. The equation for dilution of the entire vial or ampule is as follows:

$$\text{ml to be added} = \frac{(\text{ desired volume unit } \times \text{ dosage available })}{(\text{ desired dosage } \times \quad 1 \quad)} - \text{ volume available}$$

SAMPLE PROBLEM   **Dosage ordered: morphine sulfate 2 mg IV push over 2 to 3 minutes. Dosage available: 8 mg/ml. The volume containing 2 mg is 0.25 ml, an impossible amount to control for bolus administration. A concentration of 1 mg per ml (or 2 mg per 2 ml) is much easier to control. How much solution will be used to dilute the vial of morphine to a concentration of 1 ml = 1 mg?**

Knowns: Unit of answer: ml to add
       Existing solution: 1 ml
       Factors: 1 ml = 1 mg
            8 mg/1

The equation is as follows:

$$\text{ml to add} = \frac{(\text{ 1 ml } \times \text{ 8 mg })}{(\text{ 1 mg } \times \text{ 1 })} - 1 \text{ ml}$$

Solve the portion within parentheses first. Subtract 1 ml from the solved portion within parentheses.

$$\text{ml to add} = \frac{\overset{(8 \text{ ml})}{(\text{ 1 ml } \times \text{ 8 })} - 1 \text{ ml}}{(\text{ 1 } \times \text{ 1 })} = 7 \text{ ml}$$

Always label, date and initial the new solution.

SAMPLE PROBLEM   **Demerol 5 mg IV push. The *Physician's Desk Reference* recommends a concentration of 10 mg/ ml for slow IV push. Dosage on hand: 50 mg per ml. How much diluting solution must be added to make entire vial dosage 10 mg/ml?**

Knowns: Unit of answer: ml to add
       Existing solution: 1 ml
       Factors: 10 mg = 1 ml
           50 mg/1

The equation is as follows:

$$\text{ml to add} = \frac{(\text{ 1 ml } \times \text{ 50 mg })}{(\text{ 10 mg } \times \text{ 1 })} - 1 \text{ ml}$$

Solve the equation.

$$\text{ml to add} = \frac{\overset{(5 \text{ ml})}{(\text{ 1 ml } \times \text{ 50 })} - 1 \text{ ml}}{(\text{ 10 } \times \text{ 1 })} = 4 \text{ ml to add}$$

Figure 16-2 shows the dilution process for this problem.

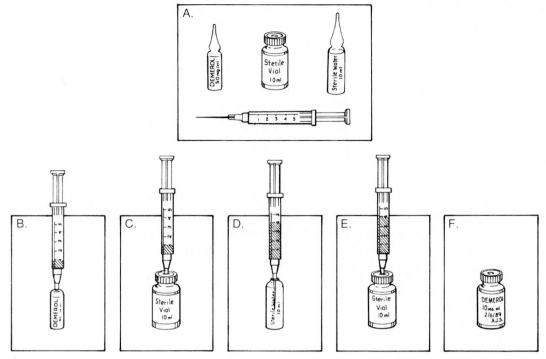

The dilution of medication process

FIGURE 16-2 The dilution of medication process. A, gather supplies. An empty sterile vial is needed to store medication. B, withdraw the 1 ml Demerol from the ampule. C, inject Demerol into empty sterile vial. D, withdraw 4 ml sterile water from ampule. E, inject sterile water from ampule. F, label vial with medication name, dosage per unit, date diluted and initials of person making the dilution.

PRACTICE PROBLEMS

Dilution of Medications

Find the volume of diluting solution to add to the existing medications to obtain the desired dosage per ml. (Answers on page 342).

11. Desired dosage: 2 mg per ml. Dosage available: 10 mg per ml. How much sterile water must be added?

12. Desired dosage: 10 mg per ml. Dosage available: 80 mg per ml. How much sterile normal saline must be added?

13. Desired dosage: 25 mg per 0.5 ml. Dosage available: 3 ml solution in vial labeled 1 ml = 100 mg. How many ml of sterile water must be added?

14. Desired dosage: 100 mcg per ml. Dosage on hand: 0.5 mg per ml. How many ml of sterile normal saline must be added?

15. Desired dosage: 1 mg per ml. Dosage on hand: 10 mg per 5 ml. How many ml of sterile water must be added?

TITRATED MEDICATIONS

Titrated medications are added to specific volumes of fluids and adjusted to infuse at the rate at which the desired effect is obtained. Medications used in titrated infusions are potent and must be monitored very closely. Minute changes in the amounts of these potent medication infusions may bring about the desired therapeutic effect. Therefore, microdrip infusion sets (60 gtt/ml) are used for almost all titrated medications. The nurse must be able to calculate drip rates ordered according to body weight and know the exact amount of medication the client is receiving per minute and/or hour. It is imperative that the nurse knows the amount of medication per milliliter, the maximum dosage, and the maximum drip rate.

Dosage Per Milliliter

The amount of medication per milliliter of infusion solution is very important in titration. The equation for dosage per ml is as follows:

$$\frac{dosage}{ml} = \frac{conversion\ factor \times total\ dosage}{if\ necessary \times total\ volume}$$

SAMPLE PROBLEM **How many micrograms of medication per milligram are in a solution of 1000 ml to which 0.1 g of medication has been added?**

Knowns: Unit of answer: mcg/ml

   Factor: 0.1 g = 1000 ml

   Conversion factors: 1 g = 1000 mg

      1 mg = 1000 mcg

The equation is as follows:

$$\frac{mcg}{ml} = \frac{1000\ mcg \times 1000\ mg \times 0.1\ g}{1\ mg \times 1\ g \times 1000\ ml}$$

Solve the equation.

$$\frac{mcg}{ml} = \frac{\overset{1}{\cancel{1000}}\ mcg \times 1000 \times 0.1}{1 \times 1 \times \underset{1}{\cancel{1000}}\ ml} = \frac{1\ mcg \times 1000 \times 0.1}{1 \times 1 \times 1\ ml} = \frac{100\ mcg}{1\ ml} = 100\ mcg/ml$$

PRACTICE PROBLEMS

Dosage per Milliliter

Show all your work. Check your answers (page 342).

16. How many mcg of medication per ml are in 500 ml of solution to which 20 mg of medication have been added?

17. How many mg of medication per ml are in 250 ml of solution to which 1 g of medication has been added?

18. If 400 mg of dopamine has been added to 500 ml normal saline, how many mcg of dopamine per ml are in this solution?

20. If 200 ml of normal saline contains 250 mg of Aminophyllin, how many mg of Aminophyllin are in 1 ml?

19. If 1000 ml 5% dextrose in water contains 10 U of pitocin, how many mU of pitocin are in 1 ml? (A mU is a milliunit. There are 1000 milliunits per unit.)

Dosage Per Minute

Recommended dosages for titrated medications are usually reported as dosage per kilogram (or pound) per minute. Therefore, it is extremely important that the nurse be aware of the dosage per minute that the client is receiving. The factors required for finding the dosage per minute are the total dosage and volume, the drop factor, the drip rate, and the conversion factors as required. The equation for dosage per minute is as follows:

$$\frac{\text{dosage}}{\text{minute}} = \frac{\text{conversion factor} \times \text{total dosage} \times \text{drop} \times \text{drip}}{\text{if necessary} \times \text{total volume} \times \text{factor} \times \text{rate}}$$

SAMPLE PROBLEM   **Mr. Gregory, a 165 lb male, is receiving intravenous dopamine to regulate his blood pressure. If 500 ml normal saline with dopamine 400 mg is infusing at 15 gtts/min through an infusion set that delivers 60 gtt/ml, what is the dosage in micrograms per minute received by Mr. Gregory?**

Knowns: Unit of Answer: mcg/min
    Factors: 500 ml = 400 mg
              60 gtt = 1 ml
              15 gtts = 1 min
    Conversion factor: 1000 mcg = 1 mg

The equation is as follows:

$$\frac{\text{mcg}}{\text{min}} = \frac{1000 \text{ mcg} \times 400 \text{ mg} \times 1 \text{ ml} \times 15 \text{ gtt}}{1 \text{ mg} \times 500 \text{ ml} \times 60 \text{ gtt} \times 1 \text{ min}}$$

Solve the equation.

$$\frac{\text{mcg}}{\text{min}} = \frac{\overset{2}{\cancel{1000}} \text{ mcg} \times \overset{100}{\cancel{400}} \times 1 \times \overset{1}{\cancel{15}}}{1 \times \underset{1}{\cancel{500}} \times \underset{\underset{1}{\cancel{15}}}{\cancel{60}} \times 1 \text{ min}} = \frac{2 \text{ mcg} \times 100 \times 1 \times 1}{1 \times 1 \times 1 \times 1 \text{ min}} = \frac{200 \text{ mcg}}{1 \text{ min}} = 200 \text{ mcg/min}$$

This means that this 165 lb man is receiving 200 mcg of dopamine per minute. This could also be written 200 mcg/165 lb/min.

SAMPLE PROBLEM   **Mrs. Fitzgerald has an infusion of 1000 ml of D5W with pitocin 10 U for induction of labor. The infusion set drop factor is 60 gtt/ml. The drip rate of the infusion is 36 gtt/min. How many mU of pitocin is Mrs. Fitzgerald receiving per minute?**

Knowns: Unit of answer: mU/min

        Factors: 10 U = 1000 ml

              60 gtt = 1 ml

              36 gtt = 1 min

Conversion factor: 1 U = 1000 mU

The equation is as follows:

$$\frac{mU}{min} = \frac{1000\ mU \times\ 10\ U \times 1\ ml \times 36\ gtt}{1\ U\ \times 1000\ ml \times 60\ gtt \times 1\ min}$$

Solve the equation.

$$\frac{mU}{min} = \frac{\cancel{1000}\ mU \times\ \cancel{10}^{1} \times 1 \times \cancel{36}^{6}}{1\ \times \cancel{1000}^{1} \times \cancel{60}_{1}^{6} \times 1\ min} = \frac{1\ mU \times 1 \times 1 \times 6}{1\ \times 1 \times 1 \times 1\ min} = \frac{6\ mU}{1\ min} = 6\ mU/min$$

PRACTICE PROBLEMS

Dosage per Minute

Show all your work. Check your answers (page 343).

21. An infusion of 1000 ml normal saline with 150 mg medication added is infusing at a rate of 24 gtt/min. The drop factor of the infusion set is 60 gtt/ml. How many mcg per minute is the client receiving?

22. An infusion of 250 ml D5NS with 4000 mcg medication is infusing at a rate of 30 gtt/min. The drop factor of the infusion set is 60 gtt/ml. How many mcg per minute is the client receiving?

23. An infusion of 500 ml of NS with 20 mg of medication is infusing at a rate of 18 gtt/min. The drop factor is 60 gtt/ml. How many mcg is the client receiving per minute?

24. An infusion of 500 ml D5W with 30 U medication is infusing at a drip rate of 26 gtt/min. The drop factor of the infusion set is 60 gtt/ml. How many mU is the client receiving per minute?

25. An infusion of 1000 ml NS with 500 mg medication is infusing at a rate of 33 gtt/min. The drop factor of the infusion set is 60 gtt/ml. How many mcg is the client receiving per minute?

26. An infusion of 1 g lidocaine in 1000 ml D5W is infusing at a rate of 84 gtt/min. The drop factor of the infusion set is 60 gtt/ml. How many mg of lidocaine is the client receiving per minute?

27. An infusion of 250 ml D5W with Nipride 50 mg is infusing at a rate of 57 gtt/min. The infusion set drop factor is 60 gtt/ml. How many mcg of Nipride is the client receiving per minute?

29. An infusion of 500 ml of D5W with 2 mg iso-proterenol is infusing at a rate of 75 gtt/min. The infusion set drop factor is 60 gtt/ml. How many mcg is the client receiving per minute?

28. Dopamine 400 mg in 250 ml normal saline is infusing at a rate of 90 gtt/min. The infusion set delivers 60 gtt/min. How many milligrams per minute are being received by the client?

30. An infusion of 1000 ml D5W with 10 U pitocin is infusing at a rate of 60 gtts/min. The infusion set delivers 60 gtt/ml. How many mU is the client receiving per minute?

Dosage Per Unit Body Weight Per Minute

The recommended dosage of some titrated medication is based on body weight. The nurse may need to know the dosage per kilogram or pound of an infusing medication. When the dosage per minute is known, it is very easy to find the dosage per unit of weight per minute. The equation for finding the dosage per kilogram per minute when the dosage per minute is known is as follows:

$$\frac{\dfrac{\text{dosage}}{\text{unit of weight}}}{\text{minute}} = \frac{\dfrac{\text{dosage}}{\text{client's weight}}}{\text{minutes}} \times \frac{\times \text{ conversion factor}}{\text{if necessary}}$$

The denominator of the fraction in the numerator of the equation will be dropped into the denominator of the equation. It may be easier to set up the problem if the fraction denominator is dropped initially. Then the equation is as follows:

$$\frac{\text{dosage}}{\text{unit of weight (/minute)}} = \frac{\text{dosage}}{\text{client's weight (}\times\text{ minute)}} \times \frac{\times \text{ conversion factor}}{\text{if necessary}}$$

Remember, the fraction denominator (weight) is multiplied by the minutes in the denominator of the equation, not written as weight/minute. Keep the 1 minute separate from the client's weight. The relationship of the numerator unit of the second factor is with the factor denominator unit, weight, not with the minute unit.

SAMPLE PROBLEM   **Mr. Gregory, a 165 pound male, is receiving 400 mg dopamine in 500 ml normal saline which is infusing at a rate of 15 gtt/min. The drop factor of the infusion set is 60 gtt/ml. What is the dosage in micrograms per pound per minute being received by Mr. Gregory?**

This is the same information as a previous sample problem on page 264, in which dosage per minute was found. The answer to that problem was that Mr. Gregory was receiving 200 mcg/min or 200 mcg/165 lb/min.

Knowns: Unit of answer: mcg/lb (/min)

Factor: 200 mcg/165 lb (× min)

The equation is as follows:

$$\frac{\text{mg}}{\text{lb (/min)}} = \frac{200 \text{ mcg}}{165 \text{ lb} \times 1 \text{ min}}$$

Solve the equation.

$$\frac{\text{mg}}{\text{lb (/min)}} = \frac{\overset{40}{\cancel{200}}\ \text{mcg}}{\underset{33}{\cancel{165}}\ \text{lb} \quad \times \quad 1 \ \text{min}} = \frac{40\ \text{mcg}}{33\ \text{lb} \quad \times \quad 1\ \text{min}} = 1.21\ \text{mcg/lb/min}$$

SAMPLE PROBLEM   **Mr. Gregory, who weighs 165 lb, has dopamine 400 mg in 500 ml normal saline infusing at a rate of 15 gtt/min using a drop factor of 60 gtt/ml.   How many micrograms per kilogram per minute is Mr. Gregory recieving?**

This is the same information as the previous sample problem. The client's weight in pounds is converted to kilograms to solve the micrograms per kilogram per minute.

Knowns: Unit of answer: mcg/kg (/min)

Factors: 200 mcg = 165 lb (× min)

Conversion factor: 1 kg = 2.2 lb

The equation is as follows:

$$\frac{\text{mcg}}{\text{kg (/min)}} = \frac{200\ \text{mcg}}{165\ \text{lb} (\times\ \text{min})} \times \frac{2.2\ \text{lb}}{1\ \text{kg}}$$

Solve the equation.

$$\frac{\text{mcg}}{\text{kg (/min)}} = \frac{\overset{8}{\cancel{200}}\ \text{mcg}}{\underset{\underset{3}{\cancel{75}}}{\cancel{165}}} \times \frac{\overset{1}{\cancel{2.2}}}{\times\ \text{min} \times\ 1\ \text{kg}} = \frac{8\ \text{mcg} \times 1}{3 \times\ \text{min} \times\ 1\ \text{kg}} = \frac{8\ \text{mcg}}{3\ \text{kg/min}} = 2.67\ \text{mcg/kg/min}$$

Dosages per unit of weight per minute when the dosage per minute is not known can be solved in one long equation. It is, however, very cumbersome and not recommended. Instead, find the dosage per minute and then the dosage per unit of weight.

PRACTICE PROBLEMS

Dosage per Unit Body Weight per Minute

Problems 31 through 38 have the same information as 21 through 28 with client weight added. (Answers on page 343.)

31. Mrs. Peabody, who weighs 110 pounds, has an infusion of 1000 ml normal saline with 150 mg of medication infusing at a drip rate of 24 gtt/min. The drop factor of the infusion set is 60 gtt/ml. How many mcg/kg/min is Mrs. Peabody receiving?

32. Mrs. Raddison has an infusion of 250 ml D5NS with 4000 mcg medication infusing at a rate of 30 gtt/min. The drop factor of the infusion set is 60 gtt/ml. Mrs. Raddison weighs 60 kilograms. How many mcg/kg/min is Mrs. Raddison receiving?

33. Mrs. Baraboo, who weighs 121 pounds, has an infusion of 500 ml of NS with 20 mg of medication. The drip rate of the IV is 18 gtt/min. The infusion set delivers 60 gtt/ml. What is the dosage in mcg/kg/min for Mrs. Baraboo?

34. Mrs. Flint has an IV of 30 U medication in 500 ml D5W infusing at 26 gtt/min. The drop factor of the infusion set is 60 gtt/ml. Mrs. Flint weighs 130 lb. How many milliunits of medication is Mrs. Flint receiving per kilogram per minute?

35. An infusion of 1000 ml NS with 500 mg medication is infusing at the rate of 33 gtt/min. The drop factor is 60 gtt/ml. The client weighs 50 kg. How many mcg of medication is the client receiving per kilogram per minute?

36. Mr. Grennon has an infusion of 1 g lidocaine in 1000 ml D5W infusing at a rate of 84 gtt/min. The drop factor is 60 gtt/ml. The client weighs 68 Kg. How many mcg is Mr. Grennon receiving per kilogram per minute?

37. Mr. Blake, who weighs 143 lb, has 50 mg Nipride in 250 ml D5W infusing at a rate of 57 gtt/min. The infusion drop factor is 60 gtt/ml. How many mcg/kg/min of Nipride is Mr. Blake receiving?

38. Mrs. Mason has 400 mg dopamine in 250 ml normal saline infusing at a rate of 90 gtt/min. The drop factor of the infusion set is 60 gtt/ml. Mrs. Mason weighs 110 lb. How many mcg per kg per min is Mrs. Mason receiving?

39. Mr. Stetman, who weighs 220 lb, has an IV of 800 mg dopamine in 250 ml normal saline infusing at 42 gtt/min. The drop factor is 60 gtt/ml. How many mcg/kg/min is Mr. Stetman receiving?

40. Mr Burns, who weighs 70 kg, has 2 g lidocaine in 1000 ml D5W infusing at the rate of 51 gtt/min. The drop factor is 60 gtt/ml. How many mcg/kg/min is Mr. Burns receiving?

Drip Rates Based On Dosage Per Body Weight Per Minute

Titrated medications are frequently ordered as *dosage per unit body weight per minute*. The nurse must be able to calculate the drip rates for these medications orders. The drop factor, total volume, total dosage, client's weight, and conversion factors as necessary are required for calculation of drip rates ordered as dosage per body weight per minute. The equation is as follows:

$$\frac{gtt}{min} = \frac{drop}{factor} \times \frac{total\ volume}{total\ dosage} \times \frac{conversion\ factor\ if}{necessary} \times \frac{\left(\dfrac{dosage}{weight\ unit} \times \dfrac{conversion\ factor\ if}{necessary} \times \dfrac{client\ weight}{1}\right)}{(1\ minute)}$$

It may be easier to set up the equation with the fraction denominator dropped into the equation denominator. Then the equation is as follows:

$$\frac{gtt}{min} = \frac{drop}{factor} \times \frac{total\ volume}{total\ dosage} \times \frac{conversion\ factor\ if}{necessary} \times \frac{dosage}{weight\ unit\ (\times\ minute)} \times \frac{conversion\ factor\ if}{necessary} \times \frac{client\ weight}{1}$$

Remember, the weight unit must be multiplied by minutes, not written as weight/minute. This preserves the relationship between the weight unit in the factor denominator and the weight unit in the numerator of the next factor.

SAMPLE PROBLEM   **Mr. Bostick, who weighs 72 kg, has an order for dopamine 5 mcg/kg/min. The intravenous solution of 250 ml D5W contains 400 mg dopamine. The drop factor is 60 gtt/ml. What is the correct drip rate for this IV medication?**

Knowns: Unit of answer: gtt/min

Factors: 60 gtt = 1 ml

   250 ml = 400 mg

   5 mcg/kg/min

   72 kg/1

Conversion factor: 1 mg = 1000 mcg

The equation is as follows:

$$\frac{gtt}{min} = \frac{60\ gtt \times 250\ ml \times \quad 1\ mg \quad \times 5\ mcg \quad\quad \times 72\ kg}{1\ ml \times 400\ mg \times 1000\ mcg \times 1\ kg \quad (\times min) \times \quad 1}$$

Solve the equation.

$$\frac{gtt}{min} = \frac{\overset{3}{\cancel{60}}\ gtt \times \overset{1}{\cancel{250}} \times \quad 1 \times \overset{1}{\cancel{5}} \quad\quad \times \overset{\overset{9}{\cancel{18}}}{\cancel{72}}}{1 \quad \times \underset{\underset{1}{\cancel{20}}}{\cancel{400}} \times \cancel{1000} \times 1\ (\times min) \times \quad 1} = \frac{3\ gtt \times 1 \times 1 \times 1 \quad\quad \times 9}{1 \quad \times 1 \times 1 \times 2(\times min) \times 1} = \frac{27}{2}\frac{gtt}{min}$$

= 13.5 gtt/min

The drip rate is 14 gtt/min.

SAMPLE PROBLEM   **Mr. Hiperted, an 80-year-old man who weighs 154 lb, is to receive nitroprusside 1 mcg/kg/min. Dosage available: nitroprusside Na 50 mg in 250 ml D5W. The drop factor of the infusion set is 60 gtt/ml. What is the drip rate for the IV.**

Knowns: Unit of answer: gtt/min

Factors: 154 lb/1

   50 mg = 250 ml

   60 gtt = 1 ml

   1 mcg/kg/min

Conversion factor: 1 mg = 1000 mcg

   1 kg = 2.2 lb

The equation is as follows:

$$\frac{gtt}{min} = \frac{60\ gtt \times 250\ ml \times \quad 1\ mg \quad \times 1\ mcg \quad\quad \times \quad 1\ kg \times 154\ lb}{1\ ml \times \quad 50\ mg \times 1000\ mcg \times 1\ kg \quad (\times\ min) \times 2.2\ lb \times \quad 1}$$

Solve the equation.

$$\frac{gtt}{min} = \frac{\overset{3}{\cancel{60}}\ gtt \times \overset{\overset{1}{\cancel{5}}}{\cancel{250}} \times \quad 1 \times 1 \quad\quad \times \quad 1 \times \overset{\overset{7}{\cancel{70}}}{\cancel{154}}}{1 \quad \times \underset{\underset{\underset{1}{\cancel{10}}}{\cancel{50}}}{\cancel{50}} \times \cancel{1000} \times 1 \quad \times\ min \times \underset{1}{\cancel{2.2}} \times \quad 1}$$

$$= \frac{3\ gtt \times 1 \times 1 \times 1 \quad\quad \times 1 \times 7}{1 \quad \times 1 \times 1 \times 1 \times min \times 1 \times 1} = \frac{21\ gtt}{1\ min} = 21\ gtt/min$$

PRACTICE PROBLEMS

Drip Rates Based on Dosage per Body Weight per Minute

Show your work. Check your answers (page 344).

41. Dosage ordered: 4 mcg/kg/min. Dosage available: 250 mg in 500 ml. Client weight: 121 lb. Drop factor: 60 gtt/ml. What is the drip rate of this IV medication?

42. Dosage ordered: 0.5 mcg/kg/min. Dosage available: 50 mg in 250 ml. Client weight: 60 kg. Drop factor: 60 gtt/ml. What is the drip rate of this IV medication?

43. Dosage ordered: Nipride 3 mcg/kg/min. Dosage available: Nipride 50 mg in 250 ml D5W. Client weight: 57 kg. Drop factor: 60 gtt/min. What is the drip rate of the IV Nipride?

44. Mr. Roper is started on dopamine at the rate of 2 mcg/kg/min. 250 ml normal saline with dopamine 400 mg is available. Mr. Roper weighs 176 lb. The infusion set drop factor is 60 gtt/ml. What is the drip rate of the dopamine infusion?

45. Dosage ordered: lidocaine 25 mcg/kg/min. Dosage available: lidocaine 2 g in 1000 ml D5W. Client weight: 99 lb. Drop factor: 60 gtt/ml. What is the drip rate of the lidocaine infusion?

Titrated Medications Using Pumps Calibrated for Milliliters Per Hour

Some pumps used for titrated medications are calibrated to deliver milliliters per hour rather than drops per minute. The conversion of minutes to hours is needed. The equation for titrated medications using milliliters per hour is as follows:

$$\frac{ml}{hr} = \frac{\text{total volume} \times \text{conversion factor if necessary} \times \left(\dfrac{\text{dosage} \times \text{conversion factor if} \times \text{client's weight}}{\text{weight unit} \times \text{necessary} \times 1} \Big/ 1\ \text{minute}\right) \times 60\ \text{min}}{\text{total dosage} \times \text{necessary} \times (\ \ \ \ \ ) \times 1\ \text{hour}}$$

Drop the denominator of the fractions in the equation numerator to simplify the equation as follows:

$$\frac{ml}{hr} = \frac{\text{total volume} \times \text{conversion factor if necessary} \times \text{dosage} \times \text{conversion factor if necessary} \times \text{client's weight} \times 60\ \text{min}}{\text{total dosage} \times \text{necessary} \times \text{weight unit} \times \text{necessary} \times 1\ (\times\ \text{minute}) \times 1\ \text{hour}}$$

SAMPLE PROBLEM   **Mr. Bostick, who weighs 72 kg, has an order for dopamine 5 mcg/kg/min. The intravenous solution of 250 ml D5W contains 400 mg dopamine. For how many milliliters per hour is the IV pump set?**

Knowns: Unit of answer: ml/h

Factors: 250 ml = 400 mg

5 mcg/kg/min

72 kg/1

Conversion factor: 1 mg = 1000 mcg

The equation is as follows:

Solve the equation.

$$\frac{ml}{h} = \frac{250\ ml \times 1\ mg \times 5\ mcg \times 72\ kg \times 60\ min}{400\ mg \times 1000\ mcg \times 1\ kg \times 1\ (\times min) \times 1\ h}$$

$$\frac{ml}{h} = \frac{\overset{1}{\cancel{250}}\ ml \times 1 \times \overset{}{5}\ mcg \times \overset{9}{\cancel{72}} \times \overset{\overset{3}{\cancel{6}}}{\cancel{60}}}{\underset{\underset{1}{\cancel{80}}}{\cancel{400}} \times \cancel{1000} \times 1\ kg \times 1\ (\times 1) \times 1\ h} = \frac{1\ ml \times 1 \times 1 \times 9 \times 3}{1 \times 2 \times 1 \times 1 \times 1 \times 1\ h}$$

$$= \frac{27\ ml}{2\ h} = 13.5\ ml/h$$

The above problem is also on page 269. Compare the answers. Note that the ml/h and the gtt/min using an infusion set that delivers 60 gtt/ml are the same quantity. This is not true if a different infusion set is used.

PRACTICE PROBLEMS

Titrated Medications using Pumps Calibrated for Milliliters per Hour

Show all your work. Check your answers (page 345).

46. Dosage ordered: 0.02 mg/kg/min. Dosage available: 100 mg in 500 ml. Client weight: 132 lb. For how many ml/h is the infusion pump set?

47. Dosage ordered: 10 mcg/kg/min. Dosage available: 500 mg in 500 ml. Client weight: 187 lb. The infusion pump is set for how many ml/h?

48. Dosage ordered: 2 mcg/kg/min. Dosage available: 250 mg in 500 ml. Client weight: 143 lb. How many ml/h will be encoded into the infusion pump?

49. Dosage ordered: sodium nitroprusside 7 mcg/kg/min. Dosage available: 50 mg sodium nitroprusside in 250 ml D5W. Client weight: 121 lb. For how many ml/h will the infusion pump be set?

50. Dosage ordered: dopamine 10 mcg/kg/min. Dosage available: 800 mg dopamine in 250 ml normal saline. Client weight: 160 lb. How many ml/h will be entered into the infusion pump's electronics?

Maximum Dosage and Drip Rate

Titrated medications are very potent and can have severe, even life-threatening, toxic effects. It is imperative that nurses know the maximum safe dosage per minute for the client's weight. As the drip rate is increased to obtain the desired effect, the maximum drip rate for the strength of the infusion solution is very important.

The maximum dosage per minute is calculated in the same manner as dosage per minute. Find the maximum dosage per unit of body weight per minute in the reference book and multiply this by the client's weight. The equations are as follows:

$$\frac{dosage}{minute} = \frac{\dfrac{dosage}{weight\ unit} \times \dfrac{conversion\ factors}{if\ necessary} \times \dfrac{client's\ weight}{1}}{\dfrac{minute}{} \times 1}$$

or

$$\frac{dosage}{minute} = \frac{dosage}{weight\ unit\ (\times\ minute)} \times \frac{conversion\ factors}{if\ necessary} \times \frac{client's\ weight}{1}$$

SAMPLE PROBLEM **Mrs. Falk has a dopamine intravenous infusion. She weighs 132 pounds. The *Physician's Desk Reference* (PDR) recommends a dosage of no more than 50 mcg/kg/min. What is the maximum dosage per minute in micrograms for Mrs. Falk?**

Knowns: Unit of answer: mcg/min

Factors: 50 mcg/kg/min

132 lb/1

Conversion factor: 1 kg = 2.2 lb

The equation is as follows:

$$\frac{mcg}{min} = \frac{50\ mcg}{1\ kg\ (\times\ 1\ min)} \times \frac{1\ kg}{2.2\ lb} \times \frac{132\ lb}{1}$$

Solve the equation.

$$\frac{mcg}{min} = \frac{50\ mcg}{1\ (\times\ min)} \times \frac{1}{\cancel{2.2}} \times \frac{\overset{60}{\cancel{132}}}{1} = \frac{50\ mcg}{1} \times \frac{1}{\times\ 1\ min} \times \frac{60}{1} \times 1 = \frac{3000\ mcg}{1\ min} = 3000\ mcg/min$$

Some maximum dosages are not based on weight. For instance, the maximum recommended dosage for pitocin is 20 microunits (0.02 units) per minute. No calculation is needed for these dosages.

PRACTICE PROBLEMS

Maximum Recommended Dosage per Minute

Show all your work. Check your answers (page 346).

51. The maximum recommended dosage is 3 mcg/kg/min. Client weight: 165 lb. What is the maximum dosage per minute?

54. The PDR recommends that Nipride is not to exceed 10 mcg/kg/min. The client weighs 198 lb. What is the maximum dosage of Nipride per minute for this client?

52. Maximum recommended dosage: 5 mcg/kg/min. Client weight: 68 kg. What is the maximum dosage per minute?

55. The PDR recommends the maximum dosage for lidocaine is 50 mg/kg/min. The client weighs 154 lb. What is the maximum recommended dosage for lidocaine per minute?

53. Maximum recommended dosage: 8 mcg/kg/min. Client weight: 187 lb. What is the maximum dosage per minute?

Maximum Drip Rates

When the maximum dosage is known, the equation for maximum drip rate is as follows:

$$\frac{gtt}{min} = \frac{drop}{factor} \times \frac{total\ volume}{total\ dosage} \times \frac{conversion\ factor}{if\ necessary} \times \frac{dosage}{per\ minute}$$

The equation for maximum drip rate when the maximum dosage is not known is

$$\frac{qtt}{min} = \frac{drop}{factor} \times \frac{total\ volume}{total\ dosage} \times \frac{conversion\ factor\ if\ necessary}{} \times \frac{dosage}{unit\ weight\ (\times\ minute)} \times \frac{conversion\ factor\ if\ necessary}{} \times \frac{client\ weight}{1}$$

SAMPLE PROBLEM **Mrs. Falk, who weighs 132 lb, has an infusion of dopamine 800 mg in 250 ml normal saline. The PDR recommends that the maximum dosage of dopamine is 50 mcg/kg/min. The drop factor is 60 gtt/min. What is the maximum drip rate for this client?**

The maximum dosage for this client (3000 mcg/min) was found in a previous sample problem.

Knowns: Unit of answer: gtt/min

Factors: 3000 mcg = 1 min

60 gtt = 1 ml

800 mg = 250 ml

Conversion factor: 1 mg = 1000 mcg

The equation is as follows:

Solve the equation.

$$\frac{gtt}{min} = \frac{60 \ gtt \times 250 \ ml \times 1 \ mg \times 3000 \ mcg}{1 \ ml \times 800 \ mg \times 1000 \ mcg \times 1 \ min}$$

$$\frac{gtt}{min} = \frac{\overset{3}{\cancel{60}} \ gtt \times \overset{25}{\cancel{250}} \times 1 \times \overset{3}{\cancel{3000}}}{1 \times \underset{\underset{4}{\cancel{40}}}{\cancel{800}} \times \underset{1}{\cancel{1000}} \times 1 \ min} = \frac{3 \ gtt \times 25 \times 1 \times 3}{1 \times 4 \times 1 \times 1 \ min} = \frac{225 \ gtt}{4 \ min} = 56.25 \ gtt/min$$

The maximum drip rate of Mrs. Falk's dopamine infusion is 57 gtt/min.

SAMPLE PROBLEM **Mrs. Slade, who weighs 51 kg, has an infusion of Nipride 50 mg in 250 ml D5W. The drop factor is 60 gtt/ml. The PDR states that the Nipride dosage is not to exceed 10 mcg/kg/min. What is the maximum drip rate for this infusion?**

Knowns: Unit of answer: gtt/min
Factors: 10 mcg/kg/min
50 mg = 250 ml
60 gtt = 1 ml
51 kg/1
Conversion factor: 1 mg = 1000 mcg
The equation is as follows:

$$\frac{gtt}{min} = \frac{60 \ gtt \times 250 \ ml \times 1 \ mg \times 10 \ mcg \times 51 \ kg}{1 \ ml \times 50 \ mg \times 1000 \ mcg \times 1 \ kg \ (\times 1 \ min) \times 1}$$

Solve the equation.

$$\frac{gtt}{min} = \frac{\overset{3}{\cancel{60}} \ gtt \times \overset{\cancel{5}}{\cancel{250}} \times 1 \times \overset{1}{\cancel{10}} \times 51}{1 \times \cancel{50} \times \cancel{1000} \times 1 \ (\times 1 \ min) \times 1}$$

$$= \frac{3 \ gtt \times 1 \times 1 \times 1 \times 51}{1 \times 1 \times 1 \times 1 \ (\times 1 \ min) \times 1} = \frac{153 \ gtt}{1 \ min} = 153 \ gtt/min$$

The maximum drip rate for Mrs. Slade's Nipride infusion is 153 gtt/min.

PRACTICE PROBLEMS

Maximum Drip Rates

Problems 56 through 58 have the same information as problems 51 through 53. (Answers on page 346.)

56. The client has a 250 ml infusion with 100 mg medication. Client weight: 165 lb. The drop factor is 60 gtt/ml. The maximum recommended dosage is 3 mcg/kg/min. What is the maximum drip rate of this infusion?

57. Mrs. Tewes has an infusion of 500 mg medication in 500 ml solution. The drop factor is 60 gtt/ml. The client weighs 68 kg. The maximum recommended dosage is 5 mcg/kg/min. What is the maximum drip rate for this infusion?

58. Mr. Barnes, who weighs 187 lb, has an infusion of 100 mg medication in 250 ml solution. The drop factor is 60 gtt/ml. The maximum recommended dosage is 8 mcg/kg/min. What is the maximum drip rate of this infusion?

59. Mrs. Harrington, who weighs 48 kg, has an infusion of 250 ml normal saline with 400 mg dopamine. The drop factor is 60 gtt/ml. The maximum recommended dosage is 50 mcg/kg/min. What is the maximum drip rate for this IV?

60. Mr. Pasch, who weighs 168 lb, has an infusion of 500 ml D5W with 1 g lidocaine infusing using a drop factor of 60 gtt/ml. The manufacturer recommends a maximum dosage of 50 mcg/kg/min. What is the maximum drip rate for this lidocaine infusion?

SELF-ASSESSMENT POSTTEST

Piggyback, Bolus and Titrated Medications

Show all your work. Check your answers (page 364).

1. IV medication order: ampicillin 500 mg IV PB q.6h. Dosage available: 500 mg in 100 ml D5W. Infusion set drop factor: 20 gtt/ml. Ampicillin is to administered in 30 min. What is the drip rate?

2. IV medication order: morphine sulfate 4 mg IV push stat. Dosage available: 10 mg/ml in 1 ml vial. Morphine by bolus should be administered over several minutes. Calculate the amount of normal saline solution to add to the morphine vial so that the entire contents yields 1 mg/ml.

3. IV medication order: lidocaine 1 g in 500 ml D5W to run at 20 mcg/kg/min. The client weighs 154 lb. The drop factor is 60 gtt/ml.
   a. What is the dosage per ml of the IV solution?

   b. What is the dosage per minute for this client?

   c. What is the drip rate of this IV medication?

   d. The only infusion pump available is calibrated for ml/h. How many ml/h is entered into the pump's electronics?

4. The maximum dosage recommended for lidocaine is 50 mcg/kg/min.
   a. What is the maximum dosage per minute for the client in problem 3?

   b. What is the maximum drip rate of this IV medication for the client in problem 3?

5. IV medication order: Aminophyllin 250 mg IV PB q.6.h. Dosage available: 250 mg in 100 ml normal saline. The drop factor is 15 gtt/ml. The IV is to infuse in 20 min. What is the drip rate?

6. An infusion of sodium nitroprusside 50 mg in 500 ml D5W is infusing at 18 gtt/min using an infusion set that delivers 60 gtt/ml. The client weighs 180 lb.
   a. What is the dosage in micrograms per minute the client is receiving?

   b. What is the dosage per kilogram per minute that this client is receiving?

.7. Mrs. Carter has an infusion of 250 ml NS with 250 mg medication infusing through an infusion pump calibrated for ml/h. The IV medication order is 150 mcg/min. The client weighs 182 lb. For how many ml/h is the pump set?

8. An infusion of 10 U pitocin in 1 liter D5W is infusing at the rate of 26 gtt/min. The drop factor is 60 gtt/ml. The maximum recommended dosage of pitocin is 20 mU per minute.
   a. What is the dosage per minute for this infusion?

   b. Is the infusing dosage within the recommended dosage for pitocin?

9. IV medication order: 12 mcg/kg/min. Client weight: 70 kg. The IV is supplied as 500 mg medication in 500 ml 5% dextrose in water. The drop factor is 60 gtt/ml. What is the drip rate of this IV medication?

10. IV medication order: dopamine 2 mcg/kg/min. Medication available: dopamine 400 mg in 250 ml NS. The drop factor is 60 gtt/ml. Client weight: 154 lb. What is the drip rate of this IV medication?

UNIT VIII POSTTEST

Intravenous Medications

Show all your work. Check your answers (page 387).

1. An IV of 500 ml normal saline contains 20 mg of an antihypertensive drug. How many micrograms of the drug are there per milliliter?

2. Mrs. Jones has an IV of 1000 ml 5% dextrose in water with 10 U pitocin infusing at 28 gtt/min using an infusion set that delivers 60 gtt/ml. How much medication is Mrs. Jones receiving per minute?

Situation: Mr. Wentworth has an intravenous medication order of Pronestyl 50 mcg/kg/min. The infusion contains 1 g Pronestyl in 500 ml D5W. The drop factor is 60 gtt/ml. Mr. Wentworth weighs 176 lb. Questions 3, 4 and 5 pertain to this infusion:

3. What is the drip rate for this IV medication?

4. How many mcg of medication is Mr. Wentworth receiving per minute?

5. What is the dosage in mcg per ml of Pronestyl in this infusion?

6. Mrs. Valdo is to receive 500 mg methicillin every 4 hours IV PB. The dosage available is methicillin 500 mg in 50 ml D5W. The drop factor is 15 gtt/ml. What is the drip rate of the IV if it is to complete in 30 min?

Situation: Mr. Brown is receiving an IV of 1000 ml normal saline with 200 mg medication which is infusing at 20 gtt/min. The drop factor of the infusion set is 60 gtt/ml. Mr. Brown weighs 67 kg. Questions 7, 8 and 9 pertain to this situation.

7. How many micrograms per minute is the patient receiving?

8. What is the dosage per kg per min that Mr. Brown is receiving?

9. The manufacturer recommends that this medication not exceed 3 mcg/kg/min. Is Mr. Brown's dosage within the recommended dosage?

Situation: Mr. Day, who weighs 187 lb, is receiving Nipride 50 mg in 500 ml 5% dextrose in water at a rate of 18 gtt/min. The drop factor of the infusion set is 60 gtt/ml. The dosage of Nipride is not to exceed 10 mcg/kg/min. Questions 10, 11 and 12 pertain to this situation.

10. How many micrograms of Nipride are there per milliliter?

11. How many micrograms is Mr. Day receiving per minute?

12. Is Mr. Day's dosage within the recommended dosage?

Situation: Mrs. Clay has an IV of 500 ml normal saline with 5 mg medication infusing at 24 gtt/min. The drop factor of the infusion set is 60 gtt/min. The maximum safe dosage is 0.08 mcg/kg/min. Mrs. Clay weighs 121 lb. Questions 13, 14 and 15 pertain to this situation.

13. How many micrograms is Mrs. Clay receiving per minute?

14. What is the maximum dosage in mcg/min Mrs. Clay could receive?

15. What would be the drip rate if the IV were infusing at the maximum safe dosage?

16. Dosage ordered: 0.2 mcg/kg/min. Client's weight: 132 lb. Medication available: 10 mg/500 ml. The infusion pump is calibrated for ml/h. For how many ml/h is the pump set?

17. Dosage ordered: 0.4 mcg/kg/min. Client's weight: 110 lb. Medication supplied: 60 mg/500 ml. Drop factor: 60 gtt/ml. What is the drip rate?

18. Dosage ordered: 12 mcg/kg/min. Client's weight: 70 kg. Medication supplied: 500 mg/500 ml. The infusion pump is calibrated for ml/h. How many ml/h are entered into the pump's electronics?

19. The drip rate of an IV of 250 ml normal saline with 100 mg medication is 46 gtt/min. The drop factor is 60 gtt/ml. How many micrograms of medication is the client receiving per minute?

20. The drip rate of an IV of 500 ml normal saline with 250 mg medication is 22 gtt/min. The drop factor is 60 gtt/ml. The client weighs 66 kg. What is the dosage in micrograms per kilogram per minute that the client is receiving?

Unit IX

Pediatric Calculations

OBJECTIVES   *At the completion of this unit, the student will have demonstrated the ability to:*

- Calculate pediatric dosages based on weight.

- Calculate pediatric dosages based on body surface area.

- Compare dosages ordered with recommended dosage ranges for pediatric clients.

- Recall Clark's, Young's, Fried's and the Surface Area Rules of pediatric dosage calculation and comparison.

- Solve pediatric intravenous fluid problems.

Medications and fluids for pediatric clients must be administered with extreme caution. Immaturity of the organ systems, especially the liver and kidneys, affects metabolism and excretion. Toxicity can develop very rapidly or unexpectedly. Knowledge of fluid and caloric requirements is important for the pediatric nurse as fluid overload and dehydration may occur.

Chapter 17

Pediatric Medications and Intravenous Fluids

The current trend in pediatric medication administration is to administer medications orally or intravenously whenever possible. Some medications, especially immunizations, must be administered intramuscularly or subcutaneously. Many medications are available in liquid form for the pediatric client.

The equation for calculation of pediatric dosages is the same as any other dosage calculation equation. To recapitulate, the equation is as follows:

$$\begin{array}{c}\text{unit and} \\ \text{amount to} \\ \text{administer}\end{array} = \dfrac{\begin{array}{c}\text{conversion} \\ \text{factor if} \\ \text{necessary}\end{array} \times \begin{array}{c}\text{amount} \\ \text{available} \\ \times \text{ dosage} \\ \text{available}\end{array} \times \begin{array}{c}\text{conversion} \\ \text{factor if} \\ \text{necessary}\end{array} \times \begin{array}{c}\text{ordered} \\ \text{dosage} \\ \times \quad 1\end{array}}{}$$

Refer to Unit IV for calculation of dosages, if necessary.

Most recommended pediatric dosages are based on body weight. Prior to administering any medication, the client's dosage is compared with the recommended dosage. Even small mistakes in medication dosages can be detrimental to infants and small children. Differences between recommended and ordered dosages are always brought to the attention of physicians and recorded on the nursing or progress notes.

Calculation of recommended dosages based on body weight is covered in Chapter 13. The equations are as follows:

Dosage per day:

$$\frac{\text{dosage}}{\text{day}} = \frac{\text{dosage} \times \text{number doses}}{1 \text{ dose} \quad \times \ 1 \text{ day}}$$

or

$$\frac{\text{dosage}}{\text{day}} = \frac{\text{dosage} \quad \times 24 \text{ hours}}{(q) \text{ hours} \times \ 1 \text{ day}}$$

Recommended dosage:

$$\text{dosage(/day)} = \frac{\begin{array}{c}\text{conversion} \\ \text{factor if} \times \\ \text{necessary} \times\end{array} \begin{array}{c}\text{dosage} \times \\ \text{unit weight} \times\end{array} \begin{array}{c}\text{conversion} \\ \text{factor if} \times \\ \text{necessary} \times\end{array} \begin{array}{c}\text{client's} \\ \text{weight} \\ 1\end{array}}{}$$

SAMPLE PROBLEM   **Mary, who weighs 22 lb, has an order for Furadantin 12.5 mg q.i.d. PO. The recommended dosage is 5 to 7 mg/kg/day. Is Mary's dosage within the recommended range?**

Solve for client's dosage per day.

Knowns: Unit of answer: mg/day

Factors: 12.5 mg = 1 dose

4 doses = 1 day

The equation for client dosage per day is:

$$\frac{\text{mg}}{\text{day}} = \frac{12.5\,\text{mg} \quad \times 4\,\text{doses}}{1\,\text{dose}\ \times 1\,\text{day}} = \frac{12.5\,\text{mg} \quad \times 4}{1 \quad \times 1\,\text{day}} = \frac{50\,\text{mg}}{1\,\text{day}} = 50\,\text{mg/day}$$

Solve for recommended dosage per day. Since this is a range, there will be two answers. Solve for minimum dosage per day.

Knowns: **Unit of answer: mg (/d)**
   Factors: **5 mg = 1 kg**
                                  22 lb/1
   Conversion factor: 1 kg = 2.2 lb

The equation for low range of the recommended dosage per day is:

$$\text{mg (/d)} = \frac{5\,\text{mg} \times\ \ 1\,\text{kg}\ \times 22\,\text{lb}}{1\,\text{kg}\ \times 2.2\,\text{lb}\ \times\ \ 1} = \frac{5\,\text{mg} \times\ \ 1 \times \overset{10}{\cancel{22}}}{1\quad \times \cancel{2.2} \times\ \ 1} = \frac{50\,\text{mg}}{1} = 50\,\text{mg (/d)}$$

Solve for maximum dosage per day.

Knowns: **Unit of answer: mg (/d)**
   Factors: **7 mg = 1 kg**
                                  22 lb/1
   Conversion factor: 1 kg = 2.2 lb

The equation for the high range of the recommended dosage per day is:

$$\text{mg (/d)} = \frac{7\,\text{mg} \times\ \ 1\,\text{kg}\ \times 22\,\text{lb}}{1\,\text{kg}\ \times 2.2\,\text{lb}\ \times\ \ 1} = \frac{7\,\text{mg} \times\ \ 1 \times \overset{10}{\cancel{22}}}{1\quad \times \cancel{2.2} \times\ \ 1} = \frac{70\,\text{mg}}{1} = 70\,\text{mg (/d)}$$

The ordered dosage, 50 mg per day, is within the recommended range of 50 to 70 mg/d.

SAMPLE PROBLEM   **Kerry, who weighs 8 lb 9 oz, has an order for Narcan 35 mcg stat. The recommended dosage is 0.01 mg/kg. Is the ordered dosage compatible with the recommended dosage?**

This is a one-time order; therefore, the only calculation that must be made is the recommended dosage calculation. Remember, there are 16 oz in each pound. Therefore, 8 lb 9 oz can be written as 8 $9/16$ lb.

Knowns: **Unit of answer: mcg**
   Factors: **0.01 mg = 1 kg**
                                  8 $9/16$ lb/1
   Conversion factors: 1 mg = 1000 mcg
                                     1 kg = 2.2 lb

The equation for recommended dosage is:

$$\text{mcg} = \frac{1000\,\text{mcg} \times 0.01\,\text{mg}\ \times\ \ 1\,\text{kg}\ \ \times 8^{9/16}\,\text{lb}}{1\,\text{mg}\ \times\ \ 1\,\text{kg}\ \times 2.2\,\text{lb}\ \times\ \ 1}$$

$$= \frac{1000\,\text{mcg} \times 0.01 \times\ \ 1 \times {}^{137}/16}{1\quad \times\ \ 1 \times 2.2 \times\ \ 1} = \frac{\overset{125}{\cancel{1000}}\,\text{mcg} \times 0.01 \times\ \ 1 \times 137}{1\quad \times\ \ 1 \times 2.2 \times \underset{2}{\cancel{16}}} = \frac{171.25\,\text{mcg}}{4.4} = 38.9\,\text{mcg}$$

Compare the ordered dosage with the recommended dosage:
   Ordered: 35 mcg   Recommended: 38.9 mcg
The ordered dosage is slightly less than the recommended dosage.

SAMPLE PROBLEM   **Tracy weighs 5725 grams. She is to be given an IV injection of Lasix. The recommended dosage is 1 mg/kg. What should Tracy's dosage be?**

Knowns: **Unit of answer: mg**

  Factors: **1 mg = 1 kg**

                      5725 g/1

  Conversion factor: 1 kg = 1000 g

The equation for the dosage is:

$$\text{mg} = \frac{1 \text{ mg} \times \quad 1 \text{ kg} \quad \times 5725 \text{ g}}{1 \text{ kg} \times 1000 \text{ gm} \times \quad 1 \text{ g}} = \frac{1 \text{ mg} \times \quad 1 \times 5725}{1 \quad \times 1000 \times \quad 1} = \frac{5725 \text{ mg}}{1000} = 5.725 \text{ mg}$$

Lasix is available in 2 ml ampules labeled 10 mg/ml. How many ml will be administered?

Knowns: **Unit of answer: ml**

  Factors: 10 mg = 1 ml

        5.7 mg/1

The equation for the amount is:

$$\text{ml} = \frac{1 \text{ ml} \times 5.7 \text{ mg}}{10 \text{ mg} \times \quad 1 \text{ mg}} = \frac{1 \text{ ml} \times 5.7}{10 \quad \times 1} = \frac{5.7 \text{ ml}}{10} = 0.57 \text{ ml}$$

PRACTICE PROBLEMS

Pediatric Dosages Based on Body Weight

Show all your work. Check your answers (page 347).

1. Bette weighs 5710 grams. She is to receive 0.1 mg medication q.8h. The recommended dosage is 0.04 to 0.06 mg per kg per day. What is the recommended dosage range for this client?

   Is Bette's dosage within the recommended range?

2. Johnnie weighs 16 lb 8 oz. He is to receive 0.6 mg/kg/day. What will his dosage be?

3. Bernie weighs 33 lb. His medication order is 6 mcg q.d. PO. The recommended dosage is 0.3 to 0.5 mcg/kg/day. What is the recommended dosage range for this client?

   Is Bernie's dosage within the recommended range?

4. Gracie's medication order is ampicillin 150 mg q.6h. The PDR lists a dosage of 50 mg/kg/day for clients up to 20 kg. Gracie weighs 26 lb. What is the recommended daily dosage for her?

What is Gracie's daily dosage?

The ordered dosage is 50 mg q.12h. PO. Is this dosage within the recommended range?

5. The recommended maintenance dosage for Dilantin is 4 to 8 mg/kg/day in two or three equally divided doses. What would be the daily dosage range for a child who weighs 43 pounds?

Dilantin suspension is available as 30 mg/5 ml. How much Dilantin will be given to this child?

DOSAGES BASED ON BODY SURFACE AREA

The dosage of some medications, such as some oncology agents, are calculated using body surface area in square meters (m^2). The client's weight and height are used to find the body surface area. A nomogram, shown in Figure 17-1, is used to find the square meters of body surface area (BSA).

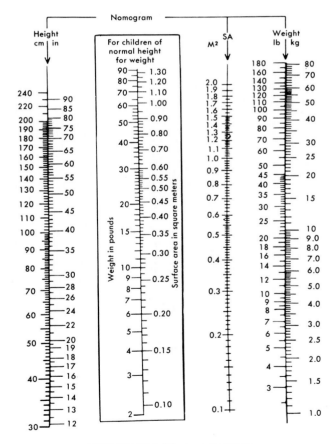

FIGURE 17-1 West nomogram

The recommended dosage is calculated according to the following equation:

$$\text{recommended dosage} = \frac{\begin{array}{c}\text{conversion}\\\text{factor if} \times\\\text{necessary} \times\end{array} \begin{array}{c}\\\text{dosage} \times\\\text{square meter} \times\end{array} \begin{array}{c}\text{client's BSA in}\\\text{square meters}\\1\end{array}}{}$$

SAMPLE PROBLEM   **4: Johnnie weighs 30 pounds and is 35 inches tall. He is to receive lomustine 130 mg per square meter every six weeks. How much will his dosage be?**

First, find the square meters of BSA on the nomogram as shown in Figure 17-2. Use a straight edge to make a straight line from 35 inches to 30 pounds. Read the square meters at the point where the line passes through the SA line, 0.59 square meters. (Note: Usually lines are not drawn on the nomogram so that the nomogram can be used again.)

Solve for dosage.

Knowns: **Unit of answer: mg**
        Factors: **130 mg = 1 m^2**
                0.59/1

The equation is as follows:

$$mg = \frac{130 \text{ mg} \times 0.59 \text{ m}^2}{1 \text{ m}^2 \times 1} = \frac{130 \text{ mg} \times 0.59}{1 \times 1} = 76.7 \text{ mg}$$

The boxed area in the nomogram is used for children whose weight and height are consistent with average height and weight. Figure 17-3 show the BSA of a child who weighs 44 pounds and is 45 inches tall. Note the arrow in the boxed area points to 44 and 0.8 square meters, as does the longer line through 44 pounds and 45 inches.

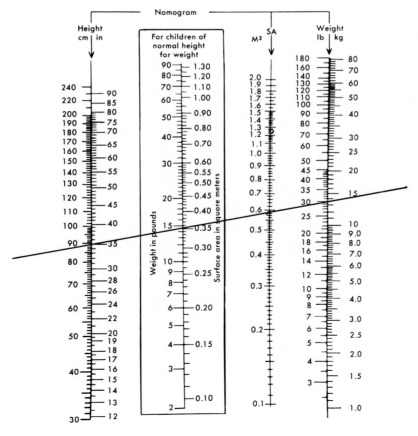

FIGURE 17-2 West nomogram for child weighing 30 pounds who is 35 inches tall

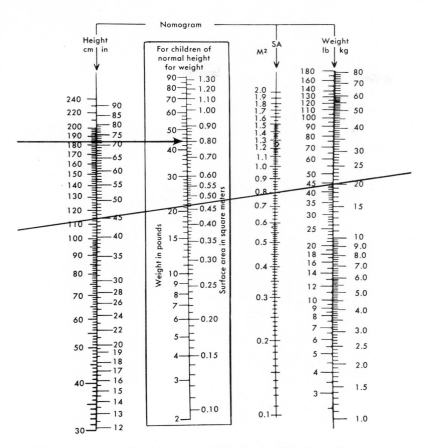

FIGURE 17-3 West nomogram for 44 pound child who is 45 inches tall

---

PRACTICE PROBLEMS

Dosages Based on Body Surface Area

(Answers on page 348.)

Situation: Missy weighs 70 pounds and is 50 inches tall. She is to receive cytarabine 200 mg per square meter BSA IV q.d. for 5 days. Questions 6 and 7 pertain to this situation.

6. Using the nomogram in Figure 17-4, find the body surface area (BSA) in square meters for Missy.

Situation: Robbie weighs 50 pounds and is 46 inches tall. He is to receive daunorubicin 25 mg IV per square meter BSA and vincristine 1.5 mg IV per square meter BSA today. Questions 8, 9 and 10 pertain to this situation.

8. Find the BSA for Robbie using the nomogram in Figure 17-4.

7. What is Missy's dosage using the square meters recorded in the SA column?

9. Find Robbie's dosage for the daunorubicin.

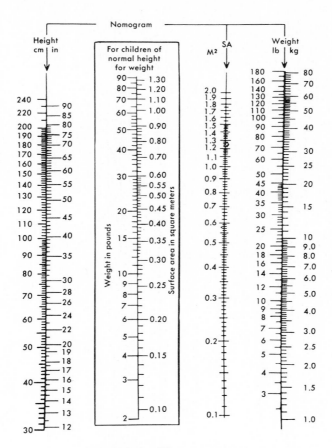

FIGURE 17-4 West nomogram

10. Find Robbie's dosage for vincristine.

PEDIATRIC DOSAGE RULES

Over the years, four rules have been developed to give a rough estimate of the acceptability of pediatric dosages. Although they are rarely used today, nurses are expected to be aware of these rules.

Clark's Rule: Gives a rough estimate of the acceptability of dosages based on the child's weight as compared to an adult dose. It presumes that the average adult weight is 150 pounds. The formula is as follows:

$$\text{child's dose} = \frac{\text{child's weight}}{150} \times \text{adult dose}$$

This could be written as follows for dimensional analysis method:

$$\text{Child's dose unit} = \frac{\text{adult dose \& unit} \times \text{child's weight in pounds}}{150 \text{ pounds} \times \qquad 1}$$

Fried's Rule: This rule provides a rough estimate of appropriateness of pediatric dosages based on the age of the child in months. It assumes that adult dosages are given when the child reaches 150 months or 12.5 years of age. The formula for Fried's rule is as follows:

$$\text{Child's dose} = \frac{\text{child's age in months}}{150} \times \text{adult dose}$$

This may be written as follows for the dimensional analysis method:

$$\text{Child's dose unit} = \frac{\text{Adult dose \& unit} \times \text{child's age in months}}{150 \text{ months} \times \qquad 1}$$

Young's Rule: This rule provides a rough estimate of an acceptable pediatric dosage based on the child's age in years. The adult's age is considered to be 12 years added to the child's age. The formula for this rule is as follows:

$$\text{Child's dose} = \frac{\text{child's age in years}}{\text{child's age in years} + 12} \times \text{adult dose}$$

This can be written in dimensional analysis equation as follows:

$$\text{Child's dose \& unit} = \frac{\text{adult dose \& unit} \times \text{child's age in years}}{\text{child's age in years} + 12 \times \qquad 1}$$

Surface Area Rule: Of the four rules, the surface area method provides the most accurate method of estimating pediatric dosages. The nomogram is used to find the child's surface area. An adult's surface area is assumed to be 1.7 square meters. The formula for this rule is as follows:

$$\text{Child's dose} = \frac{\text{child's body surface area in m}^2}{1.7} \times \text{adult dose}$$

This formula in dimensional analysis is:

$$\text{Child's dose unit} = \frac{\text{adult dose \& unit} \times \text{child's body surface area in m}^2}{1.7 \text{ m}^2 \times \qquad 1}$$

Do not memorize these rules; pharmaceutical companies provide information on pediatric dosages. Nurses are expected to know, however, that Clark's Rule is based on the child's weight, Fried's and Young's Rules are based on the child's age in months and years, respectively, and the Surface Area Rule is based on the child's body surface area in square meters.

PEDIATRIC INTRAVENOUS FLUID CALCULATIONS

Pediatric clients receiving intravenous fluids must be monitored very closely. Infusion pumps are usually used to aid this monitoring. Two types of infusion pumps are in use today. One is set to deliver a specific number of drops per minute; microdrip (minidrip) infusion sets delivering 60 drops per milliliter are used with this pump. The other pump is a precision-controlled syringe pump that delivers very small amounts of solution over a specific time frame. This pump uses calibrations of volume per hour.

The infusion sets most commonly used in pediatrics have calibrated volume control chambers, called *burets* or *volutrols*, which provide additional safety. Specific amounts of fluid, usually the fluid to infuse in one hour, are run into this chamber, pictured in Figure 17-5.

Pediatric infusions are usually ordered in milliliters per hour. Remember, calculation of intravenous fluid drip rates requires the volume per time frame and the drop factor of the infusion set. The drip rate is always recorded as drops per minute. The equation is as follows:

$$\text{gtt/min} = \frac{\text{drop} \times \text{IV fluid} \times \text{amount hours to}}{\text{factor} \times \text{time IV is} \times \text{minutes if}}$$
$$\text{to infuse} \qquad \text{necessary}$$

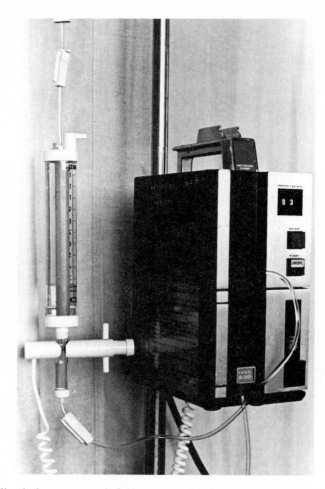

FIGURE 17-5 Pediatric intravenous infusion set and infusion pump. The infusion set has a volume control chamber (buret). The infusion pump is calibrated for drip rates. (From Whaley, L.F., and Wong, D.L.: Nursing care of infants and children, ed. 3, St. Louis, 1987, The C.V. Mosby Co.)

SAMPLE PROBLEM   **IV order: D5NS 25 ml per hour. Infusion set drop factor: 60 gtt/ml. What is the drip rate?**

Knowns: Unit of answer: gtt/min

Factors: 60 gtt = 1 ml

25 ml = 1 h

Conversion factor: 1 h = 60 min

The equation is as follows:

$$\frac{gtt}{min} = \frac{60\ gtt \times 25\ ml \times 1\ h}{1\ ml \times 1\ h \times 60\ min} = \frac{\overset{1}{\cancel{60}}\ gtt \times 25 \times 1}{1 \times 1 \times \underset{1}{\cancel{60}}\ min} = \frac{25\ gtt}{1\ min} = 25\ gtt/min$$

Pediatric intravenous medications may be administered by the same methods as adult intravenous medications, continuous drip, bolus, piggyback, and titrations. In addition, medications compatible with the infusion solution may be added to the buret and run for short periods of time. The amount of total fluid in the buret must be compatible with the amount of fluid to be infused during the time frame this medication is to infuse.

SAMPLE PROBLEM   **IV medication order: gentamycin 20 mg q.8h. per buret over 30 minutes. IV fluid order: D5W 50 ml/h. The drop factor is 60 gtt/ml. How much total fluid should be in the buret for the IV medication to infuse in 30 minutes?**

Knowns: **Unit of answer: ml**

Factor: **50 ml = 1 hr**

                30 min/1

Conversion factor: 1 h = 60 min

The equation is as follows:

$$
ml = \frac{50\ ml \times 1\ h \times 30\ min}{1\ h \times 60\ min \times 1} = \frac{\overset{25}{\cancel{50}}\ ml \times 1 \times \overset{1}{\cancel{30}}}{1 \times \underset{\underset{1}{2}}{\cancel{60}} \times 1} = \frac{25\ ml \times 1 \times 1}{1 \times 1 \times 1} = \frac{25\ ml}{1} = 25\ ml
$$

PRACTICE PROBLEMS

Pediatric Intravenous Infusion Calculations

Show all your work. Check your answers (page 348).

11. Mary has the following orders: (1) 5% dextrose in 0.45% normal saline 60 ml/h IV and (2) ampicillin 100 mg IV via buret q.6h. The drop factor of the buret infusion set is 60 gtt/ml.
What is the drip rate for this infusion?

How many ml solution should be in the buret for the ampicillin to infuse in 20 minutes?

12. Marla is to receive D5W 80 ml/h IV. She has an order for Kantrex 60 mg IV q.8h. per buret. The drop factor is 60 gtt/ml.
What is the drip rate for this IV?

How much solution should be in the buret for the Kantrex to infuse in 30 minutes?

13. An IV is infusing at 100 ml/h. How much solution is put in the buret for a medication that is to infuse in 40 minutes?

14. D5W 1000 ml is infusing at 75 ml/h. The drop factor of the infusion set is 60 gtt/ml. What is the drip rate?

15. An IV is infusing at 50 ml/h through an infusion set that delivers 60 gtt/ml. What is the drip rate?

PEDIATRIC MEDICATIONS AND INTRAVENOUS FLUIDS

Show all your work. Check your answers (page 366).

Situation: Dosage ordered: Polycillin 225 mg q.8h. PO. Dosage available: Polycillin 250 mg per 5 ml. Client weight: 30 lb. Recommended dosage: 50 mg/kg/d. Questions 1, 2 and 3 pertain to this situation.

1. How many ml will the child receive at each dose?

2. What is the child's daily dosage?

3. What is the recommended daily dosage for a child of this weight?

Situation: Dosage ordered: methotrexate 30 mg IM twice weekly. Dosage available: 25 mg/ml. Recommended dosage: 30 mg/square meter. The child weighs 52 lb and is 50 inches tall. (This child is considered to be of normal height and weight.) Questions 4, 5 and 6 pertain to this situation.

4. Using the West nomogram in Figure 17-4, find the child's body surface area in square meters.

5. How many ml of methotrexate will be given?

6. What is the recommended dosage for a child with this body surface area?

7. Cindy is to receive 200,000 U Mycostatin q.i.d. PO for thrush. Dosage available: Mycostatin 100,000 U/ml. How many ml will Cindy receive at each dose?

Match the following.
8. Clark's Rule___   a. Based on body surface area.
9. Fried's Rule___   b. Based on age in months.
10. Young's Rule___   c. Based on body weight.
   d. Based on age in years.

Situation: Dosage ordered: 90 mcg b.i.d. PO. Dosage available: 1 mg/ml. Recommended dosage: 25 mcg/kg/d. Client weight: 16 lb 4 oz. Questions 11, 12 and 13 pertain to this situation.

11. What is the recommended daily dosage for this child?

12. What is the daily dosage ordered?

13. How many ml will the client receive at each dose?

14. Carolyn is to receive 100 mg b.i.d. PO. The medication is available in 60 ml bottles labeled 125 mg = 5 ml. How many ml will Carolyn receive per dose?

15. Dosage ordered: V-Cillin K 100,000 U PO q.i.d. Dosage available: V-Cillin K 200,000 U/5 ml. How many ml will the client receive?

Situation: Candy is to receive vincristine sulfate 2 mg/square meter weekly IV. Dosage available: Vincristine 1 mg/ml. Candy's BSA is 0.8 square meters.

16. How much vincristine should she receive?

17. How many ml will Candy receive each week?

Situation: Shirley is to receive 75 mg PO q.6h. The recommended dosage is 100 mg/kg/d. Shirley weighs 6 lb 10 ounces. The medication is available in 100 ml bottles labeled 125 mg = 5 ml.

18. What is the recommended dosage per day for a child of Shirley's weight?

19. What is Shirley's daily dosage?

20. How many ml will Shirley receive?

Situation: Three-month-old Allene weighs 12 pounds. She is NPO and has an IV infusing at 35 ml/hr. The drop factor is 60 gtt/ml. She receives 60 mg Lincocin q.6h. IV via buret to infuse in 30 minutes. Questions 21 and 22 pertain to this situation.

21. What is the drip rate of the IV?

22. How much total solution will be in the buret for the Lincocin to infuse in 30 minutes?

23. Lincocin is available in 2 ml vials labeled 300 mg/ml. How many ml of Lincocin will be added to the buret?

Situation: the recommended dosage of a medication is 15 mg/kg/d in four divided doses. Cindy weighs 44 lb. The medication is available as 150 mg/5 ml. Questions 24 and 25 pertain to this situation.

24. How many mg will Cindy receive at each dose?

25. How many ml will Cindy receive at each dose?

UNIT IX POSTTEST

PEDIATRIC CALCULATIONS

Show all your work. Check your answers (page 389).

Carol weighs 15 lb 2 oz. Her medication order is ampicillin 60 mg q.4h. The recommended dosage for ampicillin is 50 mg per kg daily. Available is ampicillin 250 mg/5 ml. Questions 1, 2, and 3 pertain to this situation.

1. How many ml of ampicillin will Carol receive at each ordered dose?

2. What is Carol's daily dosage of ampicillin?

3. What is Carol's recommended dosage?

Georgie, who weighs 33 lb, has an IV of D5W which is to infuse at 60 ml/h. The infusion set contains a buret and delivers 60 gtt/ml. Georgie has a medication order for Garamycin 30 mg q.8h. IV per buret. Garamycin is supplied as 10 mg/ml. The recommended range for Garamycin is 6 to 7.5 mg/kg/day. Questions 4, 5, 6, 7 and 8 pertain to this situation.

4. What is the maximum recommended dosage for Georgie's weight?

5. What is the minimum recommended dosage for Georgie's weight?

6. Is Georgie's dosage within the recommended range?

7. Garamycin is to be infused in 30 minutes. How much total solution is to be added to the buret for the Garamycin infusion?

8. How many ml of Garamycin will be added to the buret?

9. Carla is to receive 20 mg of a medication per square meter body surface. Her body surface area is 0.74 square meters. How many mg should she receive?

Situation: Barbara weighs 33 lb. Her medication order: 25 mg q.6h. The recommended dosage is 5 to 7 mg/kg/day. Questions 10, 11, 12, and 13 pertain to this situation.

10. What is the minimum dosage for Barbara?

11. What is the maximum dosage for Barbara?

12. Is Barbara's dosage within the recommended range?

13. Donna is NPO and has an IV of D5NS infusing at 50 ml/h. The infusion set delivers 60 gtt/ml. What is the drip rate of the IV.

Situation: Joan weighs 10 lb 5 oz. She is to receive 200 mcg/kg/day in 3 divided doses. Questions 14 and 15 pertain to this situation.

14. How many mcg should Joan receive per day?

15. How many mcg should Joan receive per dose?

Situation: Patti weighs 13 lb 12 oz. She has an IV of D5W infusing at 25 ml/h. Her medication order is 12.5 mg q.6h. IV via buret. The recommended dosage of the medication is 7 to 8 mg/kg/day. Questions 16 through 20 pertain to this situation.

16. What is the maximum recommended dosage?

17. What is the minimum recommended dosage?

18. What is Patti's daily dosage?

19. Is Patti's dosage within the recommended range?

20. What is the drip rate of Patti's IV using an infusion set with a drop factor of 60 gtt/ml?

GLOSSARY

addends: numbers to be added together.

ampule: a glass medication container that cannot be resealed after opening.

common fraction: part of a whole written with a numerator and denominator.

complex fraction: common fraction with a common fraction in the numerator and/or denominator.

constant: a quantity that remains the same in a problem.

conversion factor: two quantities and their units of measurement that are always equal to each other.

decimal fraction: part of a whole using the decimal point to indicate powers of tenths for the denominator, while the numerator is written after the decimal point.

denominator: the bottom number of a common fraction. Indicates the number of parts into which the whole is divided.

difference: the amount by which one quantity is greater or less than another; the amount that remains after one quantity is subtracted from another.

dividend: the quantity divided by the divisor. May be written as the numerator of a common fraction.

divisor: the quantity by which another quantity is divided. May be written as the denominator in a common fraction.

dosage: the amount of medication to be given. Expressed in a weight unit of measurement, such as grains or grams.

dose: the amount of medication to be given at one time or at stated intervals.

equivalent: equal to.

factor: two related quantities and their units of measurement that are equal to each other in a particular problem.

fraction: part of a whole.

improper fraction: common fraction in which the numerator is equal to or larger than the denominator. Indicates an amount equal to or greater than 1.

infusion: introduction of intravenous fluids by gravity flow.

intramuscular: within a muscle. Usually refers to medications administered directly into the muscle.

intravenous: within a vein. Usually implies medications or fluids administered directly into the vein.

inversion of fraction: to turn upside down so that the numerator becomes the denominator. Used in division of fractions.

least common denominator: the smallest number that is evenly divisible by all the denominators within a problem.

minuend: the quantity from which the subtrahend is subtracted.

mixed number: combination of a whole number and a common fraction.

multiplicand: the quantity to be multiplied.

multiplier: the quantity by which the multiplicand is multiplied.

numerator: the top number of a common fraction, indicating the number of parts of the whole related to the denominator, the total number of parts of the whole.

parenteral: medications or fluids administered intradermally or into a vein, or muscle, or subcutaneous tissue.

percentage: hundredths of a whole.

product: the result obtained by multiplication.

proper fraction: common fraction in which the numerator is smaller than the denominator.

quotient: the quantity resulting from division of one quantity by another.

ratio: the relationship between two quantities. A common fraction expressed with the numerator followed by a colon and the denominator.

reconstitution: the addition of solution to a medication in powder form.

reduction of fraction to its lowest terms: to change the numerator and denominator of a fraction to the lowest possible quantities without changing its value by dividing both the numerator and denominator by the same number.

subtrahend: the quantity subtracted from the minuend.

sum: the answer in addition. Sometimes called the total.

vial: a glass container with a self-sealing rubber stopper. May contain single or multiple medication doses.

APPENDIX A

EQUIVALENTS AMONG MEASUREMENT SYSTEMS APPROXIMATE AND ACTUAL

| | *Metric* | | *English*
Household and Apothecary | |
	Approximate	*Actual*	*Approximate*	*Actual*
Weight		1 kg = 1000 g	2.2 lb	2.2046 lb
	455 g	453.5924 g		1 lb = 16 oz
	30 g	28.35 g		1 oz
		1 g = 1000 mg	15 gr	15.432356 gr
	60 mg	64.7989 mg		1 gr
		1 mg = 1000 mcg	1/60 gr	0.015432 gr
		1 mcg		0.000015 gr
Volume		0.06161 ml or cc		1 mx
		1 ml or cc	15–16 mx	16.23 mx
	4 to 5 ml or cc	5 ml	1 tsp = 1 dram	tsp
	4 to 5 ml or cc	3.6967 ml or cc		1 dram
		15 ml or cc		1 Tbsp = 3 tsp
	30 ml or cc	29.5737 ml or cc		1 oz = 2 Tbsp
	250 or 240 ml	236.5896 ml or cc		1 C = 8 oz
	500 or 480 ml	473.1792 ml or cc		1 pt = 2 C
	1000 or 960 ml	946.358 ml or cc		1 qt = 2 pt
	4000 ml	3785.434 ml or cc		1 gal = 4 qt
Length		1 meter = 100 cm	39 inches	39.37 inches
	2.5 cm	2.54 cm		1 inch
		1 cm = 10 mm	0.39 inch	0.3937 inch
		1 mm	0.039 inch	0.03937 inch

APPENDIX B

TEMPERATURE CONVERSION BETWEEN CELSIUS AND FAHRENHEIT

Most thermometers in the United States use the Fahrenheit scale. Agencies that record temperatures in Celsius use thermometers in the Celsius scale. Conversion between Celcius (C) and Fahrenheit (F) is rare but may occasionally be necessary. Temperature is expressed in degrees, (°).

Water freezes at 0°C and 32°F and boils at 100°C and 220°F. For each five degrees of Celsius temperature, there are nine degrees on the Fahrenheit scale. Therefore, the conversion factor for the Celsius scale to the Fahrenheit scale is 5 to 9 or 5C°/9F°. The scale is adjusted by 32 degrees to account for the difference between the freezing points on the two scales.

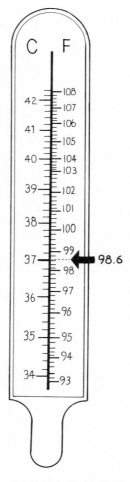

FIGURE A-1 Comparison of Celsius and Fahrenheit temperatures. Normal body temperature is indicated by the arrow.

Conversion from Celsius to Fahrenheit is as follows:

$$\text{Fahrenheit}° = \frac{(9° \text{ Fahrenheit} \times \text{Celsius} °) + 32°}{(5° \text{ Celsius} \quad \times \quad 1 \,)} \text{ or } F° = \frac{(9° \text{ F} \times C°) + 32°}{(5° \text{ C} \times 1)}$$

Convert 38°C to F. The equation is as follows:

$$F° = \frac{(9° \text{ F} \times 38° \text{ C}) + 32°}{(5° \text{ C} \times 1} = \frac{(9° \text{ F} \times 38) + 32°}{(5 \quad \times 1)} = \frac{(342° \text{ F}) + 32°}{(\quad 5 \quad)} = \frac{68.4° \text{ F} + 32°}{1} = 100.4°\text{F}$$

Conversion from Fahrenheit to Celsius is as follows:

$$\text{Celsius}° = \frac{5° \text{ Celsius} \quad \times (\text{Fahrenheit}° - 32°)}{9° \text{ Fahrenheit} \times \quad 1} \text{ or } C° = \frac{5° \text{ C} \times (F° - 32)}{9°\text{F} \times \quad 1}$$

Convert 98.6°F to C. The equation is as follows:

$$C° = \frac{5° \text{ C} \times (98.6° \text{ F} - 32°)}{9° \text{ F} \times \quad 1} = \frac{5° \text{ C} \times (66.6° \text{ F})}{9° \text{ F} \times \quad 1} = \frac{5° \text{ C} \times 66.6}{9 \quad \times \quad 1} = \frac{333° \text{ C}}{9} = 37° \text{ C}$$

Remember, portions within parentheses are solved first.

APPENDIX C

CHEMICAL SYMBOLS USED IN ADMINISTRATION OF MEDICATIONS AND TREATMENTS

SYMBOL	ELEMENT	EXAMPLE OF USE
Al	aluminum	antacid aluminum hydroxide, AlOH
As	arsenic	treatment of parasites and skin disorders
Ba	barium	opaque contrast medium for X-rays such as Ba enema
Bi	bismuth	relief of gastrointestinal inflammation
Br	bromine	central nervous system depressant rarely used today
Ca	calcium	essential element for bone formation
C	carbon	carbon dioxide CO_2
Cl	chlorine	disinfectant as hypochlorite
Co	cobalt	radioisotope Co-60 used for radiation therapy
Cu	copper	trace element necessary for bone formation
F	fluorine	prevention of tooth decay
Ga	gallium	radioisotope used for diagnosis of soft tissue tumors
Au	gold	used cautiously for treatment of rheumatoid arthritis
He	helium	used to facilitate delivery of oxygen to lungs
H	hydrogen	water, H_2O
I	iodine	used in diagnosis and treatment of thyroid diseases
Fe	iron	used to treat anemia
Pb	lead	shield for X-rays
Li	lithium	mood stabilizer for treatment of manic-depression
Mg	magnesium	antacid, cathartic
Mn	manganese	occurs in body tissue in small amounts
Hg	mercury	in thermometers and mercurial sphygmomanometers
Mo	molybdenum	essential trace element
N	nitrogen	occurs in all proteins
O	oxygen	oxygen, O_2
P	phosphorus	essential element for bone formation and cell metabolism
K	potassium	essential electrolyte
Ra	radium	needles and seeds used to treat malignancies
Se	selenium	radioisotope used in nuclear medicine
Ag	silver	chemical cautery
Na	sodium	essential electrolyte
S	sulfur	used most often as a sulfate, SO_4
Ta	tantalum	wire sutures, prosthesis
Tc	technetium	radioisotope in nuclear medicine
Tl	thallium	radioisotope used in diagnosis
Ti	titanium	ointment to protect skin from sun
V	vanadium	salts used to treat several diseases
Xe	xenon	isotope used for diagnosis
Zn	zinc	trace element

APPENDIX D

CONVERSION BETWEEN STANDARD AND MILITARY TIME

Some agencies use the 24-hour clock (military time) for all schedules and charting requiring the recording of time. The use of military time eliminates the confusion of A.M. and P.M. times of the same value and the need to use different colors of ink for charting on each shift.

The 24-hour clock (military) times consist of four digits. The first two digits are the hour and the last two are the minutes. Calculation of time using the 24-hour clock involves the following rules:

- Hours with less than 2 digits are preceded by zeroes.
  Example: 9 A.M. is 0900 hours

- Hours after 12 noon are calculated by adding 12 to the actual time.
  Example: 3:15 P.M. is 1515 hours (12 + 3:15)

- Midnight is the end of the 24-hour clock and is recorded as 2400 hours

- Time after midnight begins with 0000 hours.
  Example: 12:01 A.M. is 0001 hours.
  Convert 7:15 P.M. to military time.
  7:15 P.M. is after 12 noon. Therefore, 12 is added to the actual time.
  7:15 + 12 = 1915 hours

- To convert military time to standard time, reverse the rules.
  Convert 0915 hours to standard time.
  0915 is a morning hour. Remove the zero preceding the 9 and insert the colon used in regular time and add the morning abbreviation.
  0915 hours = 9:15 A.M.

APPENDIX E

ENCOURAGED OR RESTRICTED FLUIDS

Fevers, respiratory infections, and a tendency to have urinary tract infections are some indications for the orders "encourage fluids" or "force fluids" to a specific amount. The nurse must ensure that a minimum of the specified amount is reached. The encouraged fluids include those given as intravenous infusions and taken orally with medications and at meals.

The easiest way to calculate oral fluids is to calculate the amount of fluids to offer per hour for a specific number of waking hours of the day. Most nurses use 12 hours as a guide, planning to offer specified amounts of fluid from breakfast until 8 or 9 P.M. Clients are seldom offered fluids at bedtime or awakened at night to encourage fluid intake unless sufficient fluids were not taken during the day. Fluid offered at bedtime may disturb the client's rest due to frequent trips to the bathroom. Intravenous fluid volumes are subtracted from the total prior to solving the equation.

The equation for finding the volume per hour for offered oral fluids is as follows:

$$\frac{\text{milliliters}}{\text{hour}} = \frac{\text{conversion factor if}}{\text{necessary}} \times \frac{(\text{ daily volume - intravenous fluids })}{(\text{ 12 hours })}$$

SAMPLE PROBLEM **The doctor's order reads "Force fluids to 3 L/day." How many ml of fluid should be offered per hour during waking hours to ensure that the client receives 3 liters of fluids each day?**

For this problem, the only hours of concern are the waking hours or 12 hours per day.

Knowns: Unit of answer: ml/h
Factors: 3 L = 12 h
Conversion factor: 1 L = 1000 ml

The equation is as follows:

$$\frac{\text{ml}}{\text{h}} = \frac{1000\,\text{ml} \times 3\,\text{L}}{1\,\text{L} \times 12\,\text{h}} = \frac{\overset{250}{\cancel{1000}}\,\text{ml} \times \overset{1}{3}}{1 \times \underset{3}{\cancel{12}}\,\text{h}} = \frac{250\,\text{ml} \times 1}{1 \times 1\,\text{h}} = \frac{250\,\text{ml}}{1\,\text{h}} = 250\,\text{ml/h}$$

After the calculations for encouraged or restricted fluids have been completed, the nurse records this on the nursing care plan. An example of the nursing order is as follows:
1. Encourage fluids to 3 L/day.
  a. Offer 250 ml q.h. oral fluids from 0800 to 2000 hrs.
  b. Client likes orange, grapefruit, tomato, and pineapple juices; hates grape juice.

SAMPLE PROBLEM   **Mr. Rogers has the following orders: 500 ml D5W q.8h. IV and encourage fluids to 3000 ml/day. How many ml per hour of oral fluids should be offered during Mr. Roger's waking hours?**

Find the daily volume of IV fluids.

Knowns: Unit of answer: ml/day

Factors: 500 ml = 8 h

24 h = 1 day

The equation for finding the volume of IV solutions is as follows:

$$\frac{ml}{d} = \frac{500\ mg \times 24\ h}{(q)8\ h \ \times\ 1\ day} = \frac{500\ mg \times \overset{3}{\cancel{24}}}{\underset{1}{\cancel{8}} \ \times\ 1\ day} = \frac{500\ mg \times 3}{1 \ \times\ 1\ day} = \frac{1500\ ml}{1\ day} = 1500\ ml/day$$

Find the oral fluid volume to offer per hour.

Knowns: Unit of answer: ml/h

Factor: 1500 ml = 12 h

Oral daily fluids: 3000 ml − 1500 ml = 1500 ml

The equation is as follows:

$$\frac{ml}{h} = \frac{\overset{125}{\cancel{1500}}\ ml}{\underset{1}{\cancel{12}}\ h} = \frac{125\ ml}{1\ h} = 125\ ml/h$$

Fluids may be restricted in persons with cardiovascular or renal problems. The doctor's order would read "restrict fluids" to a specific amount per day maximum. Fluids are not offered to the patient and may be restricted when requested. The maximum fluid intake includes intravenous solutions and all fluids taken with meals and medications. Intravenous fluids and fluids for scheduled medications must be subtracted from the total allowance.

Restricted fluids are usually calculated so that 2/3 of the daily fluid allowance is ingested on the day shift and 1/3 on the evening shift. Any liquids taken during the night shift are subtracted from the day shift amount. Some nurses do calculate restricted fluids using 1/2 the allowance for day shift and 1/4 each for evening and night shift. Since clients tend to sleep at night, it is probably preferable to use 2/3 of the allowance for the day shift.

SAMPLE PROBLEM   **Mrs. Jones has the following order: Restrict fluids to 500 ml/day. She is receiving 6 pills each day and requires an ounce of water to swallow each pill. She receives no fluids with her meals. Calculate the amount of fluids Mrs. Jones may receive on the day shift using 2/3 allowance.**

Find the amount of fluid required for medications.

Knowns: Unit of answer: ml

Conversion factor: 30 ml = 1 oz

Factors: 6 doses = 1 day

1 oz/dose

The equation is as follows:

$$\frac{ml}{d} = \frac{30\ ml \ \times 1\ oz \ \times 6\ doses}{1\ oz \ \times 1\ dose \times 1\ day} = \frac{30\ ml \ \times 1 \times 6}{1 \ \times 1 \times 1} = \frac{180\ ml}{1\ day} = 180\ ml/day$$

Find the fluid volume for the day shift.

Knowns: Unit of answer: ml/day shift (ds)   **Factors: 2/3 d = 1 day shift (ds)**
Daily oral fluids: 500 ml − 180 ml = 320 ml/day   **320 ml = 1 day**

$$\frac{ml}{ds} = \frac{320\,ml \times 2/3\,day}{1\,day \times 1\,ds} = \frac{320\,ml \times 2/3}{\times 1\,ds} = \frac{320\,ml \times 2}{1 \times 3\,ds} = \frac{640\,ml}{3\,ds} = 213.3\,ml/ds$$

The nursing care plan reflects this calculation.
1. Restrict fluids to 500 ml/d as follows:
    a. Day shift fluids: 215 ml
    b. Evening shift fluids: 105 ml
    c. Maximum fluids with medications: 30 ml/tablet

APPENDIX F

CALCULATION OF KILOCALORIES

A kilocalorie (Calorie) is 1000 times the amount of heat required to raise the temperature of 1 gram of water 1 degree Celsius. The calculation of kilocalories, abbreviated Cal or kcal, may be necessary for certain clients, including diabetics, those on weight reduction diets, or those who are undernourished. Calories are calculated in three ways: (1) conversion of grams of carbohydrate, protein, or fat to Calories, (2) use of a food Calorie list for each food, and (3) conversion to Calories using the American Diabetic Association exchange list.

CONVERSION OF GRAMS TO KILOCALORIES

Conversion of grams to Calories requires conversion factors of kilocalories (Calories) per gram. The conversion factors are as follows:

Carbohydrate (CHO):   4 Calories per gram
Protein (prot):   4 Calories per gram
Fat: 9 Calories per gram

The equations for calculation of kilocalories when the grams are known are as follows:

For carbohydrates and proteins: For Fats:

$$Cal = \frac{4\,Cal}{1g} \times \frac{g\ CHO\ or\ prot}{\times\ 1}$$ $$Cal = \frac{9\ Cal \times g\ fat}{1\ g \times 1}$$

SAMPLE PROBLEM   **The client on a low fat diet consumed the following at lunch: 80 g CHO, 30 g protein and 5 g fat. How many calories did the client consume for this meal?**

Knowns: Unit of answer: Cal
Conversion factors: 4 Cal = 1 g CHO
                      4 Cal = 1 g prot
                      9 Cal = 1 g fat
Factors: 80 g CHO/1
          30 g prot/1
          5 g fat/1

The equation for this problem is as follows:

$$Cal = \frac{4\ Cal}{1\ g\ CHO} \times \frac{80\ g\ CHO}{1} = \frac{4\ Cal}{1} \times \frac{80}{1} = \frac{320\ Cal}{1} = 320\ Cal$$

$$Cal = \frac{4\ Cal}{1\ g\ prot} \times \frac{30\ g\ prot}{1} = \frac{4\ Cal}{1} \times \frac{30}{1} = \frac{120\ Cal}{1} = 120\ Cal$$

$$Cal = \frac{9\ Cal}{1\ g\ fat} \times \frac{5\ g\ fat}{1} = \frac{9\ Cal}{1} \times \frac{5}{1} = \frac{45\ Cal}{1} = 45\ Cal$$

Total =   485 Cal

Some clients receiving intravenous infusions are on very strict diets. The Calories in the intravenous solutions are calculated and subtracted from the oral Calorie daily allowance.

SAMPLE PROBLEM   **Mr. Douglas is on a strict 2000 Calorie diet. He is receiving 2 IVs per day, each of which has 50 grams of dextrose. How many Calories may he take orally while the IVs are infusing?**

Calculate the Calories in the IVs.
Knowns: Unit of answer: Cal
Factor: 50 + 50 = 100 g CHO/1
Conversion factor: 4 Cal = 1 g CHO

The equation is as follows:

$$\text{Cal} = \frac{4\,\text{Cal}}{1\,\text{g CHO} \times} \frac{\times\,100\,\text{g CHO}}{1} = \frac{4\,\text{Cal}}{1} \frac{\times\,100}{\times\,1} = \frac{400\,\text{Cal}}{1} = 400\,\text{Cal}$$

Subtract the intravenous Calories from the Calories allowed each day.

$$\text{Cal} = 2000\,\text{Cal} - 400\,\text{Cal} = 1600\,\text{Calories orally allowed.}$$

When the grams of carbohydrate, protein, and fat are not known, Calories can be calculated using a food Calorie count list. After the Calorie count of each food is found on the list, the Calories are added together. This is a time-consuming process. An easier way is to use the food exchange list of the American Diabetic Association.

CALCULATIONS OF KILOCALORIES USING AN EXCHANGE LIST

The exchange system consists of six categories of foods, each of which has a standard amount of carbohydrate (CHO), protein, and fat per exchange. An exchange list designates the foods and appropriate volumes within each group. Table F-1 contains the composition and Caloric value of each type of exchange. Do not memorize this table.

Each Calorie diet has a specific amount of each exchange group per day, divided into meals and snacks.

The health care professional on the unit estimates the amount of each exchange that the client has consumed and calculates the Calories from this amount. This calculation is very simple. Multiply the calories per exchange by the number of exchanges consumed.

TABLE F-1   Food Exchange Composition and Kilocalories

| Exchange | Weight in Grams | | | Kilocalories |
	CHO	Protein	Fat	
Milk	12	8	10	170
Vegetable	5	2		28
Fruit	10			40
Bread	15	2		68
Meat		7	5	73
Fat			5	45

From *Exchange lists for meal planning.* New York, 1986, American Diabetic Association.

SAMPLE PROBLEM **Calculate the following breakfast Calorie count for the following exchanges:**

1 Fruit	2 Fat
1 1/2 Bread	1 Milk
1 1/2 Meat	

Calculation of this breakfast is shown in Figure A-3.

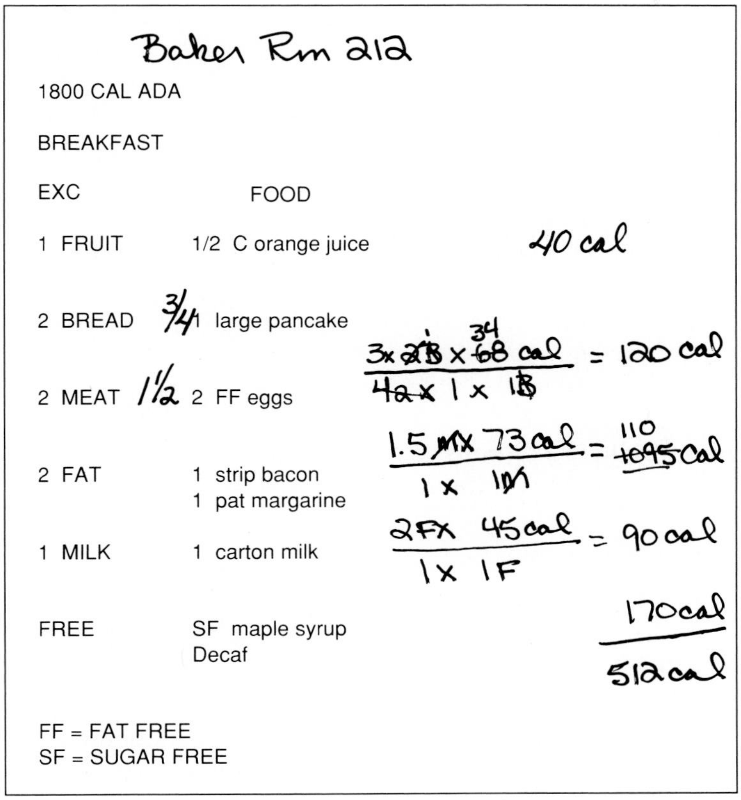
Baker Rm 212

1800 CAL ADA

BREAKFAST

EXC	FOOD	
1 FRUIT	1/2 C orange juice	40 cal
2 BREAD 3/4	1 large pancake	$\frac{3 \times 2B \times 68 \text{ cal}}{4 \times 1 \times 1B}$ = 120 cal
2 MEAT 1 1/2	2 FF eggs	$\frac{1.5 M \times 73 \text{ cal}}{1 \times 1M}$ = 110 cal
2 FAT	1 strip bacon 1 pat margarine	$\frac{2F \times 45 \text{ cal}}{1 \times 1F}$ = 90 cal
1 MILK	1 carton milk	170 cal
FREE	SF maple syrup Decaf	512 cal

FF = FAT FREE
SF = SUGAR FREE

FIGURE A-3 Diet sheet with completed calorie count.

APPENDIX G

PEDIATRIC INTAKE AND OUTPUT

Intake and output is usually a routine order for neonates in a newborn nursery and many clients on pediatric units. Output for healthy infants is usually recorded by making a notation each time the infant voids. Infants who are premature or ill may require actual measurement of output. This is accomplished by recording the dry diaper weight in grams on the intake and output record prior to putting the diaper on or under the infant. This weight is subtracted from the wet diaper weight after the infant voids. The answer is converted to milliliters. Remember, in solutions 1 gram water = 1 milliliter = 1 cubic centimeter.

SAMPLE PROBLEM   **The dry diaper weight is 22 grams. The wet diaper weight is 35 grams. What is the output of the infant at this voiding?**

Wet diaper weight − dry diaper weight = output in grams
Convert grams to milliliters.

$$35 \text{ g} - 22 \text{ g} = 13 \text{ g}$$
$$13 \text{ g} = 13 \text{ ml output}$$

Most nurseries and pediatric units use prepackaged formulas. The labels show the total amount, and a convenient scale of ounces and milliliters or cubic centimeters is on the bottle. To find the intake of a formula-feeding infant, subtract the amount remaining from the total amount of the formula. The trend is to record amounts in milliliters, although some agencies use ounces.

Breast-fed infants are weighed immediately before and after feeding in the same clothing to assess milk intake. The before-feeding weight is subtracted from the after-feeding weight to find the amount of breast milk consumed. If the infant voids during feeding, the diaper is changed after the infant is weighed. Some agencies used metric scales, while others use avoirdupois scales. If metric scales are used, the weight in grams is converted to milliliters.

SAMPLE PROBLEM   **Baby Mary weighs 9 pounds, 12 ³/₄ ounces immediately before she is fed. Immediately after feeding, she weighs 10 pounds, 1 ¹/₄ ounces. How many ounces of breast milk has Mary received?**

Knowns: a.c. weight: **9 lb 12 ³/₄ oz**
                   p.c. weight: **10 lb 1 ¹/₄ oz**
Conversion factor: 1 lb = 16 oz

$$10 \text{ lb } 1 \, ^{1}/_{4} \text{ oz} = 9 \text{ lb } 17 \, ^{1}/_{4} \text{ oz} = 9 \text{ lb } 16 \, ^{5}/_{4} \text{ oz}$$
$$\underline{-9 \text{ lb } 12 \, ^{3}/_{4} \text{ oz} = 9 \text{ lb } 12 \, ^{3}/_{4} \text{ oz} = 9 \text{ lb } 12 \, ^{3}/_{4} \text{ oz}}$$
$$4 \, ^{2}/_{4} \text{ oz} = 4 \, ^{1}/_{2} \text{ ounces}$$

The equation for converting ounces to milliliters is as follows:

$$\text{ml} = \frac{30 \text{ ml} \times 4.5 \text{ oz}}{1 \text{ oz} \times 1} = \frac{30 \text{ ml} \times 4.5}{1 \times 1} = \frac{135 \text{ ml}}{1} = 135 \text{ ml}$$

APPENDIX H

FLUID AND KILOCALORIE REQUIREMENT

Infants and small children may become dehydrated or overhydrated easily. Therefore, assessment of daily fluid intake is an important function of the pediatric nurse. Table H-1 shows the daily fluid requirements for infants and children.

Daily fluid requirements are based on the pediatric client's weight. Fluid requirements are high during infancy. As the child grows older, fluid requirements decrease. The equation for calculating fluid requirements is as follows:

$$\text{ml (/day)} = \frac{\text{ml} \times}{\text{kg}} \frac{\text{Conversion} \quad \text{client's}}{\text{factor if} \times \text{weight}} \frac{}{\text{necessary} \times \quad 1}$$

Because fluid requirements are expressed as a range, both the minimum and maximum amounts must be calculated.

SAMPLE PROBLEM   **Five-month-old Maureen weighs 17 pounds. What is her daily fluid requirement range?**

Table H.1 shows that a five month infant requires 140 to 160 ml per kg.
Solve for the range minimum.
Knowns: Unit of answer: ml
Conversion factor: 1 kg = 2.2 lb
Factors: 140 ml = 1 kg
        17 lb/1
The equation is as follows:

$$\text{ml (/day)} = \frac{140\,\text{ml} \times \quad 1\,\text{kg} \times 17\,\text{lb}}{1\,\text{kg} \times 2.2\,\text{lb} \times \quad 1} = \frac{\overset{70}{\cancel{140}}\,\text{ml} \times \quad \frac{1 \times 17}{\cancel{2.2} \times \quad 1}}{1 \qquad 1.1} = \frac{1190\,\text{ml}}{1.1} = 1081\,\text{ml}$$

TABLE H-1   Average Daily Fluid and Caloric Requirements

Age	Weight in Grams Fluids ml/kg/day	Kilocalories Cal/kg/day
Newborn	80-100	
Infant		
first 6 months	140-160	115
second 6 months	125-145	105
Toddler	115-135	100
Preschooler	100-110	85
Children	90-100	85
Preadolescent	70-85	55
Adolescent	40-60	40

From Whaley, L.F. & Wong, D.L.: *Nursing care of infants and children*, St. Louis: 1987, The C.V. Mosby Co., 109, 1159.

Solve for the range maximum.
Knowns: Unit of answer: ml
Conversion factor: 1 kg = 2.2 lb
Factors: 160 ml = 1 kg
          17 lb/1

The equation is as follows:

$$\text{ml (/day)} = \frac{160 \text{ ml} \times 1 \text{ kg} \times 17 \text{ lb}}{1 \text{ kg} \times 2.2 \text{ lb} \times} = \frac{\overset{80}{\cancel{100}} \text{ml} \times 1 \times 17}{1 \times \underset{1.1}{\cancel{2.2}} \times 1} = \frac{1360 \text{ ml}}{1.1} = 1233 \text{ ml}$$

Assessment of daily fluid intake involves comparing the pediatric client's daily fluid intake with the daily requirements.

SAMPLE PROBLEM **Maureen's fluid intake for the past 24 hours is as follows: 3 ½ ounces, 2 ½ ounces, 6 ounces, 3 ounces, 5 ounces, and 4 ounces. Was her fluid intake of 24 ounces adequate?**

Convert the 24 ounces to milliliters.
Knowns: Unit of answer: ml
Conversion factor: 1 oz = 30 ml
Factor: 24 oz

$$\text{ml (/d)} = \frac{30 \text{ ml} \times 24 \text{ oz}}{1 \text{ oz} \times 1} = \frac{720 \text{ ml}}{1} = 720 \text{ ml}$$

Compare Maureen's fluid intake, 720 ml, with the fluid requirement range, 1081 to 1233 ml. Maureen's fluid intake is not adequate.

Pediatric clients require a minimum amount of kilocalories to sustain growth. It is necessary to assess Caloric intake, especially for clients who do not thrive. Table H.1 shows the average Caloric requirement for growth. Full strength formulas contain 20 kilocalories per ounce. Breast milk also contains about 20 Calories per ounce.

SAMPLE PROBLEM **Four-month-old Mark has gained little weight in the past month. He now weighs 15 pounds. His formula intake for the past 24 hours was 32 ounces. Is his Caloric intake adequate?**

Table H.1 shows that a 4 month old requires 115 Calories/kilogram.
Calculate the daily Caloric requirement.
Knowns: Unit of answer: Cal
Conversion factor: 1 kg = 2.2 lb
Factors: 115 Cal = 1 kg
          15 lb/1

$$\text{Cal (/day)} = \frac{115 \text{ Cal} \times 1 \text{ kg} \times 15 \text{ lb}}{1 \text{ kg} \times 2.2 \text{ lb} \times 1} = \frac{115 \text{ Cal} \times 1 \times 15}{1 \times 2.2 \times 1} = \frac{1725 \text{ Cal}}{2.2} = 784 \text{ Cal}$$

Calculate Mark's Caloric intake.
Knowns: Unit of answer: Cal
Factors: 20 Cal = 1 oz
          32 oz/1

$$\text{Cal (/day)} = \frac{20 \text{ Cal} \times 32 \text{ oz}}{1 \text{ oz} \times 1} = \frac{20 \text{ Cal} \times 32}{1 \times 1} = \frac{640 \text{ Cal}}{1} = 640 \text{ Cal}$$

Mark's Caloric intake, 640 Calories, is less than the daily requirement, 784 Calories.

SAMPLE PROBLEM   **Three-month-old Ronny, who weighs 11 pounds, was admitted to the pediatric unit with a diagnosis of failure to thrive. His breast milk intake was calculated at 930 ml. Is his Caloric intake adequate?**

Solve for Ronny's daily Caloric requirement.
Knowns: Unit of answer: Cal (/day)
Conversion factor: 1 kg = 2.2 lb
Factors: 115 Cal = 1 kg
11 lb/1

$$\text{Cal (/day)} = \frac{115\,\text{Cal} \times 1\,\text{kg} \times 11\,\text{lb}}{1\,\text{kg} \times 2.2\,\text{lb} \times 1} = \frac{115\,\text{Cal} \times 1 \times \overset{1}{\cancel{11}}}{1 \times \underset{0.2}{\cancel{2.2}} \times 1} = \frac{115\,\text{Cal}}{0.2} = 575\,\text{Cal}$$

Solve for Ronny's Caloric intake for the last 24 hours.
Knowns: Unit of answer: Cal (/d)
**   Conversion factor: 1 oz = 30 ml**
Factors: 20 Cal = 1 oz
**   930 ml/1**

$$\text{Cal (/day)} = \frac{20\,\text{Cal} \times 1\,\text{oz} \times 930\,\text{ml}}{1\,\text{oz} \times 30\,\text{ml} \times 1} = \frac{20\,\text{Cal} \times 1 \times \overset{31}{\cancel{930}}}{1 \times \underset{1}{\cancel{30}} \times 1} = \frac{620\,\text{Cal}}{1} = 620\,\text{Cal}$$

Ronny's Caloric intake, 620 Calories, is greater than the daily requirement, 575 Calories. Therefore, his Caloric intake is adequate.

APPENDIX I

FORMULA PREPARATION

Formulas are available in prepackaged bottles, as concentrates, and as powders. Concentrates and powders have mixing instructions for full-strength formula. Sometimes, the order is for half-strength formula. Full-strength prepared formulas are diluted with equal parts of water to make half-strength formulas. Concentrates and powders must be diluted according to the instructions.

SAMPLE PROBLEM   **Formula order is for half-strength Similac. Full-strength formula is made from 1 scoop Similac powder to each 2 ounces of water. How much Similac powder will be used to make 6 ounces of half-strength formula?**

If 1 scoop powder makes 2 ounces full-strength formula, then 1 scoop powder makes 4 ounces half-strength formula.

Knowns: **Unit of answer: scoop**

Factors: **1 scoop = 4 ounces**

             6 ounces/1

$$\text{scoop} = \frac{1\ \text{scoop} \times 6\ \text{oz}}{4\ \text{oz} \qquad \times 1} = \frac{1\ \text{scoop} \times \overset{3}{\cancel{6}}}{\underset{2}{\cancel{4}} \qquad \times 1} = \frac{3\ \text{scoops}}{2} = 1\,^{1}/_{2}\ \text{scoops}.$$

This could also have been solved by multiplying the full-strength formula preparation by one-half as in the following equation:

$$\text{scoop} = \frac{1\ \text{scoop} \times 6\ \text{oz} \qquad \times 1}{2\ \text{oz} \qquad \times 1 \qquad \times 2} = \frac{1\ \text{scoop} \times \overset{3}{\cancel{6}} \times 1}{\underset{1}{\cancel{2}} \qquad \times 1 \times 2} = \frac{3\ \text{scoops}}{2} = 1\,^{1}/_{2}\ \text{scoops}$$

Water is added to the powder in a quantity sufficient to make 6 ounces.

SAMPLE PROBLEM   **Formula order: Similac one-half strength. Full-strength formula is made from equal parts of Similac concentrate and water. How much formula concentrate is needed to make 6 ounces of half-strength formula?**

If equal parts of formula concentrate and water are used, then 1 ounce of Similac concentrate makes 2 ounces of formula.

Knowns: **Unit of answer: oz concentrate (conc)**

Factors: **1 oz conc = 2 oz formula (form)**

             6 oz/1

             1/2

The equation is as follows:

$$\text{oz conc} = \frac{1\,\text{oz conc} \times 6\,\text{oz form} \times 1}{2\,\text{oz form} \times 1 \qquad \times 2} = \frac{1\,\text{oz conc} \times \overset{3}{\cancel{6}} \times 1}{\underset{1}{\cancel{2}} \qquad \times 1 \times 2} = \frac{3\,\text{oz conc}}{2} = 1\,{}^{1}\!/_{2}\,\text{oz conc}$$

Water is added to the concentrate in a quantity sufficient to make 6 ounces.

Answers

PRACTICE PROBLEM ANSWERS

UNIT I: THE FOUNDATIONS OF DIMENSIONAL ANALYSIS

Chapter 1: Roman Numerals

1. XXV $= 25$
2. iiss $= 2\frac{1}{2}$
3. XIV $= 14$
4. XXXVI $= 36$
5. viiss $= 7\frac{1}{2}$
6. $14\frac{1}{2} =$ xivss
7. $9\frac{1}{2} =$ ixss
8. $15 =$ XV, xv
9. $29 =$ XXIX, xxix
10. $4 =$ IV, iv

Chapter 2: Common Fractions

1. 1/4, 1/5, 1/6: Least common denominator $= 60$
2. 1/3, 1/6, 2/9: Least common denominator $= 18$
3. 1/8, 2/5, 1/4: Least common denominator $= 40$
4. 3/8, 5/6, 7/12: Least common denominator $= 24$
5. 1/2, 2/3, 3/4: Least common denominator $= 12$
6. 1/4, 1/5, 1/6: Least common denominator $= 60$

$1/4 = 15/60$: $60 \div 4 = 15$; $\dfrac{15 \times 1}{15 \times 4} = \dfrac{15}{60}$

$1/5 = 12/60$: $60 \div 5 = 12$; $\dfrac{12 \times 1}{12 \times 5} = \dfrac{12}{60}$

$1/6 = 10/60$: $60 \div 6 = 10$; $\dfrac{10 \times 1}{10 \times 6} = \dfrac{10}{60}$

7. 1/3, 1/6, 2/9: Least common denominator $= 18$

$1/3 = 6/18$: $18 \div 3 = 6$; $\dfrac{6 \times 1}{6 \times 3} = \dfrac{6}{18}$

$1/6 = 3/18$: $18 \div 6 = 3$; $\dfrac{3 \times 1}{3 \times 6} = \dfrac{3}{18}$

$2/9 = 4/18$: $18 \div 9 = 2$; $\dfrac{2 \times 2}{2 \times 9} = \dfrac{4}{18}$

8. 1/8, 2/5, 1/4: Least common denominator $= 40$

$1/8 = 5/40$: $40 \div 8 = 5$; $\dfrac{5 \times 1}{5 \times 8} = \dfrac{5}{40}$

$2/5 = 16/40$: $40 \div 5 = 8$; $\dfrac{8 \times 2}{8 \times 5} = \dfrac{16}{40}$

$1/4 = 10/40$: $40 \div 4 = 10$; $\dfrac{10 \times 1}{10 \times 4} = \dfrac{10}{40}$

9. 3/8, 5/6, 7/12: Least common denominator $= 24$

$3/8 = 9/24$: $24 \div 8 = 3$; $\dfrac{3 \times 3}{3 \times 8} = \dfrac{9}{24}$

$5/6 = 20/24$: $24 \div 6 = 4$; $\dfrac{4 \times 5}{4 \times 6} = \dfrac{20}{24}$

$7/12 = 14/24$: $24 \div 12 = 2$; $\dfrac{2 \times 7}{2 \times 12} = \dfrac{14}{24}$

10. 1/2, 2/3, 3/4: Least common denominator $= 12$

$1/2 = 6/12$: $12 \div 2 = 6$; $\dfrac{6 \times 1}{6 \times 2} = \dfrac{6}{12}$

$2/3 = 8/12$: $12 \div 3 = 4$; $\dfrac{4 \times 2}{4 \times 3} = \dfrac{8}{12}$

$3/4 = 9/12$: $12 \div 4 = 3$; $\dfrac{3 \times 3}{3 \times 4} = \dfrac{9}{12}$

11. $19/6 = 3\frac{1}{6}$:

$$\begin{array}{r} 3\frac{1}{6} \\ 6\overline{)19} \\ \underline{18} \\ 1 \end{array}$$

12. $2\dfrac{20}{5} = 6$: $2 + \dfrac{4}{5\,\overline{)\,20}} = 6$

$$\begin{array}{r} \underline{20} \\ 0 \end{array}$$

13. $43/8 = 5\dfrac{3}{8}$:

$$\begin{array}{r} 5\frac{3}{8} \\ 8\overline{)43} \\ \underline{40} \\ 3 \end{array}$$

14. $8/20 = 2/5$: $\dfrac{8 \div 4}{20 \div 4} = \dfrac{2}{5}$

15. $5\dfrac{5}{4} = 6\dfrac{1}{4}$: $5 + \dfrac{1\frac{1}{4}}{4\,\overline{)\,5}} = 6\frac{1}{4}$

$$\begin{array}{r} \underline{4} \\ 1 \end{array}$$

16. $5\dfrac{3}{4} = 23/4$: $\dfrac{(5 \times 4) + 3}{4} = \dfrac{20 + 3}{4} = \dfrac{23}{4}$

17. $2\dfrac{1}{3} = 7/3$: $\dfrac{(2 \times 3) + 1}{3} = \dfrac{6 + 1}{3} = \dfrac{7}{3}$

18. $8\dfrac{1}{2} = 17/2$: $\dfrac{(8 \times 2) + 1}{2} = \dfrac{16 + 1}{2} = \dfrac{17}{2}$

19. $5\dfrac{3}{4} = 4\dfrac{7}{4}$: $5 - 1\dfrac{(1 \times 4) + 3}{4} = 4\dfrac{4 + 3}{4} = 4\dfrac{7}{4}$

20. $2\dfrac{1}{3} = 1\dfrac{4}{3}$: $2 - 1\dfrac{(1 \times 3) + 1}{3} = 1\dfrac{3 + 1}{3} = 1\dfrac{4}{3}$

21. 1/8, 11/12, 5/6, 3/4   Least common denominator: 24

$1/8 = 3/24$: $24 \div 8 = 3$; $\dfrac{3 \times 1}{3 \times 8} = \dfrac{3}{24}$

$11/12 = 22/24$: $24 \div 12 = 2$; $\dfrac{2 \times 11}{2 \times 12} = \dfrac{22}{24}$

$5/6 = 20/24$: $24 \div 6 = 4$; $\dfrac{4 \times 5}{4 \times 6} = \dfrac{20}{24}$

$3/4 = 18/24$: $24 \div 4 = 6$; $\dfrac{6 \times 3}{6 \times 4} = \dfrac{18}{24}$

$$\begin{array}{r} 3 \\ 22 \\ 20 \\ \underline{+24} \\ 63 \\ \hline 24 \end{array}$$

$= 24\overline{)63}\ \dfrac{15 \div 3}{24 \div 3} = 2\frac{5}{8}$

$$\begin{array}{r} \underline{48} \\ 15 \end{array}$$

22. 1/6, 1/10, 3/5   Least common denominator: 30

$1/6 = 5/30$: $30 \div 6 = 5$; $\dfrac{5 \times 1}{5 \times 6} = \dfrac{5}{30}$

$1/10 = 3/30$: $30 \div 10 = 3$; $\dfrac{3 \times 1}{3 \times 10} = \dfrac{3}{30}$

$3/5 = 18/30$: $30 \div 5 = 6$; $\dfrac{6 \times 3}{6 \times 5} = \dfrac{+30}{18}$

$$\dfrac{26 \div 2}{30 \div 2} = \dfrac{13}{15}$$

23. 8/9, 2/3, 1/2   Least common denominator: 18

$8/9 = 16/18$: $18 \div 9 = 2$; $\dfrac{2 \times 8}{2 \times 9} = \dfrac{16}{18}$

$2/3 = 12/18$: $18 \div 3 = 6$; $\dfrac{6 \times 2}{6 \times 3} = \dfrac{12}{18}$

$1/2 = 9/18$: $18 \div 2 = 9$; $\dfrac{9 \times 1}{9 \times 2} = \dfrac{+18}{9}$

$$\dfrac{37}{18} = 18\overline{)37} \quad 2\tfrac{1}{18}$$
$$\dfrac{36}{1}$$

24. $2^{9}/_{10}$, $1^{4}/_{5}$, $3^{1}/_{4}$ Least common denominator: 20

$2^{9}/_{10} = 2^{18}/_{20}$: $20 \div 10 = 2$; $2 + \dfrac{2 \times 9}{2 \times 10} = 2\dfrac{18}{20}$

$1^{4}/_{5} = 1^{16}/_{20}$: $20 \div 5 = 4$; $1 + \dfrac{4 \times 4}{4 \times 5} = 1\dfrac{16}{20}$

$3^{1}/_{4} = 3^{5}/_{20}$: $20 \div 4 = 5$; $3 + \dfrac{5 \times 1}{5 \times 4} = 3\dfrac{+5}{20}$

$$6\dfrac{39}{20}$$
$$= 6 + 20\overline{)39}\,1\tfrac{19}{20} = 7\tfrac{19}{20}$$
$$\dfrac{20}{19}$$

25. 1/3, 1/7, 1/9   Least common denominator: 63

$1/3 = 21/63$: $63 \div 3 = 21$; $\dfrac{21 \times 1}{21 \times 3} = \dfrac{21}{63}$

$1/7 = 9/63$: $63 \div 7 = 9$; $\dfrac{9 \times 1}{9 \times 7} = \dfrac{9}{63}$

$1/9 = 7/63$: $63 \div 9 = 7$; $\dfrac{7 \times 1}{7 \times 9} = \dfrac{+7}{63}$

$$\dfrac{37}{63}$$

26.
$$2\tfrac{5}{8}$$
$$-1\tfrac{3}{8}$$
$$\overline{1\tfrac{2}{8}} = 1\dfrac{2 \div 2}{8 \div 2} = 1\dfrac{1}{4}$$

27. $5\tfrac{3}{16} - 2\tfrac{7}{8}$ Least common denominator: 16

$5\tfrac{3}{16} = 5 - 1\dfrac{(1 \times 16) + 3}{16} = 4\tfrac{19}{16}$

$-2\tfrac{7}{8} = 2 \qquad \dfrac{7 \times 2}{8 \times 2} = -2\tfrac{14}{16}$

$$2\tfrac{5}{16}$$

28. $2\tfrac{5}{6} - 1\tfrac{2}{3}$ Least common denominator: 6

$2\tfrac{5}{6} = \qquad = 2\tfrac{5}{6}$

$-1\tfrac{2}{3} = 1\dfrac{(2 \times 2)}{2 \times 3} = -1\tfrac{4}{6}$

$$1\tfrac{1}{6}$$

29.
$$4 = 3\tfrac{16}{16}$$
$$-3\tfrac{15}{16} = -3\tfrac{15}{16}$$
$$\overline{\tfrac{1}{16}}$$

30. $5\tfrac{1}{4} - 3\tfrac{15}{16}$ Least common denominator: 16

$5\tfrac{1}{4} = 5\dfrac{(4 \times 1)}{4 \times 4} = 5\tfrac{4}{16} = 5 - 1\dfrac{(16 \times 1) + 4}{16} = 4\tfrac{20}{16}$

$-3\tfrac{15}{16} \qquad\qquad\qquad\qquad\qquad\qquad\qquad -3\tfrac{15}{16}$

$$1\tfrac{5}{16}$$

31. $1/4 \times 3/5 \times 1/3 = \dfrac{1 \times \cancel{3}\,^{1} \times 1}{4 \times 5 \times \cancel{3}\,_{1}} = \dfrac{1}{20}$

32. $2\tfrac{1}{2} \times 1\tfrac{3}{8} \times 6\tfrac{1}{3} = \dfrac{[(2 \times 2) + 1] \times [(1 \times 8) + 3] \times [(6 \times 3) + 1]}{2 \quad \times \quad 8 \quad \times \quad 3}$

$= \dfrac{5 \times 11 \times 19}{2 \times 8 \times 3} = \dfrac{1045}{48} = 48\overline{)1045}\,21\tfrac{37}{48}$

$$\dfrac{96}{85}$$
$$\dfrac{48}{37}$$

33. $3 \times 1/3 \times 1\tfrac{3}{16} = \dfrac{3 \times 1 \times [(1 \times 16) + 3]}{1 \times 3 \times 16} = \dfrac{\cancel{3}\,^{1} \times 1 \times 19}{1 \times \cancel{3}\,_{1} \times 16}$

$= \dfrac{19}{16} = 16\overline{)19}\,1\tfrac{3}{16}$

$$\dfrac{16}{3}$$

34. $3\tfrac{1}{4} \times \tfrac{2}{5} \times 4 = \dfrac{[(3 \times 4) + 1] \times 2 \times 4}{4 \times 5 \times 1} = \dfrac{13 \times 2 \times \cancel{4}\,^{1}}{\cancel{4}\,_{1} \times 5 \times 1}$

$= \dfrac{26}{5} = 5\overline{)26}\,5\tfrac{1}{5}$

$$\dfrac{25}{1}$$

35. $\tfrac{1}{3} \times \tfrac{1}{3} \times \tfrac{1}{3} = \dfrac{1 \times 1 \times 1}{3 \times 3 \times 3} = \dfrac{1}{27}$

36. $2\tfrac{1}{3} \div \tfrac{6}{7} = \dfrac{(2 \times 3) + 1}{3} \div \tfrac{6}{7} = \tfrac{7}{3} \div \tfrac{6}{7} = \dfrac{7 \times 7}{3 \times 6}$

$= \dfrac{49}{18} = 18\overline{)49}\,2\tfrac{13}{18}$

$$\dfrac{36}{13}$$

37. $\tfrac{1}{3} \div \tfrac{1}{3} = \dfrac{1 \times 3}{3 \times 1} = \dfrac{3}{3} = 1$

38. $6 \div \tfrac{1}{8} = \tfrac{6}{1} \div \tfrac{1}{8} = \dfrac{6 \times 8}{1 \times 1} = \dfrac{48}{1} = 48$

39. $3/8 \div 1\tfrac{1}{3} = \tfrac{3}{8} \div \dfrac{(1 \times 3) + 1}{3} = \tfrac{3}{8} \div \tfrac{4}{3} = \dfrac{3 \times 3}{8 \times 4} = \dfrac{9}{32}$

40. $3/7 \div 3 = \tfrac{3}{7} \div \tfrac{3}{1} = \dfrac{\cancel{3}\,^{1} \times 1}{7 \times \cancel{3}\,_{1}} = \dfrac{1}{7}$

Chapter 3: Decimal Fractions

1. $\dfrac{3}{12} = 12\overline{)3.00}\,0.25$

$$\dfrac{2\,4}{60}$$
$$\dfrac{60}{0}$$

2. $4/1000 = 0.004. = 0.004$

3. $2\tfrac{4}{9} = 2 + 9\overline{)4.0000}\,0.4444 = 2.4444$

$$\dfrac{3\,6}{40}$$
$$\dfrac{36}{40}$$
$$\dfrac{36}{40}$$
$$\dfrac{36}{4}$$

4. $0.326 = \dfrac{\overset{163}{\cancel{326}}}{\underset{500}{\cancel{1000}}} = \dfrac{163}{500}$

5. $0.15 = \dfrac{\overset{3}{\cancel{15}}}{\underset{20}{\cancel{100}}} = \dfrac{3}{20}$

6. $102 + 1.02 + 10.2 =$

$$
\begin{array}{r}
102.00 \\
1.02 \\
+\ 10.20 \\
\hline
113.22
\end{array}
$$

7. $1.05 + 10 + 10.30 =$

$$
\begin{array}{r}
1.05 \\
10.00 \\
+\ 10.30 \\
\hline
21.35
\end{array}
$$

8. $16.9 + 19.243 + 170.23 + 1.982 =$

$$
\begin{array}{r}
16.900 \\
19.243 \\
170.230 \\
+\ 1.982 \\
\hline
208.355
\end{array}
$$

9. $1.03 + 5.2 + 3.13 =$

$$
\begin{array}{r}
1.03 \\
5.20 \\
+\ 3.13 \\
\hline
9.36
\end{array}
$$

10. $13.6 + 18.25 + 2.003 =$

$$
\begin{array}{r}
13.600 \\
18.250 \\
+\ 2.003 \\
\hline
33.853
\end{array}
$$

11. $214.5 - 138.24 =$

$$
\begin{array}{r}
0\ \ 4 \\
214.50 \\
-\ 138.24 \\
\hline
76.26
\end{array}
$$

12. $9.24 - 8.98 =$

$$
\begin{array}{r}
8\ 1 \\
9.24 \\
-\ 8.98 \\
\hline
0.26
\end{array}
$$

13. $26.0 - 8.3333 =$

$$
\begin{array}{r}
15\ 999 \\
26.0000 \\
-\ 8.3333 \\
\hline
17.6667
\end{array}
$$

14. $3.1 - 1.0504 =$

$$
\begin{array}{r}
099 \\
3.1000 \\
-\ 1.0504 \\
\hline
2.0496
\end{array}
$$

15. $32.98 - 3.89 =$

$$
\begin{array}{r}
2\ \ 8 \\
32.98 \\
-\ 3.89 \\
\hline
29.09
\end{array}
$$

16.

$$
\begin{array}{r}
22.9 \\
\times\ 15 \\
\hline
1145 \\
229\ \ \\
\hline
3435
\end{array}
$$
;   1 decimal point space $= 343.5$

17.

$$
\begin{array}{r}
4.0005 \\
\times\ 4.005 \\
\hline
200025 \\
00000 \\
00000 \\
160020\ \ \ \ \ \\
\hline
160220025
\end{array}
$$
;   7 decimal point spaces $= 16.0220025$

18. $6.000 \times 0.34 = 6 \times 0.34$

$$
\begin{array}{r}
= 0.34 \\
\times\ 6 \\
\hline
204
\end{array}
$$
;   2 decimal point spaces $= 2.04$

19.

$$
\begin{array}{r}
1.02 \\
\times\ 25.2 \\
\hline
204 \\
510\ \ \\
204\ \ \ \ \\
\hline
25704
\end{array}
$$
;   3 decimal point spaces $= 25.704$

20.

$$
\begin{array}{r}
0.98 \\
\times\ 9.8 \\
\hline
784 \\
882\ \ \\
\hline
9604
\end{array}
$$
;   3 decimal point spaces $= 9.604$

21.

$$
0.25 \overline{)0.40\cdot 0} \quad \begin{array}{r} 1.6 \end{array}
$$

$$
\begin{array}{r}
25 \\
\hline
15\ 0 \\
15\ 0 \\
\hline
0
\end{array}
$$

22. $15.4 \overline{)26.9\cdot 860}$ $\dfrac{1.752}{} = 1.75$

$$
\begin{array}{r}
15\ 4 \\
\hline
11\ 5\ 8 \\
10\ 7\ 8 \\
\hline
8\ 06 \\
7\ 70 \\
\hline
360 \\
308 \\
\hline
52
\end{array}
$$

23. $25.06 \overline{)823.00\cdot 000}$ $\dfrac{32.841}{} = 32.84$

$$
\begin{array}{r}
751\ 8 \\
\hline
71\ 20 \\
50\ 12 \\
\hline
21\ 08\ 0 \\
20\ 04\ 8 \\
\hline
1\ 03\ 20 \\
1\ 00\ 24 \\
\hline
2\ 960 \\
2\ 506 \\
\hline
454
\end{array}
$$

24. $18.5 \overline{)26.8\cdot 000}$ $\dfrac{1.448}{} = 1.45$

$$
\begin{array}{r}
18\ 5 \\
\hline
8\ 3\ 0 \\
7\ 4\ 0 \\
\hline
9\ 00 \\
7\ 40 \\
\hline
1\ 600 \\
1\ 480 \\
\hline
120
\end{array}
$$

25. $22.08 \overline{)560.00\cdot 000}$ $\dfrac{25.362}{} = 25.36$

$$
\begin{array}{r}
44\ 16 \\
\hline
118\ 40 \\
110\ 40 \\
\hline
8\ 00\ 0 \\
6\ 62\ 4 \\
\hline
1\ 37\ 60 \\
1\ 32\ 48 \\
\hline
5\ 120 \\
4\ 416 \\
\hline
704
\end{array}
$$

Chapter 4: Percentages

1. $0.42 = 0.42 \times 100 = 42\%$
2. $1.05 = 1.05 \times 100 = 105\%$
3. $0.0275 = 0.0275 \times 100 = 2.75\%$
4. $13\frac{1}{2}\% = 13 + \dfrac{0.5}{2 \overline{)1.0}} = 13.5\% \div 100 = 0.135$
   $\quad\quad\quad\quad\quad\quad 1\ 0$

5. $\frac{3}{4}\% = \dfrac{0.75}{4 \overline{)3.00}} = 0.75\% \div 100 = 0.0075$
   $\quad\quad\quad 2\ 8$
   $\quad\quad\quad\ \ 20$
   $\quad\quad\quad\ \ \underline{20}$

6. $\frac{6}{7} = \dfrac{0.857}{7 \overline{)6.000}} = 0.857 \times 100 = 85.7\%$
   $\quad\quad 5\ 6$
   $\quad\quad\ \ 40$
   $\quad\quad\ \ \underline{35}$
   $\quad\quad\ \ 50$
   $\quad\quad\ \ \underline{49}$
   $\quad\quad\ \ \ 1$

7. $\frac{2}{15} = \dfrac{0.133}{15 \overline{)2.000}} = 0.133 \times 100 = 13.3\%$
   $\quad\quad\quad 1\ 5$
   $\quad\quad\quad\ 50$
   $\quad\quad\quad\ \underline{45}$
   $\quad\quad\quad\ 50$
   $\quad\quad\quad\ \underline{45}$

8. $\frac{7}{10} = 0.7 \times 100 = 70\%$

9. $12\% = \dfrac{\cancel{12}}{\cancel{100}} = 3 = {}^{3}\!/_{25}$
   $\quad\quad\quad\ 25$

10. $55\% = \dfrac{\cancel{55}}{\cancel{100}} = 11 = {}^{11}\!/_{20}$
    $\quad\quad\quad\ 20$

11. 20% of $120 = 120 \times 0.2\ (0.20) = 24.0 = 24$
12. 2% of $21 = 21 \times 0.02 = 0.42$
13. $12\frac{1}{2}\%$ of $100 = 12 + \dfrac{0.5}{2 \overline{)1.0}} = 12.5\% \times 100$
    $\quad\quad\quad\quad\quad\quad\quad 1\ 0$
    $\quad\quad\quad = 0.125 \times 100 = 12.5$

14. Answer: interest plus account balance in dollars
    Interest: 6%   Account balance : $250.35
    $(6\% \times \$250.35) + \$250.35 = \quad \$250.35$
    $\quad\quad\quad\quad\quad\quad\quad\quad\quad\quad\quad\quad \underline{\times\ 0.06}$
    $\quad\quad\quad\quad\quad\quad\quad\quad\quad\quad\quad\quad \$15.0210$
    $= \$15.02 + \$250.35 = \$265.37$
    $(6\% + 100\%) \times 250.35 = \quad \$250.35$
    $\quad\quad\quad\quad\quad\quad\quad\quad\quad\quad\quad \underline{\times\ 1.06}$
    $\quad\quad\quad\quad\quad\quad\quad\quad\quad\quad\quad 150210$
    $\quad\quad\quad\quad\quad\quad\quad\quad\quad\quad\quad 00000$
    $\quad\quad\quad\quad\quad\quad\quad\quad\quad\quad\quad \underline{25035}$
    $\quad\quad\quad\quad\quad\quad\quad\quad\quad\quad\quad 2653710 = \$265.3710$
    $\quad\quad\quad\quad\quad\quad\quad\quad\quad\quad\quad\quad\quad\quad = \$265.37$

15. Answer: number of parts to equal 10% increase
    % increase: 10%   Number parts: 1260
    $10\% + 1260 = 0.1 \times 1260 = 126.0 = 126$ more computer parts

Chapter 5: Equations Written as Fractions

Numbers in parentheses indicate multiplication of numerators and denominators without cancellation.

1. $\dfrac{\overset{1}{\cancel{6}} \times \overset{1}{\cancel{3}} \times \overset{3}{6} \times \overset{1}{\cancel{5}}}{\underset{2}{\cancel{10}} \times \underset{2}{\cancel{10}} \times \underset{1}{\cancel{3}} \times \underset{5}{\cancel{15}}} = \dfrac{1 \times 1 \times 3 \times 1}{1 \times 2 \times 1 \times 5} = \dfrac{3}{10} = 0.3$ \hfill (450/1500)

2. $\dfrac{\overset{1}{\cancel{6}} \times \overset{1}{\cancel{12}} \times \overset{1}{5} \times \overset{2}{\cancel{16}}}{\underset{1}{\cancel{10}} \times \underset{1}{\cancel{4}} \times \underset{1}{\cancel{6}} \times \underset{1}{\cancel{6}}} = \dfrac{1 \times 1 \times 1 \times 2}{1 \times 1 \times 1 \times 1} = \dfrac{2}{1} = 2$ \hfill (2880/1440)

3. $\dfrac{\overset{1}{\cancel{2}} \times \overset{1}{\cancel{7}} \times \overset{5}{\cancel{25}} \times \overset{1}{\cancel{9}}}{\underset{1}{\cancel{6}} \times \underset{1}{\cancel{3}} \times \underset{3}{\cancel{21}} \times \underset{4}{\cancel{20}}} = \dfrac{1 \times 1 \times 5 \times 1}{1 \times 1 \times 3 \times 4} = \dfrac{5}{12} = 0.41\overline{6} = 0.42$ \hfill (3150/7560)

4. $\dfrac{\overset{2}{\cancel{8}} \times 16 \times \overset{4}{\cancel{24}} \times \overset{1}{\cancel{9}}}{\underset{1}{\cancel{6}} \times \underset{3}{\cancel{27}} \times \underset{1}{\cancel{4}} \times 5} = \dfrac{2 \times 16 \times 4 \times 1}{1 \times 3 \times 1 \times 5} = \dfrac{128}{15} = 8.5\overline{3} = 8.53$ \hfill (27648/3240)

5. $\dfrac{\overset{2}{\cancel{6}} \times \overset{1}{5} \times \overset{8}{\cancel{120}} \times \overset{4}{\cancel{60}}}{\underset{1}{1} \times \underset{5}{\cancel{25}} \times \underset{1}{\cancel{15}} \times \underset{1}{\cancel{3}}} = \dfrac{2 \times 1 \times 8 \times 4}{1 \times 1 \times 1 \times 1} = \dfrac{64}{1} = 64$ \hfill (216000/3375)

6. $\dfrac{1/2 \times 5 \times 6 \times 2}{1 \times 4 \times 7 \times 15} = \dfrac{1 \times \overset{1}{\cancel{5}} \times \overset{1}{\cancel{6}} \times \overset{1}{\cancel{2}}}{\underset{1}{\cancel{2}} \times 1 \times \underset{2}{\cancel{4}} \times 7 \times \underset{1}{\cancel{15}}} = \dfrac{1 \times 1 \times 1 \times 1}{1 \times 1 \times 2 \times 7 \times 1} = \dfrac{1}{14} = 0.071 = 0.07$ \hfill (60/2) \hfill (420)

7. $\dfrac{4\,2/3 \times 30 \times 9 \times 2}{2 \times 7 \times 8 \times 1} = \dfrac{14/3 \times 30 \times 9 \times 2}{2 \times 7 \times 8 \times 1} = \dfrac{14 \times 30 \times 9 \times 2}{3 \times 2 \times 7 \times 8 \times 1} = \dfrac{1 \times 5 \times 9 \times 1}{1 \times 1 \times 1 \times 2 \times 1} = \dfrac{45}{2} = 22.5$ $\qquad \dfrac{(7560/3)}{112}$

8. $\dfrac{1\,1/4 \times 2 \times 1 \times 2}{1 \times 3 \times 5 \times 1} = \dfrac{5/4 \times 2 \times 1 \times 2}{1 \times 3 \times 5 \times 1} = \dfrac{5 \times 2 \times 1 \times 2}{4 \times 1 \times 3 \times 5 \times 1} = \dfrac{1 \times 1 \times 1 \times 1}{1 \times 1 \times 3 \times 1 \times 1} = \dfrac{1}{3} = 0.33$ $\qquad \dfrac{(20/4)}{15}$

9. $\dfrac{3/5 \times 5 \times 2 \times 9}{1 \times 4 \times 18 \times 1} = \dfrac{3 \times 5 \times 2 \times 9}{5 \times 1 \times 4 \times 18 \times 1} = \dfrac{3 \times 1 \times 1 \times 1}{1 \times 1 \times 2 \times 2 \times 1} = \dfrac{3}{4} = 0.75$ $\qquad \dfrac{(270/5)}{(72)}$

10. $\dfrac{6/7 \times 5 \times 9 \times 30}{2 \times 25 \times 6 \times 4} = \dfrac{6 \times 5 \times 9 \times 30}{7 \times 2 \times 25 \times 6 \times 4} = \dfrac{1 \times 1 \times 9 \times 3}{7 \times 1 \times 1 \times 1 \times 4} = \dfrac{27}{28} = 0.964 = 0.96$ $\qquad \dfrac{(8100/7)}{(1200)}$

11. $\dfrac{4 \times 1 \times 18 \times 9}{1/6 \times 24 \times 27 \times 8} = \dfrac{6 \times 4 \times 1 \times 18 \times 9}{1 \times 24 \times 27 \times 8} = \dfrac{1 \times 1 \times 1 \times 3 \times 1}{1 \times 4 \times 1 \times 1} = \dfrac{3}{4} = 0.75$ $\qquad \dfrac{(648)}{(5184/6)}$

12. $\dfrac{9 \times 1 \times 8 \times 1}{3/4 \times 8 \times 7 \times 3} = \dfrac{4 \times 9 \times 1 \times 8 \times 1}{3 \times 8 \times 7 \times 3} = \dfrac{1 \times 1 \times 1 \times 4 \times 1}{1 \times 1 \times 7 \times 1} = \dfrac{4}{7} = 0.571 = 0.57$ $\qquad \dfrac{(72)}{(504/4)}$

13. $\dfrac{1 \times 4 \times 7 \times 5}{3 \times 21 \times 10 \times 1\,4/7} = \dfrac{1 \times 4 \times 7 \times 5}{3 \times 21 \times 10 \times 11/7} = \dfrac{1 \times 4 \times 7 \times 5 \times 7}{3 \times 21 \times 10 \times 11} = \dfrac{1 \times 2 \times 1 \times 1 \times 7}{3 \times 3 \times 1 \times 11} = \dfrac{14}{99} = 0.141 = 0.14$ $\qquad \dfrac{(140)}{(69307)}$

14. $\dfrac{5 \times 9 \times 15 \times 2}{2/3 \times 4 \times 60 \times 1} = \dfrac{3 \times 5 \times 9 \times 15 \times 2}{2 \times 4 \times 60 \times 1} = \dfrac{1 \times 1 \times 9 \times 15 \times 1}{1 \times 4 \times 4 \times 1} = \dfrac{135}{16} = 8.437 = 8.44$ $\qquad \dfrac{(1350)}{(480/3)}$

15. $\dfrac{2 \times 3 \times 6 \times 3}{1\,1/2 \times 6 \times 9 \times 8} = \dfrac{2 \times 3 \times 6 \times 3}{3/2 \times 6 \times 9 \times 8} = \dfrac{2 \times 2 \times 3 \times 6 \times 3}{3 \times 6 \times 9 \times 8} = \dfrac{1 \times 1 \times 1 \times 1 \times 1}{1 \times 1 \times 3 \times 2} = \dfrac{1}{6} = 0.166 = 0.17$ $\qquad \dfrac{(108)}{(1296/2)}$

16. $\dfrac{0.5 \times 3 \times 1/6 \times 5}{4 \times 5 \times 8 \times 3} = \dfrac{0.5 \times 3 \times 1 \times 5}{4 \times 5 \times 6 \times 8 \times 3} = \dfrac{0.5 \times 1 \times 1 \times 1}{4 \times 1 \times 2 \times 8 \times 3} = \dfrac{0.5}{192} = 0.0026 = 0.003$ $\qquad \dfrac{(7.5/6)}{(480)}$

17. $\dfrac{10 \times \left(\dfrac{110 \times 1}{1 \times 2.2}\right) \times 33}{1 \times 1 \times 4} = \dfrac{10 \times 110 \times 1 \times 33}{1 \times 1 \times 2.2 \times 1 \times 4} = \dfrac{5 \times 25 \times 1 \times 33}{1 \times 1 \times 1 \times 1 \times 1} = \dfrac{4125}{1} = 4125$ $\qquad \dfrac{(36300/2.2)}{(4)}$

18. $\dfrac{2 \times (3\,1/2 + 1/4) \times 4}{1 \times 9 \times 0.3} = \dfrac{2 \times 15 \times 4}{1 \times 4 \times 9 \times 0.3} = \dfrac{1 \times 5 \times 2}{1 \times 1 \times 3 \times 0.3} = \dfrac{10}{0.9} = 11.111 = 11.11$ $\qquad \dfrac{(120/4)}{(2.7)}$

$[3\,2/4 + 1/4 = 3\,3/4 = 15/4]$

19. $\dfrac{1 \times 5 \times 7 \times 24}{4/7 \times 21 \times 4 \times 1} = \dfrac{\overset{1}{\cancel{7}} \times 1 \times 5 \times 7 \times \overset{\overset{\overset{1}{\cancel{2}}}{\cancel{6}}}{\cancel{24}}}{\underset{1}{\cancel{4}} \times \underset{3}{\cancel{21}} \times \underset{2}{\cancel{4}} \times 1} = \dfrac{1 \times 1 \times 5 \times 7 \times 1}{1 \times 1 \times 2 \times 1} = \dfrac{35}{2} = 17.5$ $\dfrac{(840)}{(336/7)}$

20. $\dfrac{2 \times 5 \times \dfrac{(110 \times 1)}{(1 \times 20)} \times 50}{1 \times 0.4 \times \qquad 1 \times 22} = \dfrac{\underset{1}{\cancel{2}} \times 5 \times \overset{1}{\cancel{110}} \times 1 \times \overset{25}{\cancel{50}}}{1 \times 0.4 \times 1 \times \underset{\underset{1}{\cancel{10}}}{\cancel{20}} \times 1 \times \underset{\underset{1}{\cancel{2}}}{\cancel{22}}} = \dfrac{1 \times 5 \times 1 \times 1 \times 25}{1 \times 0.4 \times 1 \times 1 \times 1 \times 1} = \dfrac{125}{0.4} = 312.5$ $\dfrac{(55000/20)}{(8.8)}$

UNIT II: INTRODUCTION TO DIMENSIONAL ANALYSIS
Chapter 6: The Dimensional Analysis Method

1. 16 tablespoons = _____ cups

$$C = \frac{1\,C \times 1\,oz \times 16\,tbsp}{8\,oz \times 2\,tbsp \times 1} = \frac{1\,C \times 1 \times \overset{2}{\cancel{16}}}{\underset{1}{\cancel{8}} \times \underset{1}{\cancel{2}} \times 1} = \frac{1\,C \times 1 \times 1}{1 \times 1 \times 1} = \frac{1\,C}{1} = 1\,C$$

2. 28 inches = _____ yards

$$yd = \frac{1\,yd \times 1\,ft \times 28\,in}{3\,ft \times 12\,in \times 1} = \frac{1\,yd \times 1 \times \overset{7}{\cancel{28}}}{3 \times \cancel{12} \times 1} = \frac{1\,yd \times 1 \times 7}{3 \times 3 \times 1} = \frac{7\,yd}{9} = 7/9\,yd$$

3. 82 ounces = _____ pounds

$$lb = \frac{1\,lb \times 82\,oz}{16\,oz \times 1} = \frac{1\,lb \times \overset{41}{\cancel{82}}}{\underset{8}{\cancel{16}} \times 1} = \frac{1\,lb \times 41}{8 \times 1} = \frac{41\,lb}{8} = 5\,1/8\,lb$$

4. 24 ounces = _____ pints

$$pt = \frac{1\,pt \times 1\,C \times 24\,oz}{2\,C \times 8\,oz \times 1} = \frac{1\,pt \times 1 \times \overset{3}{\cancel{24}}}{2 \times \underset{1}{\cancel{8}} \times 1} = \frac{1\,pt \times 1 \times 3}{2 \times 1 \times 1} = \frac{3\,pt}{2} = 1\,1/2\,pt$$

5. 8 3/4 pounds = _____ ounces

$$oz = \frac{16\,oz \times 8\,3/4\,lb}{1\,lb \times 1} = \frac{16\,oz \times 35/4}{1 \times 1} = \frac{\overset{4}{\cancel{16}}\,oz \times 35}{1 \times \underset{1}{\cancel{4}} \times 1} = \frac{4\,oz \times 35}{1 \times 1 \times 1} = \frac{140\,oz}{1} = 140\,oz$$

6. Unit of answer: $ Factors: 3 lb = $1.04 5 5/8 lb/1

$$\$ = \frac{\$1.04 \times 5\,5/8\,lb}{3\,lb \times 1} = \frac{\$1.04 \times 45/8}{3 \times 1} = \frac{\overset{0.13}{\cancel{\$1.04}} \times \overset{15}{\cancel{45}}}{\underset{1}{\cancel{3}} \times 1 \times \underset{1}{\cancel{8}}} = \frac{\$0.13 \times 15}{1 \times 1} = \frac{\$1.95}{1} = \$1.95$$

7. Unit of answer: $ Factors: $15,000 = 100% 11%/1

$$\$ = \frac{\$15,000 \times 11\%}{100\% \times 1} = \frac{\overset{150}{\cancel{\$15,000}} \times 11}{\underset{1}{\cancel{100}} \times 1} = \frac{\$150 \times 11}{1 \times 1} = \frac{\$1650}{1} = \$1650$$

8. This problem asks for a comparison of 80 kilometers per hour and 55 miles per hour. If 55 mi/h is equal to or less than 80 km/h, the driver is not speeding. For this comparison, mi/h can be converted to km/h or km/h can be converted to mi/h.
Unit of answer: km/h (m/h)   Factor: 55mi/h (80km/h)   Conversion factor: 1 km = 0.6 mi

$$\frac{km}{h} = \frac{1\,km \times 55\,mi}{0.6\,mi \times 1\,h} = \frac{1\,km \times 55}{0.6 \times 1\,h} = \frac{55\,km}{0.6\,h} = \frac{91.666\,km}{1\,h} = 91.67\,km/h$$

91.67 km/h > 80km/h (the speed limit). Therefore, the driver is speeding.

$$\frac{mi}{h} = \frac{0.6\,mi \times 80\,km}{1\,km \times 1\,h} = \frac{0.6\,mi \times 80}{1 \times 1\,h} = \frac{48\,mi}{1\,h} = 48\,mi/h$$

48 mi/h (the speed limit) is less than 55 mi/h. Therefore, the driver is speeding.

9. Unit of answer: $ Factors: $128.50 = 100% 115%/1 The new tax is 115% of the old tax.

$$\$ = \frac{\$128.50 \times 115\,\%}{100\,\% \times 1} = \frac{\overset{64.25}{\cancel{\$128.50}} \times \overset{23}{\cancel{115}}}{\underset{\underset{10}{\cancel{20}}}{\cancel{100}} \times 1} = \frac{\$64.25 \times 23}{10 \times 1} = \frac{\$1477.75}{10} = \$147.775 = \$147.78$$

10. Unit of answer: sq yd   Factor: 189 sq ft/1   Conversion factor: 1 sq yd = 9 sq ft

$$sq\,yd = \frac{1\,sq\,yd \times 189\,sq\,ft}{9\,sq\,ft \times 1} = \frac{1\,sq\,yd \times \overset{21}{\cancel{189}}}{\underset{1}{\cancel{9}} \times 1} = \frac{21\,sq\,yd}{1} = 21\,sq\,yd$$

11. 36 mi = _____ km

$$km = \frac{1\ km \times 36\ mi}{0.6\ mi \times 1} = \frac{1\ km \times \overset{6}{\cancel{36}}}{\underset{1}{\cancel{0.6}} \times 1}\ \underset{(0.1)}{} = \frac{6\ km}{1}\ \underset{(0.1)}{} = 6\ km\ (60\ km)$$

The error is in cancellations of 0.6 by 6. The corrections are in parentheses.

12. 25 yd = _____ rd

$$rd = \frac{1\ rd \times 3\ ft \times 25\ yd}{16\ 2/3\ ft \times 1\ yd \times 1} = \frac{1\ rd \times 3 \times 25}{50/3 \times 1 \times 1} = \frac{50 \times 1\ rd \times \overset{1}{\cancel{3}} \times 25}{\underset{1}{\cancel{3}} \times 1 \times 1} = \frac{1250\ rd}{1} = 1250\ rd$$

This answer is illogical. A rod is larger than a yard. Therefore, the number of rods must be less than the number of yards. The error is not inverting the proper fraction. The correct equation is as follows:

$$\frac{3 \times 1\ rd \times 3 \times \overset{1}{\cancel{25}}}{\underset{2}{\cancel{50}} \times 1 \times 1} = \frac{3 \times 1\ rd \times 3 \times 1}{2 \times 1 \times 1} = \frac{9\ rd}{2} = 4\ 1/2\ rd$$

13. What is this month's interest on a loan of $300 with an interest rate of 20% per year?

$$\$ = \frac{\$300 \times 20\ \% \times 1\ yr \times 1\ mo}{100\% \times 1\ yr \times 12\ mo \times 1} = \frac{\overset{3}{\cancel{\$300}} \times \overset{4\,(5)}{\cancel{20}} \times 1 \times 1}{\underset{1}{\cancel{100}} \times 1 \times \underset{3}{\cancel{12}} \times 1} = \frac{\overset{(15)}{\$12}}{3} = \$4.00\ (\$5.00)$$

The error is in cancellations of 20 by 4. The corrections are in parentheses.

14. 2 gal = _____ oz

$$oz = \frac{8\ oz \times 2\ C \times 2\ pt \times 4\ qt \times 2\ gal}{1\ C \times 1\ pt \times 1\ qt \times 1\ gal \times 1} = \frac{8\ oz \times 2 \times 2 \times 4 \times 2}{1 \times 1 \times 1 \times 1 \times 1} = \frac{\overset{(256)}{108}\ oz}{1} = 108\ oz\ (256\ oz)$$

The error is in multiplication of the numerator. The corrections are in parentheses.

15. Three dozen eggs cost $1.39. How much will 84 eggs cost?

$$\$ = \frac{\$1.39 \times 1\ dozen \times 84\ eggs}{3\ dozen \times 12\ eggs \times 1} = \frac{\$1.39 \times 1 \times \overset{7}{\cancel{84}}}{3 \times \underset{1}{\cancel{12}} \times 1} = \frac{\$9.73}{3}\ \underset{}{\overset{(3.243)}{}} = \$3.333 = \$3.33\ (\$3.24)$$

The error is in division of numerator by denominator. Corrections are in parentheses.

UNIT III: SYSTEMS OF MEASUREMENT

Chapter 7: The English Measurement Systems

1. $\frac{1}{2}\ \overline{3}$ = _____ T

$$T = \frac{2T \times \frac{1}{2}oz}{1oz \times 1} = \frac{2T \times \frac{1}{2}}{1 \times 1} = \frac{\overset{1}{\cancel{2}}T \times 1}{1 \times \underset{1}{\cancel{2}} \times 1} = \frac{1T \times 1}{1 \times 1 \times 1} = \frac{1T}{1} = 1T$$

2. 2 qt = _____ oz

$$oz = \frac{8oz \times 2C \times 2pt \times 2qt}{1C \times 1pt \times 1qt \times 1} = \frac{8oz \times 2 \times 2 \times 2}{1 \times 1 \times 1 \times 1} = \frac{64oz}{1} = 64oz$$

3. 4 tbs = _____ tsp

$$tsp = \frac{3tsp \times 4tbs}{1tbs \times 1} = \frac{3tsp \times 4}{1 \times 1} = \frac{12tsp}{1} = 12tsp$$

4. 12 $\overline{3}$ = _____ tsp

$$tsp = \frac{1tsp \times 12dr}{1dr \times 1} = \frac{1tsp \times 12}{1 \times 1} = \frac{12tsp}{1} = 12\ tsp$$

5. 5 C = _____ oz

$$oz = \frac{8oz \times 5C}{1C \times 1} = \frac{8oz \times 5}{1 \times 1} = \frac{40oz}{1} = 40oz$$

6. 6 pt = _____ qt

$$qt = \frac{1qt \times 6pt}{2pt \times 1} = \frac{1qt \times \overset{3}{\cancel{6}}}{\underset{1}{\cancel{2}} \times 1} = \frac{1qt \times 3}{1 \times 1} = \frac{3qt}{1} = 3qt$$

7. 7 $\overline{3}$ = _____ $\overline{3}$

$$dr = \frac{1dr \times 3tsp \times 2T \times 7oz}{1tsp \times 1T \times 1oz \times 1} = \frac{1dr \times 3 \times 2 \times 7}{1 \times 1 \times 1 \times 1} = \frac{42dr}{1} = 42\ dr$$

8. 30 oz = _____ qt

$$qt = \frac{1qt \times 1pt \times 1C \times 30oz}{2pt \times 2C \times 8oz \times 1} = \frac{1qt \times 1 \times 1 \times \overset{15}{\cancel{30}}}{\underset{2}{\cancel{2}} \times 2 \times 8 \times 1} = \frac{1qt \times 1 \times 1 \times 15}{1 \times 2 \times 8 \times 1}$$
$$= \frac{15qt}{16} = \frac{15}{16}qt$$

9. 18 $\overline{3}$ = _____ lb

$$lb = \frac{1lb \times 18oz}{16oz \times 1} = \frac{1lb \times \overset{9}{\cancel{18}}}{\underset{8}{\cancel{16}} \times 1} = \frac{1lb \times 9}{8 \times 1} = \frac{9lb}{8} = 1\frac{1}{8}lb$$

10. 7 oz = _____ C

$$C = \frac{1C \times 7oz}{8oz \times 1} = \frac{1C \times 7}{8 \times 1} = \frac{7C}{8} = \frac{7}{8}C$$

11. 6 $\overline{3}$ = _____ tbsp

$$tbsp = \frac{2tbsp \times 6oz}{1oz \times 1} = \frac{2tbsp \times 6}{1 \times 1} = \frac{12tbsp}{1} = 12\ tbsp$$

12. 12 oz = _____ pt

$$pt = \frac{1pt \times 1C \times 12oz}{2C \times 8oz \times 1} = \frac{1pt \times 1 \times \overset{3}{\cancel{12}}}{\underset{2}{\cancel{2}} \times \cancel{8} \times 1} = \frac{1pt \times 1 \times 3}{2 \times 2 \times 1} = \frac{3pt}{4} = \frac{3}{4}pt$$

13. 4 C = _____ Tbsp

$$Tbsp = \frac{2Tbsp \times 8oz \times 4C}{1oz \times 1C \times 1} = \frac{2Tbsp \times 8 \times 4}{1 \times 1 \times 1} = \frac{64Tbsp}{1} = 64Tbsp$$

14. $12 \, \overline{3} =$ _____ tbsp

$$\text{tbsp} = \frac{1\text{tbsp} \times 1\text{tsp} \times 12\text{dr}}{3\text{tsp} \times 1\text{dr} \times 1} = \frac{1\text{tbsp} \times 1 \times \cancel{12}^4}{\cancel{3} \times 1 \times 1}$$

$$= \frac{1\text{tbsp} \times 1 \times 4}{1 \times 1 \times 1} = \frac{4\text{tbsp}}{1} = 4\text{tbsp}$$

15. $1\frac{1}{2}$ qt = _____ C

$$C = \frac{2C \times 2\text{pt} \times 1\frac{1}{2}\text{qt}}{1\text{pt} \times 1\text{qt} \times 1} = \frac{2C \times 2 \times \frac{3}{2}}{1 \times 1 \times 1}$$

$$= \frac{\cancel{2}C \times 2 \times 3}{1 \times 1 \times \cancel{2} \times 1} = \frac{1C \times 2 \times 3}{1 \times 1 \times 1 \times 1} = \frac{6C}{1} = 6C$$

16. 60 oz = _____ qt

$$\text{qt} = \frac{1\text{qt} \times 1\text{pt} \times 1C \times 60}{2\text{pt} \times 2C \times 8\text{oz} \times 1} = \frac{1\text{qt} \times 1 \times 1 \times \cancel{60}^{\overset{15}{\cancel{30}}}}{\cancel{2} \times \cancel{2} \times 8 \times 1} = \frac{1\text{qt} \times 1 \times 1 \times 15}{1 \times 1 \times 8 \times 1}$$

$$= \frac{15\text{qt}}{8} = 1\frac{7}{8}\text{qt}$$

17. 21" = _____ '

$$\text{ft} = \frac{1\text{ft} \times 21\text{in}}{12\text{in} \times 1} = \frac{1\text{ft} \times \cancel{21}^7}{\cancel{12}_4 \times 1} = \frac{1\text{ft} \times 7}{4 \times 1} = \frac{7\text{ft}}{4} = 1\frac{3}{4}\text{ft}$$

18. $6\frac{1}{2}$ lb = _____ oz

$$\text{oz} = \frac{16\text{oz} \times 6\frac{1}{2}\text{lb}}{1\text{lb} \times 1} = \frac{16\text{oz} \times \frac{13}{2}}{1 \times 1} = \frac{\cancel{16}^8\text{oz} \times 13}{1 \times \cancel{2}_1} = \frac{8\text{oz} \times 13}{1 \times 1}$$

$$= \frac{104\text{oz}}{1} = 104\text{oz}$$

19. $24 \, \overline{3} =$ _____ lb

$$\text{lb} = \frac{1\text{lb} \times 24\text{oz}}{16\text{oz} \times 1} = \frac{1\text{lb} \times \cancel{24}^3}{\cancel{16}_2 \times 1} = \frac{1\text{lb} \times 3}{2 \times 1} = \frac{3\text{lb}}{2} = 1\frac{1}{2}\text{lb}$$

20. $3\frac{1}{6}$ ft = _____ in

$$\text{in} = \frac{12\text{in} \times 3\frac{1}{6}\text{ft}}{1\text{ft} \times 1} = \frac{12\text{in} \times \frac{19}{6}}{1 \times 1} = \frac{\cancel{12}^2\text{in} \times 19}{1 \times \cancel{6}_1} = \frac{2\text{in} \times 19}{1 \times 1} = \frac{38\text{in}}{1}$$

$$= 38\text{in}$$

In this answer, the dropped fraction denominator, 6, was substituted for the 1 in the equation denominator. This is correct because $6 \times 1 = 6$.

Chapter 8: The Metric System

Alternate solutions are shown in parentheses

1. 4 g = _____ mg

$$\text{mg} = \frac{1000 \, \text{mg} \times 4 \, \text{g}}{1 \, \text{g} \times 1} = \frac{1000 \, \text{mg} \times 4}{1 \times 1} = \frac{4000 \, \text{mg}}{1}$$

$$= 4000 \, \text{mg}$$

2. 2000 mcg = _____ g

$$\text{g} = \frac{1 \, \text{g} \times 1 \, \text{mg} \times 2000 \, \text{mcg}}{1000 \, \text{mg} \times 1000 \, \text{mcg} \times 1} = \frac{1 \, \text{g} \times 1 \times \cancel{2000}^2}{\cancel{1000}_1 \times 1000 \times 1}$$

$$= \frac{1 \, \text{g} \times 1 \times 2}{1 \times 1000 \times 1} = \frac{2 \, \text{g}}{1000} = 0.002 \, \text{g}$$

3. 250 g = _____ kg

$$\text{g} = \frac{1 \, \text{kg} \times 250 \, \text{g}}{1000 \, \text{g} \times 1} = \frac{1 \, \text{kg} \times 250}{1000 \times 1} = \frac{250 \, \text{kg}}{1000} = 0.25 \, \text{kg}$$

$$\left(\frac{1 \, \text{kg} \times \cancel{250}^{0.25}}{\cancel{1000}_1 \times 1} = \frac{1 \, \text{kg} \times 0.25}{1 \times 1} = \frac{0.25 \, \text{kg}}{1} = 0.25 \, \text{kg} \right)$$

4. 0.04 g = _____ mg

$$\text{mg} = \frac{1000 \, \text{mg} \times 0.04 \, \text{g}}{1 \, \text{g} \times 1} = \frac{1000 \, \text{mg} \times 0.04}{1 \times 1} = \frac{40 \, \text{mg}}{1}$$

$$= 40 \, \text{mg}$$

5. 0.5 mg = _____ mcg

$$\text{mcg} = \frac{1000 \, \text{mcg} \times 0.5 \, \text{mg}}{1 \, \text{mg} \times 1} = \frac{1000 \, \text{mcg} \times 0.5}{1 \times 1}$$

$$= \frac{500 \, \text{mcg}}{1} = 500 \, \text{mcg}$$

6. 35 mcg = _____ mg

$$\text{mg} = \frac{1 \, \text{mg} \times 35 \, \text{mcg}}{1000 \, \text{mcg} \times 1} = \frac{1 \, \text{mg} \times 35}{1000 \times 1} = \frac{35 \, \text{mg}}{1000}$$

$$= 0.035 \, \text{mg}$$

$$\left(\frac{1 \, \text{mg} \times \cancel{35}^{0.035}}{\cancel{1000}_1 \times 1} = \frac{1 \, \text{mg} \times 0.035}{1 \times 1} = \frac{0.035 \, \text{mg}}{1} = 0.035 \, \text{mg} \right)$$

7. 0.002 mg = _____ mcg

$$\text{mg} = \frac{1000 \, \text{mg} \times 0.002 \, \text{g}}{1 \times 1} = \frac{1000 \, \text{mg} \times 0.002}{1 \times 1}$$

$$= \frac{2 \, \text{mg}}{1} = 2 \, \text{mg}$$

8. 0.75 mg = _____ mcg

$$\text{mcg} = \frac{1000 \, \text{mcg} \times 0.75 \, \text{mg}}{1 \, \text{mg} \times 1} = \frac{1000 \, \text{mcg} \times 0.75}{1 \times 1}$$

$$= \frac{750 \, \text{mcg}}{1} = 750 \, \text{mcg}$$

9. 3050 g = _____ kg

$$\text{kg} = \frac{1 \, \text{kg} \times 3050 \, \text{g}}{1000 \, \text{g} \times 1} = \frac{1 \, \text{kg} \times \cancel{3050}^{3.05}}{\cancel{1000}_1 \times 1} =$$

$$\frac{1 \, \text{kg} \times 3.05}{1 \times 1}$$

$$= \frac{3.05 \, \text{kg}}{1} = 3.05 \, \text{kg}$$

10. 6.3 kg = _____ g

$$\text{g} = \frac{1000 \, \text{g} \times 6.3 \, \text{kg}}{1 \, \text{kg} \times 1} = \frac{1000 \, \text{g} \times 6.3}{1 \times 1} = \frac{6300 \, \text{g}}{1} = 6300 \, \text{g}$$

11. 3 m = _____ cm

$$\text{cm} = \frac{100 \, \text{cm} \times 3 \, \text{m}}{1 \, \text{m} \times 1} = \frac{100 \, \text{cm} \times 3}{1 \times 1} = \frac{300 \, \text{cm}}{1} = 300 \, \text{cm}$$

12. 15 mm = _____ cm

$$\text{cm} = \frac{1 \, \text{cm} \times 15 \, \text{mm}}{10 \, \text{mm} \times 1} = \frac{1 \, \text{cm} \times \cancel{15}^{1.5}}{\cancel{10}_1 \times 1} = \frac{1.5 \, \text{cm}}{1} = 1.5 \, \text{cm}$$

13. 6 cm = _____ mm

$$\text{mm} = \frac{10 \, \text{mm} \times 6 \, \text{cm}}{1 \, \text{cm} \times 1} = \frac{10 \, \text{mm} \times 6}{1 \times 1} = \frac{60 \, \text{mm}}{1} = 60 \, \text{mm}$$

14. 22 mm = _____ cm

$$\text{cm} = \frac{1 \, \text{cm} \times 22 \, \text{mm}}{10 \, \text{mm} \times 1} = \frac{1 \, \text{cm} \times \cancel{22}^{2.2}}{\cancel{10}_1 \times 1} = \frac{1 \, \text{cm} \times 2.2}{1 \times 1}$$

$$= \frac{2.2 \, \text{cm}}{1} = 2.2 \, \text{cm}$$

15. 0.1 cm = _____ mm

$$\text{mm} = \frac{10 \, \text{mm} \times 0.1 \, \text{cm}}{1 \, \text{cm} \times 1} = \frac{10 \, \text{mm} \times 0.1}{1 \times 1} = \frac{1 \, \text{mm}}{1} = 1 \, \text{mm}$$

16. $0.5\ \text{L} = \underline{\hspace{1cm}} \text{cc}$

$$cc = \frac{1\ cc\ \times 1000\ ml \times 0.5\ L}{1\ ml \times\quad 1\ L\quad \times\quad 1} = \frac{1\ cc\ \times 1000 \times 0.5}{1\quad \times\quad 1\quad \times\ 1} = \frac{500\ cc}{1} = 500\ cc$$

Logically, if 1 ml = 1 cc, then 1000 ml = 1000 cc. Therefore, 1000 cc = 1 L

This conversion factor can be used to omit 1 step in the equation.

This conversion factor is used in solving problem 25.

17. $750\ \text{ml} = \underline{\hspace{1cm}} \text{L}$

$$L = \frac{1\ L\ \times 750\ ml}{1000\ ml \times\quad 1} = \frac{1\ L \times \overset{0.75}{\cancel{750}}}{\cancel{1000} \times\ 1} = \frac{0.75\ L}{1} = 0.75\ L$$

18. $250\ \text{ml} = \underline{\hspace{1cm}} \text{cc}$

$$cc = \frac{1\ cc\ \times 250\ ml}{1\ ml \times\quad 1} = \frac{1\ cc\ \times 250}{1\quad \times\ 1} = \frac{250\ cc}{1} = 250\ cc$$

Logically, if 1 ml = 1 cc, then 250 ml = 250 cc.

19. $1.8\ \text{ml} = \underline{\hspace{1cm}} \text{cc}$

$$cc = \frac{1\ cc\ \times 1.8\ ml}{1\ ml \times\quad 1} = \frac{1\ cc\ \times 1.8}{1\quad \times\ 1} = \frac{1.8\ cc}{1} = 1.8\ cc$$

20. $1.5\ \text{L} = \underline{\hspace{1cm}} \text{cc}$

$$cc = \frac{1000\ cc \times 1.5\ L}{1\ L\quad \times\quad 1} = \frac{1000\ cc \times 1.5}{1\quad \times\quad 1} = \frac{1500\ cc}{1} = 1500\ cc$$

Chapter 9: Conversion Among Measurement Systems

1. $gr\ ii = \underline{\hspace{1cm}} mg$

$$mg = \frac{60\ mg \times gr\ 2}{1\ gr \times\quad 1} = \frac{60\ mg \times 2}{1\quad \times 1} = \frac{120\ mg}{1}$$
$$= 120\ mg$$

$$mg = \frac{1000\ mg \times gr\ 2}{15\ gr \times\quad 1} = \frac{\overset{200}{\cancel{1000}}\ mg \times 2}{\underset{3}{\cancel{15}}\quad \times 1} = \frac{400\ mg}{3}$$
$$= 133.3\ mg$$

2. $0.3\ g = \underline{\hspace{1cm}} gr$

$$gr = \frac{15\ gr \times 0.3\ g}{1\ g \times\quad 1} = \frac{15\ gr \times 0.3}{1\quad \times\ 1} = \frac{4.5\ gr}{1} = 4\tfrac{1}{2}\ gr$$

$$gr = \frac{1\ gr\ \times 1000\ mg \times 0.3\ g}{60\ mg \times\quad 1\ g\quad \times\quad 1} = \frac{1\ gr\ \times \overset{50}{\cancel{1000}} \times \overset{0.1}{\cancel{0.3}}}{\underset{\underset{1}{\cancel{6}}}{\cancel{60}}\quad \times\quad 1 \times 1}$$

$$= \frac{5\ gr}{1} = 5\ gr$$

3. $gr\ 1/300 = \underline{\hspace{1cm}} mcg$

$$mcg = \frac{1000\ mcg \times 60\ mg\ \times gr\ \tfrac{1}{300}}{1\ mg\quad \times\ 1\ gr\quad \times 1}$$
$$= \frac{\overset{10}{\cancel{1000}}\ mcg \times \overset{20}{\cancel{60}} \times\quad 1}{1\quad \times\ 1 \times \underset{\underset{1}{\cancel{6}}}{\cancel{300}}} = \frac{200\ mcg}{1} = 200\ mcg$$

$$mcg = \frac{1000\ mcg \times 1000\ mg\ \times \tfrac{1}{300}\ gr}{1\ mg\quad \times\quad 15\ g\quad \times 1}$$
$$= \frac{\overset{10}{\cancel{1000}}\ mcg \times \overset{200}{\cancel{1000}} \times\quad 1}{1\quad \times\ \underset{3}{\cancel{15}} \times \underset{3}{\cancel{300}}} = \frac{2000\ mcg}{9} = 222.2\ mcg$$

4. $45\ kg = \underline{\hspace{1cm}} lb$

$$lb = \frac{2.2\ lb\ \times 45\ kg}{1\ kg \times\quad 1} = \frac{2.2\ lb\ \times 45}{1\quad \times\ 1} = \frac{99\ lb}{1} = 99\ lb$$

5. $200\ mcg = gr \underline{\hspace{1cm}}$

$$gr = \frac{1\ gr\ \times\quad 1\ mg\ \times 200\ mcg}{60\ mg\ \times 1000\ mcg \times\quad 1} = \frac{1\ gr\quad \times\quad 1 \times \cancel{200}}{60\quad \times \underset{5}{\cancel{1000}} \times\ 1}$$

$$= \frac{1\ gr}{300} = gr\ 1/300$$

$$gr = \frac{15\ gr\quad \times\quad 1\ mg\ \times 200\ mcg}{1000\ mg\ \times 1000\ mcg \times\quad 1} = \frac{\overset{3}{\cancel{15}}\ gr\quad \times\ 1 \times \overset{1}{\cancel{200}}}{\underset{5}{\cancel{1000}}\quad \times \underset{200}{\cancel{1000}} \times\ 1}$$

$$= \frac{3\ gr}{1000} = 3/1000\ gr$$

6. $gr\ viiss = \underline{\hspace{1cm}} g$

$$g = \frac{1\ g\ \times gr\ 7\tfrac{1}{2}}{15\ gr \times\quad 1} = \frac{1\ g\ \times \tfrac{15}{2}}{15\quad \times 1} = \frac{1\ g\ \times \overset{1}{\cancel{15}}}{\underset{1}{\cancel{15}}\quad \times\ 2} = \frac{1\ g}{2} = 0.5\ g$$

7. $6\ lb\ 6\ oz = \underline{\hspace{1cm}} g$

$$g = \frac{1000\ g\ \times\ 1\ kg \times 6\tfrac{3}{8}\ lb}{1\ kg \times 2.2\ lb \times\ 1} = \frac{1000\ g\ \times\quad 1 \times \tfrac{51}{8}}{1\quad \times 2.2 \times 1} = \frac{\overset{125}{\cancel{1000}}\ g\quad \times\ 1 \times 51}{1\quad \times 2.2 \times \underset{1}{\cancel{8}}} = \frac{6375\ g}{2.2} = 2897.7\ g$$

8. $0.04\ g = \underline{\hspace{1cm}} gr$

$$gr = \frac{15\ gr \times 0.04\ g}{1\ g \times\quad 1} = \frac{15\ gr \times 0.04}{1\quad \times\ 1} = \frac{0.6\ gr}{1} = 3/5\ gr$$

9. $154\ lb = \underline{\hspace{1cm}} kg$

$$kg = \frac{1\ kg \times 154\ lb}{2.2\ lb \times\quad 1} = \frac{1\ kg \times \overset{70}{\cancel{154}}}{\underset{1}{\cancel{2.2}}\quad \times\ 1} = \frac{70\ kg}{1} = 70\ kg$$

10. $gr\ XX = \underline{\hspace{1cm}} mg$

$$mg = \frac{60\ mg \times gr\ 20}{1\ gr \times\quad 1} = \frac{60\ mg \times 20}{1\quad \times\ 1} = \frac{1200\ mg}{1}$$
$$= 1200\ mg$$

$$mg = \frac{1000\ mg \times 20\ gr}{15\ gr \times\quad 1} = \frac{1000\ mg \times \overset{4}{\cancel{20}}}{\underset{3}{\cancel{15}}\quad \times\ 1} = \frac{4000\ mg}{3}$$
$$= 1333.3\ mg$$

11. 10 kg = _____ lb

$$lb = \frac{2.2\,lb \times 10\,kg}{1\,kg \times 1} = \frac{2.2\,lb \times 10}{1 \times 1} = \frac{22\,lb}{1} = 22\,lb$$

12. 0.6 mg = _____ gr

$$gr = \frac{1\,gr \times 0.6\,mg}{60\,mg \times 1} = \frac{1\,gr \times 0.6}{60 \times 1} = \frac{gr\;\;0.1}{10}$$

$$= gr\;\;1/100$$

$$gr = \frac{15\,gr \times 0.6\,mg}{1000\,mg \times 1} = \frac{15\,gr \times 0.6}{1000 \times 1} = \frac{gr\;\;0.9}{100}$$

$$= gr\;\;9/1000$$

13. gr $\frac{1}{150}$ = _____ mg

$$mg = \frac{60\,mg \times gr\;\frac{1}{150}}{1\,gr \times 1} = \frac{60\,mg \times \frac{1}{150}}{1 \times 1} = \frac{60\,mg \times 1}{1 \times 150}$$

$$= \frac{2\,mg}{5} = 0.4\,mg$$

$$mg = \frac{1000\,mg \times gr\;\frac{1}{150}}{15\,gr \times 1} = \frac{1000\,mg \times \frac{1}{150}}{15 \times 1} = \frac{1000\,mg \times 1}{15 \times 150}$$

$$= \frac{4\,mg}{9} = 0.44\,mg$$

14. 7 lb 14 oz = _____ kg

$$kg = \frac{1\,kg \times 7\frac{7}{8}\,lb}{2.2\,lb \times 1} = \frac{1\,kg \times \frac{63}{8}}{2.2 \times 1} = \frac{1\,kg \times 63}{2.2 \times 8} = \frac{63\,kg}{17.6} = 3.5795\,kg = 3.58\,kg$$

15. 60 mcg = _____ gr

$$gr = \frac{1\,gr \times 1\,mg \times 60\,mcg}{60\,mg \times 1000\,mcg \times 1} = \frac{1\,gr \times 1 \times 60}{60 \times 1000 \times 1} = \frac{1\,gr}{1000} = gr\;\;1/1000$$

16. 250 g = _____ oz

$$oz = \frac{16\,oz \times 2.2\,lb \times 1\,kg \times 250\,g}{1\,lb \times 1\,kg \times 1000\,g \times 1} = \frac{16\,oz \times 2.2 \times 1 \times 250}{1 \times 1 \times 1000 \times 1} = \frac{8.8\,oz}{1} = 8\;4/5\,oz$$

17. gr $\frac{1}{6}$ = _____ mg

$$mg = \frac{60\,mg \times gr\;\frac{1}{6}}{1\,gr \times 1} = \frac{60\,mg \times \frac{1}{6}}{1 \times 1} = \frac{60\,mg \times 1}{1 \times 6} = \frac{10\,mg}{1}$$

$$= 10\,mg$$

$$mg = \frac{1000\,mg \times gr\;\frac{1}{6}}{15\,gr \times 1} = \frac{1000\,mg \times \frac{1}{6}}{15 \times 1} = \frac{1000\,mg \times 1}{15 \times 6}$$

$$= \frac{100\,mg}{9} = 11.1\,mg$$

18. 0.4 mg = _____ gr

$$gr = \frac{1\,gr \times 0.4\,mg}{60\,mg \times 1} = \frac{1\,gr \times 0.4}{60 \times 1} = \frac{gr\;\;0.1}{15} = gr\;\;1/150$$

19. 4.8 kg = _____ lb

$$lb = \frac{2.2\,lb \times 4.8\,kg}{1\,kg \times 1} = \frac{2.2\,lb \times 4.8}{1 \times 1} = \frac{10.56\,lb}{1} = 10\;14/25\,lb$$

20. 0.8 g = _____ gr

$$gr = \frac{15\,gr \times 0.8\,g}{1\,g \times 1} = \frac{15\,gr \times 0.8}{1 \times 1} = \frac{12\,gr}{1} = 12\,gr$$

21. 8 inches = _____ cm

$$cm = \frac{2.5\,cm \times 8\,in}{1\,in \times 1} = \frac{2.5\,cm \times 8}{1 \times 1} = \frac{20\,cm}{1} = 20\,cm$$

22. 96 cm = _____ in

$$in = \frac{1\,in \times 96\,cm}{2.5\,cm \times 1} = \frac{1\,in \times 96}{2.5 \times 1} = \frac{96\,in}{2.5} = 38\;2/5\,in$$

23. 28 cm = _____ in

$$in = \frac{1\,in \times 28\,cm}{2.5\,cm \times 1} = \frac{1\,in \times 28}{2.5 \times 1} = \frac{28\,in}{2.5} = 11\;1/5\,in$$

24. 42 in = _____ m

$$m = \frac{1\,m \times 42\,in}{39\,in \times 1} = \frac{1\,m \times 42}{39 \times 1} = \frac{14\,m}{13} = 1.077\,m$$

25. 10 cm = _____ in

$$in = \frac{1\,in \times 10\,cm}{2.5\,cm \times 1} = \frac{1\,in \times 10}{2.5 \times 1} = \frac{4\,in}{1} = 4\,in$$

26. 16 in = _____ mm

$$mm = \frac{10\ mm \times 2.5\ cm \times 16\ in}{1\ cm \times 1\ in \times 1} = \frac{10\ mm \times 2.5 \times 16}{1 \times 1 \times 1} = \frac{400\ mm}{1} = 400\ mm$$

27. 112 mm = _____ in

$$in = \frac{1\ in \times 1\ cm \times 112\ mm}{2.5\ cm \times 10\ mm \times 1} = \frac{1\ in \times 1 \times \overset{56}{\cancel{112}}}{2.5 \times \underset{5}{\cancel{10}} \times 1} = \frac{56\ in}{12.5} = 4\ 12/25\ in$$

28. $1\frac{1}{2}$ in = _____ mm

$$mm = \frac{10\ mm \times 2.5\ cm \times 1\frac{1}{2}\ in}{1\ cm \times 1\ in \times 1} = \frac{10\ mm \times 2.5 \times \frac{3}{2}}{1 \times 1 \times 1} = \frac{\overset{5}{\cancel{10}}\ mm \times 2.5 \times 3}{1 \times 1 \times \underset{1}{\cancel{2}}} = \frac{37.5\ mm}{1} = 37.5\ mm$$

29. 12.5 mm = _____ in

$$in = \frac{1\ in \times 1\ cm \times 12.5}{2.5\ cm \times 10\ mm \times 1} = \frac{1\ in \times 1 \times \overset{\overset{1}{\cancel{5}}}{\cancel{12.5}}}{\underset{1}{\cancel{2.5}} \times \underset{2}{\cancel{10}} \times 1} = \frac{1\ in}{2} = 1/2\ in$$

30. 3 in = _____ cm

$$cm = \frac{2.5\ cm \times 3\ in}{1\ in \times 1} = \frac{2.5\ cm \times 3}{1 \times 1} = \frac{7.5\ cm}{1} = 7.5\ cm$$

31. $7\frac{1}{2}$ minims = _____ cc

$$cc = \frac{1\ cc \times 7\frac{1}{2}\ mx}{15\ mx \times 1} = \frac{1\ cc \times \frac{15}{2}}{15 \times 1} = \frac{1\ cc \times \overset{1}{\cancel{15}}}{\underset{1}{\cancel{15}} \times 2}$$
$$= \frac{1\ cc}{2} = 0.5\ cc$$

$$cc = \frac{1\ cc \times 7\frac{1}{2}\ mx}{16\ mx \times 1} = \frac{1\ cc \times \frac{15}{2}}{16 \times 1} = \frac{1\ cc \times 15}{16 \times 2}$$
$$= \frac{15\ cc}{32} = 0.468\ cc = 0.47\ cc$$

32. $1\frac{1}{2}$ oz = _____ cc

$$cc = \frac{30\ cc \times 1\frac{1}{2}\ oz}{1\ oz \times 1} = \frac{30\ cc \times \frac{3}{2}}{1 \times 1} = \frac{\overset{15}{\cancel{30}}\ cc \times 3}{1 \times \underset{1}{\cancel{2}}} = \frac{45\ cc}{1} = 45\ cc$$

33. 3 pt = _____ ml

$$ml = \frac{500\ ml \times 3\ pt}{1\ pt \times 1} = \frac{500\ ml \times 3}{1 \times 1} = \frac{1500\ ml}{1} = 1500\ ml \qquad ml = \frac{30\ ml \times 16\ oz \times 3\ pt}{1\ oz \times 1\ pt \times 1} = \frac{30\ ml \times 16 \times 3}{1 \times 1 \times 1} = \frac{1440\ ml}{1} = 1440\ ml$$

34. 6 ml = _____ minims

$$mx = \frac{15\ mx \times 6\ ml}{1\ ml \times 1} = \frac{15\ mx \times 6}{1 \times 1} = \frac{90\ mx}{1} = 90\ mx \qquad mx = \frac{16\ mx \times 6\ ml}{1\ ml \times 1} = \frac{16\ mx \times 6}{1 \times 1} = \frac{96\ mx}{1} = 96\ mx$$

35. 15 cc = _____ tsp

$$tsp = \frac{1\ tsp \times 15\ cc}{5\ ml \times 1} = \frac{1\ tsp \times \overset{3}{\cancel{15}}}{\underset{1}{\cancel{5}} \times 1} = \frac{3\ tsp}{1} = 3\ tsp \qquad tsp = \frac{1\ tsp \times 15\ cc}{4\ ml \times 1} = \frac{1\ tsp \times 15}{4 \times 1} = \frac{15\ tsp}{4} = 3\ 3/4\ tsp$$

36. 6 drams = _____ ml

$$ml = \frac{5\ ml \times 6\ dr}{1\ dr \times 1} = \frac{5\ ml \times 6}{1 \times 1} = \frac{30\ ml}{1} = 30\ ml \qquad ml = \frac{4\ ml \times 6\ dr}{1\ dr \times 1} = \frac{4\ ml \times 6}{1 \times 1} = \frac{24\ ml}{1} = 24\ ml$$

37. 12 Tbsp = _____ cc

$$cc = \frac{15\ cc \times 12\ Tbsp}{1\ Tbsp \times 1} = \frac{15\ cc \times 12}{1 \times 1} = \frac{180\ cc}{1} = 180\ cc$$

38. 45 ml = _____ Tbsp

$$Tbsp = \frac{1\ Tbsp \times 45\ ml}{15\ ml \times 1} = \frac{1\ Tbsp \times \overset{3}{\cancel{45}}}{\underset{1}{\cancel{15}} \times 1} = \frac{3\ Tbsp}{1} = 3\ Tbsp$$

39. $\frac{1}{2}$ pt = _____ ml

$$ml = \frac{500\ ml \times \frac{1}{2}\ pt}{1\ pt \times 1} = \frac{500\ ml \times \frac{1}{2}}{1 \times 1} = \frac{\overset{250}{\cancel{500}}\ ml \times 1}{1 \times \underset{1}{\cancel{2}}}$$
$$= \frac{250\ ml}{1} = 250\ ml$$

$$ml = \frac{30\ ml \times 16\ oz \times \frac{1}{2}\ pt}{1\ oz \times 1\ pt \times 1} = \frac{30\ ml \times 16 \times \frac{1}{2}}{1 \times 1 \times 1} = \frac{30\ ml \times \overset{8}{\cancel{16}} \times 1}{1 \times 1 \times \underset{1}{\cancel{2}}}$$
$$= \frac{240\ ml}{1} = 240\ ml$$

40. $\frac{1}{4}$ qt = _____ ml

$$ml = \frac{1000 \text{ ml} \times \frac{1}{4}\text{ qt}}{1 \text{ qt} \times 1} = \frac{1000 \text{ ml} \times \frac{1}{4}}{1 \times 1} = \frac{\overset{250}{\cancel{1000}} \text{ ml} \times 1}{1 \times \cancel{4}}$$

$$= \frac{240 \text{ ml}}{1} = 240 \text{ ml}$$

$$ml = \frac{30 \text{ ml} \times 32 \text{ oz} \times \frac{1}{4}\text{ qt}}{1 \text{ oz} \times 1 \text{ qt} \times 1} = \frac{30 \text{ ml} \times 32 \times \frac{1}{4}}{1 \times 1 \times 1} = \frac{30 \text{ ml} \times \overset{8}{\cancel{32}} \times 1}{1 \times 1 \times \cancel{4}}$$

$$= \frac{250 \text{ ml}}{1} = 250 \text{ ml}$$

Calculating Fluid Intake

41–44. Knowns: Unit of Answers: ml

Conversion factors: 1 C = 250 ml (8 oz)   1 pt = 500 ml (16 oz)   1 Coffee cup = 5 oz
1 oz = 30 ml

$\frac{1}{2}$ cup orange juice

$$ml = \frac{30 \text{ ml} \times 8 \text{ oz} \times \frac{1}{2}\text{ C}}{1 \text{ oz} \times 1 \text{ C} \times 1} = \frac{30 \text{ ml} \times \overset{4}{\cancel{8}} \times 1}{1 \times 1 \times \cancel{2}} = \quad 120 \text{ ml}$$

$$ml = \frac{250 \text{ ml} \times \frac{1}{2}\text{ C}}{1 \text{ C} \times 1}$$

1 $\frac{1}{2}$ slices buttered wheat toast: not fluid intake
1 cup coffee

$$ml = \frac{30 \text{ ml} \times 5 \text{ oz}}{1 \text{ oz} \times 1} = \frac{30 \text{ ml} \times 5}{1 \times 1} = \frac{150 \text{ ml}}{1} = \quad 150 \text{ ml}$$

$$= \frac{\overset{125}{\cancel{250}} \text{ ml} \times 1}{1 \times \cancel{2}} = \frac{125 \text{ ml}}{1} = 125 \text{ ml}$$

$$150 \text{ ml}$$

1 cup raisin bran: not fluid intake
$\frac{1}{2}$ of a half-pint milk

$$ml = \frac{500 \text{ ml} \times (\frac{1}{2} \times \frac{1}{2}\text{ pt})}{1 \text{ pt} \times 1} = \frac{\overset{125}{\underset{\cancel{250}}{\cancel{500}}} \text{ ml} \times 1 \times 1}{1 \times \cancel{2} \times \cancel{2}}$$

$$ml = \frac{30 \text{ ml} \times \overset{\overset{4}{\cancel{8}}}{\cancel{16}} \text{ oz} \times 1 \times 1 \text{ pt}}{1 \text{ oz} \times 1 \text{ pt} \times \cancel{2} \times \cancel{2}} = \frac{120 \text{ ml}}{1} = \quad 120 \text{ ml}$$

$$= \frac{125 \text{ ml}}{1} = 125 \text{ ml}$$

Total: $\overline{\quad 390 \text{ ml}}$ $\overline{\quad 400 \text{ ml}}$

45–48. Knowns: Unit of Answers: cc

Conversion factors: 1 Tbsp = 15 cc   1 Coffee cup = 5 oz   1 pt = 500 cc (16 oz)

4 oz fresh fruit: not fluid intake
$\frac{1}{2}$ C lettuce and tomato salad: not fluid intake
5 Tbsp cream of chicken soup

$$cc = \frac{15 \text{ cc} \times 5 \text{ Tbsp}}{1 \text{ Tbsp} \times 1} = \frac{15 \text{ cc} \times 5}{1 \times 1} = \frac{75 \text{ cc}}{1} = 75 \text{ cc}$$

$$75 \text{ cc}$$

3 oz roast beef: not fluid intake
$\frac{1}{4}$ C broccoli: not fluid intake
$\frac{1}{2}$ pt milk

$$cc = \frac{30 \text{ cc} \times 16 \text{ oz} \times 1 \text{ pt}}{1 \text{ pt} \times 1 \text{ pt} \times 2} = \frac{30 \text{ cc} \times \overset{8}{\cancel{16}} \times 1}{1 \times 1 \times \cancel{2}} = \quad 240 \text{ cc}$$

$$cc = \frac{500 \text{ cc} \times \frac{1}{2}\text{ pt}}{1 \text{ pt} \times 1} = \frac{\overset{250}{\cancel{500}} \text{ cc} \times 1}{1 \times \cancel{2}}$$

1 cup coffee

$$cc = \frac{30 \text{ cc} \times 5 \text{ oz}}{1 \text{ oz} \times 1} = \frac{30 \text{ cc} \times 5}{1 \times 1} = \frac{150 \text{ cc}}{1} = \quad 150 \text{ cc}$$

$$= \frac{250 \text{ cc}}{1} = 250 \text{ cc}$$

$$150 \text{ cc}$$

Total: $\overline{\quad 465 \text{ cc}}$ $\overline{\quad 475 \text{ cc}}$

49–57. Knowns: Unit of answers: ml

Conversion factors: 1 C = 250 ml (8 oz)   1 pt = 500 ml (16 oz)

1 qt = 1000 ml (32 oz)   1 Tbsp = 15 ml

1 glass = 1 C   1 oz = 30 ml

$\frac{1}{2}$ C orange juice

$$ml = \frac{30\ ml \times 8\ oz \times \frac{1}{2}\ C}{1\ oz \times 1\ C \times 1} = \frac{30\ ml \times \overset{4}{\cancel{8}} \times 1}{1 \times 1 \times 1 \times \underset{1}{\cancel{2}}} = 120\ ml$$

$$ml = \frac{250\ ml \times \frac{1}{2}\ C}{1\ C \times 1} = \frac{\overset{125}{\cancel{250}}\ ml \times 1}{1 \times 1 \times \underset{1}{\cancel{2}}} = 125\ ml$$

$\frac{1}{2}$ pint container of milk

$$ml = \frac{30\ ml \times 16\ oz \times \frac{1}{2}\ pt}{1\ oz \times 1\ pt \times 1} = \frac{30\ ml \times \overset{8}{\cancel{16}} \times 1}{1 \times 1 \times 1 \times \underset{1}{\cancel{2}}} = 240\ ml$$

$$ml = \frac{500\ ml \times \frac{1}{2}\ pt}{1\ pt \times 1} = \frac{\overset{250}{\cancel{500}}\ ml \times 1}{1 \times 1 \times \underset{1}{\cancel{2}}} = 250\ ml$$

$\frac{1}{2}$ quart water

$$ml = \frac{30\ ml \times 32\ oz \times \frac{1}{2}\ qt}{1\ oz \times 1\ qt \times 1} = \frac{30\ ml \times \overset{16}{\cancel{32}} \times 1}{1 \times 1 \times 1 \times \underset{1}{\cancel{2}}} = 480\ ml$$

$$ml = \frac{1000\ ml \times \frac{1}{2}\ qt}{1\ qt \times 1} = \frac{\overset{500}{\cancel{1000}}\ ml \times 1}{1 \times 1 \times \underset{1}{\cancel{2}}} = 500\ ml$$

$\frac{1}{2}$ cup strawberry ice cream

$$ml = \frac{30\ ml \times 8\ oz \times \frac{1}{2}\ C}{1\ oz \times 1\ C \times 1} = \frac{30\ ml \times \overset{4}{\cancel{8}} \times 1}{1 \times 1 \times 1 \times \underset{1}{\cancel{2}}} = 120\ ml$$

$$ml = \frac{250\ ml \times \frac{1}{2}\ C}{1\ C \times 1} = \frac{\overset{125}{\cancel{250}}\ ml \times 1}{1 \times 1 \times \underset{1}{\cancel{2}}} = 125\ ml$$

7 Tbsp creamed soup

$$ml = \frac{15\ ml \times 7\ T}{1\ T \times 1} = \frac{15\ ml \times 7}{1 \times 1} = 105\ ml$$

$$105\ ml$$

$\frac{1}{2}$ glass water

$$ml = \frac{30\ ml \times 8\ oz \times \frac{1}{2}\ C}{1\ oz \times 1\ C \times 1} = \frac{30\ ml \times \overset{4}{\cancel{8}} \times 1}{1 \times 1 \times 1 \times \underset{1}{\cancel{2}}} = 120\ ml$$

$$ml = \frac{250\ ml \times \frac{1}{2}\ C}{1\ C \times 1} = \frac{\overset{125}{\cancel{250}}\ ml \times 1}{1 \times 1 \times \underset{1}{\cancel{2}}} = 125\ ml$$

1 glass iced tea

$$ml = \frac{30\ ml \times 8\ oz \times 1\ C}{1\ oz \times 1\ C \times 1} = \frac{30\ ml \times 8 \times 1}{1 \times 1 \times 1} = 240\ ml$$

$$ml = \frac{250\ ml \times 1\ C}{1\ C \times 1} = \frac{250\ ml \times 1}{1 \times 1} = 250\ ml$$

12 oz. Dr. Pepper

$$ml = \frac{30\ ml \times 12\ oz}{1\ oz \times 1} = \frac{30\ ml \times 12}{1 \times 1} = 360\ ml$$

$$360\ ml$$

Total: $\overline{1785\ ml}$ $\overline{1840\ ml}$

58–60. Knowns: Unit of answers: ml

Conversion factors: 1 oz = 30 ml   1 qt = 1000 ml (32 oz)

1 T = 15 ml

2 popsicles, 3 oz each

$$ml = \frac{30\ ml \times 3\ oz \times 2\ pop}{1\ oz \times 1\ pop \times 1} = \frac{30\ ml \times 3 \times 2}{1 \times 1 \times 1} = 180\ ml$$

$$180\ ml$$

1 sliced apple: not fluid intake

6 Tbsp jello

$$ml = \frac{15\ ml \times 6\ T}{1\ T \times 1} = \frac{15\ ml \times 6}{1 \times 1} = 90\ ml$$

$$90\ ml$$

$\frac{1}{2}$ cup dry cereal: not fluid intake

$\frac{1}{4}$ quart lemonade

$$ml = \frac{30\ ml \times 32\ oz \times \frac{1}{4}\ qt}{1\ oz \times 1\ qt \times 1} = \frac{30\ ml \times \overset{8}{\cancel{32}} \times 1}{1 \times 1 \times 1 \times \underset{1}{\cancel{4}}} = 240\ ml$$

$$ml = \frac{1000\ ml \times \frac{1}{4}\ qt}{1\ qt \times 1} = \frac{\overset{250}{\cancel{1000}}\ ml \times 1}{1 \times 1 \times \underset{1}{\cancel{4}}} = 250\ ml$$

Total: $\overline{510\ ml}$ $\overline{520\ ml}$

UNIT IV: DOSAGE CONVERSIONS AND CALCULATIONS

Chapter 10: Interpretation of Medication Orders and Labels

1. Ampicillin 250 mg PO q.i.d. = ampicillin 250 milligrams by mouth four times a day
2. Garamycin 80 mg IV PB q.8h. = Garamycin 80 milligrams intravenous piggyback every 8 hours.
3. Demerol and Phenergan 50 mg aa IM stat. = Demerol and Phenergan 50 milligrams of each intramuscularly immediately.
4. Nitroglycerine ung 1 inch to chest q.d. = Nitroglycerine ointment 1 inch to chest every day.
5. 1000 ml D5W c̄ KCl 20 mEq IV to run 8 h; then KVO with D5NS = 1000 milliliters 5% dextrose in water with potassium chloride 20 milliequivalents intravenously to run 8 hours; then keep vein open with 5% dextrose in normal saline.
6. MOM 30 ml c̄ cascara 5 ml PO q.o.d. SOS = milk of magnesia 30 milliliters with cascara 5 milliliters by mouth every other day if necessary once only.

7. Pantapon gr $\frac{1}{3}$ s.c. preop on call = Pantapon grains 1/3 subcutaneously preoperatively on call.

8. Mylanta $\bar{3}$ I PO t.i.d. p.c. = Mylanta 1 ounce by mouth three times a day after meals.

9. Donnatal tab I PO q.i.d. a.c. & h.s. = Donnatal 1 tablet by mouth four times a day before meals and at bedtime.

10. SSKI gtts 10 in orange juice q.s. to 60 ml PO q.6h. = saturated solution of potassium iodide 10 drops in orange juice in a quantity sufficient to make 60 milliliters by mouth every 6 hours.

11. Neodecadron gtt. i OS q.h. wa & q.2h. at noc = Neodecadron 1 drop in left eye every hour while awake and every 2 hours at night.

12. Calomine lotion to rash L leg ad lib = Calomine lotion to rash on left leg as desired.

13. Lasix 20 mg IV bid = Lasix 20 milligrams intravenously twice a day.

14. ephinephrine 1:1000 0.3 ml s.c. stat. = epinephrine 1:1000, 0.3 milliliters subcutaneously immediately.

15. Dyazide cap i PO b.i.d. = Dyazide 1 capsule by mouth twice a day.

16. boric acid 5% gtt. i OU t.i.d. = 5% boric acid 1 drop in both eyes three times a day.

17. Irrigate O.D. c̄ 50 ml NS ASAP = irrigate right eye with 50 milliliters of normal saline as soon as possible.

18. nitroglycerine 0.4 mg SL PRN = nitroglycerine 0.4 milligrams sublingually as needed (when required).

19. Procaine penicillin 300,000 U IM q.d. = Procaine penicillin 300,000 units intramuscularly every day.

20. ASA gr V PO q.d. = aspirin 5 grains by mouth every day.

21. Dalmane 30 mg PO h.s. = Dalmane 30 mg by mouth at bedtime. Therefore, only 1 dose daily or 30 mg daily.

22. Robinul 2 mg PO q.i.d. a.c. & h.s. = Robinul 2 mg by mouth <u>four times a day</u> before meals and at bedtime.
Factors: 2 mg = 1 dose; 4 doses = 1 day

$$\frac{mg}{d} = \frac{2\ mg \times 4\ doses}{1\ dose \times} = \frac{2\ mg \times 4}{1 \times 1\ d} = \frac{8\ mg}{1\ d} = 8\ mg/d$$

23. Pen Vee K 400,000 U q.6h. PO = Pen Vee K 400,000 units <u>every 6 hours</u> by mouth.
Factors: 400,000 U = (q) 6 h; 24 h = 1 d

$$\frac{U}{d} = \frac{400,000\ U \times 24\ h}{(q)6\ h \times 1\ d} = \frac{400,000\ U \times \overset{4}{\cancel{24}}}{\underset{1}{\cancel{6}} \times 1\ d} = \frac{1,600,000\ U}{1\ d} = 1,600,000\ U/d$$

24. Phenergan 50 mg IM q.8h. = Phenergan 50 mg intramuscularly <u>every 8 hours</u>.
Factors: 50 mg = (q) 8 h; 24 h = 1 d

$$\frac{mg}{d} = \frac{50\ mg \times 24\ h}{(q)8\ h \times 1\ d} = \frac{50\ mg \times \overset{3}{\cancel{24}}}{\underset{1}{\cancel{8}} \times 1\ d} = \frac{150\ mg}{1\ d} = 150\ mg/d$$

25. Solu-cortef 100 mg IV q.3h. = Solu-cortef 100 mg intravenously <u>every 3 hours</u>.
Factors: 100 mg = (q) 3 h; 24 h = 1 d

$$\frac{mg}{d} = \frac{100\ mg \times 24\ h}{(q)3\ h \times 1\ d} = \frac{100\ mg \times \overset{8}{\cancel{24}}}{\underset{1}{\cancel{3}} \times 1\ d} = \frac{800\ mg}{1\ d} = 800\ mg/d$$

26. Conversion factor: 1 gr = 60 mg (15 gr = 1000 mg); Factor: gr 7.5/1

$$mg = \frac{60\ mg \times gr\ 7.5}{1\ gr \times} = \frac{60\ mg \times 7.5}{1 \times 1} = \frac{450\ mg}{1} = 450\ mg$$

$$mg = \frac{1000\ mg \times gr\ 7.5}{15\ gr \times 1} = \frac{1000\ mg \times \overset{1}{\cancel{7.5}}}{\underset{2}{\cancel{15}} \times 1} = \frac{1000\ mg}{2} = 500\ mg$$

7 1/2 gr = 450 or 500 mg; therefore, the correct label is aspirin 500 mg.

27. Conversion factor: gr 1 = 60 mg (15 gr = 1000 mg); Factor: gr 1/150/1

$$mg = \frac{60\ mg \times gr\ 1/150}{1\ gr \times 1} = \frac{\overset{2}{\cancel{60}}\ mg \times 1}{1 \times 1 \times \underset{5}{\cancel{150}}} = \frac{2\ mg}{5} = 0.4\ mg\ (400\ mcg)$$

$$mg = \frac{1000\ mg \times gr\ 1/150}{15\ gr \times 1} = \frac{\overset{\overset{4}{\cancel{20}}}{\cancel{1000}}\ mg \times 1}{\underset{3}{\cancel{15}} \times 1 \times \underset{3}{\cancel{150}}} = \frac{4\ mg}{9} = 0.444\ mg\ (444\ mcg)$$

1/150 gr = 0.4 or 0.444 mg (400 or 444 mcg). The correct label is 400 mcg/0.5 ml.

For the remainder of the problems, the conversion of 1 gr = 60 mg is used for amounts of 1 grain or less, while 15 gr = 1000 mg is used for amounts larger than 1 grain.

28. Conversion factor: 1 gr = 60 mg; Factor: gr 1/100/1

$$mg = \frac{60\ mg \times gr\ 1/100}{1\ gr \times 1} = \frac{\overset{6}{\cancel{60}}\ mg \times 1}{1 \times 1 \times \underset{1}{\cancel{100}}} = \frac{6\ mg}{10} = 0.6\ mg$$

1/100 gr = 0.6 mg. The correct label is 0.6 mg (600 mcg) tablet.

29. Conversion factors: 1 gr = 60 mg; Factor: gr 1/5/1

$$mg = \frac{60\ mg\ \times\ gr\ 1/5}{1\ gr\ \times\quad 1} = \frac{\overset{12}{\cancel{60}}\ mg\ \times\quad 1}{1\quad \times\ 1 \times\ \underset{1}{\cancel{5}}} = \frac{12\ mg}{1} = 12\ mg$$

1/5 gr = 12 mg (13.3 mg if conversion factor of 15 gr = 1000 mg used). The correct label to choose is morphine sulfate 15 mg/ml, of which only a portion will be given.

30. Conversion factor: 1000 mg = 1 g; Factor: 0.5 g/1

$$mg = \frac{1000\ mg\ \times\ 0.5\ g}{1\ g\ \times\quad 1} = \frac{1000\ mg\ \times\ 0.5}{1\quad \times\quad 1} = \frac{500\ mg}{1}$$

0.5 grams = 500 mg. The correct label is 500 mg.

31. The ordered amount, 0.4 mg, is the same as one of the labels. The correct label is atropine 0.4 mg/ml.

32. Conversion factor: 1 g = 1000 mg; Factor: 0.1 g/1

$$mg = \frac{1000\ mg\ \times\ 0.1\ g}{1\ g\ \times\quad 1} = \frac{1000\ mg\ \times\ 0.1}{1\quad \times\quad 1} = \frac{100\ mg}{1} = 100\ mg$$

The label to choose is Pyridium 100 mg tablet.

33. Factors: 1/100 gr/1 Conversion factor: 1 gr = 60 mg

$$mg = \frac{60\ mg\ \times\ gr\ 1/100}{1\ gr\ \times\quad 1} = \frac{\overset{6}{\cancel{60}}\ mg\ \times\ 1}{1\quad \times\ 1 \times\ \underset{10}{\cancel{100}}} = \frac{6\ mg}{10} = 0.6\ mg$$

The correct label to choose is 1 mg/ml. Only a portion of this will be given.

34. Factors: 0.250 g/1. Conversion factor: 1 g = 1000 mg

$$mg = \frac{1000\ mg\ \times\ 0.250\ g}{1\ g\ \times\quad 1} = \frac{1000\ mg\ \times\ 0.250}{1\quad \times\quad 1} = \frac{250\ mg}{1} = 250\ mg$$

The correct label to choose is 250 mg cap.

35. Order of Lanoxin 125 mcg PO q.d. is the same as the label, Lanoxin 125 mcg tab.

Chapter 11: Calculation of Oral Medication Dosages

Dosages are calculated for the specific dose only. Therefore, the number of doses per day, i.e. bid, tid, q4h, etc., was extraneous information in these problems.

1. Factors: 4 mg = 1 tab; 16 mg/1

$$tab = \frac{1\ tab \times 16\ mg}{4\ mg \times\ 1} = \frac{1\ tab \times \overset{4}{\cancel{16}}}{\cancel{4}\quad \times\ 1} = \frac{4\ tab}{1} = 4\ tab$$

2. Factors: 1 cap = 0.1 g; gr 3/1   Conversion factor: 1 g = 15 gr

$$cap = \frac{1\ cap \times\ 1\ g\ \times gr\ 3}{0.1\ g\ \times 15\ gr \times\ 1} = \frac{1\ cap \times\ 1 \times \overset{1}{\cancel{3}}}{0.1\quad \times \underset{5}{\cancel{15}} \times 1} = \frac{1\ cap}{0.5} = 2\ caps$$

3. Factors: 1 tab = 400 U; 200 U/1

$$tab = \frac{1\ tab \times 200\ U}{400\ U\ \times\quad 1} = \frac{1\ tab \times \overset{1}{\cancel{200}}}{\underset{2}{\cancel{400}}\quad \times\ 1} = \frac{1\ tab}{2} = 1/2\ tab$$

4. Factors: 1 tab = 0.5 g; 250 mg/1   Conversion factor: 1 g = 1000 mg

$$tab = \frac{1\ tab \times\quad 1\ g\quad \times 250\ mg}{0.5\ g\quad \times 1000\ mg \times\quad 1} = \frac{1\ tab \times\quad 1 \times \overset{1}{\cancel{250}}}{0.5\quad \times \underset{4}{\cancel{1000}} \times\ 1} = \frac{1\ tab}{2} = 1/2\ tab$$

5. Factors: 1 tab = 250 mg; 1 g/1   Conversion factor: 1 g = 1000 mg

$$tab = \frac{1\ tab \times 1000\ mg \times 1\ g}{250\ mg \times\quad 1\ g\quad \times 1} = \frac{1\ tab \times \overset{4}{\cancel{1000}} \times 1}{\underset{1}{\cancel{250}}\quad \times\quad 1 \times 1} = \frac{4\ tab}{1} = 4\ tab$$

6. Factors: 1 tab = 4mg; $\frac{1}{8}$ gr/1   Conversion Factor: 1 gr = 60 mg

$$tab = \frac{1\ tab \times 60\ mg \times gr\ \frac{1}{8}}{4\ mg \times 1\ gr \times\quad 1} = \frac{1\ tab \times \overset{15}{\cancel{60}} \times 1}{\underset{1}{\cancel{4}}\quad \times\ 1 \times 8} = \frac{15\ tab}{8} = 1\frac{7}{8} = 2\ tab$$

7. Factors: 1 tab = 100 mcg; 0.25 mg/1   Conversion factor: 1 mg = 1000 mcg

$$tab = \frac{1\ tab\quad \times 1000\ mcg \times 0.25\ mg}{100\ mcg \times\quad 1\ mg\quad \times\ 1} = \frac{1\ tab \times \overset{10}{\cancel{1000}} \times 0.25}{\underset{1}{\cancel{100}}\quad \times\quad 1 \times\quad 1} = = 2.5\ tab$$

8. Factors: 1 tab = 0.1 g; gr 1.5/1   Conversion factor: 1 g = 15 gr

$$\text{tab} = \frac{1\ \text{tab} \times \ 1\ \text{g}\ \times \text{gr}\ 1.5}{0.1\ \text{g}\ \ \times 15\ \text{gr} \times \ \ \ 1} = \frac{1\ \text{tab} \times \ \ 1 \times \overset{0.1}{\cancel{1.5}}}{0.1\ \ \ \times \cancel{15} \times \ 1} = \frac{0.1\ \text{tab}}{0.1} = 1\ \text{tab}$$

9. Factors: 1 cap = 120 mcg; $\frac{1}{500}$ gr/1   Conversion factors: 1 gr = 60 mg; 1 mg = 1000 mcg

$$\text{cap} = \frac{1\ \text{cap}\ \times 1000\ \text{mcg} \times 60\ \text{mg} \times \text{gr}\ \frac{1}{500}}{120\ \text{mcg} \times \ \ \ \ 1\ \text{mg} \times 1\ \text{gr} \times \ \ \ 1} = \frac{1\ \text{cap} \times \overset{\overset{1}{\cancel{2}}}{\cancel{1000}} \times \overset{1}{\cancel{60}} \times \ \ 1}{\underset{\underset{1}{\cancel{2}}}{\cancel{120}} \ \ \times \ 1 \times 1 \times \cancel{500}} = \frac{1\ \text{cap}}{1} = 1\ \text{cap}$$

10. Factors: 1 tab = 0.05 g; 25 mg/1   Conversion factor: 1000 mg = 1 g

$$\text{tab} = \frac{1\ \text{tab} \times \ \ \ 1\ \text{g}\ \ \times 25\ \text{mg}}{0.05\ \text{g}\ \ \times 1000\ \text{mg} \times \ 1} = \frac{1\ \text{tab} \times \ \ \ 1 \times \overset{1}{\cancel{25}}}{0.05\ \ \times \underset{40}{\cancel{1000}} \times \ 1} = \frac{1\ \text{tab}}{2} = 1/2\ \text{tab}$$

11. Factors: 1 tab = 0.5 mg; 0.75 mg/1

$$\text{tab} = \frac{1\ \text{tab} \times 0.75\ \text{mg}}{0.5\ \text{mg} \times \ 1} = \frac{1\ \text{tab} \times \overset{3}{\cancel{0.75}}}{\underset{2}{\cancel{0.5}} \ \times \ 1} = \frac{3\ \text{tab}}{2} = 1\ 1/2\ \text{tab}$$

12. Factors: 1 cap = 250 mg; 500 mg/1

$$\text{cap} = \frac{1\ \text{cap} \times 500\ \text{mg}}{250\ \text{mg} \times \ 1} = \frac{1\ \text{tab} \times \overset{2}{\cancel{500}}}{\underset{1}{\cancel{250}} \ \times \ 1} = \frac{2\ \text{cap}}{1} = 2\ \text{cap}$$

13. Factors: 1 tab = 325 mg; 10 gr/1 Conversion factor: 15 gr = 1000 mg

$$\text{tab} = \frac{1\ \text{tab} \times 1000\ \text{mg} \times 10\ \text{gr}}{325\ \text{mg} \times \ \ 15\ \text{gr} \times 1} = \frac{1\ \text{tab} \times \overset{40}{\cancel{1000}} \times \overset{2}{\cancel{10}}}{\underset{13}{\cancel{325}} \ \times \underset{3}{\cancel{15}} \times \ 1} = \frac{80\ \text{tab}}{39} = 2\frac{2}{39} = 2\ \text{tabs}$$

14. Factors: 1 tab = 125 mg; 250 mg/1

$$\text{tab} = \frac{1\ \text{tab} \times 250\ \text{mg}}{125\ \text{mg} \times \ 1} = \frac{1\ \text{tab} \times \overset{2}{\cancel{2250}}}{\underset{1}{\cancel{125}} \ \times \ 1} = \frac{2\ \text{tab}}{1} = 2\ \text{tabs}$$

15. Factors: 1 tab = 0.75 mg; 750 mcg/1; Conversion factor: 1mg = 1000 mcg

$$\text{tab} = \frac{1\ \text{tab} \times \ \ \ \ 1\ \text{mg}\ \ \times 750\ \text{mcg}}{0.75\ \text{mg} \times 1000\ \text{mcg} \times \ \ \ 1} = \frac{1\ \text{tab} \times \ \ \ 1 \times \overset{\overset{1}{\cancel{10}}}{\cancel{750}}}{\underset{0.01}{\cancel{0.75}} \ \times \underset{100}{\cancel{1000}} \times \ \ 1} = \frac{1\ \text{tab}}{1} = 1\ \text{tab}$$

16. Factors: 1 cap = 30 mg; 60 mg/1

$$\text{cap} = \frac{1\ \text{cap} \times 60\ \text{mg}}{30\ \text{mg} \times \ 1} = \frac{1\ \text{cap} \times \overset{2}{\cancel{60}}}{\underset{1}{\cancel{30}} \ \times \ 1} = \frac{2\ \text{cap}}{1} = 2\ \text{cap}$$

17. Factors: 1 tab = 400 mg; 1 g/1 Conversion factor: 1 g = 1000 mcg

$$\text{tab} = \frac{1\ \text{tab} \times 1000\ \text{mg} \times 1\ \text{g}}{400\ \text{mg} \times \ \ \ 1\ \text{g}\ \ \times \ 1} = \frac{1\ \text{tab} \times \overset{5}{\cancel{1000}} \times \ 1}{\underset{2}{\cancel{400}} \ \ \times \ 1 \times 1} = \frac{5\ \text{tab}}{2} = 2\frac{1}{2}\ \text{tab}$$

18. Factors: 1 tab = 300 mg; gr 5/1 Conversion factor: 1 gr = 60 mg

$$\text{tab} = \frac{1\ \text{tab} \times 60\ \text{mg} \times \text{gr}\ 5}{300\ \text{mg} \times \ 1\ \text{gr}\ \times \ \ \ 1} = \frac{1\ \text{tab} \times \overset{1}{\cancel{60}} \times \overset{1}{\cancel{5}}}{\underset{\underset{1}{\cancel{5}}}{\cancel{300}} \ \ \times \ 1 \times 1} = \frac{1\ \text{tab}}{1} = 1\ \text{tab}$$

19. Factors: 1 cap = 25 mg; 50 mg/1

$$\text{cap} = \frac{1\ \text{cap} \times 50\ \text{mg}}{25\ \text{mg} \times \ 1} = \frac{1\ \text{cap} \times \overset{2}{\cancel{50}}}{\underset{1}{\cancel{25}} \ \times \ 1} = \frac{2\ \text{cap}}{1} = 2\ \text{cap}$$

20. Factors: 1 cap = 15 mg; 15 mg/1
    The ordered dosage and label dosage are the same; therefore, 1 cap will be given.

21. Dosage ordered: Coumadin 13 mg PO q.d. Combination of two 5 mg tabs and one and one-half 2 mg tabs uses the fewest number of tablets.

22. Dosage ordered: Thorazine 35 mg PO q.i.d. Combination of one 10 mg and one 25 mg tab is the only way to obtain 35 mg.

23. Dosage ordered: Coumadin 3.5 mg h.s. PO. Combination of one 2.5 mg tablet and one-half 2 mg tablet uses the fewest number of tablets.

24. Dosages ordered: Decadron 1.25 mg b.i.d. PO × 2 d. Combination of one 0.75 mg tab and one 0.5 mg tab uses the fewest number of tablets.

25. Dosage ordered: Synthroid 0.125 mg PO q AM. Combination of one 50 mcg (0.05 mg) and one 75 mcg (0.075 mg) tab uses the fewest number of tablets.

26. Factors: 5 ml (cc) = 0.5 g; $\frac{3}{4}$ gr/1 Conversion factor: 1 g = 15 gr

$$cc = \frac{5\ cc \times 1\ g \times gr\frac{3}{4}}{0.5\ g \times 15\ gr \times 1} = \frac{5\ cc \times 1 \times 3}{0.5 \times 15 \times 4} = \frac{1\ cc}{2} = 0.5\ cc$$

27. Factors: 1 ml = 300 mg; 75 mg/1

$$ml = \frac{1\ ml \times 75\ mg}{300\ mg \times 1} = \frac{1\ ml \times 75}{300 \times 1} = \frac{1\ ml}{4} = 0.25\ ml$$

28. Factors: 5 ml = 50 mcg; $\frac{1}{300}$ gr/1 Conversion factors: 1 gr = 60 mg; 1 mg = 1000 mcg; 1 tsp = 5 ml

$$tsp = \frac{1\ tsp \times 5\ ml \times 1000\ mcg \times 60\ mg \times gr\frac{1}{300}}{5\ ml \times 50\ mcg \times 1\ mg \times 1\ gr \times 1} = \frac{1\ tsp \times 5 \times 1000 \times 60 \times 1}{5 \times 50 \times 1 \times 1 \times 300} = \frac{4\ tsp}{1} = 4\ tsp$$

29. Factors: 150 mg/ml; 1.5 g/1 Conversion factors: 1 dram = 5 ml; 1 g = 1000 mg

$$dram = \frac{1\ dram \times 1\ ml \times 1000\ mg \times 1.5\ g}{5\ ml \times 150\ mg \times 1\ g \times 1\ g} = \frac{2\ drams}{1} = 2\ drams$$

30. Factors: 200 mcg/ml; 0.4 mg/1 Conversion factor: 1 mg = 1000 mcg

$$ml = \frac{1\ ml \times 1000\ mcg \times 0.4\ mg}{200\ mcg \times 1\ mg \times 1} = \frac{1\ ml \times 1000 \times 0.4}{200 \times 1 \times 1} = \frac{2\ ml}{1} = 2\ ml$$

31. Factors: 300 mcg = 1 ml; $\frac{1}{100}$ gr/1 Conversion factors: gr 1 = 60 mg; 1 mg = 1000 mcg

$$ml = \frac{1\ ml \times 1000\ mcg \times 60\ mg \times gr\frac{1}{100}}{300\ mcg \times 1\ mg \times 1\ gr \times 1} = \frac{1\ ml \times 1000 \times 60 \times 1}{300 \times 1 \times 1 \times 100} = \frac{2\ ml}{1} = 2\ ml$$

32. Factors: 100 mg = 5 ml; $\frac{1}{8}$ gr/1 Conversion factors: 1 gr = 60 mg

$$ml = \frac{5\ ml \times 60\ mg \times gr\frac{1}{8}}{100\ mg \times 1\ gr \times 1} = \frac{5 \times 60 \times 1}{100 \times 1 \times 8} = \frac{3\ ml}{8} = 0.375\ ml$$

33. Factors: 1 g = 1 ml; 0.25 g/1 Conversion factor: 1 cc = 1 ml.

$$cc = \frac{1\ cc \times 0.25\ g}{1\ g \times 1} = \frac{1\ cc \times 0.25}{1 \times 1} = \frac{0.25\ cc}{1} = 0.25\ cc$$

34. Factors: 5 ml = 0.5 g; 3 gr/1 Conversion factor: 1 g = 15 gr

$$ml = \frac{5\ ml \times 1\ g \times 3\ gr}{0.5\ g \times 15\ gr \times 1} = \frac{5\ ml \times 1 \times 3}{0.5 \times 15 \times 1} = \frac{1\ ml}{0.5} = 2\ ml$$

35. Factors: 1 mg = 5 ml; 600 mcg Conversion factors: 1 ml = 1 cc; 1 mg = 1000 mcg

$$cc = \frac{5\ cc \times 600\ mcg \times 5\ cc \times 1\ mg}{1\ mg \times 1000\ mcg \times 1} = \frac{5\ cc \times 1 \times 600}{1 \times 1000 \times 1} = \frac{3\ cc}{1} = 3\ cc$$

36. Factors: 200 mg = 5 ml; 400 mg/l

$$ml = \frac{5\ ml\ \times 400\ mg}{200\ mg \times 1} = \frac{5\ ml \times \overset{2}{\cancel{400}}}{\underset{1}{\cancel{200}}\ \times\ 1} = \frac{10\ ml}{1} = 10\ ml$$

37. Factors: 125 mg/5 ml; 250 mg/l

$$ml = \frac{5\ ml\ \times 250\ mg}{125\ mg \times 1} = \frac{5\ ml \times \overset{2}{\cancel{250}}}{\underset{1}{\cancel{125}}\ \times\ 1} = \frac{10\ ml}{1} = 10\ ml$$

38. Factors: 125 mg = 5 ml; 100 mg/l   Conversion factor: 1 cc = 1 ml

$$cc = \frac{5\ cc\ \times 100\ mg}{125\ mg \times 1} = \frac{\overset{1}{\cancel{5}}\ cc \times \overset{4}{\cancel{100}}}{\underset{\underset{1}{5}}{\cancel{125}}\ \times\ 1} = \frac{4\ cc}{1} = 4\ cc$$

39. Factors: 12.5 mg = 5 ml; 50 mg/l   Conversion factor: 1 tsp = 5 ml

$$tsp = \frac{1\ tsp \times\ \ \ 5\ ml \times 50\ mg}{5\ ml \times 12.5\ mg \times 1} = \frac{1\ tsp\ \times\ \overset{1}{\cancel{5}} \times \overset{4}{\cancel{50}}}{\underset{1}{\cancel{5}}\ \ \times \underset{1}{\cancel{12.5}} \times 1} = \frac{4\ tsp}{1} = 4\ tsp$$

40. Factors: 400,000 U = 5 ml; 400,000 U/l   Conversion factor: 1 tsp = 5 ml

$$tsp = \frac{1\ tsp \times\ \ \ \ \ 5\ ml \times 400,000\ U}{5\ ml \times 400,000\ U\ \times\ \ \ \ \ \ 1} = \frac{1\ tsp\ \times\ \ \overset{1}{\cancel{5}} \times \overset{1}{\cancel{400,000}}}{\underset{1}{\cancel{5}}\ \ \times \underset{1}{\cancel{400,000}} \times\ \ \ 1} = \frac{1\ tsp}{1} = 1\ tsp$$

Logically, if 1 tsp = 5 ml and 5 ml = 400,000 U, then 1 tsp = 400,000 U.

41. Factors: 40 mEq = 15 ml; 20 mEq/l

$$ml = \frac{15\ ml\ \ \times 20\ mEq}{40\ mEq \times 1} = \frac{15\ ml \times \overset{1}{\cancel{20}}}{\underset{2}{\cancel{40}}\ \times\ 1} = \frac{15\ ml}{2} = 7.5\ ml$$

42. Factors: 100,000 U = 1 ml; 100,000 U
    The ordered dosage and the label dosage are the same. Therefore, 1 ml is given.

43. Factors: 250 mg = 5 ml; 250 mg. Conversion factor: 1 cc = 1 ml.

$$cc = \frac{5\ cc\ \ \times 250\ mg}{250\ mg \times 1} = \frac{5\ cc \times \overset{1}{\cancel{250}}}{\cancel{250}\ \times\ 1} = \frac{5\ cc}{1} = 5\ cc$$

44. Factors: 20 mg = 1 ml; $\frac{1}{4}$ gr/l   Conversion factor: 1 gr = 60 mg

$$ml = \frac{1\ ml\ \times 60\ mg \times gr\ \frac{1}{4}}{20\ mg \times\ 1\ gr \times\ \ \ \ 1} = \frac{1\ ml \times \overset{3}{\cancel{60}} \times 1}{\underset{1}{\cancel{20}}\ \ \times\ 1 \times 4} = \frac{3\ ml}{4} = 0.75\ ml$$

45. Factors: 300 mg = 5 ml; 600 mg/l; 8 mEq = 300 mg

$$ml = \frac{5\ ml\ \ \ \times\ \ \ 8\ mEq \times 600\ mg}{8\ mEq \times\ 300\ mg\ \ \times\ \ \ 1} = \frac{5\ ml\ \times\ \ \overset{1}{\cancel{8}} \times \overset{2}{\cancel{600}}}{\underset{1}{\cancel{8}}\ \ \ \times \underset{1}{\cancel{300}} \times\ 1} = \frac{10\ ml}{1} = 10\ ml$$

Chapter 12: Calculation of Parenteral Medication Dosages

1. Factors: 50 mg = 1 ml; 35 mg/l

$$ml = \frac{1\ ml\ \ \times\ 35mg}{50\ mg\ \times\ 1} = \frac{1\ ml\ \times\ \overset{7}{\cancel{35}}}{\underset{10}{\cancel{50}}\ \ \times\ 1} = \frac{7\ ml}{10} = 0.7\ ml$$

2. Factors: 75 mg = 1 ml; gr 2/l   Conversion factor: 15 gr = 1000 mg

$$ml = \frac{1\ ml\ \ \times\ 1000\ \ mg\ \times\ gr\ 2}{75\ mg\ \times\ \ \ 15\ gr\ \ \times\ \ \ 1} = \frac{1\ ml\ \times\ \overset{\overset{8}{\cancel{40}}}{\cancel{1000}} \times\ 2}{\underset{3}{\cancel{75}}\ \ \times\ \underset{3}{\cancel{15}} \times 1} = \frac{16\ ml}{9} = 1.77\ ml\ = 1.8\ ml$$

3. Factors: 250 mg = 1 ml; 100 mg

$$ml = \frac{1\ ml\ \ \times\ 100\ \ mg}{250\ \ mg\ \times\ \ \ \ 1} = \frac{1\ ml\ \times\ \overset{2}{\cancel{100}}}{\underset{5}{\cancel{250}}\ \ \times\ 1} = \frac{2\ ml}{5} = 0.4\ ml$$

4. Factors: 1.5 mg = 1 ml; 200 mcg   Conversion factors: 1 mg = 1000 mg; 15 (16) mx = 1 ml

$$mx = \frac{15 \ mx \times 1 \ ml \times 1 \ mg \times 200 \ mcg}{1 \ ml \times 1.5 \ mg \times 1000 \ mcg \times 1} = \frac{\overset{1}{\cancel{15}} \ mx \times 1 \times 1 \times \overset{2}{\cancel{200}}}{1 \times \underset{0.1}{\cancel{1.5}} \times \underset{10}{\cancel{1000}} \times 1} = \frac{2 \ mx}{1} = 2 \ mx$$

$$mx = \frac{16 \ mx \times 1 \ ml \times 1 \ mg \times 200 \ mcg}{1 \ ml \times 1.5 \ mg \times 1000 \ mcg \times 1} = \frac{\overset{1}{\cancel{16}} \ mx \times 1 \times 1 \times \overset{2}{\cancel{200}}}{1 \times 1.5 \times \underset{10}{\cancel{1000}} \times 1} = \frac{32 \ mx}{15} = 2.13 \ mx$$

5. Factors: 0.1 g = 1 ml; 250 mg   Conversion factor: 1 g = 1000 mg

$$ml = \frac{1 \ ml \times 1 \ g \times 250 \ mg}{0.1 \ g \times 1000 \ mg \times 1} = \frac{1 \ ml \times 1 \times \overset{1}{\cancel{250}}}{0.1 \times \underset{4}{\cancel{1000}} \times 1} = \frac{1 \ ml}{0.4} = 2.5 \ ml$$

6. Factors: 500 mcg = 1 ml; 1/150 gr/1   Conversion Factors: 1 gr = 60 mg; 1mg = 1000 mcg

$$ml = \frac{1 \ ml \times 1000 \ mcg \times 60 \ mg \times gr \ 1/150}{500 \ mcg \times 1 \ mg \times 1 \ gr \times 1} = \frac{1 \ ml \times \overset{2}{\cancel{1000}} \times \overset{2}{\cancel{60}} \times 1}{\underset{1}{\cancel{500}} \times 1 \times 1 \times \underset{5}{\cancel{150}}} = \frac{4 \ ml}{5} = 0.8 \ ml$$

7. Factors: 1 g = 10 ml; 1 gr/1   Conversion factor: 1 g = 15 gr; 1 ml = 15 (16) mx

$$mx = \frac{15 \ mx \times 10 \ ml \times 1 \ g \times 1 \ gr}{1 \ ml \times 1 \ g \times 15 \ gr \times 1} = \frac{\overset{1}{\cancel{15}} \ mx \times 10 \times 1 \times 1}{1 \times 1 \times \underset{1}{\cancel{15}} \times 1} = \frac{10 \ mx}{1} = 10 \ mx$$

$$mx = \frac{16 \ mx \times 10 \ ml \times 1 \ g \times 1 \ gr}{1 \ ml \times 1 \ g \times 15 \ gr \times 1} = \frac{16 \ mx \times \overset{2}{\cancel{10}} \times 1 \times 1}{1 \times 1 \times \underset{3}{\cancel{15}} \times 1} = \frac{32 \ mx}{3} = 10.67 \ mx$$

8. Factors: 1,000,000 U = 1 ml; 400,000 U/1

$$ml = \frac{1 \ ml \times 400,000 \ U}{1,000,000 \ U \times 1} = \frac{1 \ ml \times \overset{4}{\cancel{400,000}}}{\underset{10}{\cancel{1,000,000}} \times 1} = \frac{4 \ ml}{10} = 0.4 \ ml$$

9. Factors: 0.6 mg = 2 ml; 1/300 gr   Conversion factor: 1 gr = 60 mg

$$ml = \frac{2 \ ml \times 60 \ mg \times gr \ 1/300}{0.6 \ mg \times 1 \ gr \times 1} = \frac{2 \ ml \times \overset{1}{\cancel{60}} \times 1}{0.6 \times 1 \times \underset{5}{\cancel{300}}} = \frac{2 \ ml}{3} = 0.67 \ ml$$

10. Factors: 500 mg = 1 ml; 0.25 g   Conversion factor: 1 g = 1000 mg

$$ml = \frac{1 \ ml \times 1000 \ mg \times 0.25 \ g}{500 \ mg \times 1 \ g \times 1} = \frac{1 \ ml \times \overset{2}{\cancel{1000}} \times 0.25}{\underset{1}{\cancel{500}} \times 1 \times 1} = \frac{0.5 \ ml}{1} = 0.5 \ ml$$

11. 5000 U/ml tubex is most appropriate. Factors: 5000 U = 1 ml; 3000 U/1

$$ml = \frac{1 \ ml \times 3000 \ U}{5000 \ U \times 1} = \frac{1 \ ml \times \overset{3}{\cancel{3000}}}{\underset{5}{\cancel{5000}} \times 1} = \frac{3 \ ml}{5} = 0.6 \ ml$$

12. Factors: gr 1 = 60 mg; 1/16 gr/1

$$mg = \frac{60 \ mg \times gr \ 1/16}{1 \ gr \times 1} = \frac{\overset{15}{\cancel{60}} \ mg \times 1}{1 \times \underset{4}{\cancel{16}}} = \frac{15 \ mg}{4} = 3.75 \ mg$$

The ampule containing 4 mg/ml is most appropriate. Factors: 4mg = 1 ml; 3.75 mg/1

$$ml = \frac{1 \ ml \times 3.75 \ mg}{4 \ mg \times 1} = \frac{1 \ ml \times 3.75}{4 \times 1} = \frac{3.75 \ ml}{4} = 0.9375 \ ml = 0.94 \ ml$$

13. Factors: 60 mg = 1 ml; 1/2 gr/1   Conversion factor: 1 gr = 60 mg

$$ml = \frac{1 \ ml \times 60 \ mg \times gr \ 1/2}{60 \ mg \times 1 \ gr \times 1} = \frac{1 \ ml \times \overset{1}{\cancel{60}} \times 1}{\underset{1}{\cancel{60}} \times 1 \times 2} = \frac{1 \ ml}{2} = 0.5 \ ml$$

14. Factors: 60 mg = 1 ml; 3/4 gr/1   Conversion factor: 1 gr = 60 mg

$$ml = \frac{1 \ ml \times 60 \ mg \times gr \ 3/4}{60 \ mg \times 1 \ gr \times 1} = \frac{1 \ ml \times \overset{1}{\cancel{60}} \times 3}{\underset{1}{\cancel{60}} \times 1 \times 4} = \frac{3 \ ml}{4} = 0.75 \ ml$$

15. Factors: 50 mg = 1 ml; 35 mg/1

$$ml = \frac{1 \ ml \ \times \ 35 \ mg}{50 \ mg \ \times \ 1} = \frac{1 \ ml \ \times \ \overset{7}{\cancel{35}}}{\underset{10}{\cancel{50}} \ \times \ 1} = \frac{7 \ ml}{10} = 0.7 \ ml$$

16. Factors: 75 mg = 1 ml; 25 mg/1

$$ml = \frac{1 \ ml \ \times \ 25 \ mg}{75 \ mg \ \times \ 1} = \frac{1 \ ml \ \times \ \overset{1}{\cancel{25}}}{\underset{3}{\cancel{75}} \ \times \ 1} = \frac{1 \ ml}{3} = 0.3\overline{3} \ ml$$

17. Factors: 1000 mcg = 1 ml; 1000 mcg/1
    1000 mcg = 1 ml; therefore 1 ml will be administered.

18. Factors: 1,200,000 U = 1 ml; 900,000 U/1

$$ml = \frac{1 \ ml \ \times \ 900,000 \ U}{1,200,000 \ U \ \times \ 1} = \frac{1 \ ml \ \times \ \overset{3}{\cancel{900,000}}}{1 \ \times \ \underset{4}{\cancel{1,200,000}}} = \frac{3 \ ml}{4} = 0.75 \ ml$$

19. Factors: 2 mg = 1 ml; 0.5 mg/1   Conversion factor: 16 mx = 1 ml

$$mx = \frac{16 \ mx \ \times \ 1 \ ml \ \times \ 0.5 \ mg}{1 \ ml \ \times \ 2 \ mg \ \times \ 1} = \frac{\overset{8}{\cancel{16}} \ \times \ 1 \ \times \ 0.5}{1 \ \times \ \underset{1}{\cancel{2}} \ \times \ 1} = \frac{4 \ mx}{1} = 4 \ mx$$

(3.75 mx if 1 ml = 15 mx)

20. Factors: 0.4 mg = 1 ml; 1/300 gr/1. Conversion factor: 1 gr = 60 mg

$$ml = \frac{1 \ ml \ \times \ 60 \ mg \ \times \ gr \ 1/300}{0.4 \ mg \ \times \ 1 \ gr \ \times \ 1} = \frac{1 \ ml \ \times \ \overset{1}{\cancel{60}} \ \times \ 1}{0.4 \ \times \ 1 \ \times \ \underset{5}{\cancel{300}}} = \frac{1 \ ml}{2} = 0.5 \ ml$$

21. Factors: 300,000 U = 1 ml; 600,000 U/1

$$ml = \frac{1 \ ml \ \times \ 600,000 \ U}{300,000 \ U \ \times \ 1} = \frac{1 \ ml \ \times \ \overset{2}{\cancel{600,000}}}{\underset{1}{\cancel{300,000}} \ \times \ 1} = \frac{2 \ ml}{1} = 2 \ ml$$

22. Factors: 5 mg = 1 ml; 2 mg/1

$$ml = \frac{1 \ ml \ \times \ 2 \ mg}{5 \ mg \ \times \ 1} = \frac{1 \ ml \ \times \ 2}{5 \ \times \ 1} = \frac{2 \ ml}{5} = 0.4 \ ml$$

23. Factors: 4 mg = 1 ml; 3 mg/1

$$ml = \frac{1 \ ml \ \times \ 3 \ mg}{4 \ mg \ \times \ 1} = \frac{1 \ ml \ \times \ 3}{4 \ \times \ 1} = \frac{3 \ ml}{4} = 0.75 \ ml$$

24. Factors: 500 mg = 2 ml; 250 mg/1

$$ml = \frac{2 \ ml \ \times \ 250 \ mg}{500 \ mg \ \times \ 1} = \frac{\overset{1}{\cancel{2}} \ ml \ \times \ \overset{1}{\cancel{250}}}{\underset{\underset{1}{2}}{\cancel{500}} \ \times \ 1} = \frac{1 \ ml}{1} = 1 \ ml$$

25. Factors: 0.2 mg = 1 ml; 300 mcg/1. Conversion factor: 1 mg = 1000 mcg

$$ml = \frac{1 \ ml \ \times \ 1 \ mg \ \times \ 300 \ mcg}{0.2 \ mg \ \times \ 1000 \ mcg \ \times \ 1} = \frac{1 \ ml \ \times \ 1 \ \times \ \overset{3}{\cancel{300}}}{0.2 \ \times \ \underset{10}{\cancel{1000}} \ \times \ 1} = \frac{3 \ ml}{2} = 1.5 \ ml$$

UNIT V: CALCULATIONS BASED ON BODY WEIGHT

Chapter 13: Dosages Based on Client Weight
Dosages Based on Body Weight

1. Factors: 5 mcg = 1 lb; 1 mg = 1000 mcg; 100 lb/1

$$mg = \frac{1 \ mg \ \times \ 5 \ mcg \ \times \ 100 \ lb}{1000 \ mcg \ \times \ 1 \ lb \ \times \ 1} = \frac{1 \ mg \ \times \ \overset{1}{\cancel{5}} \ \times \ \overset{1}{\cancel{100}}}{\underset{\underset{2}{10}}{\cancel{1000}} \ \times \ 1 \ \times \ 1} = \frac{1 \ mg}{2} = 0.5 \ mg$$

2. Factors: 20 mcg = 1 kg; 1 mg = 1000 mcg; 50 kg/1

$$mg = \frac{1 \ mg \ \times \ 20 \ mcg \ \times \ 50 \ kg}{1000 \ mcg \ \times \ 1 \ kg \ \times \ 1} = \frac{1 \ mg \ \times \ \overset{1}{\cancel{20}} \ \times \ \overset{1}{\cancel{50}}}{\underset{\underset{1}{50}}{\cancel{1000}} \ \times \ 1 \ \times \ 1} = \frac{1 \ mg}{1} = 1 \ mg$$

3. Factors: 4 mcg = 1 kg; 1 kg = 2.2 lb; 176 lb/1

$$\text{mcg} = \frac{4\ \text{mcg} \times 1\ \text{kg} \times 176\ \text{lb}}{1\ \text{kg} \times 2.2\ \text{lb} \times 1} = \frac{4\ \text{mcg} \times 1 \times \overset{80}{\cancel{176}}}{1 \times \underset{1}{\cancel{2.2}} \times 1} = \frac{320\ \text{mcg}}{1} = 320\ \text{mcg}$$

4. Factors: 0.5 mg = 1 kg; 12 kg/l

$$\text{mg} = \frac{0.5\ \text{mg} \times 12\ \text{kg}}{1\ \text{kg} \times 1} = \frac{0.5\ \text{mg} \times 12}{1 \times 1} = \frac{6\ \text{mg}}{1} = 6\ \text{mg}$$

5. Factors: 25 mg = 1 lb; 1 kg = 2.2 lb; 85 kg/l

$$\text{mg} = \frac{25\ \text{mg} \times 2.2\ \text{lb} \times 85\ \text{kg}}{1\ \text{lb} \times 1\ \text{kg} \times 1} = \frac{25\ \text{mg} \times 2.2 \times 85}{1 \times 1 \times 1} = \frac{4675\ \text{mg}}{1} = 4675\ \text{mg}$$

6. Factors: 1 mg = 1000 mcg; 30 mcg = 1 kg; 1 kg = 2.2 lb; 88 lb/1

$$\text{mg} = \frac{1\ \text{mg} \times 30\ \text{mcg} \times 1\ \text{kg} \times 88\ \text{lb}}{1000\ \text{mcg} \times 1\ \text{kg} \times 2.2\ \text{lb} \times 1} = \frac{1\ \text{mg} \times \overset{3}{\cancel{30}} \times 1 \times \overset{\overset{4}{\cancel{40}}}{\cancel{88}}}{\underset{\underset{10}{\cancel{100}}}{\cancel{1000}} \times 1 \times 2.2 \times 1} = \frac{12\ \text{mg}}{10} = 1.2\ \text{mg}$$

7. Factors: 1 g = 1000 mg; 0.3 mg = 1 kg; 1 kg = 2.2 lb; 231 lb/1

$$\text{g} = \frac{1\ \text{g} \times 0.3\ \text{mg} \times 1\ \text{kg} \times 231\ \text{lb}}{1000\ \text{mg} \times 1\ \text{kg} \times 2.2\ \text{lb} \times 1} = \frac{1\ \text{g} \times 0.3 \times 1 \times \overset{105}{\cancel{231}}}{1000 \times 1 \times \underset{1}{\cancel{2.2}} \times 1} = \frac{31.5\ \text{g}}{1000} = 0.0315\ \text{g}$$

8. Factors: 10 mcg = 1 kg; 24 kg/l

$$\text{mcg} = \frac{10\ \text{mcg} \times 24\ \text{kg}}{1\ \text{kg} \times 1} = \frac{10\ \text{mcg} \times 24}{1 \times 1} = \frac{240\ \text{mcg}}{1} = 240\ \text{mcg}$$

9. Factors: 0.15 mcg = 1 kg; 1 kg = 2.2 lb; 198 lb/1

$$\text{mcg} = \frac{0.15\ \text{mcg} \times 1\ \text{kg} \times 198\ \text{lb}}{1\ \text{kg} \times 2.2\ \text{lb} \times 1} = \frac{0.15\ \text{mcg} \times 1 \times \overset{90}{\cancel{198}}}{1 \times \underset{1}{\cancel{2.2}} \times 1} = \frac{13.5\ \text{mcg}}{1} = 13.5\ \text{mcg}$$

10. Factors: 1 mg = 1000 mcg; 0.03 mg = 1 kg; 1 kg = 2.2 lb; 121 lb/1

$$\text{mcg} = \frac{1000\ \text{mcg} \times 0.03\ \text{mg} \times 1\ \text{kg} \times 121\ \text{lb}}{1\ \text{mg} \times 1\ \text{kg} \times 2.2\ \text{lb} \times 1} = \frac{1000\ \text{mcg} \times 0.03 \times 1 \times \overset{55}{\cancel{121}}}{1 \times 1 \times \underset{1}{\cancel{2.2}} \times 1} = \frac{1650\ \text{mcg}}{1}$$

$$= 1650\ \text{mcg}$$

Calculation of Dosages Based on Body Weight

11. Factors: 50 mg = 1 tab; 1 mg = 1 kg; 1 kg = 2.2 lb; 110 lb/1

$$\text{tab} = \frac{1\ \text{tab} \times 1\ \text{mg} \times 1\ \text{kg} \times 110\ \text{lb}}{50\ \text{mg} \times 1\ \text{kg} \times 2.2\ \text{lb} \times 1} = \frac{1\ \text{tab} \times 1 \times 1 \times \overset{\overset{1}{\cancel{50}}}{\cancel{110}}}{\underset{1}{\cancel{50}} \times 1 \times \underset{1}{\cancel{2.2}} \times 1} = \frac{1\ \text{tab}}{1} = 1\ \text{tab}$$

12. Factors: 1 ml = 15 (16) mx; 0.5 mg = 1 ml; 1 mg = 1000 mcg; 6 mcg = 1 kg; 121 lb/1

$$\text{mx} = \frac{15\ \text{mx} \times 1\ \text{ml} \times 1\ \text{mg} \times 6\ \text{mcg} \times 1\ \text{kg} \times 121\ \text{lb}}{1\ \text{ml} \times 0.5\ \text{mg} \times 1000\ \text{mcg} \times 1\ \text{kg} \times 2.2\ \text{lb} \times 1} = \frac{\overset{3}{\cancel{15}}\ \text{mx} \times 1 \times 1 \times \overset{3}{\cancel{6}} \times 1 \times \overset{11}{\cancel{121}}}{1 \times \underset{0.1}{\cancel{0.5}} \times \underset{100}{\cancel{1000}} \times 1 \times 2.2 \times 1} = \frac{99\ \text{mx}}{10} = 9.9\ \text{mx}$$

$$\text{mx} = \frac{16\ \text{mx} \times 1\ \text{ml} \times 1\ \text{mg} \times 6\ \text{mcg} \times 1\ \text{kg} \times 121\ \text{lb}}{1\ \text{ml} \times 0.5\ \text{mg} \times 1000\ \text{mcg} \times 1\ \text{kg} \times 2.2\ \text{lb} \times 1} = \frac{\overset{2}{\cancel{16}}\ \text{mx} \times 1 \times 1 \times 6 \times 1 \times \overset{11}{\cancel{121}}}{1 \times \underset{0.1}{\cancel{0.5}} \times \underset{125}{\cancel{1000}} \times 1 \times 2.2 \times 1}$$

$$= \frac{132\ \text{mx}}{12.5} = 10.56\ \text{mx}$$

13. Factors: 0.01 ml = 1 kg; 1 kg = 2.2 lb; 180 lb/1

$$\text{ml} = \frac{0.01\ \text{ml} \times 1\ \text{kg} \times 180\ \text{lb}}{1\ \text{kg} \times 2.2\ \text{lb} \times 1} = \frac{0.01\ \text{ml} \times 1 \times \overset{90}{\cancel{180}}}{1 \times \underset{1.1}{\cancel{2.2}} \times 1} = \frac{0.9\ \text{ml}}{1.1} = 0.818\ \text{ml} = 0.82\ \text{ml}$$

14. Factors: 1 mg = 1000 mcg; 10 mcg = 1 kg; 1 kg = 2.2 lb; 66 lb/1

$$\text{mg} = \frac{1\ \text{mg} \times 10\ \text{mcg} \times 1\ \text{kg} \times 66\ \text{lb}}{1000\ \text{mcg} \times 1\ \text{kg} \times 2.2\ \text{lb} \times 1} = \frac{1\ \text{mg} \times \overset{1}{\cancel{10}} \times 1 \times \overset{3}{\cancel{66}}}{\underset{\underset{10}{\cancel{100}}}{\cancel{1000}} \times 1 \times 2.2 \times 1} = \frac{3\ \text{mg}}{10} = 0.3\ \text{mg (/day)}$$

Factors: 1 tab = 0.1 mg; 0.3 mg = 1 day; 3 doses = 1 d

$$\text{tab} = \frac{1\,\text{tab}\ \times 0.3\,\text{mg}\ \times 1\,\text{day}}{0.1\,\text{mg}\ \times\ 1\,\text{day}\ \times 3\,\text{doses}} = \frac{1\,\text{tab}\ \times \cancel{0.3} \times 1}{\cancel{0.1}\ \times\ 1 \times \cancel{3}\,\text{doses}} = \frac{1\,\text{tab}}{1\,\text{dose}} = 1\,\text{tab/dose}$$

15. Factors: 1 ml = 15 (16) mx; 250 mg = 1 ml; 20 mg = 1 kg; 1 kg = 2.2 lb; $19\frac{1}{4}\ (\frac{77}{4})$ lb/1

$$\text{mx} = \frac{15\,\text{mx} \times\ 1\,\text{ml} \times 20\,\text{mg} \times\ 1\,\text{kg}\ \times 19\frac{1}{4}\,\text{lb}}{1\,\text{ml}\ \times 250\,\text{mg} \times\ 1\,\text{kg}\ \times 2.2\,\text{lb}\ \times\ 1} = \frac{\cancel{15}\,\text{mx} \times\ 1 \times \overset{1}{\cancel{20}} \times\ 1 \times \overset{7}{\cancel{77}}}{1\ \times \underset{\underset{5}{50}}{\cancel{250}} \times\ 1 \times \underset{0.2}{2.2} \times \underset{2}{\cancel{4}}} = \frac{21\,\text{mx}}{2} = 10.5\,\text{mx}$$

$$\text{mx} = \frac{16\,\text{mx} \times\ 1\,\text{ml} \times 20\,\text{mg} \times\ 1\,\text{kg}\ \times 19\frac{1}{4}\,\text{lb}}{1\,\text{ml}\ \times 250\,\text{mg} \times\ 1\,\text{kg}\ \times 2.2\,\text{lb}\ \times\ 1} = \frac{\overset{4}{\cancel{16}}\,\text{mx} \times\ 1 \times \overset{1}{\cancel{20}} \times\ 1 \times \overset{7}{\cancel{77}}}{1\ \times \underset{25}{\cancel{250}} \times\ 1 \times \underset{\underset{0.1}{0.2}}{2.2} \times \underset{1}{\cancel{4}}} = \frac{28\,\text{mx}}{2.5} = 11.2\,\text{mx}$$

16. Factors: 3 mcg = 1 kg; 1 kg = 2.2 lb; 198 lb/1; 3 doses = 1 day

$$\text{mcg} = \frac{3\,\text{mcg} \times\ 1\,\text{kg}\ \times 198\,\text{lb}}{1\,\text{kg}\ \times 2.2\,\text{lb}\ \times\ 1} = \frac{3\,\text{mcg} \times\ 1 \times \overset{90}{\cancel{198}}}{1\ \times \underset{1}{\cancel{2.2}} \times\ 1} = \frac{270\,\text{mcg}}{1} = 270\ \text{mcg daily dosage}$$

$$\frac{\text{mcg}}{\text{dose}} = \frac{270\,\text{mcg} \times 1\,\text{day}}{1\,\text{day}\ \times 3\,\text{doses}} = \frac{\overset{90}{\cancel{270}}\,\text{mcg} \times 1}{1\ \times \underset{1}{\cancel{3}}\,\text{doses}} = \frac{90\,\text{mcg}}{1\,\text{dose}} = 90\,\text{mcg/dose}$$

17. Factors: 10 U = 1 kg; 1 kg = 2.2 lb; 8 lb 15 oz = $8\frac{15}{16}\ (\frac{143}{16})$ lb/1; 50 U = 1 ml; 1 ml = 15 (16) mx

$$\text{mx} = \frac{15\,\text{mx} \times\ 1\,\text{ml} \times 10\,\text{U}\ \times\ 1\,\text{kg}\ \times 8\frac{15}{16}\,\text{lb}}{1\,\text{ml}\ \times 50\,\text{U}\ \times\ 1\,\text{kg}\ \times 2.2\,\text{lb}\ \times\ 1} = \frac{\overset{3}{\cancel{15}}\,\text{mx} \times\ 1 \times \overset{1}{\cancel{10}} \times\ 1 \times \overset{65}{\cancel{143}}}{1\ \times \underset{\underset{1}{\cancel{5}}}{\cancel{50}} \times\ 1 \times \underset{1}{\cancel{2.2}} \times 16} = \frac{195\,\text{mx}}{16} = 12.19\,\text{mx}$$

$$\text{mx} = \frac{16\,\text{mx} \times\ 1\,\text{ml} \times 10\,\text{U}\ \times\ 1\,\text{kg} \times 8\frac{15}{16}\,\text{lb}}{1\,\text{ml}\ \times 50\,\text{U}\ \times\ 1\,\text{kg} \times 2.2\,\text{lb}\ \times\ 1} = \frac{\overset{1}{\cancel{16}}\,\text{mx} \times\ 1 \times \overset{1}{\cancel{10}} \times\ 1 \times \overset{13}{\cancel{143}}}{1\ \times \underset{\underset{1}{\cancel{5}}}{\cancel{50}} \times\ 1 \times \underset{1}{\cancel{2.2}} \times \cancel{16}} = \frac{13\,\text{mx}}{1} = 13\,\text{mx}$$

18. Factors: 25 mg = 1 kg; 141 lb/1; 1 kg = 2.2 lb; 1 tab = 200 mg; 4 doses = 1 day

$$\frac{\text{tab}}{\text{dose}} = \frac{1\,\text{tab} \times 25\,\text{mg} \times\ 1\,\text{kg}\ \times 141\,\text{lb}\ \ \times 1\,\text{day}}{200\,\text{mg} \times\ 1\,\text{kg}\ \times 2.2\,\text{lb}\ \times\ 1\,(\times\,\text{day}) \times 4\,\text{doses}} = \frac{1\,\text{tab} \times \overset{1}{\cancel{25}} \times\ 1 \times 141\ \ \ \times 1}{\underset{8}{\cancel{200}}\ \ \ \times\ 1 \times 2.2 \times\ \ 1\,(\times 1)\ \times 4\,\text{doses}}$$

$$= \frac{141\ \text{tab}}{70.4\ \text{doses}} = \frac{2.002\ \text{tab}}{1\ \text{doses}} = 2\,\text{tab/dose}$$

19. Factors: 50 mcg = 1 kg; 1 kg = 2.2 lb; 220 lb/1; 2.5 mg = 1 tab; 1000 mcg = 1 mg

$$\text{tab} = \frac{1\,\text{tab} \times\ \ 1\,\text{mg}\ \times 50\,\text{mcg} \times\ 1\,\text{kg}\ \times 220\,\text{lb}}{2.5\,\text{mg}\ \times 1000\,\text{mcg} \times\ 1\,\text{kg}\ \times 2.2\,\text{lb}\ \times\ 1} = \frac{1\,\text{tab} \times\ \ 1 \times \overset{1}{\cancel{50}} \times\ 1 \times \overset{\overset{2}{\cancel{100}}}{\cancel{220}}}{\underset{1}{\cancel{2.5}}\ \ \ \times \underset{\underset{1}{20}}{\cancel{1000}} \times\ 1 \times \underset{1}{\cancel{2.2}} \times\ 1} = \frac{2\,\text{tabs}}{1} = 2\,\text{tabs}$$

20. Factors: 1 g = 1000 mg; 15 mg = 1 lb; 134 lb/1; 1 g = 5 ml; 1 tsp = 5 ml

$$\text{tsp} = \frac{1\,\text{tsp} \times 5\,\text{ml} \times\ \ 1\,\text{g}\ \times 15\,\text{mg} \times 134\,\text{lb}}{5\,\text{ml} \times 1\,\text{g}\ \ \times 1000\,\text{mg} \times\ 1\,\text{lb}\ \times\ 1} = \frac{1\,\text{tsp} \times\ \overset{1}{\cancel{5}}\ \times\ \ 1 \times \overset{3}{\cancel{15}} \times \overset{67}{\cancel{134}}}{\underset{1}{\cancel{5}}\,\text{ml} \times\ 1 \times \underset{\underset{100}{200}}{\cancel{1000}} \times\ 1 \times\ \ 1} = \frac{201\,\text{tsp}}{100} = 2.01\,\text{tsp} = 2\,\text{tsp}$$

21. Factors: 0.03 mg = 1 kg; 1 kg = 2.2 lb; 1 tab = 2 mg; $149\frac{1}{2}$ lb/1

$$\text{tab} = \frac{1\,\text{tab} \times 0.03\,\text{mg} \times\ \ 1\,\text{kg}\ \times 149.5\,\text{lb}}{2\,\text{mg} \times\ \ \ 1\,\text{kg}\ \times 2.2\,\text{lb}\ \times\ 1} = \frac{1\,\text{tab} \times 0.03 \times\ \ 1 \times 149.5}{2\ \ \ \times\ \ 1 \times 2.2 \times\ \ 1} = \frac{4.485\,\text{tab}}{4.4} = 1.01\,(1)\,\text{tab}$$

22. Factors: 1 tab = 50 mg; 2.5 mg = 1 kg; 1 kg = 2.2 lb; 154 lb/1;

$$\text{tab} = \frac{1\,\text{tab} \times 2.5\,\text{mg} \times\ \ 1\,\text{kg}\ \times 154\,\text{lb}}{50\,\text{mg} \times\ \ 1\,\text{kg}\ \times 2.2\,\text{lb}\ \times\ 1} = \frac{1\,\text{tab} \times \overset{0.1}{\cancel{2.5}} \times\ \ 1 \times \overset{\overset{35}{\cancel{70}}}{\cancel{154}}}{\underset{\underset{1}{2}}{\cancel{50}}\ \ \ \times\ 1 \times \underset{1}{\cancel{2.2}} \times\ 1} = \frac{3.5\,\text{tabs}}{1} = 3.5\,\text{tabs}$$

23. Factors: 5 mg = 1 kg; 1 kg = 2.2 lb; $57\frac{1}{2}$ lb/1; 5 mg = 1 ml; 4 doses = 1 d

$$mg = \frac{5\,mg \times 1\,kg \times 57.5\,lb}{1\,kg \times 2.2\,lb \times 1} = \frac{5\,mg \times 1 \times 57.5}{1 \times 2.2 \times 1} = \frac{287.5\,mg}{2.2} = 130.68\,mg\ daily\ dosage$$

$$ml = \frac{1\,ml \times 130.68\,mg \times 1\,day}{5\,mg \times 1\,day \times 4\,doses} = \frac{1\,ml \times 130.68 \times 1}{5 \times 1 \times 4\,doses} = \frac{130.68\,ml}{20\,doses} = 6.53\ (6.5)\ ml/dose$$

24. Factors: 25 mg = 1 kg; 1 kg = 2.2 lb; 132 lb/1; 1 cap = 500 mg

$$cap = \frac{1\,cap \times 25\,mg \times 1\,kg \times 132\,lb}{500\,mg \times 1\,kg \times 2.2\,lb \times 1} = \frac{1\,cap \times \overset{1}{\cancel{25}} \times 1 \times \overset{\overset{3}{\cancel{60}}}{\cancel{132}}}{\underset{\underset{1}{20}}{\cancel{500}} \times 1 \times \underset{1}{\cancel{2.2}} \times 1} = \frac{3\,caps}{1} = 3\,caps$$

25. Factors: 200 IU = 1 kg; 1 kg = 2.2 lb; 110 lb/1

$$IU = \frac{200\,IU \times 1\,kg \times 110\,lb}{1\,kg \times 2.2\,lb \times 1} = \frac{200\,IU \times 1 \times \overset{50}{\cancel{110}}}{1 \times \underset{1}{\cancel{2.2}} \times 1} = \frac{10000\,IU}{1} = 10,000\,IU$$

26. Factors: Recommended dosage: 30 mg = 1 kg; 1 kg = 2.2 lb; 176 lb/1

$$mg = \frac{30\,mg \times 1\,kg \times 176\,lb}{1\,kg \times 2.2\,lb \times 1} = \frac{30\,mg \times 1 \times \overset{80}{\cancel{176}}}{1 \times \underset{1}{\cancel{2.2}} \times 1} = \frac{2400\,mg}{1} = 2400\,mg\ dosage\ recommended$$

Factors: Ordered dosage: 300 mg = (q) 4 h; 24 h = 1 d

$$\frac{mg}{d} = \frac{300\,mg \times 24\,h}{(q)4\,h \times 1\,d} = \frac{300\,mg \times \overset{6}{\cancel{24}}}{\underset{1}{\cancel{4}} \times 1\,d} = \frac{1800\,mg}{1\,d} = 1800\,mg/d\ ordered$$

Recommended dosage > ordered dosage by 600 mg/d

27. Factors: Recommended: 1.5 g/1; 1 g = 1000 mg

$$mg = \frac{1000\,mg \times 1.5\,g}{1\,g \times 1} = \frac{1000\,mg \times 1.5}{1 \times 1} = \frac{1500\,mg}{1} = 1500\,mg\ (/d)\ recommended$$

Factors: 500 mg = 1 dose; 3 doses = 1 d

$$\frac{mg}{d} = \frac{500\,mg \times 3\,doses}{1\,dose \times 1\,d} = \frac{500\,mg \times 3}{1 \times 1\,d} = \frac{1500\,mg}{d} = 1500\,mg/d\ ordered$$

The ordered dosage is equal to the recommended dosage

28. Factors: Recommended: 1 mg = 1000 mcg; 2 mcg = 1 kg; 1 kg = 2.2 lb; 136 lb/1

$$mg = \frac{1\,mg \times 2\,mcg \times 1\,kg \times 136\,lb}{1000\,mcg \times 1\,kg \times 2.2\,lb \times 1} = \frac{1\,mg \times \overset{1}{\cancel{2}} \times 1 \times 136}{1000 \times 1 \times \underset{1.1}{\cancel{2.2}} \times 1} = \frac{136\,mg}{1100}$$

$$= 0.1236\,mg$$

Ordered dosage of 0.125 mg/d is slightly greater than the recommended dosage of 0.124 mg/d by 0.001 mg

29. Factors: Recommended: 2 mg = 1 kg; 1 kg = 2.2 lb; 165 lb/1

$$mg = \frac{2\,mg \times 1\,kg \times 165\,lb}{1\,kg \times 2.2\,lb \times 1} = \frac{2\,mg \times 1 \times \overset{75}{\cancel{165}}}{1 \times \underset{1}{\cancel{2.2}} \times 1} = \frac{150\,mg}{1} = 150\,mg\ (/d)\ recommended$$

Factors: Ordered: 50 mg = (q) 8 h; 24 h = 1 d

$$\frac{mg}{d} = \frac{50\,mg \times 24\,h}{(q)8\,h \times 1\,d} = \frac{50\,mg \times \overset{3}{\cancel{24}}}{\underset{1}{\cancel{8}} \times 1\,d} = \frac{150\,mg}{1\,d} = 150\,mg/d$$

The ordered dosage is equal to the recommended dosage.

30. Factors: Recommended: 5g/d

Factors: Ordered: 1 g = 1 dose; 4 doses = 1 d

$$\frac{g}{d} = \frac{1\,g \times 4\,doses}{1\,dose \times 1\,d} = \frac{1\,g \times 4}{1 \times 1\,d} = \frac{4\,g}{1\,d} = 4\,g/d\ ordered$$

The recommended dosage is greater than the ordered dosage by 1 g.

31. Factors: Recommended: 100 to 150 mg/d

Factors: Ordered: 25 mg = (q) 4 h; 24 h = 1 d

$$\frac{mg}{d} = \frac{25\,mg \times 24\,h}{(q)4\,h \times 1\,d} = \frac{25\,mg \times \overset{6}{\cancel{24}}}{\underset{1}{\cancel{4}} \times 1\,d} = \frac{150\,mg}{1\,d} = 150\,mg/d$$

The ordered dosage is within the recommended dosage range.

32. Factors: Recommended minimum: 10 mg = 1 kg; 98 kg/1

$$mg = \frac{10\ mg \times 98\ kg}{1\ kg \times 1} = \frac{10\ mg \times 98}{1 \times 1} = \frac{980\ mg}{1} = 980\ mg\ (/d)$$

Factors: Recommended maximum: 15 mg = 1 kg; 98 kg/1

$$mg = \frac{15\ mg \times 98\ kg}{1\ kg \times 1} = \frac{15\ mg \times 98}{1 \times 1} = \frac{1470\ mg}{1} = 1470\ mg\ (/d)$$

Factors: Ordered: 250 mg = (q) 6 h; 24 h = 1 d

$$mg = \frac{250\ mg \times 24\ h}{(q)6\ h \times 1\ d} = \frac{250\ mg \times \overset{4}{\cancel{24}}}{\underset{1}{\cancel{6}} \times 1\ d} = \frac{1000\ mg}{1\ d} = 1000\ mg/d$$

The ordered dosage is within the recommended range.

33. Factors: Recommended: 2 to 5 mg/d

Factors: Ordered: 1 mg = 1000 mcg; 750 mcg = (q) 3 h; 24 h = 1 d

$$\frac{mg}{d} = \frac{1\ mg \times 750\ mcg \times 24\ h}{1000\ mcg \times (q)3\ h \times 1\ d} = \frac{1\ mg \times \overset{75}{\cancel{750}} \times \overset{8}{\cancel{24}}}{\underset{100}{\cancel{1000}} \times \underset{1}{\cancel{3}} \times 1\ d} = \frac{600\ mg}{100\ d} = 6\ mg/d$$

The ordered dosage exceeds the recommended dosage by 1 mg.

34. Factors: Recommended minimum: 10 mcg = 1 kg; 1 kg = 2.2 lb; 176 lb/1

$$mcg = \frac{10\ mcg \times 1\ kg \times 176\ lb}{1\ kg \times 2.2\ lb \times 1} = \frac{10\ mcg \times 1 \times \overset{80}{\cancel{176}}}{1 \times \underset{1}{\cancel{2.2}} \times 1} = \frac{800\ mcg}{1} = 800\ mcg\ (/d)$$

Factors: Recommended maximum: 15 mcg = 1 kg; 1 kg = 2.2 lb; 176 lb/1

$$mcg = \frac{15\ mcg \times 1\ kg \times 176\ lb}{1\ kg \times 2.2\ lb \times 1} = \frac{15\ mcg \times 1 \times \overset{80}{\cancel{176}}}{1 \times \underset{1}{\cancel{2.2}} \times 1} = \frac{1200\ mcg}{1} = 1200\ mcg$$

Factors: Ordered: 1 mg = 1000 mcg; 1 gr = 60 mg; $\frac{1}{300}$ gr = 1 dose; 4 doses = 1 d

$$\frac{mcg}{d} = \frac{1000\ mcg \times 60\ mg \times gr\ \frac{1}{300} \times 4\ doses}{1\ mg \times 1\ gr \times 1\ dose \times 1\ d} = \frac{\overset{200}{\cancel{1000}}\ mcg \times \overset{1}{\cancel{60}} \times 1 \times 4}{1 \times 1 \times \underset{\underset{1}{5}}{\cancel{300}} \times 1\ d} = 800\ mcg/d$$

The ordered daily dosage is within the recommended dosage range.

35. Factors: Recommended minimum: 20 mg = 1 kg; 1 kg = 2.2 lb; 110 lb/1

$$mg = \frac{20\ mg \times 1\ kg \times 110\ lb}{1\ kg \times 2.2\ lb \times 1} = \frac{20\ mg \times 1 \times \overset{50}{\cancel{110}}}{1 \times \underset{1}{\cancel{2.2}} \times 1} = \frac{1000\ mg}{1} = 1000\ mg\ (/d)$$

Factors: Recommended maximum: 30 mg = 1 kg; 1 kg = 2.2 lb; 110 lb/1

$$mg = \frac{30\ mg \times 1\ kg \times 110\ lb}{1\ kg \times 2.2\ lb \times 1} = \frac{30\ mg \times 1 \times \overset{50}{\cancel{110}}}{1 \times \underset{1}{\cancel{2.2}} \times 1} = \frac{1500\ mg}{1} = 1500\ mg\ (/d)$$

Factors: Ordered: 400 mg = 1 dose; 3 doses = 1 d

$$\frac{mg}{d} = \frac{400\ mg \times 3\ doses}{1\ dose \times 1\ d} = \frac{400\ mg \times 3}{1 \times 1\ d} = \frac{1200\ mg}{1\ d} = 1200\ mg/d$$

The ordered dosage is within the recommended range.

36. Factors: Recommended: 0 to 3 g = 1 d

Factors: Ordered: 1 g = 1000 mg; 500 mg = (q) 4 h; 24 h = 1 d

$$\frac{g}{d} = \frac{1\ g \times 500\ mg \times 24\ h}{1000\ mg \times (q)4\ h \times 1\ d} = \frac{1\ g \times \overset{1}{\cancel{500}} \times \overset{3}{\cancel{6}\cancel{24}}}{\underset{\underset{1}{2}}{\cancel{1000}} \times \underset{1}{\cancel{4}} \times 1\ d} = \frac{3\ g}{1\ d} = 3\ g/d$$

The ordered dosage is within the recommended range.

37. Factors: Recommended: 0 to 1 mg = 1 lb; 1 kg = 2.2 lb; 70 kg/1

$$mg = \frac{1\ mg \times 2.2\ lb \times 70\ kg}{1\ lb \times 1\ kg \times 1} = \frac{1\ mg \times 2.2 \times 70}{1 \times 1 \times 1} = \frac{154\ mg}{1} = 154\ mg\ (/d)$$

Factors: Ordered: 1 g = 1000 mg; 0.5 g = 1 dose; 2 doses = 1 d

$$\frac{mg}{d} = \frac{1000\ mg \times 0.5\ g \times 2\ doses}{1\ g \times 1\ dose \times 1\ d} = \frac{1000\ mg \times 0.5 \times 2}{1 \times 1 \times 1\ d} = \frac{1000\ mg}{1\ d} = 1000\ mg/d$$

Ordered dosage exceeds the recommended range.

38. Factors: Maximum: 5 mcg = 1 kg; 1 kg = 2.2 lb; 165 lb/1

$$\text{mcg} = \frac{5\,\text{mcg} \times 1\,\text{kg} \times 165\,\text{lb}}{1\,\text{kg} \times 2.2\,\text{lb} \times 1} = \frac{5\,\text{mcg} \times 1 \times \overset{75}{\cancel{165}}}{1 \times \cancel{2.2} \times 1} = \frac{375\,\text{mcg}}{1} = 375\,\text{mcg}$$

Factors: Minimum: 2 mcg = 1 kg; 1 kg = 2.2 lb; 165 lb/1

$$\text{mcg} = \frac{2\,\text{mcg} \times 1\,\text{kg} \times 165\,\text{lb}}{1\,\text{kg} \times 2.2\,\text{lb} \times 1} = \frac{2\,\text{mcg} \times 1 \times \overset{75}{\cancel{165}}}{1 \times \cancel{2.2} \times 1} = \frac{150\,\text{mcg}}{1} = 150\,\text{mcg}$$

Factors: 1 mg = 1000 mcg; 0.15 mg = 1 dose; 2 doses = 1 d

$$\frac{\text{mcg}}{\text{d}} = \frac{1000\,\text{mcg} \times 0.15\,\text{mg} \times 2\,\text{doses}}{1\,\text{mg} \times 1\,\text{dose} \times 1\,\text{d}} = \frac{1000\,\text{mcg} \times 0.15 \times 2}{1 \times 1 \times 1\,\text{d}} = \frac{300\,\text{mcg}}{1\,\text{d}} = 300\,\text{mcg/d}$$

The ordered dosage is within the recommended dosage range.

39. Factors: Recommended: 5 to 10 g/d

Factors: Ordered: 1 g = 15 gr; 30 gr = 1 dose; 4 doses = 1 d

$$\frac{\text{g}}{\text{d}} = \frac{1\,\text{g} \times 30\,\text{gr} \times 4\,\text{doses}}{15\,\text{gr} \times 1\,\text{dose} \times 1\,\text{d}} = \frac{1\,\text{g} \times \overset{2}{\cancel{30}} \times 4}{\cancel{15} \times 1 \times 1\,\text{d}} = \frac{8\,\text{g}}{1\,\text{d}} = 8\,\text{g/d}$$

The ordered dosage is within the recommended range.

40. Factors: Minimum: 50 mcg = 1 kg; 1 kg = 2.2 lb; 132 lb/1

$$\text{mcg} = \frac{50\,\text{mcg} \times 1\,\text{kg} \times 132\,\text{lb}}{1\,\text{kg} \times 2.2\,\text{lb} \times 1} = \frac{50\,\text{mcg} \times 1 \times \overset{60}{\cancel{132}}}{1 \times \cancel{2.2} \times 1} = \frac{3000\,\text{mcg}}{1} = 3000\,\text{mcg/d}$$

Factors: Maximum: 60 mcg = 1 kg; 1 kg = 2.2 kg; 132 lb/1

$$\text{mcg} = \frac{60\,\text{mcg} \times 1\,\text{kg} \times 132\,\text{lb}}{1\,\text{kg} \times 2.2\,\text{lb} \times 1} = \frac{60\,\text{mcg} \times 1 \times \overset{60}{\cancel{132}}}{1 \times \cancel{2.2} \times 1} = \frac{3600\,\text{mcg}}{1} = 3600\,\text{mcg/d}$$

Factors: Ordered: 1 mg = 1000 mcg; 1.2 mg = 1 dose; 3 doses = 1 d

$$\frac{\text{mcg}}{\text{d}} = \frac{1000\,\text{mcg} \times 1.2\,\text{mg} \times 3\,\text{doses}}{1\,\text{mg} \times 1\,\text{dose} \times 1\,\text{d}} = \frac{1000\,\text{mcg} \times 1.2 \times 3}{1\,\text{mg} \times 1 \times 1\,\text{d}} = \frac{3600\,\text{mcg}}{1\,\text{d}} = 3600\,\text{mcg/d}$$

The ordered dosage is within the recommended range.

UNIT VI: SOLUTIONS

Chapter 14: Calculation of Solutes and Solvents

1. Factors: 500 ml = 100%; 0.9%/1

$$\text{ml (salt)} = \frac{500\,\text{ml} \times 0.9\,\%}{100\,\% \times 1} = \frac{\overset{5}{\cancel{500}}\,\text{ml} \times 0.9}{\cancel{100} \times 1} = \frac{4.5\,\text{ml}}{1} = 4.5\,\text{ml salt}$$

ml (water) = 500 ml − 4.5 ml = 495.5 ml approximately or add water q.s. to 500 ml.

2. Factors: 100 ml = 100%; 5%/1

$$\text{ml} = \frac{100\,\text{ml} \times 5\,\%}{100\,\% \times 1} = \frac{\overset{1}{\cancel{100}}\,\text{ml} \times 5}{\cancel{100} \times 1} = \frac{5\,\text{ml}}{1} = 5\,\text{ml}$$

3. Factors: 800 ml = 100%; 20%/1

$$\text{ml} = \frac{800\,\text{ml} \times 20\,\%}{100\,\% \times 1} = \frac{\overset{8}{\cancel{800}}\,\text{ml} \times 20}{\cancel{100} \times 1} = \frac{160\,\text{ml}}{1} = 160\,\text{ml}$$

4. Factors: 1 tsp = 5 ml; 1500 ml = 100%; 0.9%/1

$$\text{tsp} = \frac{1\,\text{tsp} \times 1500\,\text{ml} \times 0.9\,\%}{5\,\text{ml} \times 100\,\% \times 1} = \frac{1\,\text{tsp} \times \overset{3}{\underset{1}{\cancel{1500}}} \times 0.9}{\cancel{5} \times \cancel{100} \times 1} = \frac{2.7\,\text{tsp}}{1} = 2.7\,\text{tsp}$$

5. Factors: 1000 ml = 1 L; 1.5 L = 100%; 0.45%/1

$$\text{ml} = \frac{1000\,\text{ml} \times 1.5\,\text{L} \times 0.45\,\%}{1\,\text{L} \times 100\,\% \times 1} = \frac{\overset{10}{\cancel{1000}}\,\text{ml} \times 1.5 \times 0.45}{1 \times \cancel{100} \times 1} = \frac{6.75\,\text{ml}}{1} = 6.75\,\text{ml}$$

6. Factors: 1 g = 4 Cal; 1 g = 1 ml; 1000 ml = 100%; 10%/1

$$\text{Cal} = \frac{4\ \text{Cal} \times 1\ \text{g} \times 1000\ \text{ml} \times 10\%}{1\ \text{g} \times 1\ \text{ml} \times 100\ \% \times 1} = \frac{4\ \text{Cal} \times 1 \times \overset{10}{\cancel{1000}} \times 10}{1 \times 1 \times \underset{1}{\cancel{100}} \times 1} = \frac{400\ \text{Cal}}{1} = 400\ \text{Cal}$$

7. Factors: dextrose: 1 g = 1 ml; 500 ml = 100%; 5%/1

$$\text{g} = \frac{1\ \text{g} \times 500\ \text{ml} \times 5\ \%}{1\ \text{ml} \times 100\ \% \times 1} = \frac{1\ \text{g} \times \overset{5}{\cancel{500}} \times 5}{1 \times \underset{1}{\cancel{100}} \times 1} = \frac{25\ \text{g}}{1} = 25\ \text{g dextrose}$$

Factors: sodium chloride: 1 g = 1 ml; 500 ml = 100%; 0.9%/1

$$\text{g} = \frac{1\ \text{g} \times 500\ \text{ml} \times 0.9\ \%}{1\ \text{ml} \times 100\ \% \times 1} = \frac{1\ \text{g} \times \overset{5}{\cancel{500}} \times 0.9}{1 \times \underset{1}{\cancel{100}} \times 1} = \frac{4.5\ \text{g}}{1} = 4.5\ \text{g sodium chloride}$$

Factors: Calories: 4 Cal = 1 g; 25 g/1

$$\text{Cal} = \frac{4\ \text{Cal} \times 25\ \text{g}}{1\ \text{g} \times 1} = \frac{4\ \text{Cal} \times 25}{1 \times 1} = \frac{100\ \text{Cal}}{1} = 100\ \text{Calories}$$

8. Factors: 4 Cal = 1 g; 1 g = 1 ml; 100 ml = 100%; 50%/1

$$\text{Cal} = \frac{4\ \text{Cal} \times 1\ \text{g} \times 100\ \text{ml} \times 50\ \%}{1\ \text{g} \times 1\ \text{ml} \times 100\ \% \times 1} = \frac{4\ \text{Cal} \times 1 \times \overset{1}{\cancel{100}} \times 50}{1 \times 1 \times \underset{1}{\cancel{100}} \times 1} = \frac{200\ \text{Cal}}{1} = 200\ \text{Cal}$$

9. Factors: 4 Cal = 1 g; 1 g = 1 ml; 1000 ml = 100%; 5%/1; 2 IVs/d

$$\text{Cal} = \frac{4\ \text{Cal} \times 1\ \text{g} \times 1000\ \text{ml} \times 5\%}{1\ \text{g} \times 1\ \text{ml} \times 100\ \% \times 1} = \frac{4\ \text{Cal} \times 1 \times \overset{10}{\cancel{1000}} \times 5}{1 \times 1 \times \underset{1}{\cancel{100}} \times 1} = \frac{200\ \text{Cal}}{1} = 200\ \text{Cal/IV}$$

200 Cal × 2 IVs/d = 400 Cal

10. Factors: dextrose: 1 g = 1 ml; 1500 ml = 100%; 2.5%/1

$$\text{g} = \frac{1\ \text{g} \times 1500\ \text{ml} \times 2.5\ \%}{1\ \text{ml} \times 100\ \% \times 1} = \frac{1\ \text{g} \times \overset{15}{\cancel{1500}} \times 2.5}{1 \times \underset{1}{\cancel{100}} \times 1} = \frac{37.5\ \text{g}}{1} = 37.5\ \text{g dextrose}$$

Factors: sodium chloride: 1 g = 1 ml; 1500 ml = 100%; 0.45%/1

$$\text{g} = \frac{1\ \text{g} \times 1500\ \text{ml} \times 0.45\ \%}{1\ \text{ml} \times 100\ \% \times 1} = \frac{1\ \text{g} \times \overset{15}{\cancel{1500}} \times 0.45}{1 \times \underset{1}{\cancel{100}} \times 1} = \frac{6.75\ \text{g}}{1} = 6.75\ \text{g}$$

11. Factors: 400 ml = 20%; 10%/1

$$\text{ml} = \frac{400\ \text{ml} \times 10\ \%}{20\ \% \times 1} = \frac{\overset{20}{\cancel{400}}\ \text{ml} \times 10}{\underset{1}{\cancel{20}} \times 1} = \frac{200\ \text{ml}}{1} = 200\ \text{ml}$$

12. Factors: 300 ml = 30%; 20%/1

$$\text{ml} = \frac{300\ \text{ml} \times 20\ \%}{30\ \% \times 1} = \frac{\overset{10}{\cancel{300}}\ \text{ml} \times 20}{\underset{1}{\cancel{30}} \times 1} = \frac{200\ \text{ml}}{1} = 200\ \text{ml}$$

13. Factors: 1 oz = 30 ml; 900 ml = 50%; 10%/1

$$\text{oz} = \frac{1\ \text{oz} \times 900\ \text{ml} \times 10\ \%}{30\ \text{ml} \times 50\ \% \times 1} = \frac{1\ \text{oz} \times \cancel{900} \times \cancel{10}}{\cancel{30} \times \cancel{50} \times 1} = \frac{6\ \text{oz}}{1} = 6\ \text{oz}$$

14. Factors: 1 oz = 30 ml; 1500 ml = 50%; 10%/1

$$\text{oz} = \frac{1\ \text{oz} \times 1500\ \text{ml} \times 10\ \%}{30\ \text{ml} \times 50\ \% \times 1} = \frac{1\ \text{oz} \times \cancel{1500} \times 10}{\cancel{30} \times \cancel{50} \times 1} = \frac{10\ \text{oz}}{1} = 10\ \text{oz}$$

15. Factors: 300 ml = 60%; 5%/1

$$\text{ml} = \frac{300\ \text{ml} \times 5\ \%}{60\ \% \times 1} = \frac{\overset{5}{\cancel{300}}\ \text{ml} \times 5}{\underset{1}{\cancel{60}} \times 1} = \frac{25\ \text{ml}}{1} = 25\ \text{ml}$$

16. Factors: 2000 ml = 20%; 100% = 1; 1/1000

$$ml = \frac{2000 \text{ ml} \times 100 \text{ \%} \times 1}{20 \text{ \%} \times 1 \times 1000} = \frac{\overset{2}{\cancel{2000}} \text{ ml} \times \overset{5}{\cancel{100}} \times 1}{\underset{1}{\cancel{20}} \times 1 \times \cancel{1000}} = \frac{10 \text{ ml}}{1} = 10 \text{ ml}$$

17. Factors: 500 ml = 50%; 1 = 100%; 1/10

$$ml = \frac{500 \text{ ml} \times 100 \text{ \%} \times 1}{50 \text{ \%} \times 1 \times 10} = \frac{\overset{10}{\cancel{500}} \text{ ml} \times \overset{10}{\cancel{100}} \times 1}{\underset{1}{\cancel{50}} \times 1 \times \cancel{10}} = \frac{100 \text{ ml}}{1} = 100 \text{ ml}$$

18. Factors: 1000 ml = 1/100; 1 = 100%; 0.5%/1

$$ml = \frac{1000 \text{ ml} \times 1 \times 0.5 \text{ \%}}{\frac{1}{100} \times 100 \text{ \%} \times 1} = \frac{\overset{1}{\cancel{100}} \times 1000 \text{ ml} \times 1 \times 0.5}{1 \times \underset{1}{\cancel{100}} \times 1} = \frac{500 \text{ ml}}{1} = 500 \text{ ml}$$

19. Factors: 200 ml = 10%; 1 = 100%; 1/10

$$ml = \frac{200 \text{ ml} \times 100 \text{ \%} \times 1}{10 \text{ \%} \times 1 \times 10} = \frac{\overset{20}{\cancel{200}} \text{ ml} \times \overset{10}{\cancel{100}} \times 1}{\underset{1}{\cancel{10}} \times 1 \times \cancel{10}} = \frac{200 \text{ ml}}{1} = 200 \text{ ml}$$

($^1/_{10}$ is the same as 10%)

20. Factors: 50 ml = 1/100; 1 = 100%; 0.05%/1

$$ml = \frac{50 \text{ ml} \times 1 \times 0.05\%}{\frac{1}{100} \times 100 \text{ \%} \times 1} = \frac{\overset{1}{\cancel{100}} \times 50 \text{ ml} \times 1 \times 0.05}{1 \times \underset{1}{\cancel{100}} \times 1} = \frac{2.5 \text{ ml}}{1} = 2.5 \text{ ml}$$

21. Factors: 1 g = 100 ml; 1 g = 1000 mg

$$\frac{mg}{ml} = \frac{1000 \text{ mg} \times 1 \text{ g}}{1 \text{ g} \times 100 \text{ ml}} = \frac{\overset{10}{\cancel{1000}} \text{ mg} \times 1}{1 \times \underset{1}{\cancel{100}} \text{ ml}} = \frac{10 \text{ mg}}{1 \text{ ml}} = 10 \text{ mg/ml}$$

22. Factors: 1 g = 40 ml; 1 g = 1000 mg

$$\frac{mg}{ml} = \frac{1000 \text{ mg} \times 1 \text{ g}}{1 \text{ g} \times 40 \text{ ml}} = \frac{\overset{25}{\cancel{1000}} \text{ mg} \times 1}{1 \times \underset{1}{\cancel{40}} \text{ ml}} = \frac{25 \text{ mg}}{1 \text{ ml}} = 25 \text{ mg/ml}$$

23. Factors: 1 g = 1000 mg; 1 g = 50 ml

$$\frac{mg}{ml} = \frac{1000 \text{ mg} \times 1 \text{ g}}{1 \text{ g} \times 50 \text{ ml}} = \frac{\overset{20}{\cancel{1000}} \text{ mg} \times 1}{1 \times \underset{1}{\cancel{50}} \text{ ml}} = \frac{20 \text{ mg}}{1 \text{ ml}} = 20 \text{ mg/ml}$$

24. Factors: 1 g = 1000 mg; 1 g = 500 ml

$$\frac{mg}{ml} = \frac{1000 \text{ mg} \times 1 \text{ g}}{1 \text{ g} \times 500 \text{ ml}} = \frac{\overset{2}{\cancel{1000}} \text{ mg} \times 1}{1 \times \underset{1}{\cancel{500}} \text{ ml}} = \frac{2 \text{ mg}}{1 \text{ ml}} = 2 \text{ mg/ml}$$

25. Factors: 1 g = 1000 mg; 1 g = 10 ml

$$\frac{mg}{ml} = \frac{1000 \text{ mg} \times 1 \text{ g}}{1 \text{ g} \times 10 \text{ ml}} = \frac{\overset{100}{\cancel{1000}} \text{ mg} \times 1}{1 \times \underset{1}{\cancel{10}} \text{ ml}} = \frac{100 \text{ mg}}{1 \text{ ml}} = 100 \text{ mg/ml}$$

UNIT VII: INTRAVENOUS FLUID ADMINISTRATION

Chapter 15: Calculations Associated with Intravenous Fluid Administration

1. Factors: 1000 ml = 10 h

$$\frac{ml}{h} = \frac{1000 \text{ ml}}{10 \text{ h}} = \frac{\overset{100}{\cancel{1000}} \text{ ml}}{\underset{1}{\cancel{10}} \text{ h}} = \frac{100 \text{ ml}}{1 \text{ h}} = 100 \text{ ml/h}$$

2. Factors: 250 ml = 4 h

$$\frac{ml}{h} = \frac{250 \text{ ml}}{4 \text{ h}} = \frac{\overset{125}{\cancel{250}} \text{ ml}}{\underset{2}{\cancel{4}} \text{ h}} = \frac{125 \text{ ml}}{2 \text{ h}} = 62.5 \text{ ml/h}$$

3. Factors: 1000 ml = 12 h; 6 h/1

$$\text{ml} = \frac{1000 \text{ ml} \times 6 \text{ h}}{12 \text{ h} \times 1} = \frac{\overset{500}{\cancel{1000}} \text{ ml} \times \overset{1}{\cancel{6}}}{\underset{\underset{1}{2}}{\cancel{12}} \times 1} = \frac{500 \text{ ml}}{1} = 500 \text{ ml}$$

If half the time has elapsed, then half the solution (500 ml) should have infused.

4. Factors: 500 ml = 8 h

$$\frac{\text{ml}}{\text{h}} = \frac{500 \text{ ml}}{8 \text{ h}} = \frac{\overset{125}{\cancel{500}} \text{ ml}}{\underset{2}{\cancel{8}} \text{ h}} = \frac{125 \text{ ml}}{2 \text{ h}} = 62.5 \text{ ml/h}$$

Factors: 62.5 ml = 1 h; 4h/1

$$\text{ml} = \frac{62.5 \text{ ml} \times 4 \text{ h}}{1 \text{ h} \times 1} = \frac{62.5 \text{ ml} \times 4}{1 \times 1} = \frac{250 \text{ ml}}{1} = 250 \text{ ml}$$

5. Factors: 1000 ml = 6 h

$$\frac{\text{ml}}{\text{h}} = \frac{1000 \text{ ml}}{6 \text{ h}} = \frac{\overset{500}{\cancel{1000}} \text{ ml}}{\underset{3}{\cancel{6}} \text{ h}} = \frac{500 \text{ ml}}{3 \text{ h}} = 166.7 \text{ ml/h}$$

In 3 hr, 500 ml should infuse.

6. Factors: 1000 ml = 12 h; 20 gtt = 1 ml; 1 hr = 60 min

$$\frac{\text{gtt}}{\text{min}} = \frac{20 \text{ gtt} \times 1000 \text{ ml} \times 1 \text{ h}}{1 \text{ ml} \times 12 \text{ h} \times 60 \text{ min}} = \frac{\overset{1}{\cancel{20}} \text{ gtt} \times \overset{250}{\cancel{1000}} \times 1}{1 \times \underset{3}{\cancel{12}} \times \underset{3}{\cancel{60}} \text{ min}} = \frac{250 \text{ gtt}}{9 \text{ min}} = 27.7 \ (28) \text{ gtt/min}$$

7. Factors: 1000 ml = 6 h; 15 gtts = 1 ml; 1 h = 60 min

$$\frac{\text{gtt}}{\text{min}} = \frac{15 \text{ gtt} \times 1000 \text{ ml} \times 1 \text{ h}}{1 \text{ ml} \times 6 \text{ h} \times 60 \text{ min}} = \frac{\overset{1}{\cancel{15}} \text{ gtt} \times \overset{\overset{125}{\cancel{250}}}{\cancel{1000}} \times 1}{1 \times \underset{3}{\cancel{6}} \times \underset{\underset{1}{\cancel{4}}}{\cancel{60}} \text{ min}} = \frac{125 \text{ gtt}}{3 \text{ min}} = 41.6 \ (42) \text{ gtt/min}$$

8. Factors: 500 ml = 6 h; 10 gtt = 1 ml; 1 h = 60 min

$$\frac{\text{gtt}}{\text{min}} = \frac{10 \text{ gtt} \times 500 \text{ ml} \times 1 \text{ h}}{1 \text{ ml} \times 6 \text{ h} \times 60 \text{ min}} = \frac{\overset{1}{\cancel{10}} \text{ gtt} \times \overset{\overset{125}{\cancel{250}}}{\cancel{500}} \times 1}{1 \times \underset{3}{\cancel{6}} \times \underset{\underset{3}{\cancel{6}}}{\cancel{60}} \text{ min}} = \frac{125 \text{ gtt}}{9 \text{ min}} = 13.8 \ (14) \text{ gtt/min}$$

9. Factors: 15 gtt = 1 ml; 100 ml = 30 min

$$\frac{\text{gtt}}{\text{min}} = \frac{15 \text{ gtt} \times 100 \text{ ml}}{1 \text{ ml} \times 30 \text{ min}} = \frac{\overset{1}{\cancel{15}} \text{ gtt} \times \overset{50}{\cancel{100}}}{1 \times \underset{\underset{1}{2}}{\cancel{30}} \text{ min}} = \frac{50 \text{ gtt}}{1 \text{ min}} = 50 \text{ gtt/min}$$

10. Factors: 500 ml = 10 h; 60 gtt = 1 ml; 1 h = 60 min

$$\frac{\text{gtt}}{\text{min}} = \frac{60 \text{ gtt} \times 500 \text{ ml} \times 1 \text{ h}}{1 \text{ ml} \times 10 \text{ h} \times 60 \text{ min}} = \frac{\cancel{60} \text{ gtt} \times \overset{50}{\cancel{500}} \times 1}{1 \times \underset{1}{\cancel{10}} \times \underset{1}{\cancel{60}} \text{ min}} = \frac{50 \text{ gtt}}{1 \text{ min}} = 50 \text{ gtt/min}$$

11. Factors: 500 ml = 5 h; 10 gtt = 1 ml; 1 h = 60 min

$$\frac{\text{gtt}}{\text{min}} = \frac{10 \text{ gtt} \times 500 \text{ ml} \times 1 \text{ h}}{1 \text{ ml} \times 5 \text{ h} \times 60 \text{ min}} = \frac{\overset{1}{\cancel{10}} \text{ gtt} \times \overset{\overset{50}{\cancel{100}}}{\cancel{500}} \times 1}{1 \times \underset{1}{\cancel{5}} \times \underset{\underset{3}{\cancel{6}}}{\cancel{60}} \text{ min}} = \frac{50 \text{ gtt}}{3 \text{ min}} = 16.6 \ (17) \text{ gtt/min}$$

12. Factors: 500 cc = 12 h; 60 gtt = 1 ml; 1 h = 60 min

$$\frac{\text{gtt}}{\text{min}} = \frac{60 \text{ gtt} \times 500 \text{ cc} \times 1 \text{ h}}{1 \text{ ml} \times 12 \text{ h} \times 60 \text{ min}} = \frac{\overset{1}{\cancel{60}} \text{ gtt} \times \overset{125}{\cancel{500}} \times 1}{1 \times \underset{3}{\cancel{12}} \times \underset{1}{\cancel{60}} \text{ min}} = \frac{125 \text{ gtt}}{3 \text{ min}} = 41.6 \ (42) \text{ gtt/min}$$

13. Factors: 1000 ml = 8 h; 15 gtt = 1 ml; 1 h = 60 min

$$\frac{\text{gtt}}{\text{min}} = \frac{15 \text{ gtt} \times 1000 \text{ ml} \times 1 \text{ h}}{1 \text{ ml} \times 8 \text{ h} \times 60 \text{ min}} = \frac{\overset{1}{\cancel{15}} \text{ gtt} \times \overset{125}{\cancel{1000}} \times 1}{1 \times \underset{1}{\cancel{8}} \times \underset{4}{\cancel{60}} \text{ min}} = \frac{125 \text{ gtt}}{4 \text{ min}} = 31.25 \ (31) \text{ gtt/min}$$

14. Factors: 1000 ml = 12 h; 10 gtt = 1 ml; 1 h = 60 min

$$\frac{\text{gtt}}{\text{min}} = \frac{10 \text{ gtt} \times 1000 \text{ ml} \times 1 \text{ h}}{1 \text{ ml} \times 12 \text{ h} \times 60 \text{ min}} = \frac{\cancel{10} \text{ gtt} \times \cancel{1000}^{\,125\, \diagup\, 250} \times 1}{1 \times \underset{3}{\cancel{12}} \times \underset{3}{\cancel{60}} \text{ min}} = \frac{125 \text{ gtt}}{9 \text{ min}} = 13.8 \ (14) \text{ gtt/min}$$

15. Factors: 50 ml = 1/2 (0.5) h; 15 gtt = 1 ml; 1 h = 60 min

$$\frac{\text{gtt}}{\text{min}} = \frac{15 \text{ gtt} \times 50 \text{ ml} \times 1 \text{ h}}{1 \text{ ml} \times 0.5 \text{ h} \times 60 \text{ min}} = \frac{\cancel{15}^{1} \text{ gtt} \times \cancel{50}^{25} \times 1}{1 \times 0.5 \times \underset{2}{\cancel{\underset{4}{\cancel{60}}}} \text{ min}} = \frac{25 \text{ gtt}}{1 \text{ min}} = 25 \text{ gtt/min}$$

16. Factors: Drip rate: 1000 ml = 10 h; 20 gtt = 1 ml; 1 h = 60 min

$$\frac{\text{gtt}}{\text{min}} = \frac{20 \text{ gtt} \times 1000 \text{ ml} \times 1 \text{ h}}{1 \text{ ml} \times 10 \text{ h} \times 60 \text{ min}} = \frac{\cancel{20}^{1} \text{ gtt} \times \cancel{1000}^{100} \times 1}{1 \times \underset{1}{\cancel{10}} \times \underset{3}{\cancel{60}} \text{ min}} = \frac{100 \text{ gtt}}{3 \text{ min}} = 33.3 \ (33) \text{ gtt/min}$$

Factors: Volume/hr: 1000 ml = 10 h

$$\frac{\text{ml}}{\text{h}} = \frac{1000 \text{ ml}}{10 \text{ h}} = \frac{\cancel{1000}^{100} \text{ ml}}{\underset{1}{\cancel{10}} \text{ h}} = \frac{100 \text{ ml}}{1 \text{ h}} = 100 \text{ ml/h}$$

Factors: Expected infused volume: 100 ml = 1 h; 5 h/1

$$\text{ml} = \frac{100 \text{ ml} \times 5 \text{ h}}{1 \text{ h} \times 1} = \frac{100 \text{ ml} \times 5}{1 \times 1} = \frac{500 \text{ ml}}{1} = 500 \text{ ml expected infused}$$

Factors: Infusion time: 1000 ml − 650 ml = 350 ml actually infused.

350 ml < 500 ml ± 25 (475 to 515); IV infusing too slowly.

Factors: Recalculation: (1000 − 350) 650 ml = (10 − 5) 5 h; 20 gtt = 1 ml; 1 h = 60 min

$$\frac{\text{gtt}}{\text{min}} = \frac{20 \text{ gtt} \times 650 \text{ ml} \times 1 \text{ h}}{1 \text{ ml} \times 5 \text{ h} \times 60 \text{ min}} = \frac{\cancel{20}^{1} \text{ gtt} \times \cancel{650}^{130} \times 1}{1 \times \underset{1}{\cancel{5}} \times \underset{3}{\cancel{60}} \text{ min}} = \frac{130 \text{ gtt}}{3 \text{ min}} = 43.3 \ (43) \text{ gtt/min}$$

17. Factors: Infusion time: 250 ml infused. Expected infused volume: 500 ml = 6 h; 1 h/1

$$\text{ml} = \frac{500 \text{ ml} \times 1 \text{ h}}{6 \text{ h} \times 1} = \frac{500 \text{ ml} \times 1}{6 \times 1} = 83.3 \text{ ml} \pm 25 \ (58 \text{ to } 108 \text{ ml}) \text{ should have infused.}$$

250 ml infused > than expected volume of 58 to 108 ml. IV infusing too rapidly.

Factors: Recalculation: 250 ml = 5 h; 10 gtt = ml; 1 h = 60 min

$$\frac{\text{gtt}}{\text{min}} = \frac{10 \text{ gtt} \times 250 \text{ ml} \times 1 \text{ h}}{1 \text{ ml} \times 5 \text{ h} \times 60 \text{ min}} = \frac{\cancel{10}^{1} \text{ gtt} \times \cancel{250}^{50} \times 1}{1 \times \underset{1}{\cancel{5}} \times \underset{6}{\cancel{60}} \text{ min}} = \frac{50 \text{ gtt}}{6 \text{ min}} = 8.3 \ (8) \text{ gtt/min}$$

18. Factors: Drip rate: 1000 ml = 10 h; 15 gtt = 1 ml; 1 h = 60 min

$$\frac{\text{gtt}}{\text{min}} = \frac{15 \text{ gtt} \times 1000 \text{ ml} \times 1 \text{ h}}{1 \text{ ml} \times 10 \text{ h} \times 60 \text{ min}} = \frac{\cancel{15}^{1} \text{ gtt} \times \cancel{1000}^{25\, \diagup\, 100} \times 1}{1 \times \underset{1}{\cancel{10}} \times \underset{4\, \diagup\, 1}{\cancel{60}} \text{ min}} = \frac{25 \text{ gtt}}{1 \text{ min}} = 25 \text{ gtt/min}$$

Factors: Infusion time: Expected infused volume: 1000 ml = 10 h; 6 h/1

$$\text{ml} = \frac{1000 \text{ ml} \times 6 \text{ h}}{10 \text{ h} \times 1} = \frac{\cancel{1000}^{100} \text{ ml} \times 6}{\underset{1}{\cancel{10}} \times 1} = \frac{600 \text{ ml}}{1} = 600 \text{ ml} \ (575 \text{ to } 625 \text{ ml}) \text{ expected infused.}$$

1000 ml − 600 ml (left in bottle) = 400 ml actually infused.

400 ml < 600 ml (575 to 625 ml). IV infusing too slowly.

Factors: Recalculation: 600 ml = (10 h − 6 h) 4 h; 15 gtt = 1 ml; 1 h = 60 min

$$\frac{\text{gtt}}{\text{min}} = \frac{15 \text{ gtt} \times 600 \text{ ml} \times 1 \text{ h}}{1 \text{ ml} \times 4 \text{ h} \times 60 \text{ min}} = \frac{\cancel{15}^{1} \text{ gtt} \times \cancel{600}^{75\, \diagup\, 150} \times 1}{1 \times \underset{1}{\cancel{4}} \times \underset{4\, \diagup\, 2}{\cancel{60}} \text{ min}} = \frac{75 \text{ gtt}}{2 \text{ min}} = 37.5 \ (38) \text{ gtt/min}$$

19. Factors: Drip rate: 1000 ml = 12 h; 60 gtt = 1 ml; 1 h = 60 min

$$\frac{\text{gtt}}{\text{min}} = \frac{60 \text{ gtt} \times 1000 \text{ ml} \times 1 \text{ h}}{1 \text{ ml} \times 12 \text{ h} \times 60 \text{ min}} = \frac{\cancel{60}^{1} \text{ gtt} \times \cancel{1000}^{250} \times 1}{1 \times \underset{3}{\cancel{12}} \times \underset{1}{\cancel{60}} \text{ min}} = \frac{250 \text{ gtt}}{3 \text{ min}} = 83.3 \ (83) \text{ gtt/min}$$

Factors: Volume/h: 1000 ml = 12 h

$$ml = \frac{1000 \text{ ml}}{12 \text{ h}} = \frac{1000 \text{ ml}}{12 \text{ h}} = 83.3 \text{ ml/h}$$

Factors: Infusion time: Volume/6 h: 1000 ml = 12 h (or 83.3 = 1 h); 6 h/1

Half the time has elapsed; therefore, half the solution should have infused. Half of the solution, 500 ml, remains in the bottle. Therefore, the IV is on time. No recalculation is necessary.

20. Factors: 1000 ml = 8 h; 20 gtt = 1 ml; 1 h = 60 min

$$\frac{\text{gtt}}{\text{min}} = \frac{20 \text{ gtt} \times 1000 \text{ ml} \times 1 \text{ h}}{1 \text{ ml} \times 8 \text{ h} \times 60 \text{ min}} = \frac{\overset{1}{\cancel{20}} \text{ gtt} \times \overset{125}{\cancel{1000}} \times 1}{1 \times \underset{1}{\cancel{8}} \times \underset{3}{\cancel{60}} \text{ min}} = \frac{125 \text{ gtt}}{3 \text{ min}} = 41.6 \ (42) \text{ gtt/min}$$

Factors: Expected infused volume/4 h: 1000 ml = 8 h; 4 h/1

$$ml = \frac{1000 \text{ ml} \times 4 \text{ h}}{8 \text{ h} \times 1} = \frac{\overset{125}{\cancel{1000}} \text{ ml} \times 4}{\underset{1}{\cancel{8}} \times 1} = \frac{500 \text{ ml}}{1} = 500 \text{ ml} \ (475 \text{ to } 515 \text{ ml})$$

Factors: Infusion time: 600 ml/4 h.

600 ml > 500 ml (475 to 515 ml). IV infusing too rapidly.

Factors: Recalculation: 400 ml = 4 h; 20 gtt = 1 ml; 1 h = 60 min

$$\frac{\text{gtt}}{\text{min}} = \frac{20 \text{ gtt} \times 400 \text{ ml} \times 1 \text{ h}}{1 \text{ ml} \times 4 \text{ h} \times 60 \text{ min}} = \frac{\overset{1}{\cancel{20}} \text{ gtt} \times \overset{100}{\cancel{400}} \times 1}{1 \times \underset{1}{\cancel{4}} \times \underset{3}{\cancel{60}} \text{ min}} \frac{100 \text{ gtt}}{3 \text{ min}} = 33.3 \ (33) \text{ gtt/min}$$

UNIT VIII: INTRAVENOUS MEDICATIONS

Chapter 16: Piggyback, Bolus and Titrated Medications

1. Factors: 50 ml = 30 min; 60 gtt = 1 ml

$$\frac{\text{gtt}}{\text{min}} = \frac{60 \text{ gtt} \times 50 \text{ ml}}{1 \text{ ml} \times 30 \text{ min}} = \frac{\overset{2}{\cancel{60}} \text{ gtt} \times 50}{1 \times \underset{1}{\cancel{30}} \text{ min}} = \frac{100 \text{ gtt}}{1 \text{ min}} = 100 \text{ gtt/min}$$

2. Factors: 100 ml = 40 min; 15 gtt = 1 ml

$$\frac{\text{gtt}}{\text{min}} = \frac{15 \text{ gtt} \times 100 \text{ ml}}{1 \text{ ml} \times 40 \text{ min}} = \frac{\overset{3}{\cancel{15}} \text{ gtt} \times \overset{25}{\cancel{100}}}{1 \times \underset{\underset{2}{8}}{\cancel{40}} \text{ min}} = \frac{75 \text{ gtt}}{2 \text{ min}} = 37.5 \ (38) \text{ gtt/min}$$

3. Factors: 50 ml = 20 min; 20 gtt = 1 ml

$$\frac{\text{gtt}}{\text{min}} = \frac{20 \text{ gtt} \times 50 \text{ ml}}{1 \text{ ml} \times 20 \text{ min}} = \frac{\overset{1}{\cancel{20}} \text{ gtt} \times 50}{1 \times \underset{1}{\cancel{20}} \text{ min}} = \frac{50 \text{ gtt}}{1 \text{ min}} = 50 \text{ gtt/min}$$

4. Factors: 150 ml = 40 min; 15 gtt = 1 ml

$$\frac{\text{gtt}}{\text{min}} = \frac{15 \text{ gtt} \times 150 \text{ ml}}{1 \text{ ml} \times 40 \text{ min}} = \frac{\overset{3}{\cancel{15}} \text{ gtt} \times \overset{75}{\cancel{150}}}{1 \times \underset{\underset{4}{8}}{\cancel{40}} \text{ min}} = \frac{225 \text{ gtt}}{4 \text{ min}} = 56.25 \ (56) \text{ gtt/min}$$

5. Factors: 100 ml = 0.5 h; 20 gtt = 1 ml; 1 h = 60 min

$$\frac{\text{gtt}}{\text{min}} = \frac{20 \text{ gtt} \times 100 \text{ ml} \times 1 \text{ h}}{1 \text{ ml} \times 0.5 \text{ h} \times 60 \text{ min}} = \frac{\overset{1}{\cancel{20}} \text{ gtt} \times \overset{20}{\cancel{100}} \times 1}{1 \times \underset{0.1}{\cancel{0.5}} \times \underset{3}{\cancel{60}} \text{ min}} = \frac{20 \text{ gtt}}{0.3 \text{ min}} = 66.6 \ (67) \text{ gtt/min}$$

6. Factors: 100 ml = 30 min; 20 gtt = 1 ml

$$\frac{\text{gtt}}{\text{min}} = \frac{20 \text{ gtt} \times 100 \text{ ml}}{1 \text{ ml} \times 30 \text{ min}} = \frac{\overset{2}{\cancel{20}} \text{ gtt} \times 100}{1 \times \underset{3}{\cancel{30}} \text{ min}} = \frac{200 \text{ gtt}}{3 \text{ min}} = 66.6 \ (67) \text{ gtt/min}$$

7. Factors: 50 ml = 20 min; 15 gtt = 1 ml

$$\frac{\text{gtt}}{\text{min}} = \frac{15 \text{ gtt} \times 50 \text{ ml}}{1 \text{ ml} \times 20 \text{ min}} = \frac{\overset{3}{\cancel{15}} \text{ gtt} \times \overset{25}{\cancel{50}}}{1 \times \underset{\underset{2}{4}}{\cancel{20}} \text{ min}} = \frac{75 \text{ gtt}}{2 \text{ min}} = 37.5 \ (38) \text{ gtt/min}$$

8. Factors: 100 ml = 30 min; 15 gtt = 1 ml

$$\frac{gtt}{min} = \frac{15 \ gtt \ \times \ 100 \ ml}{1 \ ml \ \times \ 30 \ min} = \frac{\overset{1}{\cancel{15}} \ gtt \ \times \ \overset{50}{\cancel{100}}}{1 \ \times \ \underset{2}{\cancel{30}} \ min} = \frac{50 \ gtt}{1 \ min} = 50 \ gtt/min$$

9. Factors: 100 ml = 15 min; 15 gtt = 1 ml

$$\frac{gtt}{min} = \frac{15 \ gtt \ \times \ 100 \ ml}{1 \ ml \ \times \ 15 \ min} = \frac{\overset{1}{\cancel{15}} \ gtt \ \times \ 100}{1 \ \times \ \underset{1}{\cancel{15}} \ min} = \frac{100 \ gtt}{1 \ min} = 100 \ gtt/min$$

10. Factors: 100 ml = 30 min; 20 gtt = 1 ml

$$\frac{gtt}{min} = \frac{20 \ gtt \ \times \ 100 \ ml}{1 \ ml \ \times \ 30 \ min} = \frac{\overset{2}{\cancel{20}} \ gtt \ \times \ 100}{1 \ \times \ \underset{3}{\cancel{30}} \ min} = \frac{200 \ gtt}{3 \ min} = 66.6 \ (67) \ gtt/min$$

11. Factors: 2 mg = 1 ml; 10 mg/1; 1 ml available

$$ml = \left(\frac{1 \ ml \ \times \ 10 \ mg}{2 \ mg \ \times \ 1}\right) - 1 \ ml = \left(\frac{1 \ ml \ \times \ \overset{5}{\cancel{10}}}{\underset{1}{\cancel{2}} \ \times \ 1}\right) - 1 \ ml = 5 \ ml - 1 \ ml = 4 \ ml$$

12. Factors: 10 mg = 1 ml; 80 mg/1; 1 ml available

$$ml = \left(\frac{1 \ ml \ \times \ 80 \ mg}{10 \ mg \ \times \ 1}\right) - 1 \ ml = \left(\frac{1 \ ml \ \times \ \overset{8}{\cancel{80}}}{\underset{1}{\cancel{10}} \ \times \ 1}\right) - 1 \ ml = 8 \ ml - 1 \ ml = 7 \ ml$$

13. Factors: 0.5 ml = 25 mg; 100 mg/1; 1 ml available

$$ml = \left(\frac{0.5 \ ml \ \times \ 100 \ mg}{25 \ mg \ \times \ 1}\right) - 1 \ ml = \left(\frac{0.5 \ ml \ \times \ \overset{4}{\cancel{100}}}{\underset{1}{\cancel{25}} \ \times \ 1}\right) - 1 \ ml = 2 \ ml - 1 \ ml = 1 \ ml$$

(If whole vial is diluted, 3 ml must be added)

14. Factors: 100 mcg = 1 ml; 1 mg = 1000 mcg; 0.5 mg/1; 1 ml available

$$ml = \left(\frac{1 \ ml \ \times \ 1000 \ mcg \ \times \ 0.5 \ mg}{100 \ mcg \ \times \ 1 \ mg \ \times \ 1}\right) - 1 \ ml = \left(\frac{1 \ ml \ \times \ \overset{10}{\cancel{1000}} \times \ 0.5}{\underset{1}{\cancel{100}} \ \times \ 1 \times \ 1}\right) - 1 \ ml = 5 \ ml - 1 \ ml = 4 \ ml$$

15. Factors: 1 ml = 1 mg; 10 mg/1; 5 ml available

$$ml = \left(\frac{1 \ ml \ \times \ 10 \ mg}{1 \ mg \ \times \ 1}\right) - 5 \ ml = \left(\frac{1 \ ml \ \times \ 10}{1 \ \times \ 1}\right) - 5 \ ml = 10 \ ml - 5 \ ml = 5 \ ml$$

16. Factors: 500 ml = 20 mg; 1 mg = 1000 mcg

$$\frac{mcg}{ml} = \frac{1000 \ mcg \ \times \ 20 \ mg}{1 \ mg \ \times \ 500 \ ml} = \frac{\overset{2}{\cancel{1000}} \ mcg \ \times \ 20}{1 \ \times \ \underset{1}{\cancel{500}} \ ml} = \frac{40 \ mcg}{1 \ ml} = 40 \ mcg/ml$$

17. Factors: 1 g = 250 ml; 1 g = 1000 mg

$$\frac{mg}{ml} = \frac{1000 \ mg \ \times \ 1 \ g}{1 \ g \ \times \ 250 \ ml} = \frac{\overset{4}{\cancel{1000}} \ mg \ \times \ 1}{1 \ \times \ \underset{1}{\cancel{250}} \ ml} = \frac{4 \ mg}{1 \ ml} = 4 \ mg/ml$$

18. Factors: 400 mg = 500 ml; 1 mg = 1000 mcg

$$\frac{mcg}{ml} = \frac{1000 \ mcg \ \times \ 400 \ mg}{1 \ mg \ \times \ 500 \ ml} = \frac{\overset{2}{\cancel{1000}} \ mcg \ \times \ 400}{1 \ \times \ \underset{1}{\cancel{500}} \ ml} = \frac{800 \ mcg}{1 \ ml} = 800 \ mcg/ml$$

19. Factors: 1000 ml = 10 U; 1000 mU = 1 U

$$\frac{mcg}{ml} = \frac{1000 \ mU \ \times \ 10 \ U}{1 \ U \ \times \ 1000 \ ml} = \frac{\overset{1}{\cancel{1000}} \ mU \ \times \ 10}{1 \ \times \ \underset{1}{\cancel{1000}} \ ml} = \frac{10 \ mU}{1 \ ml} = 10 \ mU/ml$$

20. Factors: 200 ml = 250 mg

$$\frac{mg}{ml} = \frac{250 \ mg}{200 \ ml} = \frac{\overset{5}{\cancel{250}} \ mg}{\underset{4}{\cancel{200}} \ ml} = \frac{5 \ mg}{4 \ ml} = 1.25 \ mg/ml$$

21. Factors: 1000 mcg = 1 mg; 150 mg = 1000 ml; 60 gtt = 1 ml; 24 gtt = min

$$\frac{mcg}{min} = \frac{1000\ mcg \times 150\ mg \times 1\ ml \times 24\ gtt}{1\ mg \times 1000\ ml \times 60\ gtt \times 1\ min} = \frac{1000\ mcg \times \overset{1}{\cancel{150}} \times 1 \times \overset{12}{\cancel{24}}}{1 \times \cancel{1000} \times \underset{\underset{1}{2}}{\cancel{60}} \times 1\ min} = \frac{60\ mcg}{1\ min} = 60\ mcg/min$$

22. Factors: 250 ml = 4000 mcg; 30 gtt = 1 min; 60 gtt = 1 ml

$$\frac{mcg}{min} = \frac{4000\ mcg \times 1\ ml \times 30\ gtt}{250\ ml \times 60\ gtt \times 1\ min} = \frac{\overset{\overset{8}{\cancel{16}}}{\cancel{4000}}\ mcg \times 1 \times \overset{1}{\cancel{30}}}{\underset{1}{\cancel{250}} \times \underset{\underset{1}{2}}{\cancel{60}} \times 1\ min} = \frac{8\ mcg}{1\ min} = 8\ mcg/min$$

23. Factors: 500 ml = 20 mg; 18 gtt = 1 min; 60 gtt = 1 ml; 1 mg = 1000 mcg

$$\frac{mcg}{min} = \frac{1000\ mcg \times 20\ mg \times 1\ ml \times 18\ gtt}{1\ mg \times 500\ ml \times 60\ gtt \times 1\ min} = \frac{1000\ mcg \times \overset{2}{\cancel{20}} \times 1 \times \overset{6}{\cancel{18}}}{1 \times \underset{1}{\cancel{500}} \times \underset{\underset{1}{3}}{\cancel{60}} \times 1\ min} = \frac{12\ mcg}{1\ min} = 12\ mcg/min$$

24. Factors: 1000 mU = 1 U; 30 U = 500 ml; 26 gtt = 1 min; 60 gtt = 1 ml

$$\frac{mU}{min} = \frac{1000\ mU \times 30\ U \times 1\ ml \times 26\ gtt}{1\ U \times 500\ ml \times 60\ gtt \times 1\ min} = \frac{1000\ mU \times \overset{\overset{1}{\cancel{2}}}{\cancel{30}} \times 1 \times 26}{1 \times \underset{1}{\cancel{500}} \times \underset{\underset{1}{2}}{\cancel{60}} \times 1\ min} = \frac{26\ mU}{1\ min} = 26\ mU/min$$

25. Factors: 1000 mcg = 1 mg; 1000 ml = 500 mg; 33 gtt = 1 min; 60 gtt = 1 ml

$$\frac{mcg}{min} = \frac{1000\ mcg \times 500\ mg \times 1\ ml \times 33\ gtt}{1\ mg \times 1000\ ml \times 60\ gtt \times 1\ min} = \frac{1000\ mcg \times \overset{25}{\cancel{500}} \times 1 \times \overset{11}{\cancel{33}}}{1 \times \cancel{1000} \times \underset{\underset{1}{3}}{\cancel{60}} \times 1\ min} = \frac{275\ mcg}{1\ min} = 275\ mcg/min$$

26. Factors: 1 g = 1000 ml; 1 g = 1000 mg; 84 gtt = 1 min; 60 gtt = 1 ml

$$\frac{mg}{min} = \frac{1000\ mg \times 1\ g \times 1\ ml \times 84\ gtt}{1\ g \times 1000\ ml \times 60\ gtt \times 1\ min} = \frac{1000\ mg \times 1 \times 1 \times \overset{7}{\cancel{84}}}{1 \times \cancel{1000} \times \underset{\underset{5}{\cancel{60}}}{} \times 1\ min} = \frac{7\ mg}{5\ min} = 1.4\ mcg/min$$

27. Factors: 250 ml = 50 mg; 57 gtt = 1 min; 60 gtt = 1 ml; 1000 mcg = 1 mg

$$\frac{mcg}{min} = \frac{1000\ mcg \times 50\ mg \times 1\ ml \times 57\ gtt}{1\ mg \times 250\ ml \times 60\ gtt \times 1\ min} = \frac{1000\ mcg \times \overset{\overset{2}{\cancel{4}}}{\cancel{50}} \times 1 \times \overset{19}{\cancel{57}}}{1 \times \underset{1}{\cancel{250}} \times \underset{\underset{\underset{1}{2}}{6}}{\cancel{60}} \times 1\ min} = \frac{190\ mcg}{1\ min} = 190\ mcg/min$$

28. Factors: 400 mg = 250 ml; 90 gtt = 1 min; 60 gtt = 1 ml

$$\frac{mg}{min} = \frac{400\ mg \times 1\ ml \times 90\ gtt}{250\ ml \times 60\ gtt \times 1\ min} = \frac{\overset{\overset{4}{\cancel{8}}}{\cancel{400}}\ mg \times 1 \times \overset{3}{\cancel{90}}}{\underset{5}{\cancel{250}} \times \underset{\underset{1}{2}}{\cancel{60}} \times 1\ min} = \frac{12\ mg}{5\ min} = 2.4\ mg/min$$

29. Factors: 500 ml = 2 mg; 1 mg = 1000 mcg; 60 gtt = 1 ml; 75 gtt = 1 min

$$\frac{mcg}{min} = \frac{1000\ mcg \times 2\ mg \times 1\ ml \times 75\ gtt}{1\ mg \times 500\ ml \times 60\ gtt \times 1\ min} = \frac{1000\ mcg \times \overset{\overset{1}{\cancel{2}}}{} \times 1 \times \overset{5}{\cancel{75}}}{1 \times \underset{1}{\cancel{500}} \times \underset{\underset{\underset{1}{2}}{4}}{\cancel{60}} \times 1\ min} = \frac{5\ mcg}{1\ min} = 5\ mcg/min$$

30. Factors: 1000 ml = 10 U; 1000 mU = 1 U; 60 gtt = 1 ml; 60 gtt = 1 min

$$\frac{mU}{min} = \frac{1000\ mU \times 10\ U \times 1\ ml \times 60\ gtt}{1\ U \times 1000\ ml \times 60\ gtt \times 1\ min} = \frac{1000\ mU \times 10 \times 1 \times \overset{1}{\cancel{60}}}{1 \times \underset{1}{\cancel{1000}} \times \underset{1}{\cancel{60}} \times 1\ min} = \frac{10\ mU}{1\ min} = 10\ mU/min$$

31. Factors: 60 mcg/min (from problem 21) = 110 lb; 1 kg = 2.2 lb;

$$\frac{mcg}{kg\ (/min)} = \frac{60\ mcg}{min \times 110\ lb \times 1\ kg} \times 2.2\ lb = \frac{\overset{6}{\cancel{60}}\ mcg}{min \times \underset{50}{\cancel{110}} \times 1\ kg} \times \overset{1}{\cancel{2.2}} = \frac{6\ mcg}{min \times 5 \times kg} = 1.2\ mcg/kg/min$$

32. Factors: 8 mcg/min (from problem 22) = 60 kg

$$\frac{mcg}{kg\ (/min)} = \frac{8\ \ mcg/min}{60\ \ \ \ kg} = \frac{\overset{2}{\cancel{8}}\ \ mcg}{min\ \times\ \underset{15}{\cancel{60}}\ \ kg} = \frac{2\ \ mcg}{min\ \times\ 15\ \ kg} = 0.133\ mcg/kg/min$$

33. Factors: 6 mcg/min (from problem 23) = 121 lb; 1 kg = 2.2 lb

$$\frac{mcg}{kg\ (/min)} = \frac{6\ \ mcg/min\ \times\ 2.2\ \ lb}{121\ \ \ \ lb\ \times\ 1\ \ kg} = \frac{6\ \ mcg\ \ \ \ \ \ \times\ \overset{1}{\cancel{2.2}}}{min\ \times\ \underset{55}{\cancel{121}}\ \times\ 1\ \ kg} = \frac{6\ \ mcg}{min\ \times\ 55\ \ kg} = 0.109\ mcg/kg/min$$

34. Factors: 26 mU/min (from problem 24) = 130 lb; 1 kg = 2.2 lb

$$\frac{mU}{kg\ (/min)} = \frac{26\ \ mU/min\ \times\ 2.2\ \ lb}{130\ \ \ \ lb\ \times\ 1\ \ kg} = \frac{\overset{13}{\cancel{26}}\ mU\ \ \ \ \ \ \times\ 2.2}{min\ \times\ \underset{65}{\cancel{130}}\ \times\ 1\ \ kg} = \frac{28.6\ \ mU}{min\ \times\ 65\ \ kg} = 0.44\ mU/kg/min$$

35. Factors: 275 mcg/min (from problem 25) = 50 kg

$$\frac{mcg}{kg\ (/min)} = \frac{275\ \ mcg/min}{50\ \ \ \ kg} = \frac{275\ \ mcg}{min\ \times\ 50\ kg} = 5.5\ mcg/kg/min$$

36. Factors: 1.4 mg/min (from problem 26) = 68 kg; 1 mg = 100 0 mcg;

$$\frac{mcg}{kg\ (/min)} = \frac{1000\ \ mcg\ \times\ 1.4\ \ mg/min}{1\ \ mg\ \times\ 68\ \ \ \ kg} = \frac{\overset{250}{\cancel{1000}}\ mcg\ \times\ 1.4}{1\ \ \ \times\ \ \ \ min\ \times\ \underset{17}{\cancel{68}}\ kg} = \frac{350\ \ mcg}{min\ \times\ 17\ \ kg} = 20.588\ mcg/kg/min$$

37. Factors: 190 mcg/min (from problem 27) = 143 lb; 1 kg = 2.2 lb

$$\frac{mcg}{kg\ (/min)} = \frac{190\ \ mcg/min\ \times\ 2.2\ \ lb}{143\ \ \ \ lb\ \times\ 1\ \ kg} = \frac{190\ \ mcg\ \ \ \ \ \ \times\ \overset{1}{\cancel{2.2}}}{min\ \times\ \underset{65}{\cancel{143}}\ \times\ 1\ \ kg} = \frac{190\ \ mcg}{min\ \times\ 65\ \ kg} = 2.92\ mcg/kg/min$$

38. Factors: 2.4 mg/min (from problem 28) = 110 lb; 1 kg = 2.2 lb; 1 mg = 1000 mcg

$$\frac{mcg}{kg\ (/min)} = \frac{1000\ \ mcg\ \times\ 2.4\ \ mg/min\ \times\ 2.2\ \ lb}{1\ \ mg\ \times\ 110\ \ \ \ lb\ \times\ 1\ \ kg} = \frac{\overset{20}{\cancel{1000}}\ mcg\ \times\ 2.4\ \ \ \ \ \ \ \ \ \ \times\ \overset{1}{\cancel{2.2}}}{1\ \ \ \times\ \ \ \ min\ \times\ \underset{\underset{1}{50}}{\cancel{110}}\ \times\ 1\ \ kg} = \frac{48\ \ mcg}{min\ \times\ \ \ kg}$$

$$= 48\ mg/kg/min$$

39. Factors: mcg/min: 1000 mcg = 1 mg; 800 mg = 250 ml; 60 gtt = 1 ml; 42 gtt = 1 min

$$\frac{mcg}{min} = \frac{1000\ \ mcg\ \times\ 800\ \ mg\ \times\ 1\ \ ml\ \times\ 42\ \ gtt}{1\ \ mg\ \times\ 250\ \ ml\ \times\ 60\ \ gtt\ \times\ 1\ \ min} = \frac{\overset{4}{\cancel{1000}}\ mcg\ \times\ \overset{40}{\cancel{800}}\ \times\ 1\ \times\ \overset{14}{\cancel{42}}}{1\ \ \ \times\ \underset{1}{\cancel{250}}\ \times\ \underset{\underset{1}{3}}{\cancel{60}}\ \times\ 1\ \ min} = \frac{2240\ \ mcg}{1\ \ min} = 2240\ mcg/min$$

Factors: mcg/kg/min: 2240 mcg/min = 220 lb; 1 kg = 2.2 lb

$$\frac{mcg}{kg\ (/min)} = \frac{2240\ \ mcg/min\ \times\ 2.2\ \ lb}{220\ \ \ \ lb\ \times\ 1\ \ kg} = \frac{2240\ \ mcg\ \ \ \ \ \ \times\ \overset{1}{\cancel{2.2}}}{min\ \times\ \underset{100}{\cancel{220}}\ \times\ 1\ \ kg} = \frac{2240\ \ mcg}{min\ \times\ 100\ \ kg} = 22.4\ mcg/kg/min$$

40. Factors: mcg/min: 2 g = 1000 ml; 60 gtt = 1 ml; 51 gtt = 1 min; 1 g = 1000 mg; 1 mg = 1000 mcg

$$\frac{mcg}{min} = \frac{1000\ \ mcg\ \times\ 1000\ \ mg\ \times\ 2\ \ g\ \times\ 1\ \ ml\ \times\ 51\ \ gtt}{1\ \ mg\ \times\ 1\ \ g\ \times\ 1000\ \ ml\ \times\ 60\ \ gtt\ \times\ 1\ \ min} = \frac{\overset{1}{\cancel{1000}}\ mcg\ \times\ \overset{50}{\cancel{1000}}\ \times\ 2\ \times\ 1\ \times\ \overset{17}{\cancel{51}}}{1\ \ \ \times\ 1\ \ \ \times\ \underset{1}{\cancel{1000}}\ \times\ \underset{\underset{1}{3}}{\cancel{60}}\ \times\ 1\ \ min}$$

$$= \frac{1700\ \ mcg}{1\ \ min} = 1700\ mcg/min$$

Factors: mcg/kg/min: 1700 mcg/min = 70 kg

$$\frac{mcg}{kg\ (/min)} = \frac{1700\ \ mcg/min}{70\ \ \ \ kg} = \frac{\overset{170}{\cancel{1700}}\ mcg}{min\ \times\ \underset{7}{\cancel{70}}\ kg} = \frac{170\ \ mcg}{min\ \times\ 7\ \ kg} = 24.285\ mcg/kg/min$$

41. Factors: 60 gtt = 1 ml; 4 mcg = 1 kg × min; 250 mg = 500 ml; 1 kg = 2.2 lb; 121 lb/1; 1 mg = 1000 mcg

$$\frac{gtt}{min} = \frac{60\ \ gtt\ \times\ 500\ \ ml\ \times\ 1\ \ mg\ \times\ 4\ \ mcg\ \times\ 1\ \ kg\ \times\ 121\ \ lb}{1\ \ ml\ \times\ 250\ \ mg\ \times\ 1000\ \ mcg\ \times\ 1\ \ kg\ \times\ min\ \times\ 2.2\ \ lb\ \times\ 1}$$

$$= \frac{\overset{3}{\cancel{60}}\ gtt\ \times\ \overset{2}{\cancel{500}}\ \times\ 1\ \times\ 4\ \ \ \ \ \ \ \ \times\ 1\ \times\ \overset{11}{\cancel{121}}}{1\ \ \ \times\ \underset{1}{\cancel{250}}\ \times\ \underset{10}{\cancel{1000}}\ \times\ 1\ \times\ min\ \times\ \underset{1}{\cancel{2.2}}\ \times\ 1} = \frac{264\ \ gtt}{10\ \ min} = 26.4\ gtt/min$$

42. Factors: 0.5 mcg = 1 kg × min; 1 mg = 1000 mcg; 50 mg = 250 ml; 60 gtt = 1 ml; 60 kg/1

$$\frac{gtt}{min} = \frac{60\ gtt \times 250\ ml \times 1\ mg \times 0.5\ mcg \times 60\ kg}{1\ ml \times 50\ mg \times 1000\ mcg \times 1\ kg \times min \times 1} = \frac{60\ gtt \times 250 \times 1 \times 0.5 \times 60}{1 \times 50 \times 1000 \times 1 \times min \times 1}$$

$$= \frac{9\ gtt}{1\ min} = 9\ gtt/min$$

43. Factors: 60 gtt = 1 ml; 250 ml = 50 mg; 3 mcg = 1 kg × min; 1 mg = 1000 mcg; 57 kg/1

$$\frac{gtt}{min} = \frac{60\ gtt \times 250\ ml \times 1\ mg \times 3\ mcg \times 57\ kg}{1\ ml \times 50\ mg \times 1000\ mcg \times 1\ kg \times min \times 1} = \frac{60\ gtt \times 250 \times 1 \times 3 \times 57}{1 \times 50 \times 1000 \times 1 \times min \times 1}$$

$$= \frac{1026\ gtt}{20\ min} = 51.3\ gtt/min$$

44. Factors: 60 gtt = 1 ml; 250 ml = 400 mg; 1 mg = 1000 mcg; 2 mcg = 1 kg × min; 1 kg = 2.2 lb; 176 lb/1

$$\frac{gtt}{min} = \frac{60\ gtt \times 250\ ml \times 1\ mg \times 2\ mcg \times 1\ kg \times 176\ lb}{1\ ml \times 400\ mg \times 1000\ mcg \times 1\ kg \times min \times 2.2\ lb \times 1}$$

$$= \frac{60\ gtt \times 250 \times 1 \times 2 \times 1 \times 176}{1 \times 400 \times 1000 \times 1 \times min \times 2.2 \times 1} = \frac{6\ gtt}{1\ min} = 6\ gtt/min$$

45. Factors: 25 mcg = 1 kg × 1 min; 2 g = 1000 ml; 1 g = 1000 mg; 1 mg = 1000 mcg; 60 g = 1 ml; 1 kg = 2.2 lb; 99 lb/1

$$\frac{gtt}{min} = \frac{60\ gtt \times 1000\ ml \times 1\ g \times 1\ mg \times 25\ mcg \times 1\ kg \times 99\ lb}{1\ ml \times 2\ g \times 1000\ mg \times 1000\ mcg \times 1\ kg \times min \times 2.2\ lb \times 1}$$

$$= \frac{60\ gtt \times 1000 \times 1 \times 1 \times 25 \times 1 \times 99}{1 \times 2 \times 1000 \times 1000 \times 1 \times min \times 2.2 \times 1} = \frac{27\ gtt}{0.8\ min} = 33.7\ (34)\ gtt/min$$

46. Factors: 0.02 mg = 1 kg × min; 1 h = 60 min; 100 mg = 500 ml; 1 kg = 2.2 lb; 132 lb/1

$$\frac{ml}{h} = \frac{500\ ml \times 0.02\ mg \times 1\ kg \times 132\ lb \times 60\ min}{100\ mg \times 1\ kg \times 1\ min \times 2.2\ lb \times 1 \times 1\ h}$$

$$= \frac{500\ ml \times 0.02 \times 1 \times 132 \times 60}{100 \times 1 \times 1 \times 2.2 \times 1 \times 1\ h} = \frac{360\ ml}{1\ h} = 360\ ml/h$$

47. Factors: 10 mcg = 1 kg × 1 min; 500 mg = 500 ml; 1 kg = 2.2 lb; 187 lb/1; 1 h = 60 min; 1 mg = 1000 mcg

$$\frac{ml}{h} = \frac{500\ ml \times 1\ mg \times 10\ mcg \times 1\ kg \times 187\ lb \times 60\ min}{500\ mg \times 1000\ mcg \times 1\ kg \times 1\ min \times 2.2\ lb \times 1 \times 1\ h}$$

$$= \frac{500\ ml \times 1 \times 10 \times 1 \times 187 \times 60}{500 \times 1000 \times 1 \times 1 \times 2.2 \times 1 \times 1\ h} = \frac{51\ ml}{1\ h} = 51\ ml/h$$

48. Factors: 2 mcg = 1 kg × 1 min; 250 mg = 500 ml; 1 mg = 1000 mcg; 1 kg = 2.2 lb; 143 lb/1; 1 h = 60 min

$$\frac{ml}{h} = \frac{500\ ml \times 1\ mg \times 2\ mcg \times 1\ kg \times 143\ lb \times 60\ min}{250\ mg \times 1000\ mcg \times 1\ kg \times 1\ min \times 2.2\ lb \times 1 \times 1\ h}$$

$$= \frac{500\ ml \times 1 \times 2 \times 1 \times 143 \times 60}{250 \times 1000 \times 1 \times 1 \times 2.2 \times 1 \times 1\ h} = \frac{78\ ml}{5\ h} = 15.6\ ml/h$$

49. Factors: 50 mg = 250 ml; 7 mcg = 1 kg × 1 min; 1 mg = 1000 mcg; 1 kg = 2.2 lb; 121 lb/1; 1 h = 60 min

$$\frac{ml}{h} = \frac{250\ ml \times 1\ mg \times 7\ mcg \times 1\ kg \times 121\ lb \times 60\ min}{50\ mg \times 1000\ mcg \times 1\ kg \times 1\ min \times 2.2\ lb \times 1 \times 1\ h}$$

$$= \frac{250\ ml \times 1 \times 7 \times 1 \times 121 \times 60}{50 \times 1000 \times 1 \times 1 \times 2.2 \times 1 \times 1\ h} = \frac{231\ ml}{2\ h} = 115.5\ ml/h$$

50. Factors: 10 mcg = 1 kg × 1 min; 800 mg = 250 ml; 1 mg = 1000 mcg; 1 kg = 2.2 lb; 160 lb/1; 1 h = 60 min

$$\frac{ml}{h} = \frac{250\ ml \times 1\ mg \times 10\ mcg \times 1\ kg \times 160\ lb \times 60\ min}{800\ mg \times 1000\ mcg \times 1\ kg \times 1\ min \times 2.2\ lb \times 1 \times 1\ h}$$

$$= \frac{250\ ml \times 1 \times 10 \times 1 \times 160 \times 60}{800 \times 1000 \times 1 \times 1 \times 2.2 \times 1 \times 1\ h} = \frac{30\ ml}{2.2\ h} = 13.6\ ml/h$$

51. Factors: 3 mcg = 1 kg × 1 min; 1 kg = 2.2 lb; 165 lb/1

$$\frac{mcg}{min} = \frac{3\ mcg \times 1\ kg \times 165\ lb}{1\ kg \times 1\ min \times 2.2\ lb \times 1} = \frac{3\ mcg \times 1 \times 165}{1 \times 1\ min \times 2.2 \times 1} = \frac{225\ mcg}{1\ min} = 225\ mcg/min$$

52. Factors: 5 mcg = 1 kg × 1 min; 68 kg/1

$$\frac{mcg}{min} = \frac{5\ mcg \times 68\ kg}{1\ kg \times 1\ min \times 1} = \frac{5\ mcg \times 68}{1 \times 1\ min \times 1} = \frac{340\ mcg}{1\ min} = 340\ mcg/min$$

53. Factors: 8 mcg = 1 kg × 1 min; 187 lb/1; 1 kg = 2.2 lb

$$\frac{mcg}{min} = \frac{8\ mcg \times 1\ kg \times 187\ lb}{1\ kg \times 1\ min \times 2.2\ lb \times 1} = \frac{8\ mcg \times 1 \times 187}{1 \times 1\ min \times 2.2 \times 1} = \frac{680\ mcg}{1\ min} = 680\ mcg/min$$

54. Factors: 10 mcg = 1 kg × 1 min; 198 lb/1; 1 kg = 2.2 lb

$$\frac{mcg}{min} = \frac{10\ mcg \times 1\ kg \times 198\ lb}{1\ kg \times 1\ min \times 2.2\ lb \times 1} = \frac{10\ mcg \times 1 \times 198}{1 \times 1\ min \times 2.2 \times 1} = \frac{900\ mcg}{1\ min} = 900\ mcg/min$$

55. Factors: 50 mg = 1 kg × 1 min; 1 kg = 2.2 lb; 154 lb

$$\frac{mg}{min} = \frac{50\ mg \times 1\ kg \times 154\ lb}{1\ kg \times 1\ min \times 2.2\ lb \times 1} = \frac{50\ mg \times 1 \times 154}{1 \times 1\ min \times 2.2 \times 1} = \frac{3500\ mg}{1\ min} = 3500\ mg/min$$

56. Factors: 225 mcg = 1 min (from problem 51); 1 mg = 1000 mcg; 100 mg = 250 ml; 60 gtt = 1 ml

$$\frac{gtt}{min} = \frac{60\ gtt \times 250\ ml \times 1\ mg \times 225\ mcg}{1\ ml \times 100\ mg \times 1000\ mcg \times 1\ min} = \frac{60\ gtt \times 250 \times 1 \times 225}{1 \times 100 \times 1000 \times 1\ min}$$

$$= \frac{135\ gtt}{4\ min} = 33.7\ (34)\ gtt/min$$

57. Factors: 340 mcg = 1 min (from problem 52) ; 500 mg = 500 ml; 60 gtt = 1 ml; 1 mg = 1000 mcg

$$\frac{gtt}{min} = \frac{60\ gtt \times 500\ ml \times 1\ mg \times 340\ mcg}{1\ ml \times 500\ mg \times 1000\ mcg \times 1\ min} = \frac{60\ gtt \times 500 \times 1 \times 340}{1 \times 500 \times 1000 \times 1\ min}$$

$$= \frac{102\ gtt}{5\ min} = 20.4\ gtt/min$$

58. Factors: 680 mcg = 1 min (from problem 53); 250 ml = 100 mg; 1 mg = 1000 mcg; 60 gtt = 1 ml

$$\frac{gtt}{min} = \frac{60\ gtt \times 250\ ml \times 1\ mg \times 680\ mcg}{1\ ml \times 100\ mg \times 1000\ mcg \times 1\ min} = \frac{60\ gtt \times 250 \times 1 \times 680}{1 \times 100 \times 1000 \times 1\ min} = \frac{102\ gtt}{1\ min} = 102\ gtt/min$$

59. Factors: 60 gtt = 1 ml; 250 ml = 400 mg; 1 mg = 1000 mcg; 50 mcg = 1 kg × 1 min; 48 kg/1

$$\frac{gtt}{min} = \frac{60\ gtt \times 250\ ml \times\quad 1\quad mg \times 50\ mcg\quad\quad\quad\quad \times\ 48\ kg}{1\ ml\ \times\ 400\ mg \times 1000\ mcg \times 1\quad kg\ \times 1\ min\ \times\quad 1}$$

$$= \frac{\overset{15}{\cancel{60}}\ gtt\ \times\ \overset{1}{\cancel{250}} \times\quad \overset{1}{1} \times\ \overset{1}{\cancel{50}}\quad\quad\quad \times\ \overset{6}{\cancel{48}}}{1\quad\times\ \underset{\underset{1}{\cancel{8}}}{400} \times\ \underset{\underset{1}{\cancel{4}}}{\cancel{1000}} \times\ 1\ \times\ 1\ min\ \times\quad 1} = \frac{90\ gtt}{1\ min} = 90\ gtt/min$$

60. Factors: 60 gtt = 1 ml; 500 ml = 1 g; 1 g = 1000 mg; 1 mg = 1000 mcg; 1 kg = 2.2 lb; 168 lb/1; 50 mcg = 1 kg × 1 min

$$\frac{gtt}{min} = \frac{60\ gtt \times 500\ ml \times\quad 1\quad g\ \times\quad 1\quad mg \times 50\ mcg\quad\quad\quad\quad \times\ 1\ kg\ \times 168\ lb}{1\ ml\ \times\quad 1\quad g\ \times 1000\ mg \times 1000\ mcg \times 1\quad kg\ \times 1\ min \times 2.2\ lb\ \times\quad 1}$$

$$= \frac{\overset{3}{\cancel{60}}\ gtt\ \times\ \overset{1}{\cancel{500}} \times\quad \overset{1}{1}\quad\times\quad \overset{1}{1} \times\ \overset{50}{\cancel{50}}\quad\quad\quad \times\ 1\ \times\ \overset{\overset{42}{\cancel{84}}}{\cancel{168}}}{1\quad\times\quad 1\quad\times\ \underset{\underset{1}{\cancel{2}}}{\cancel{1000}} \times\ \underset{\underset{1}{\cancel{50}}}{1000} \times\ 1\ \times\ 1\ min\ \times\ \underset{1.1}{\cancel{2.2}} \times\quad 1} = \frac{126\ gtt}{1.1\ min} = 114.5\ (115)\ gtt/min$$

UNIT IX: PEDIATRIC CALCULATIONS

Chapter 17: Pediatric Medications and Intravenous Fluids

1. Factors: Maximum dosage: 0.06 mg = 1 kg; 1 kg = 1000 g; 5710 g/1

$$mg\ (/d) = \frac{0.06\ mg \times\quad 1\ kg\ \times 5710\ g}{1\ kg\ \times 1000\ g\quad\times\quad 1} = \frac{0.06\ mg \times\quad 1 \times \overset{571}{\cancel{5710}}}{1\ mg \times \underset{100}{\cancel{1000}} \times\quad 1} = \frac{34.26\ mg}{100} = 0.3426\ mg$$

Factors: Minimum dosage: 0.04 mg = 1 kg; 1 kg = 1000 g; 5710 g/1

$$mg\ (/d) = \frac{0.04\ mg \times\quad 1\ kg\ \times 5170\ g}{1\ kg\ \times 1000\ g\quad\times\quad 1} = \frac{0.04\ mg \times\quad 1 \times \overset{571}{\cancel{5710}}}{1\quad\times \underset{100}{\cancel{1000}} \times\quad 1} = \frac{22.84\ mg}{100} = 0.2284\ mg$$

Factors: Bette's dosage: 0.1 mg = (q) 8h; 24 h = 1 d

$$\frac{mg}{d} = \frac{0.1\ mg \times 24\ h}{(q)\ 8h\ \times\ 1\ d} = \frac{0.1\ mg \times \overset{3}{\cancel{24}}}{\underset{1}{\cancel{8}}\quad\times\ 1\ d} = \frac{0.3\ mg}{1\ d} = 0.3\ mg/d;\ \text{within recommended range}$$

2. Factors: 0.6 mg = 1 kg; 1 kg = 2.2 lb; 16 lb 8 oz (16 ½ or 16.5 lb)/1

$$mg = \frac{0.6\ mg \times\quad 1\ kg\ \times 16.5\ lb}{1\ kg\ \times 2.2\ lb\ \times\quad 1\ lb} = \frac{\overset{0.3}{\cancel{0.6}}\ mg \times\quad 1 \times 16.5}{1\ mg \times \underset{1.1}{\cancel{2.2}} \times\quad 1} = \frac{4.95\ mg}{1.1} = 4.5\ mg$$

3. Factors: Minimum: 0.3 mcg = 1 kg; 1 kg = 2.2 lb; 33 lb/1

$$mcg\ (/d) = \frac{0.3\ mcg \times\quad 1\ kg\ \times 33\ lb}{1\ kg\ \times 2.2\ lb\ \times\quad 1} = \frac{0.3\ mcg \times\quad 1 \times \overset{3}{\cancel{33}}}{1\quad\times \underset{0.2}{\cancel{2.2}} \times\quad 1} = \frac{0.9\ mcg}{0.2} = 4.5\ mcg$$

Factors: Maximum: 0.5 mcg = 1 kg; 1 kg = 2.2 lb; 33 lb/1

$$mcg\ (/d) = \frac{0.5\ mcg \times\quad 1\ kg\ \times 33\ lb}{1\ kg\ \times 2.2\ lb\ \times\quad 1} = \frac{0.5\ mcg \times\quad 1 \times \overset{3}{\cancel{33}}}{1\ mcg \times \underset{0.2}{\cancel{2.2}} \times\quad 1} = \frac{1.5\ mcg}{0.2} = 7.5\ mcg$$

Factors: Bernie's dosage: 6 mcg q.d. within recommended range.

4. Factors: Maximum: 50 mg = 1 kg; 1 kg = 2.2 lb; 26 lb/1

$$mg\ (/d) = \frac{50\ mg \times\quad 1\ kg\ \times 26\ lb}{1\ kg\ \times 2.2\ lb\ \times\quad 1} = \frac{50\ mg \times\quad 1 \times \overset{13}{\cancel{26}}}{1\quad\times \underset{1.1}{\cancel{2.2}} \times\quad 1} = \frac{650\ mg}{1.1\ mg} = 590.909\ mg$$

Factors: Gracie's dosage: 150 mg = (q) 6 h; 24 h = 1 d

$$mg = \frac{150\ mg \times 24\ h}{(q)6\ h\ \times\ 1\ d} = \frac{150\ mg \times \overset{4}{\cancel{24}}}{\underset{1}{\cancel{6}}\quad\times\ 1} = \frac{600\ mg}{1\ d} = 600\ mg/d$$

Ordered dosage exceeds recommended dosage by 9 mg.

5. Factors: Minimum: 4 mg = 1 kg; 1 kg = 2.2 lb; 43 lb/1

$$\text{mg (/d)} = \frac{4\text{ mg} \times 1\text{ kg} \times 42\text{ lb}}{1\text{ kg} \times 2.2\text{ lb} \times 1} = \frac{\overset{2}{\cancel{4}}\text{ mg} \times 1 \times 43}{1 \times \underset{1.1}{\cancel{2.2}} \times 1} = \frac{86\text{ mg}}{1.1} = 78.18\text{ mg}$$

Factors: Maximum: 8 mg = 1 kg; 1 kg = 2.2 lb; 43 lb

$$\text{mg (/d)} = \frac{8\text{ mg} \times 1\text{ kg} \times 43\text{ lb}}{1\text{ kg} \times 2.2\text{ lb} \times 1} = \frac{\overset{4}{\cancel{8}}\text{ mg} \times 1 \times 43}{1 \times \underset{1.1}{\cancel{2.2}} \times 1} = \frac{172\text{ mg}}{1.1} = 156.36\text{ mg}$$

Factors: Client's mg/dose: 50 mg = (q) 8h; 24 h = 1 d

$$\frac{\text{mg}}{\text{d}} = \frac{50\text{ mg} \times 24\text{ h}}{(q)\,8\text{ h} \times 1\text{ d}} = \frac{50\text{ mg} \times \overset{3}{\cancel{24}}}{\underset{1}{\cancel{8}} \times 1\text{ d}} = \frac{150\text{ mg}}{1\text{ d}} = 150\text{ mg/d}$$

Ordered dosage is within the recommended range.

Factors: 30 mg = 5 ml; 50 mg/1

$$\text{ml} = \frac{5\text{ ml} \times 50\text{ mg}}{30\text{ mg} \times 1\text{ mg}} = \frac{5\text{ ml} \times \overset{5}{\cancel{50}}}{\underset{3}{\cancel{30}} \times 1} = \frac{25\text{ ml}}{3} = 8.3\text{ ml}$$

6. Missy's BSA is 1.06 square meters.

7. Factors: 200 mg = 1 m^2; 1.06 m^2/1

$$\text{mg} = \frac{200\text{ mg} \times 1.06\text{ m}^2}{1\text{ m}^2 \times 1} = \frac{200\text{ mg} \times 1.06}{1 \times 1} = \frac{212\text{ mg}}{1} = 212\text{ mg}$$

8. Robbie's BSA is 0.86 square meters.

9. Factors: 25 mg = 1 m^2; 0.86 m^2/1

$$\text{mg} = \frac{25\text{ mg} \times 0.86\text{ m}^2}{1\text{ m}^2 \times 1} = \frac{25\text{ mg} \times 0.86}{1 \times 1} = \frac{21.5\text{ mg}}{1} = 21.5\text{ mg}$$

10. Factors: 1.5 mg = 1 m^2; 0.86 m^2/1

$$\text{mg} = \frac{1.5\text{ mg} \times 0.86\text{ m}^2}{1\text{ m}^2 \times 1} = \frac{1.5\text{ mg} \times 0.86}{1 \times 1} = \frac{1.29\text{ mg}}{1} = 1.29\text{ mg}$$

11. Factors: Drip rate: 60 gtt = 1 ml; 60 ml = 1 h; 1 h = 60 min

$$\frac{\text{gtt}}{\text{min}} = \frac{60\text{ gtt} \times 60\text{ ml} \times 1\text{ h}}{1\text{ ml} \times 1\text{ h} \times 60\text{ min}} = \frac{60\text{ gtt} \times \overset{1}{\cancel{60}} \times 1}{1 \times 1 \times \underset{1}{\cancel{60}}\text{ min}} = \frac{60\text{ gtt}}{1\text{ min}} = 60\text{ gtt/min}$$

Factors: buret solution: 60 ml = 1 h; 1 h = 60 min; 20 min/1

$$\text{ml} = \frac{60\text{ ml} \times 1\text{ h} \times 20\text{ min}}{1\text{ h} \times 60\text{ min} \times 1} = \frac{\overset{1}{\cancel{60}}\text{ ml} \times 1 \times 20}{1 \times \underset{1}{\cancel{60}} \times 1} = \frac{20\text{ ml}}{1} = 20\text{ ml}$$

12. Factors: Drip rate: 60 gtt = 1 ml; 80 ml = 1 h; 1 h = 60 min

$$\frac{\text{gtt}}{\text{min}} = \frac{60\text{ gtt} \times 80\text{ ml} \times 1\text{ h}}{1\text{ ml} \times 1\text{ h} \times 60\text{ min}} = \frac{\overset{1}{\cancel{60}}\text{ gtt} \times 80 \times 1}{1 \times 1 \times \underset{1}{\cancel{60}}\text{ min}} = \frac{80\text{ gtt}}{1\text{ min}} = 80\text{ gtt/min}$$

Factors: buret solution: 80 ml = 1 h; 1 h = 60 min; 30 min/1

$$\text{ml} = \frac{80\text{ ml} \times 1\text{ h} \times 30\text{ min}}{1\text{ h} \times 60\text{ min} \times 1} = \frac{\overset{40}{\cancel{80}}\text{ ml} \times 1 \times \overset{1}{\cancel{30}}}{1 \times \underset{\underset{1}{\cancel{2}}}{\cancel{60}} \times 1} = \frac{40\text{ ml}}{1} = 40\text{ ml}$$

13. Factors: 100 ml = 1 h; 1 h = 60 min; 40 min/1

$$\text{ml} = \frac{100\text{ ml} \times 1\text{ h} \times 40\text{ min}}{1\text{ h} \times 60\text{ min} \times 1} = \frac{\overset{5}{\cancel{100}}\text{ ml} \times 1 \times 40}{1 \times \underset{3}{\cancel{60}} \times 1} = \frac{200\text{ ml}}{3} = 66.7\text{ ml}$$

14. Factors: 60 gtt = 1 ml; 75 ml = 1 h; 1 h = 60 min

$$\frac{\text{gtt}}{\text{min}} = \frac{60\text{ gtt} \times 75\text{ ml} \times 1\text{ h}}{1\text{ ml} \times 1\text{ h} \times 60\text{ min}} = \frac{\overset{1}{\cancel{60}}\text{ gtt} \times 75 \times 1}{1 \times 1 \times \underset{1}{\cancel{60}}\text{ min}} = \frac{75\text{ gtt}}{1\text{ min}} = 75\text{ gtt/min}$$

15. Factors: 60 gtt = 1 ml; 50 ml = 1 h; 1 h = 60 min

$$\frac{\text{gtt}}{\text{min}} = \frac{60\text{ gtt} \times 50\text{ ml} \times 1\text{ h}}{1\text{ ml} \times 1\text{ h} \times 60\text{ min}} = \frac{\overset{1}{\cancel{60}}\text{ gtt} \times 50 \times 1}{1 \times 1 \times \underset{1}{\cancel{60}}\text{ min}} = \frac{50\text{ gtt}}{1\text{ min}} = 50\text{ gtt/min}$$

SELF-ASSESSMENT POSTTEST ANSWERS

UNIT I: MATHEMATICAL KNOWLEDGE BASE

Chapter 1: Roman Numerals

1. XIX = 19
2. xxivss = 24 1/2
3. xxiii = 23
4. xvi = 6
5. XV = 15
6. ivss = 4 1/2
7. VII = 7
8. iiiss = 3 1/2
9. XXIX = 29
10. XXXVI = 36
11. 25 = XXV or xxv
12. 12 = XII or xii
13. 26 = XXVI or xxvi
14. 8 = VIII or viii
15. 7 1/2 = viiss
16. 14 = XIV or xiv
17. 34 = XXXIV or xxxiv
18. 2 1/2 = iiss
19. 39 = XXXIX or xxxix
20. 18 = XVIII or xviii

Chapter 2: Fractions

1. Two and thirty-eight seventy-fifths = 2 38/75
2. Three twenty-fifths = 3/25
3. Sixty-seven one-thousandths = 67/1000
4. 1:5 = 1/5
5. 1/7, 1/8, 1/4 Least common denominator = 56
6. 7/10, 4/5, 3/4 Least common denominator = 20
7. 3 1/4 + 1 1/2 + 4 2/3 + 1 5/6

Least common denominator = 12

$$3\frac{1}{4} = 3\frac{3 \times 1}{3 \times 4} = 3\frac{3}{12}$$

$$1\frac{1}{2} = 1\frac{6 \times 1}{6 \times 2} = 1\frac{6}{12}$$

$$4\frac{2}{3} = 4\frac{4 \times 2}{4 \times 3} = 4\frac{8}{12}$$

$$1\frac{5}{6} = 1\frac{2 \times 5}{2 \times 6} = 1\frac{10}{12}$$

$$9\frac{27}{12} = 9\frac{9}{4} = 9 + 2\frac{1}{4} = 11\frac{1}{4}$$

8. 5/8 + 3/4 + 7/16 + 1/2 Least common denominator = 16

$$\frac{5}{8} = \frac{2 \times 5}{2 \times 8} = \frac{10}{16}$$

$$\frac{3}{4} = \frac{4 \times 3}{4 \times 4} = \frac{12}{16}$$

$$\frac{7}{16} = \frac{7}{16}$$

$$\frac{1}{2} = \frac{8 \times 1}{8 \times 2} = \frac{8}{16}$$

$$\frac{37}{16}$$

$$= 16\overline{)37}^{\,2\frac{5}{16}}$$
$$\underline{32}$$
$$5$$

9. 8/9 - 1/2 Least common denominator = 18

$$\frac{8}{9} = \frac{2 \times 8}{2 \times 9} = \frac{16}{18}$$

$$\frac{1}{2} = \frac{9 \times 1}{9 \times 2} = -\frac{9}{18}$$

$$\frac{7}{18}$$

10. 5 5/7 - 3 20/21 Least common denominator = 21

$$5\frac{5}{7} = 5\frac{3 \times 5}{3 \times 7} = 5\frac{15}{21} = 5 - 1\frac{(21 \times 1) + 15}{21} = \quad 4\frac{36}{21}$$

$$3\frac{20}{21} \qquad\qquad\qquad\qquad\qquad\qquad -3\frac{20}{21}$$

$$1\frac{16}{21}$$

11. 3 1/8 - 1 1/2 Least common denominator = 8

$$3\frac{1}{8} = 3 - 1\frac{(8 \times 1) + 1}{8} = 2\frac{9}{8}$$

$$1\frac{1}{2} = \frac{4 \times 1}{4 \times 2} = -1\frac{4}{8}$$

$$1\frac{5}{8}$$

12. 1 5/8 - 3/4 Least common denominator = 8

$$1\frac{5}{8} = 1 - 1\frac{(8 \times 1) + 5}{8} = \frac{13}{8}$$

$$\frac{3}{4} = \frac{2 \times 3}{2 \times 4} = -\frac{6}{8}$$

$$\frac{7}{8}$$

13. $1/3 \times 1/4 \times 2/3 = \dfrac{1 \times 1 \times \overset{1}{\cancel{2}}}{3 \times \underset{2}{\cancel{4}} \times 3} = \dfrac{1 \times 1 \times 1}{3 \times 2 \times 3} = \dfrac{1}{18}$

14. $3 \times 2/3 \times 1/3 = \dfrac{\overset{1}{\cancel{3}} \times 2 \times 1}{1 \times \underset{1}{\cancel{3}} \times 3} = \dfrac{1 \times 2 \times 1}{1 \times 1 \times 3} = \dfrac{2}{3}$

15. $2 1/2 \times 1/6 \times 4 1/3 = \dfrac{\left[(2 \times 2) + 1\right] \times 1 \times \left[(4 \times 3) + 1\right]}{2 \times 6 \times 3}$

$$= \frac{5 \times 1 \times 13}{2 \times 6 \times 3} = \frac{65}{36}$$

$$= 36\overline{)65}^{\,1\frac{29}{36}}$$
$$\underline{36}$$
$$29$$

16. $1/6 \times 1 1/2 \times 4 = \dfrac{1 \times \left[(1 \times 2) + 1\right] \times 4}{6 \times 2 \times 1} = \dfrac{1 \times \overset{1}{\cancel{3}} \times \overset{\overset{1}{\cancel{2}}}{\cancel{4}}}{\underset{2}{\cancel{6}} \times \underset{1}{\cancel{2}} \times 1}$

$$= \frac{1 \times 1 \times 1}{1 \times 1 \times 1} = \frac{1}{1} = 1$$

17. $1/4 \div 1/4 = \dfrac{1 \times \cancel{4}}{\cancel{4} \times 1} = \dfrac{1}{1} = 1$

18. $1/4 \div 4 = \dfrac{1}{4} \div \dfrac{4}{1} = \dfrac{1 \times 1}{4 \times 4} = \dfrac{1}{16}$

19. $6 \div 1\frac{1}{3} = \dfrac{6}{1} \div \dfrac{(1 \times 3) + 1}{3} = \dfrac{6}{1} \div \dfrac{4}{3} = \dfrac{\overset{3}{\cancel{6}} \times 3}{1 \times \underset{2}{\cancel{4}}} = \dfrac{3 \times 3}{1 \times 2} =$

$$\frac{9}{2} = 4\frac{1}{2}$$

20. $2\frac{1}{2} \div \dfrac{1}{6} = \dfrac{(2 \times 2) + 1}{2} \div \dfrac{1}{6} = \dfrac{5 \times \overset{3}{\cancel{6}}}{\underset{1}{\cancel{2}} \times 1} = \dfrac{5 \times 3}{1 \times 1} = \dfrac{15}{1} = 15$

Chapter 3: Decimal Fractions

1. Four ten-thousandths = 0.0004
2. Two and three-hundredths = 2.03
3. 4/10 = 0.4
4.
$$3/7 = 7\overline{)3.000} = 0.43$$
$$\begin{array}{r} 0.428 \\ \underline{2\ 8} \\ 20 \\ \underline{14} \\ 60 \\ \underline{56} \\ 4 \end{array}$$

5. 1 7/1000 = 1 + 0.007. = 1.007 = 1.01
6. 37/12 = $12\overline{)37.000}$ = 3.08
$$\begin{array}{r} 3.083 \\ \underline{36} \\ 1\ 00 \\ \underline{96} \\ 40 \\ \underline{36} \\ 4 \\ 2 \end{array}$$

7. $0.016 = \dfrac{16}{1000} = \dfrac{2}{125}$
   125

8. 1.13 = 1 13/100
9. 1.3087 + 1.63 + 4.631 + 4 = 1.3087
$$\begin{array}{r} 1.6300 \\ 4.6310 \\ \underline{4.0000} \\ 11.5697 \end{array}$$

10. 0.25 + 0.5 + 0.341 + 1.00 = 0.250
$$\begin{array}{r} 0.500 \\ 0.341 \\ \underline{1.000} \\ 2.091 \end{array}$$

11. 13.0896 − 6.10556 =
$$\begin{array}{r} 2\quad5 \\ 13.08960 \\ \underline{-\ 6.10556} \\ 6.98404 \end{array}$$

12. 1 − 0.534 =
$$\begin{array}{r} 0\ 99 \\ 1.000 \\ \underline{-0.534} \\ 0.466 \end{array}$$

13.
$$\begin{array}{r} 2.54 \\ \underline{\times\ 3.2} \\ 508 \\ \underline{762} \\ 8128 \end{array}$$ = (3 decimal places) = 8.128

14.
$$\begin{array}{r} 0.06 \\ \underline{\times 0.005} \\ 00030 \end{array}$$ = (5 decimal places) = 0.0003

15.
$$\begin{array}{r} 1.98 \\ \underline{\times\quad 6.2} \\ 396 \\ \underline{1188} \\ 12276 \end{array}$$ = (3 decimal places) = 12.276

16.
$$\begin{array}{r} 33.05 \\ \underline{\times\quad 0.5} \\ 16525 \end{array}$$ = (3 decimal places) = 16.525

17. $0.05\overline{)26.00}$ = 520.
$$\begin{array}{r} 5\ 20. \\ \underline{25} \\ 1\ 0 \\ \underline{1\ 0} \\ 00 \end{array}$$

18. $0.007\overline{)21.087.24}$ = 3012.46
$$\begin{array}{r} 3\ 012.462 \\ \underline{21} \\ 08 \\ \underline{7} \\ 17 \\ \underline{14} \\ 32 \\ \underline{28} \\ 44 \\ \underline{42} \\ 20 \\ 14 \end{array}$$

19. $0.5\overline{)0.6.3487}$ = 1.27
$$\begin{array}{r} 1.2697 \\ \underline{5} \\ 13 \\ \underline{10} \\ 34 \\ \underline{30} \\ 48 \\ \underline{45} \\ 37 \\ \underline{35} \\ 2 \end{array}$$

20. $0.56\overline{)3.40.000006}$ = 6.07
$$\begin{array}{r} 6.071428 \\ \underline{3\ 36} \\ 400 \\ \underline{392} \\ 80 \\ \underline{56} \\ 240 \\ \underline{224} \\ 160 \\ \underline{112} \\ 486 \\ \underline{448} \\ 38 \end{array}$$

Chapter 4: Percentages

1. 0.27 = 0.27 × 100 = 27%
2. 1.055 = 1.055 × 100 = 105.5%
3. 0.13 = 0.13 × 100 = 13%
4. 0.44 = 0.44 × 100 = 44%
5. 7.5% = 7.5 ÷ 100 = 0.075
6. 28% = 28 ÷ 100 = 0.28
7. 27/100 = 0.27 × 100 = 27%
8. 18/21 = $21\overline{)18.000}$ = 0.86 × 100 = 86%
$$\begin{array}{r} 0.857 \\ \underline{16\ 8} \\ 1\ 20 \\ \underline{1\ 05} \\ 150 \\ \underline{147} \\ 3 \end{array}$$

9. 3/5 = $5\overline{)3.0}$ = 0.6 × 100 = 60%
$$\begin{array}{r} 0.6 \\ \underline{3\ 0} \\ 0 \end{array}$$

10. 11/20 = $20\overline{)11.00}$ = 0.55 × 100 = 55%
$$\begin{array}{r} 0.55 \\ \underline{10\ 0} \\ 1\ 00 \\ \underline{1\ 00} \\ 0 \end{array}$$

11. 16% = 16/100 = $\dfrac{\cancel{16}}{\cancel{100}}$ = 4/25
   25

12. 18% = 18/100 = $\frac{9}{\cancel{18}}$ = 9/50
$\frac{\cancel{18}}{\cancel{100}}$
50

13. 15% of 200 = 200 × (15 ÷ 100) =   200
        ×0.15
        1000
        200
        3000 (2 decimal places) = 30.

14. 25% of 15 = 15 × (25 ÷ 100) =   15
        ×0.25
        75
        30
        375 (2 decimal places) = 3.75

15. 33% of 60 = 60 × (33 ÷ 100) =   60
        ×0.33
        180
        180
        1980 (2 decimal places) = 19.80

16. 8% of 150 = 150 × (8 ÷ 100) =   150
        ×0.08
        1200 (2 decimal places) = 12.

17. 105% of 400 = 400 × (105 ÷ 100) =   400
        ×1.05
        2000
        000
        400
        42000 (2 decimal places) = 420.

18. 30% of 6 = 6 × (30 ÷ 100) = 6 × 0.3
        = 18(1 decimal place) = 1.8
19. Answer: Sales tax amount in dollars
    Cost: $19.95 Tax: 6 3/8%
        0.375
    Decimal fraction = (6 + 8)$\overline{3.00}$) ÷ 100
        2 4
        60
        56
        40
        40
    = 6.38 ÷ 100 = 0.0638
        $19.95
        ×0.0638
        15960
        5985
        11970
        1272810 (6 decimal places)
    = 1.272810 = $1.27

20. Answer: cost + tax in dollars
    Cost: $19.95   Tax: $1.27

    $19.95
    + 1.27
    $21.22

Chapter 5: Equations Written As Fractions

(Answers in parentheses are the multiplication of numerators and denominators without cancellation.)

1. $\dfrac{\overset{3}{\cancel{6}} \times 12 \times \overset{0.1}{\cancel{0.5}} \times \overset{1}{\cancel{3}}}{\underset{1}{\cancel{2}} \times \underset{\underset{1}{3}}{\cancel{15}} \times 1 \times 1} = \dfrac{3 \times 12 \times 0.1 \times 1}{1 \times 1 \times 1 \times 1} = \dfrac{3.6}{1} = 3.6\,(108/30)$

2. $\dfrac{1/6 \times 50 \times 20 \times 3}{1 \times 8 \times 9 \times 5} = \dfrac{1 \times \overset{5}{\cancel{50}} \times \overset{5}{20} \times \overset{1}{\cancel{3}}}{\underset{3}{\cancel{6}} \times 1 \times \underset{2}{\cancel{8}} \times \underset{3}{\cancel{9}} \times \cancel{5}} = \dfrac{1 \times 5 \times 5 \times 1}{3 \times 1 \times 2 \times 3 \times 1} = \dfrac{25}{18} = 1.388 = 1.39\left(\dfrac{3006/6}{360}\right)$

3. $\dfrac{30 \times 1 \times 1 \times 5/6}{1 \times 2.2 \times 20 \times 1} = \dfrac{\overset{5}{\cancel{30}} \times 1 \times 1 \times \overset{1}{\cancel{5}}}{1 \times 2.2 \times \cancel{20} \times 1 \times \cancel{6}} = \dfrac{5 \times 1 \times 1 \times 1}{1 \times 2.2 \times 4 \times 1 \times 1} = \dfrac{5}{8.8} = 0.568 = 0.57\left(\dfrac{150/6}{44}\right)$

4. $\dfrac{22 \times 5/6 \times 3 \times 1}{1 \times 2.2 \times 4 \times 0.5} = \dfrac{\overset{1}{\cancel{22}} \times \overset{1}{\cancel{5}} \times \overset{1}{\cancel{3}} \times 1}{1 \times \underset{0.1}{\cancel{2.2}} \times \underset{2}{\cancel{6}} \times 4 \times \underset{0.1}{\cancel{0.5}}} = \dfrac{1}{0.08} = 12.5\left(\dfrac{330/6}{4.4}\right)$

5. $\dfrac{3/8 \times 5 \times 25 \times 15}{1 \times 6 \times 50 \times 1} = \dfrac{\overset{1}{\cancel{8}} \times 5 \times \overset{1}{\cancel{25}} \times 15}{8 \times 1 \times \underset{2}{\cancel{6}} \times \underset{2}{\cancel{50}} \times 1} = \dfrac{1 \times 5 \times 1 \times 15}{8 \times 1 \times 2 \times 2 \times 1} = \dfrac{75}{32} = 2.343 = 2.34\left(\dfrac{5625/8}{300}\right)$

6. $\dfrac{2 \times 3 \times 1 \times 9}{1 \times 1/6 \times 13 \times 5} = \dfrac{2 \times 3 \times 6 \times 1 \times 9}{1 \times 1 \times 13 \times 5} = \dfrac{324}{65} = 4.984 = 4.98\left(\dfrac{54}{65/6}\right)$

7. $\dfrac{1/150 \times 1 \times 1000 \times 16}{1 \times 15 \times 2 \times 1} = \dfrac{1 \times 1 \times \overset{\overset{20}{\cancel{100}}}{\cancel{1000}} \times \overset{8}{16}}{\underset{15}{\cancel{150}} \times 1 \times \underset{3}{\cancel{15}} \times \underset{1}{2} \times 1} = \dfrac{160}{45} = 3.555 = 3.56\left(\dfrac{16000/150}{30}\right)$

8. $\dfrac{15 \times \overset{(92 \times 1)}{(1 \times 2.2)} \times 5.5 \times 3/10}{1 \times 1 \times 5 \times 2} = \dfrac{\overset{3}{\cancel{15}} \times \overset{23}{\cancel{92}} \times 1 \times \overset{1}{\cancel{5.5}} \times 3}{1 \times 1 \times \underset{\underset{1}{2}}{\cancel{2.2}} \times 1 \times \cancel{5} \times 2 \times \cancel{10}} = \dfrac{3 \times 23 \times 1 \times 1 \times 3}{1 \times 1 \times 1 \times 1 \times 1 \times 2 \times 1}$

$= \dfrac{207}{2} = 103.5\left(\dfrac{22770/22}{10}\right)$

9. $\dfrac{0.4 \times 1 \times 15}{1 \times 1.5 \times 1/6} = \dfrac{\overset{4}{\cancel{0.4}} \times 1 \times \overset{1}{\cancel{15}} \times 6}{1 \times \underset{\underset{1}{\cancel{0.1}}}{\cancel{1.5}} \times 1} = \dfrac{4 \times 1 \times 1 \times 6}{1 \times 1 \times 1} = \dfrac{24}{1} = 24\left(\dfrac{6}{1.5/6}\right)$

10. $\dfrac{\overset{1}{\cancel{5}} \times 1 \times \overset{1}{\cancel{3}} \times 16}{1 \times \underset{3}{\cancel{15}} \times \underset{5}{\cancel{10}} \times 1} = \dfrac{1 \times 1 \times 1 \times 16}{1 \times 3 \times 5 \times 1} = \dfrac{16}{15} = 1.066 = 1.07\left(\dfrac{160}{150}\right)$

UNIT II: INTRODUCTION TO DIMENSIONAL ANALYSIS

Chapter 6: The Dimensional Analysis Method

1. 90 kilometers/hour = _____ miles/hour

$\dfrac{\text{mi}}{\text{h}} = \dfrac{0.6 \text{ mi} \times 90 \text{ km}}{1 \text{ km} \times 1 \text{ h}} = \dfrac{0.6 \text{ mi} \times 90}{1 \times 1 \text{ h}} = \dfrac{54 \text{ mi}}{1 \text{ h}} = 54 \text{ mi/h}$

2. 1/4 quart = _____ ounces

$\text{oz} = \dfrac{8 \text{ oz} \times 2 \text{ C} \times 2 \text{ pt} \times 1/4 \text{ qt}}{1 \text{ C} \times 1 \text{ pt} \times 1 \text{ qt} \times 1} = \dfrac{8 \text{ oz} \times 2 \times 2 \times 1/4}{1 \times 1 \times 1 \times 1} = \dfrac{\overset{2}{\cancel{8}} \text{ oz} \times 2 \times 2 \times 1}{1 \times 1 \times 1 \times \underset{1}{\cancel{4}} \times 1}$

$= \dfrac{2 \text{ oz} \times 2 \times 2 \times 1}{1 \times 1 \times 1 \times 1 \times 1} = \dfrac{8 \text{ oz}}{1} = 8 \text{ oz}$

3. 18 teaspoons = _____ tablespoons

$\text{tbsp} = \dfrac{1 \text{ tbsp} \times 18 \text{ tsp}}{3 \text{ tsp} \times 1} = \dfrac{1 \text{ tbsp} \times \overset{6}{\cancel{18}}}{\underset{1}{\cancel{3}} \times 1} = \dfrac{1 \text{ tbsp} \times 6}{1 \times 1} = \dfrac{6 \text{ tbsp}}{1} = 6 \text{ tbsp}$

4. 8 1/8 pounds = _____ ounces

$\text{oz} = \dfrac{16 \text{ oz} \times 8\,1/8 \text{ lb}}{1 \text{ lb} \times 1} = \dfrac{16 \text{ oz} \times 65/8}{1 \times 1} = \dfrac{\overset{2}{\cancel{16}} \text{ oz} \times 65}{1 \times \underset{1}{\cancel{8}} \times 1} = \dfrac{2 \text{ oz} \times 65}{1 \times 1 \times 1} = \dfrac{130 \text{ oz}}{1} = 130 \text{ oz}$

5. 6 tablespoons = _____ ounces

$\text{oz} = \dfrac{1 \text{ oz} \times 6 \text{ tbsp}}{2 \text{ tbsp} \times 1} = \dfrac{1 \text{ oz} \times \overset{3}{\cancel{6}}}{\underset{1}{\cancel{2}} \times 1} = \dfrac{1 \text{ oz} \times 3}{1 \times 1} = \dfrac{3 \text{ oz}}{1} = 3 \text{ oz}$

6. Unit of answer: dollars   Factors: \$1200 = 100%; 5.5%/1

$\$ = \dfrac{\$1200 \times 5.5\%}{100\% \times 1} = \dfrac{\overset{12}{\cancel{\$1200}} \times 5.5}{\underset{1}{\cancel{100}} \times 1} = \dfrac{\$66}{1} = \$66$

7. Unit of answer: dollars; Factors: \$212.53 = 100%; 16%/1; Conversion factor: 1 yr = 12 mo

$\$ = \dfrac{\$212.53 \times 16\% \times 1 \text{ yr} \times 1 \text{ mo}}{100\% \times 1 \text{ yr} \times 12 \text{ mo} \times 1} = \dfrac{\overset{2.1253}{\cancel{\$212.53}} \times \overset{4}{\cancel{16}} \times 1 \times 1}{\underset{1}{\cancel{100}} \times 1 \times \underset{3}{\cancel{12}} \times 1} = \dfrac{\$2.1253 \times 4 \times 1 \times 1}{1 \times 1 \times 3 \times 1}$

$\dfrac{\$8.5012}{3} = \$2.833 = \$2.83$

8. This problem asks for a comparison of 65 mi/h to 100 km/h to find if the driver is speeding. The rate of km/h can be changed to mi/h or mi/h can be changed to km/h.

Unit of answer: km/h (mi/h); Factor: 65 mi/h (100 km/h); Conversion factor: 1 km = 0.6 mi

$\dfrac{\text{km}}{\text{h}} = \dfrac{1 \text{ km} \times 65 \text{ mi}}{0.6 \text{ mi} \times 1 \text{ h}} = \dfrac{1 \text{ km} \times 65}{0.6 \times 1 \text{ h}} = \dfrac{65 \text{ km}}{0.6 \text{ h}} = 108.33 \text{ km/h}$

The speed limit is 108.3 km/h. The driver is not speeding because 100 km/h < 108.3 km/h.

$\dfrac{\text{mi}}{\text{h}} = \dfrac{0.6 \text{ mi} \times 100 \text{ km}}{1 \text{ km} \times 1 \text{ h}} = \dfrac{0.6 \text{ mi} \times 100}{1 \times 1 \text{ h}} = \dfrac{60 \text{ mi}}{1 \text{ h}} = 60 \text{ mi/h}$

The driver is going 60 mi/h in a 65 mi/h zone. The driver is not speeding.

9. Unit of answer: km; Factor: 26 mi/1; Conversion factor: 1 km = 0.6 mi

$\text{km} = \dfrac{1 \text{ km} \times 26 \text{ mi}}{0.6 \text{ mi} \times 1} = \dfrac{1 \text{ km} \times \overset{13}{\cancel{26}}}{\underset{0.3}{\cancel{0.6}} \times 1} = \dfrac{1 \text{ km} \times 13}{0.3 \times 1} = \dfrac{13 \text{ km}}{0.3} = 43.3 \text{ km}$

10. Unit of answer: handbags (hb); Factors: 28 handbags = 100%; (100% + 25%)/1 or 125%/1

$$\text{handbags} = \frac{28 \text{ hb} \times 125 \text{ \%}}{100 \text{ \%} \times 1} = \frac{\overset{7}{\cancel{28}} \text{ hb} \times \overset{5}{\cancel{125}}}{\underset{\underset{1}{\cancel{25}}}{\cancel{100}} \times 1} = \frac{7 \text{ hb} \times 5}{1 \times 1} = \frac{35 \text{ hb}}{1} = 35 \text{ handbags}$$

UNIT III: CONVERSIONS WITHIN AND AMONG MEASUREMENT SYSTEMS

Chapter 7: The English Measurement Systems

1. 39 in = _____ ft

$$\text{ft} = \frac{1 \text{ ft} \times 39 \text{ in}}{12 \text{ in} \times 1} = \frac{1 \text{ ft} \times \overset{13}{\cancel{39}}}{\underset{4}{\cancel{12}} \times 1} = \frac{1 \text{ ft} \times 13}{4 \times 1} = \frac{13 \text{ ft}}{4} = 3\frac{1}{4} \text{ ft}$$

2. 45 oz = _____ lb

$$\text{lb} = \frac{1 \text{ lb} \times 45 \text{ oz}}{16 \text{ oz} \times 1} = \frac{1 \text{ lb} \times 45}{16 \times 1} = \frac{45 \text{ lb}}{16} = 2\frac{13}{16} \text{ lb}$$

3. 3 pt = _____ oz

$$\text{oz} = \frac{8 \text{ oz} \times 2 \text{ C} \times 3 \text{ pt}}{1 \text{ C} \times 1 \text{ pt} \times 1} = \frac{8 \text{ oz} \times 2 \times 3}{1 \times 1 \times 1} = \frac{48 \text{ oz}}{1} = 48 \text{ oz}$$

4. 24 T = _____ C

$$\text{C} = \frac{1 \text{ C} \times 1 \text{ oz} \times 24 \text{ T}}{8 \text{ oz} \times 2 \text{ T} \times 1} = \frac{1 \text{ C} \times 1 \times \overset{3}{\cancel{24}}}{\underset{1}{\cancel{8}} \times 2 \times 1} = \frac{1 \text{ C} \times 1 \times 3}{1 \times 2 \times 1} = \frac{3 \text{ C}}{2} = 1\frac{1}{2} \text{ C}$$

5. 5 qt = _____ oz

$$\text{oz} = \frac{8 \text{ oz} \times 2 \text{ C} \times 2 \text{ pt} \times 5 \text{ qt}}{1 \text{ C} \times 1 \text{ pt} \times 1 \text{ qt} \times 1} = \frac{8 \text{ oz} \times 2 \times 2 \times 5}{1 \times 1 \times 1 \times 1} = \frac{160 \text{ oz}}{1} = 160 \text{ oz}$$

6. 30 oz = _____ lb

$$\text{lb} = \frac{1 \text{ lb} \times 30 \text{ oz}}{16 \text{ oz} \times 1} = \frac{1 \text{ lb} \times \overset{15}{\cancel{30}}}{\underset{8}{\cancel{16}} \times 1} = \frac{1 \text{ lb} \times 15}{8 \times 1} = \frac{15 \text{ lb}}{8} = 1\frac{7}{8} \text{ lb}$$

7. $2\frac{5}{8}$ ft = _____ in

$$\text{in} = \frac{12 \text{ in} \times 2\frac{5}{8}\text{ft}}{1 \text{ ft} \times 1} = \frac{12 \text{ in} \times {}^{21}/_{8}}{1 \times 1} = \frac{\overset{3}{\cancel{12}} \text{ in} \times 21}{1 \times \underset{2}{\cancel{8}}} = \frac{3 \text{ in} \times 21}{1 \times 2} = \frac{63 \text{ in}}{2} = 31\frac{1}{2} \text{ in}$$

8. 29 oz = _____ pt

$$\text{pt} = \frac{1 \text{ pt} \times 1 \text{ C} \times 29 \text{ oz}}{2 \text{ C} \times 8 \text{ oz} \times 1} = \frac{1 \text{ pt} \times 1 \times 29}{2 \times 8 \times 1} = \frac{29 \text{ pt}}{16} = 1\frac{13}{16} \text{ pt}$$

9. 15/16 lb = _____ oz

$$\text{oz} = \frac{16 \text{ oz} \times {}^{15}/_{16} \text{ lb}}{1 \text{ lb} \times 1} = \frac{\overset{1}{\cancel{16}} \text{ oz} \times 15}{1 \times \underset{1}{\cancel{16}}} = \frac{1 \text{ oz} \times 15}{1 \times 1} = \frac{15 \text{ oz}}{1} = 15 \text{ oz}$$

10. 24 tsp = _____ C

$$\text{C} = \frac{1 \text{ C} \times 1 \text{ oz} \times 1 \text{ T} \times 24 \text{ tsp}}{8 \text{ oz} \times 2 \text{ T} \times 3 \text{ tsp} \times 1} = \frac{1 \text{ C} \times 1 \times 1 \times \overset{\overset{1}{\cancel{3}}}{\cancel{24}}}{\underset{1}{\cancel{8}} \times 2 \times \underset{1}{\cancel{3}} \times 1} = \frac{1 \text{ C} \times 1 \times 1 \times 1}{1 \times 2 \times 1 \times 1} = \frac{1 \text{ C}}{2} = \frac{1}{2} \text{ C}$$

11. 64 oz = _____ pt

$$\text{pt} = \frac{1 \text{ pt} \times 1 \text{ C} \times 64 \text{ oz}}{2 \text{ C} \times 8 \text{ oz} \times 1} = \frac{1 \text{ pt} \times 1 \times \overset{\overset{4}{\cancel{32}}}{\cancel{64}}}{\underset{1}{\cancel{2}} \times \underset{1}{\cancel{8}} \times 1} = \frac{1 \text{ pt} \times 1 \times 4}{1 \times 1 \times 1} = \frac{4 \text{ pt}}{1} = 4 \text{ pt}$$

12. 26 oz = _____ lb

$$\text{lb} = \frac{1 \text{ lb} \times 26 \text{ oz}}{16 \text{ oz} \times 1} = \frac{1 \text{ lb} \times \overset{13}{\cancel{26}}}{\underset{8}{\cancel{16}} \times 1} = \frac{1 \text{ lb} \times 13}{8 \times 1} = \frac{13 \text{ lb}}{8} = 1\frac{5}{8} \text{ lb}$$

13. 14 C = _____ qt

$$\text{qt} = \frac{1 \text{ qt} \times 1 \text{ pt} \times 14 \text{ C}}{2 \text{ pt} \times 2 \text{ C} \times 1} = \frac{1 \text{ qt} \times 1 \times \cancel{14}^{\,7}}{\cancel{2}_{1} \times 2 \times 1} = \frac{1 \text{ qt} \times 1 \times 7}{1 \times 2 \times 1} = \frac{7 \text{ qt}}{2} = 3\frac{1}{2}\text{ qt}$$

14. 14 tsp = _____ oz

$$\text{oz} = \frac{1 \text{ oz} \times 1 \text{ T} \times 14 \text{ tsp}}{2 \text{ pt} \times 3 \text{ tsp} \times 1} = \frac{1 \text{ oz} \times 1 \times \cancel{14}^{\,7}}{\cancel{2}_{1} \times 3 \times 1} = \frac{1 \text{ oz} \times 1 \times 7}{1 \times 3 \times 1} = \frac{7 \text{ oz}}{3} = 2\frac{1}{3}\text{ oz}$$

15. $3\frac{1}{2}$ C = _____ oz

$$\text{oz} = \frac{8 \text{ oz} \times 3^{1}/_{2} \text{ C}}{1 \text{ C} \times 1} = \frac{8 \text{ oz} \times {}^{7}/_{2}}{1 \times 1} = \frac{\cancel{8}^{\,4} \text{ oz} \times 7}{1 \times \cancel{2}_{1}} = \frac{4 \text{ oz} \times 7}{1 \times 1} = \frac{28 \text{ oz}}{1} = 28\text{ oz}$$

16. $4\frac{1}{6}$ feet = _____ in

$$\text{in} = \frac{12 \text{ in} \times 4^{1}/_{6} \text{ ft}}{1 \text{ ft} \times 1} = \frac{12 \text{ in} \times {}^{25}/_{6}}{1 \times 1} = \frac{\cancel{12}^{\,2} \text{ in} \times 25}{1 \times \cancel{6}_{1}} = \frac{2 \text{ in} \times 25}{1 \times 1} = \frac{50 \text{ in}}{1} = 50\text{ in}$$

17. 27 T = _____ pt

$$\text{pt} = \frac{1 \text{ pt} \times 1 \text{ C} \times 1 \text{ oz} \times 27 \text{ T}}{2 \text{ C} \times 8 \text{ oz} \times 2 \text{ T} \times 1} = \frac{1 \text{ pt} \times 1 \times 1 \times 27}{2 \times 8 \times 2 \times 1} = \frac{27 \text{ pt}}{32} = \frac{27}{32}\text{ pt}$$

18. 12 ℥ = _____ lb

$$\text{lb} = \frac{1 \text{ lb} \times 12 \text{ oz}}{16 \text{ oz} \times 1} = \frac{1 \text{ lb} \times \cancel{12}^{\,3}}{\cancel{16}_{4} \times 1} = \frac{1 \text{ lb} \times 3}{4 \times 1} = \frac{3 \text{ lb}}{4} = \frac{3}{4}\text{ lb}$$

19. 6 C = _____ ℥

$$\text{oz} = \frac{8 \text{ oz} \times 6 \text{ C}}{1 \text{ C} \times 1} = \frac{8 \text{ oz} \times 6}{1 \times 1} = \frac{48 \text{ oz}}{1} = 48\text{ oz}$$

20. 20 ℨ = _____ tsp

$$\text{tsp} = \frac{1 \text{ tsp} \times 20 \text{ dr}}{1 \text{ dr} \times 1} = \frac{1 \text{ tsp} \times 20}{1 \times 1} = \frac{20 \text{ tsp}}{1} = 20\text{ tsp}$$

Chapter 8: The Metric System

1. 44 mcg = _____ mg

$$\text{mg} = \frac{1 \text{ mg} \times 44 \text{ mcg}}{1000 \text{ mcg} \times 1} = \frac{1 \text{ mg} \times 44}{1000 \times 1} = \frac{44 \text{ mg}}{1000} = 0.044\text{ mg}$$

2. 180 mm = _____ cm

$$\text{cm} = \frac{1 \text{ cm} \times 180 \text{ mm}}{10 \text{ mm} \times 1} = \frac{1 \text{ cm} \times \cancel{180}^{\,18}}{\cancel{10}_{1} \times 1} = \frac{1 \text{ cm} \times 18}{1 \times 1} = \frac{18 \text{ cm}}{1} = 18\text{ cm}$$

3. 0.75 L = _____ cc

$$\text{cc} = \frac{1000 \text{ cc} \times 0.75 \text{ L}}{1 \text{ L} \times 1} = \frac{1000 \text{ cc} \times 0.75}{1 \times 1} = \frac{750 \text{ cc}}{1} = 750\text{ cc}$$

4. 26 mg = _____ g

$$\text{g} = \frac{1 \text{ g} \times 26 \text{ mg}}{1000 \text{ mg} \times 1} = \frac{1 \text{ g} \times 26}{1000 \times 1} = \frac{26 \text{ g}}{1000} = 0.026\text{ g}$$

5. 450 g = _____ kg

$$\text{kg} = \frac{1 \text{ kg} \times 450 \text{ g}}{1000 \text{ g} \times 1} = \frac{1 \text{ kg} \times \cancel{450}^{\,45}}{\cancel{1000}_{100} \times 1} = \frac{45 \text{ kg}}{100} = 0.45\text{ kg}$$

6. 1500 mcg = _____ g

$$\text{g} = \frac{1 \text{ g} \times 1 \text{ mg} \times 1500 \text{ mcg}}{1000 \text{ mg} \times 1000 \text{ mcg} \times 1} = \frac{1 \text{ g} \times 1 \times \cancel{1500}^{\,1.5}}{1000 \times \cancel{1000}_{1} \times 1} = \frac{1.5 \text{ g}}{1000} = 0.0015\text{ g}$$

7. 3 g = _____ mg

$$\text{mg} = \frac{1000 \text{ mg} \times 3 \text{ g}}{1 \text{ g} \times 1} = \frac{1000 \text{ mg} \times 3}{1 \times 1} = \frac{3000 \text{ mg}}{1} = 3000\text{ mg}$$

8. 0.51 kg = _____ g

$$\text{g} = \frac{1000 \text{ g} \times 0.51 \text{ kg}}{1 \text{ kg} \times 1} = \frac{1000 \text{ g} \times 0.51}{1 \times 1} = \frac{510 \text{ g}}{1} = 510\text{ g}$$

9. 0.06 mg = _____ mcg

$$\text{mcg} = \frac{1000 \text{ mcg} \times 0.06 \text{ mg}}{1 \text{ mg} \times 1} = \frac{1000 \text{ mcg} \times 0.06}{1 \times 1} = \frac{60 \text{ mcg}}{1} = 60\text{ mcg}$$

10. 5.5 kg = _____ g

$$g = \frac{1000 \ \ g \ \ \times \ 5.5 \ \ kg}{1 \ \ kg \ \times \ 1} = \frac{1000 \ \ g \ \times \ 5.5}{1 \ \times \ 1} = \frac{5500 \ \ g}{1} = 5500 \, g$$

11. 12 cc = _____ ml

1 cc = 1 ml; therefore, 12 cc = 12 ml

12. 12 g = _____ mg

$$mg = \frac{1000 \ \ mg \ \times \ 12 \ \ g}{1 \ \ g \ \times \ 1} = \frac{1000 \ \ mg \ \times \ 12}{1 \ \times \ 1} = \frac{12000 \ \ mg}{1} = 12000 \, mg$$

13. 2.5 kg = _____ g

$$g = \frac{1000 \ \ g \ \times \ 2.5 \ \ kg}{1 \ \ kg \ \times \ 1} = \frac{1000 \ \ g \ \times \ 2.5}{1 \ \times \ 1} = \frac{2500 \ \ g}{1} = 2500 \, g$$

14. 53 mcg = _____ mg

$$mg = \frac{1 \ \ mg \ \times \ 53 \ \ mcg}{1000 \ \ mcg \ \times \ 1} = \frac{1 \ \ mg \ \times \ 53}{1 \ \times \ 1} = \frac{53 \ \ mg}{1000} = 0.053 \, mg$$

15. 8 cm = _____ mm

$$mm = \frac{10 \ \ mm \ \times \ 8 \ \ cm}{1 \ \ cm \ \times \ 1} = \frac{10 \ \ mm \ \times \ 8}{1 \ \times \ 1} = \frac{80 \ \ mm}{1} = 80 \, mm$$

16. 225 ml = _____ L

$$L = \frac{1 \ \ L \ \times \ 225 \ \ ml}{1000 \ \ ml \ \times \ 1} = \frac{1 \ \ L \ \times \ 225}{1000 \ \times \ 1} = \frac{225 \ \ L}{1000} = 0.225 \, L$$

17. 1200 mg = _____ mcg

$$mcg = \frac{1000 \ \ mcg \ \times \ 1200 \ \ mg}{1 \ \ mg \ \times \ 1} = \frac{1000 \ \ mcg \ \times \ 1200}{1 \ \times \ 1} = 1,200,000 \, mcg$$

18. 1500 ml = _____ L

$$L = \frac{1 \ \ L \ \times \ 1500 \ \ ml}{1000 \ \ ml \ \times \ 1} = \frac{1 \ \ L \ \times \ \overset{1.5}{\cancel{1500}}}{\underset{1}{\cancel{1000}} \ \times \ 1} = \frac{1.5 \ \ L}{1} = 1.5 \, L$$

19. 0.005 g = _____ mcg

$$mcg = \frac{1000 \ \ mcg \ \times \ 1000 \ \ mg \ \times \ 0.005 \ \ g}{1 \ \ mg \ \times \ 1 \ \ g \ \times \ 1} = \frac{1000 \ \ mcg \ \times \ 1000 \ \times \ 0.005}{1 \ \times \ 1 \ \times \ 1} = \frac{5000 \ \ mcg}{1} = 5000 \, mcg$$

20. 0.4 L = _____ ml

$$ml = \frac{1000 \ \ ml \ \times \ 0.4 \ \ L}{1 \ \ L \ \times \ 1} = \frac{1000 \ \ ml \ \times \ 0.4}{1 \ \times \ 1} = \frac{400 \ \ ml}{1} = 400 \, ml$$

Chapter 9: Conversions Among Measurement Systems

1. gr 1/300 = _____ mg

$$mg = \frac{60 \ \ mg \ \times \ gr \ 1/300}{1 \ \ gr \ \times \ 1} = \frac{\overset{1}{\cancel{60}} \ \ mg \ \times \ 1}{1 \ \times \ \underset{5}{\cancel{300}}} = \frac{1 \ \ mg \ \times \ 1}{1 \ \times \ 5}$$

$$= \frac{1 \ \ mg}{5} = 0.2 \, mg$$

$$mg = \frac{1000 \ \ mg \ \times \ gr \ 1/300}{15 \ \ gr \ \times \ 1} = \frac{\overset{2}{\cancel{1000}} \ \ mg \ \times \ 1}{\underset{3}{\cancel{15}} \ \times \ \underset{3}{\cancel{300}}}$$

$$= \frac{2 \ \ mg \ \times \ 1}{3 \ \times \ 3} = \frac{2 \ \ mg}{9} = 0.22 \, mg$$

2. 200 mcg = _____ gr

$$gr = \frac{1 \ \ gr \ \times \ 1 \ \ mg \ \times \ 200 \ \ mcg}{60 \ \ mg \ \times \ 1000 \ \ mcg \ \times \ 1}$$

$$= \frac{1 \ \ gr \ \times \ 1 \ \times \ \overset{1}{\cancel{200}}}{60 \ \times \ \underset{5}{\cancel{1000}} \ \times \ 1} = \frac{1 \ \ gr \ \times \ 1 \ \times \ 1}{60 \ \times \ 5 \ \times \ 1}$$

$$= \frac{1 \ \ gr}{300} = gr \ 1/300$$

$$gr = \frac{15 \ \ gr \ \times \ 1 \ \ mg \ \times \ 200 \ \ mcg}{1000 \ \ mg \ \times \ 1000 \ \ mcg \ \times \ 1}$$

$$= \frac{\overset{3}{\cancel{15}} \ \ gr \ \times \ 1 \ \times \ \overset{1}{\cancel{200}}}{1000 \ \times \ \underset{\cancel{5}}{1000} \ \times \ 1} = \frac{3 \ \ gr \ \times \ 1 \ \times \ 1}{1000 \ \times \ 1 \ \times \ 1}$$

$$= \frac{3 \ \ gr}{1000} = gr \ 3/1000$$

3. 25 minims = _____ cc

$$cc = \frac{1 \ \ cc \ \times \ 25 \ \ mx}{15 \ \ mx \ \times \ 1} = \frac{1 \ \ cc \ \times \ \overset{5}{\cancel{25}}}{\underset{3}{\cancel{15}} \ \times \ 1} = \frac{1 \ \ cc \ \times \ 5}{3 \ \times \ 1}$$

$$= \frac{5 \ \ cc}{3} = 1.67 \, cc$$

$$cc = \frac{1 \ \ cc \ \times \ 25 \ \ mx}{16 \ \ mx \ \times \ 1} = \frac{1 \ \ cc \ \times \ 25}{16 \ \times \ 1} = \frac{25 \ \ cc}{16}$$

$$= 1.56 \, cc$$

4. gr viiss = _____ g

$$g = \frac{1 \ \ g \ \times \ gr \ 7.5}{15 \ \ gr \ \times \ 1} = \frac{1 \ \ g \ \times \ \overset{0.5}{\cancel{7.5}}}{\underset{1}{\cancel{15}} \ \times \ 1} = \frac{1 \ \ g \ \times \ 0.5}{1 \ \times \ 1} = \frac{0.5 \ \ g}{1} = 0.5 \, g$$

5. 7 lb 8 oz = _____ kg

$$kg = \frac{1 \ \ kg \ \times \ 7.5 \ \ lb}{2.2 \ \ lb \ \times \ 1} = \frac{1 \ \ kg \ \times \ 7.5}{2.2 \ \times \ 1} = \frac{7.5 \ \ kg}{2.2} = 3.41 \, kg$$

6. 55 kg = _____ lb

$$lb = \frac{2.2 \text{ lb} \times 55 \text{ kg}}{1 \text{ kg} \times 1} = \frac{2.2 \text{ lb} \times 55}{1 \times 1} = \frac{121 \text{ lb}}{1} = 121 \text{ lb}$$

7. 35 mm = _____ in

$$in = \frac{1 \text{ in} \times 1 \text{ cm} \times 35 \text{ mm}}{2.5 \text{ cm} \times 10 \text{ mm} \times 1} = \frac{1 \text{ in} \times 1 \times \overset{7}{\cancel{35}}}{\underset{0.5}{\cancel{2.5}} \times 10 \times 1} = \frac{1 \text{ in} \times 1 \times 7}{0.5 \times 10 \times 1} = \frac{7 \text{ in}}{5} = 1\frac{2}{5} \text{ in}$$

8. 0.4 mg = _____ gr

$$gr = \frac{1 \text{ gr} \times 0.4 \text{ mg}}{60 \text{ mg} \times 1} = \frac{1 \text{ gr} \times \overset{1}{\cancel{0.4}}}{\underset{150}{\cancel{60}} \times 1} = \frac{1 \text{ gr}}{150}$$

$$= \text{gr } 1/150$$

$$gr = \frac{15 \text{ gr} \times 0.4 \text{ mg}}{1000 \text{ mg} \times 1} = \frac{\overset{3}{\cancel{15}} \text{ gr} \times \overset{1}{\cancel{0.4}}}{\underset{\underset{500}{200}}{\cancel{1000}} \times 1} = \frac{3 \text{ gr}}{500}$$

$$= \text{gr } 3/500$$

9. gr XXX = _____ mg

$$mg = \frac{1000 \text{ mg} \times \text{gr } 30}{15 \text{ gr} \times 1} = \frac{1000 \text{ mg} \times \overset{2}{\cancel{30}}}{\underset{1}{\cancel{15}} \times 1}$$

$$= \frac{1000 \text{ mg} \times 2}{1 \times 1} = \frac{2000 \text{ mg}}{1} = 2000 \text{ mg}$$

$$mg = \frac{60 \text{ mg} \times \text{gr } 30}{1 \text{ gr} \times 1} = \frac{60 \text{ mg} \times 30}{1 \times 1}$$

$$= \frac{1800 \text{ mg}}{1} = 1800 \text{ mg}$$

10. 0.75 ml = _____ minims

$$mx = \frac{15 \text{ mx} \times 0.75 \text{ ml}}{1 \text{ ml} \times 1} = \frac{15 \text{ mx} \times 0.75}{1 \times 1} = \frac{11.25 \text{ mx}}{1}$$

$$= 11.25 \text{ mx}$$

$$mx = \frac{16 \text{ mx} \times 0.75 \text{ ml}}{1 \text{ ml} \times 1} = \frac{16 \text{ mx} \times 0.75}{1 \times 1} = \frac{12 \text{ mx}}{1} = 12 \text{ mx}$$

11. gr 1/600 = _____ mcg

$$mcg = \frac{1000 \text{ mcg} \times 60 \text{ mg} \times \text{gr } 1/600}{1 \text{ mg} \times 1 \text{ gr} \times 1} = \frac{\overset{10}{\cancel{1000}} \text{ mcg} \times \overset{10}{\cancel{60}} \times 1}{1 \times 1 \times \underset{\underset{1}{\cancel{6}}}{\cancel{600}}} = \frac{10 \text{ mcg} \times 10 \times 1}{1 \times 1 \times 1} = \frac{100 \text{ mcg}}{1} = 100 \text{ mcg}$$

12. 2 g = _____ gr

$$gr = \frac{15 \text{ gr} \times 2 \text{ g}}{1 \text{ g} \times 1} = \frac{15 \text{ gr} \times 2}{1 \times 1} = \frac{30 \text{ gr}}{1} = 30 \text{ gr}$$

13. 4 lb 5 oz = _____ g

$$g = \frac{1000 \text{ g} \times 1 \text{ kg} \times 4^{5/16} \text{ lb}}{1 \text{ kg} \times 2.2 \text{ lb} \times 1} = \frac{\overset{\overset{125}{\cancel{500}}}{\cancel{1000}} \text{ g} \times 1 \times 69}{1 \times \underset{1.1}{\cancel{2.2}} \times \underset{4}{\cancel{16}}} = \frac{8625 \text{ g}}{4.4} = 1960.23 \text{ g}$$

14. 45 mg = _____ gr

$$gr = \frac{1 \text{ gr} \times 45 \text{ mg}}{60 \text{ mg} \times 1} = \frac{1 \text{ gr} \times \overset{3}{\cancel{45}}}{\underset{4}{\cancel{60}} \times 1} = \frac{1 \text{ gr} \times 3}{4 \times 1}$$

$$= \frac{3 \text{ gr}}{4} = \text{gr} \frac{3}{4}$$

$$gr = \frac{15 \text{ gr} \times 45 \text{ mg}}{1000 \text{ mg} \times 1} = \frac{\overset{3}{\cancel{15}} \text{ gr} \times \overset{9}{\cancel{45}}}{\underset{\underset{40}{200}}{\cancel{1000}} \times 1} = \frac{27 \text{ gr}}{40} = \text{gr} \frac{27}{40}$$

15. gr iiss = _____ g

$$g = \frac{1 \text{ g} \times \text{gr } 2.5}{15 \text{ gr} \times 1} = \frac{1 \text{ g} \times \overset{0.5}{\cancel{2.5}}}{\underset{3}{\cancel{15}} \times 1} = \frac{1 \text{ gr} \times 0.5}{3 \times 1} = \frac{0.5 \text{ g}}{3} = 0.167 \text{ g}$$

16. 6 mg = _____ gr

$$gr = \frac{1 \text{ gr} \times 6 \text{ mg}}{60 \text{ mg} \times 1} = \frac{1 \text{ gr} \times \overset{1}{\cancel{6}}}{\underset{10}{\cancel{60}} \times 1} = \frac{1 \text{ gr} \times 1}{10 \times 1}$$

$$= \frac{1 \text{ gr}}{10} = \text{gr } 1/10$$

$$gr = \frac{15 \text{ gr} \times 6 \text{ mg}}{1000 \text{ mg} \times 1} = \frac{\overset{3}{\cancel{15}} \text{ gr} \times \overset{3}{\cancel{6}}}{\underset{\underset{100}{200}}{\cancel{1000}} \times 1} = \frac{3 \text{ gr} \times 3}{100 \times 1}$$

$$= \frac{9 \text{ gr}}{100} = \text{gr } 9/100$$

17-20. 1/3 C creamed broccoli soup

$$ml = \frac{250 \text{ ml} \times 1/3 \text{ C}}{1 \text{ C} \times 1} = \frac{250 \text{ ml} \times 1}{1 \times 3} = \frac{250 \text{ ml}}{3} = 83 \text{ ml}$$

$$ml = \frac{30 \text{ ml} \times 8 \text{ oz} \times 1/3 \text{ C}}{1 \text{ oz} \times 1 \text{ C} \times 1} = \frac{\overset{10}{\cancel{30}} \text{ ml} \times 8 \times 1}{1 \times 1 \times \cancel{3}_{1}}$$

$$= \frac{80 \text{ ml}}{1} = 80 \text{ ml}$$

1 C lettuce and tomato salad: not fluid intake

2 slices roast beef: not fluid intake

1/2 C oven-browned potatoes: not fluid intake

1/2 pint milk

$$ml = \frac{500 \text{ ml} \times 1/2 \text{ pt}}{1 \text{ pt} \times 1} = \frac{\overset{250}{\cancel{500}} \text{ ml} \times 1}{1 \times \cancel{2}_{1}} = \frac{250 \text{ ml}}{1} = 250 \text{ ml}$$

$$ml = \frac{30 \text{ ml} \times 16 \text{ oz} \times 1/2 \text{ pt}}{1 \text{ oz} \times 1 \text{ pt} \times 1} = \frac{30 \text{ ml} \times \overset{8}{\cancel{16}} \times 1}{1 \times 1 \times \cancel{2}_{1}}$$

$$= \frac{240 \text{ ml}}{1} = 240 \text{ ml}$$

1/2 C sliced fresh fruit: not fluid intake

2 glasses iced tea

$$ml = \frac{250 \text{ ml} \times 2 \text{ C}}{1 \text{ C} \times 1} = \frac{250 \text{ ml} \times 2}{1 \times 1} = \frac{500 \text{ ml}}{1} = \underline{500 \text{ ml}}$$

$$ml = \frac{30 \text{ ml} \times 8 \text{ oz} \times 2 \text{ C}}{1 \text{ oz} \times 1 \text{ C} \times 1} = \frac{30 \text{ ml} \times 8 \times 2}{1 \times 1 \times 1}$$

$$= \frac{480 \text{ ml}}{1} = \underline{480 \text{ ml}}$$

Total   833 ml   800 ml

UNIT IV: DOSAGE CONVERSIONS AND CALCULATIONS

Chapter 10: Interpretation Of Medication Orders And Labels

1. Esidrex 50 mg PO b.i.d. = Esidrex 50 milligrams by mouth twice a day.
2. 1000 cc D5NS IV q.8h. = 1000 cubic centimeters 5% dextrose in normal saline intravenously every 8 hours.
3. Pyridium 200 mg PO t.i.d. = Pyridium 200 milligrams by mouth 3 times a day.
4. Morphine sulfate gr 1/8 sub q q.4h. p.r.n. = morphine sulfate grains 1/8 subcutaneously every 4 hours as needed (when required).
5. Phenobarbital gr 1/2 PO q.i.d. = phenobarbital 1/2 grain by mouth 4 times a day.
6. Demerol 75 mg c Vistaril 25 mg IM q.4h. PRN = Demerol 75 milligrams with Vistaril 25 mg intramuscularly every 4 hours as needed (when required).
7. Digoxin 0.25 mg q.d. PO = digoxin 0.25 milligrams every day by mouth.
8. Bicillin 1,200,000 U IM stat. = Bicillin 1,200,000 units intramuscularly immediately.
9. Amphogel 30 cc PO q.2h. = Amphogel 30 cubic centimeters by mouth every 2 hours.
10. 1000 ml D5W c KCl 20 mEq IV q.8h. = 1000 milliliters 5% dextrose in water with potassium chloride 20 milliequivalents intravenously every 8 hours.
11. Unit of answer: mg/d; Factors: 500 mg = (q) 4 h; 24 h = 1 d

$$\frac{mg}{d} = \frac{500 \text{ mg} \times 24 \text{ h}}{(q)4 \text{ h} \times 1 \text{ d}} = \frac{500 \text{ mg} \times \overset{6}{\cancel{24}}}{\cancel{4}_{1} \times 1 \text{ d}} = \frac{500 \text{ mg} \times 6}{1 \times 1 \text{ d}} = \frac{3000 \text{ mg}}{1 \text{ d}} = 3000 \text{ mg/d}$$

12. Unit of answer: mg/d; Factors: 250 mg = 1 dose; 4 doses = 1 d

$$\frac{mg}{d} = \frac{250 \text{ mg} \times 4 \text{ doses}}{1 \text{ dose} \times 1 \text{ d}} = \frac{250 \text{ mg} \times 4}{1 \times 1 \text{ d}} = \frac{1000 \text{ mg}}{1 \text{ d}} = 1000 \text{ mg/d}$$

13. Unit of answer: mg/d; Factors: 50 mg = 1 dose; 2 doses = 1 d

$$\frac{mg}{d} = \frac{50 \text{ mg} \times 2 \text{ doses}}{1 \text{ dose} \times 1 \text{ d}} = \frac{50 \text{ mg} \times 2}{1 \times 1 \text{ d}} = \frac{100 \text{ mg}}{1 \text{ d}} = 100 \text{ mg/d}$$

14. Unit of answer: gr/d; Factors: gr X = (q) 3 h; 24 h = 1 d

$$\frac{gr}{d} = \frac{10 \text{ gr} \times 24 \text{ h}}{(q)3 \text{ h} \times 1 \text{ d}} = \frac{10 \text{ gr} \times \overset{8}{\cancel{24}}}{\cancel{3}_{1} \times 1 \text{ d}} = \frac{10 \text{ gr} \times 8}{1 \times 1 \text{ d}} = \frac{80 \text{ gr}}{1 \text{ d}} = 80 \text{ gr/d}$$

15. Medication order: Atropine 0.2 mg s.c. noc Labels: Atropine 400 mcg (0.4 mg)/ml and 1 mg/ml
    400 mcg (0.4 mg)/ml is the label to choose.
16. Medication order: nitroglycerine gr 1/200 SL p.r.n. Labels: Nitroglycerine 0.3 mg tab and 0.4 mg tab.

$$mg = \frac{60 \text{ mg} \times \text{gr } 1/200}{1 \text{ gr} \times 1} = \frac{\overset{3}{\cancel{60}} \text{ mg} \times 1}{1 \times \underset{10}{\cancel{200}}} = \frac{3 \text{ mg} \times 1}{1 \times 10} = \frac{3 \text{ mg}}{10} = 0.3 \text{ mg}$$

The label to choose is 0.3 mg.

17. Medication order: morphine sulfate gr 1/4 s.c. stat. Labels: morphine sulfate 10 mg/ml and 15 mg/ml

$$mg = \frac{60 \text{ mg} \times \text{gr } 1/4}{1 \text{ gr} \times 1} = \frac{\overset{15}{\cancel{60}} \text{ mg} \times 1}{1 \times \cancel{4}_{1}} = \frac{15 \text{ mg} \times 1}{1 \times 1} = \frac{15 \text{ mg}}{1} = 15 \text{ mg}$$

The label to choose is 15 mg.

18. Medication order: acetaminophen gr V PO q.4h. p.r.n. Labels: acetaminophen 325 mg tab and 500 mg tab.

$$mg = \frac{60 \ mg \ \times \ 5 \ gr}{1 \ gr \ \times \ 1} = \frac{60 \ mg \ \times \ 5}{1 \ \times \ 1} = \frac{300 \ mg}{1} = 300 \ mg$$

The label to choose is 325 mg tab.

19. Medication order: morphine sulfate gr 1/7 IM q.4h. p.r.n. Labels: morphine sulfate 10 mg/ml and 15 mg/ml

$$mg = \frac{60 \ mg \ \times \ gr \ 1/7}{1 \ gr \ \times \ 1} = \frac{60 \ mg \ \times \ 1}{1 \ \times \ 7} = \frac{60 \ mg}{7} = 8.57 \ mg$$

The correct label to choose is 10 mg/ml.

20. Medication order: amoxicillin 0.5 g q.6h. PO Labels: amoxicillin 250 mg tab and 500 mg tab.

$$mg = \frac{1000 \ mg \ \times \ 0.5 \ g}{1 \ g \ \times \ 1} = \frac{1000 \ mg \ \times \ 0.5}{1 \ \times \ 1} = \frac{500 \ mg}{1} = 500 \ mg$$

The correct label to choose is 500 mg tab.

Chapter 11: Calculation Of Oral Medication Dosages

1. Factors: 1 tab = 400,000 U; 200,000 U/1

$$tab = \frac{1 \ tab \ \times \ 200,000 \ U}{400,000 \ U \ \times \ 1} = \frac{1 \ tab \ \times \ \overset{1}{\cancel{200,000}}}{\underset{2}{\cancel{400,000}} \ \times \ 1} = \frac{1 \ tab}{2} = \frac{1}{2} \ tab$$

2. Factors: 100 mcg = 5 ml (cc); 0.25 mg/1. Conversion factor: 1 mg = 1000 mcg

$$cc = \frac{5 \ cc \ \times \ 1000 \ mcg \ \times \ 0.25 \ mg}{100 \ mcg \ \times \ 1 \ mg \ \times \ 1} = \frac{5 \ cc \ \times \ \overset{10}{\cancel{1000}} \times \ 0.25}{\underset{1}{\cancel{100}} \ \times \ 1 \times \ 1} = \frac{12.5 \ cc}{1} = 12.5 \ cc$$

3. Factors: 0.25 g = 5 ml; 100 mg/1. Conversion factor: 1 g = 1000 mg

$$ml = \frac{5 \ ml \ \times \ 1 \ g \ \times \ 100 \ mg}{0.25 \ g \ \times \ 1000 \ mg \ \times \ 1} = \frac{\overset{1}{\cancel{5}} \ ml \ \times \ 1 \ \times \ \overset{1}{\cancel{100}}}{\underset{0.05}{\cancel{0.25}} \ \times \ \underset{10}{\cancel{1000}} \times \ 1} = \frac{1 \ ml}{0.5} = 2 \ ml$$

4. Dosage ordered: Coumadin 12 mg PO q.d. Combinations of two 5 mg tab plus one 2 mg tab or one 7.5 mg tab, one 2.5 mg tab and one 2 mg tab use the fewest number of tablets.

5. Factors: 1 tab = 2 mg; 1/60 gr/1. Conversion factor: 1 gr = 60 mg

$$tab = \frac{1 \ tab \ \times \ 60 \ mg \ \times \ gr \ 1/60}{2 \ mg \ \times \ 1 \ gr \ \times \ 1} = \frac{1 \ tab \ \times \ \overset{1}{\cancel{60}} \times \ 1}{2 \ \times \ 1 \times \ \underset{1}{\cancel{60}}} = \frac{1 \ tab}{2} = \frac{1}{2} \ tab$$

6. Factors: 400 mcg = 1 tab; 0.6 mg/1. Conversion factor: 1 mg = 1000 mcg.

$$tab = \frac{1 \ tab \ \times \ 1000 \ mcg \ \times \ 0.6 \ mg}{400 \ mcg \ \times \ 1 \ mg \ \times \ 1} = \frac{1 \ tab \ \times \ \overset{5}{\cancel{1000}} \times \ 0.6}{\underset{2}{\cancel{400}} \ \times \ 1 \times \ 1} = \frac{3 \ tabs}{2} = 1\frac{1}{2} \ tabs$$

7. Factors: 10 mg = 1 ml; 1/3 gr/1. Conversion factor: 1 gr = 60 mg

$$ml = \frac{1 \ ml \ \times \ 60 \ mg \ \times \ gr \ 1/3}{10 \ mg \ \times \ 1 \ gr \ \times \ 1} = \frac{1 \ ml \ \times \ \overset{2}{\cancel{60}} \times \ 1}{\underset{1}{\cancel{10}} \ \times \ 1 \times \ \underset{1}{\cancel{3}}} = \frac{2 \ ml}{1} = 2 \ ml$$

8. Factors: 1 tab = 400 mcg; 1/300 gr/1. Conversion factors: 1 gr = 60 mg; 1 mg = 1000 mcg

$$tab = \frac{1 \ tab \ \times \ 1000 \ mcg \ \times \ 60 \ mg \ \times \ gr \ 1/300}{400 \ mcg \ \times \ 1 \ mg \ \times \ 1 \ gr \ \times \ 1} = \frac{1 \ tab \ \times \ \overset{1}{\cancel{1000}} \times \ \overset{1}{\cancel{60}} \times \ 1}{\underset{2}{\cancel{400}} \ \times \ 1 \times \ 1 \times \ \underset{1}{\cancel{300}}} = \frac{1 \ tab}{2} = \frac{1}{2} \ tab$$

9. Factors: 1 ml = 25 mcg; 0.2 mg/1. Conversion factor: 1 mg = 1000 mcg

$$ml = \frac{1 \ ml \ \times \ 1000 \ mcg \ \times \ 0.2 \ mg}{25 \ mcg \ \times \ 1 \ mg \ \times \ 1} = \frac{1 \ ml \ \times \ \overset{40}{\cancel{1000}} \times \ 0.2}{\underset{1}{\cancel{25}} \ \times \ 1 \times \ 1} = \frac{8 \ ml}{1} = 8 \ ml$$

10. Factors: 1 tab = 4 mg; 1/30 gr/1. Conversion factor: 1 gr = 60 mg

$$tab = \frac{1 \ tab \ \times \ 60 \ mg \ \times \ gr \ 1/30}{4 \ mg \ \times \ 1 \ gr \ \times \ 1} = \frac{1 \ tab \ \times \ \overset{15}{\cancel{60}} \times \ 1}{\underset{1}{\cancel{4}} \ \times \ 1 \times \ \underset{2}{\cancel{30}}} = \frac{1 \ tab}{2} = \frac{1}{2} \ tab$$

11. Factors: 1 tab = 25 mcg; 0.05 mg/1 Conversion factor: 1 mg = 1000 mcg

$$\text{tab} = \frac{1 \text{ tab } \times \ 1000 \text{ mcg } \times \ 0.05 \text{ mg}}{25 \text{ mcg } \times \quad 1 \quad \times \quad 1} = \frac{1 \text{ tab } \times \ \overset{40}{\cancel{1000}} \times \ 0.05}{\underset{1}{\cancel{25}} \quad \times \quad 1 \ \times \quad 1} = \frac{2 \text{ tab}}{1} = 2 \text{ tab}$$

12. Factors: 1 tab = 0.1 g; gr 3/1 Conversion factor: 1 g = 15 gr

$$\text{tab} = \frac{1 \text{ tab } \times \ 1 \text{ g } \times \ 3 \text{ gr}}{0.1 \text{ g } \times \ 15 \text{ gr } \times \ 1} = \frac{1 \text{ tab } \times \ 1 \times \overset{1}{\cancel{3}}}{0.1 \quad \times \ \underset{5}{\cancel{15}} \times \ 1} = \frac{1 \text{ tab}}{0.5} = 2 \text{ tab}$$

13. Factors: 5 ml (cc) = 0.25 mg; 30 mcg/1. Conversion factor: 1 mg = 1000 mcg

$$\text{cc} = \frac{5 \text{ cc } \times \quad 1 \text{ mg } \times \ 30 \text{ mcg}}{0.25 \text{ mg } \times \ 1000 \text{ mcg } \times \quad 1} = \frac{\overset{1}{\cancel{5}} \text{ cc } \times \quad 1 \times \overset{3}{\cancel{30}}}{0.25 \quad \times \ \underset{\underset{20}{200}}{\cancel{1000}} \times \ 1} = \frac{3 \text{ cc}}{5} = 0.6 \text{ cc}$$

14. Factors: 5 ml (1 tsp) = 0.5 g; 7.5 gr/1 Conversion factor: 1 g = 15 gr

$$\text{tsp} = \frac{1 \text{ tsp } \times \ 1 \text{ g } \times \ 7.5 \text{ gr}}{0.5 \text{ g } \times \ 15 \text{ gr } \times \ 1} = \frac{1 \text{ tsp } \times \quad 1 \times \overset{\overset{1}{\cancel{15}}}{\cancel{7.5}}}{\underset{1}{\cancel{0.5}} \quad \times \ \underset{1}{\cancel{15}} \times \ 1} = \frac{1 \text{ tsp}}{1} = 1 \text{ tsp}$$

15. Factors: 1 tab = 40 mg; 1/3 gr/1 Conversion factor: 1 gr = 60 mg

$$\text{tab} = \frac{1 \text{ tab } \times \ 60 \text{ mg } \times \ \text{gr } 1/3}{40 \text{ mg } \times \ 1 \text{ gr } \times \quad 1} = \frac{1 \text{ tab } \times \ \overset{3}{\cancel{60}} \times \overset{1}{\cancel{3}}}{\underset{2}{\cancel{40}} \quad \times \ 1 \times \underset{1}{\cancel{3}}} = \frac{1 \text{ tab}}{2} = \frac{1}{2} \text{ tab}$$

16. Factors: 1 tab = 20 mg; 50 mg/1

$$\text{tab} = \frac{1 \text{ tab } \times \ 50 \text{ mg}}{20 \text{ mg } \times \ 1} = \frac{1 \text{ tab } \times \ \overset{5}{\cancel{50}}}{\underset{2}{\cancel{20}} \quad \times \ 1} = \frac{5 \text{ tab}}{2} = 2\frac{1}{2} \text{ tab}$$

17. Factors: 1 cap = 0.1 g; 400 mg/1 Conversion factor: 1 g = 1000 mg

$$\text{cap} = \frac{1 \text{ cap } \times \quad 1 \text{ g } \quad \times \ 400 \text{ mg}}{0.1 \text{ g } \times \ 1000 \text{ mg } \times \quad 1} = \frac{1 \text{ cap } \times \quad 1 \times \overset{4}{\cancel{400}}}{0.1 \quad \times \ \underset{10}{\cancel{1000}} \times \ 1} = \frac{4 \text{ cap}}{1} = 4 \text{ cap}$$

18. Factors: 5 ml (1 tsp) = 500 mg; 250 mg/1

$$\text{tsp} = \frac{1 \text{ tsp } \times \ 250 \text{ mg}}{500 \text{ mg } \times \ 1} = \frac{1 \text{ tsp } \times \ \overset{1}{\cancel{250}}}{\underset{2}{\cancel{500}} \quad \times \ 1} = \frac{1 \text{ tsp}}{2} = \frac{1}{2} \text{ tsp}$$

19. Factors: 1 tab = 500 mg; 1.25 g/1 Conversion factor: 1 g = 1000 mg

$$\text{tab} = \frac{1 \text{ tab } \times \ 1000 \text{ mg } \times \ 1.25 \text{ g}}{500 \text{ mg } \times \quad 1 \text{ g } \times \quad 1} = \frac{1 \text{ tab } \times \ \overset{2}{\cancel{1000}} \times \ 1.25}{\underset{1}{\cancel{500}} \quad \times \quad 1 \ \times \quad 1} = \frac{2.5 \text{ tab}}{1} = 2\frac{1}{2} \text{ tab}$$

20. Factors: 1 ml = 2 mg; 1/30 gr/1. Conversion factor: 1 gr = 60 mg

$$\text{ml} = \frac{1 \text{ ml } \times \ 60 \text{ mg } \times \ \text{gr } 1/30}{2 \text{ mg } \times \ 1 \text{ gr } \times \quad 1} = \frac{1 \text{ ml } \times \ \overset{\overset{1}{\cancel{30}}}{\cancel{60}} \times \quad 1}{\underset{1}{\cancel{2}} \quad \times \ 1 \times \underset{1}{\cancel{30}}} = \frac{1 \text{ ml}}{1} = 1 \text{ ml}$$

Chapter 12: Calculation Of Parenteral Medication Dosages

1. Factors: 12.5 mg = 1 ml; 35 mg/1

$$\text{ml} = \frac{1 \text{ ml } \times \ 35 \text{ mg}}{12.5 \text{ mg } \times \ 1} = \frac{1 \text{ ml } \times \ \overset{7}{\cancel{35}}}{\underset{2.5}{\cancel{12.5}} \quad \times \ 1} = \frac{7 \text{ ml}}{2.5} = 2.8 \text{ ml}$$

2. Factors: 300 mg = 1 ml; 200 mg/l. Conversion factor: 15 (16) mx = 1 ml

$$mx = \frac{15 \text{ mx} \times 1 \text{ ml} \times 200 \text{ mg}}{1 \text{ ml} \times 300 \text{ mg} \times 1} = \frac{\overset{5}{\cancel{15}} \text{ mx} \times 1 \times \overset{2}{\cancel{200}}}{1 \times \underset{\underset{1}{\cancel{3}}}{\cancel{300}} \times 1} = \frac{10 \text{ mx}}{1} = 10 \text{ mx}$$

$$mx = \frac{16 \text{ mx} \times 1 \text{ ml} \times 200 \text{ mg}}{1 \text{ ml} \times 300 \text{ mg} \times 1} = \frac{16 \text{ mx} \times 1 \times \overset{2}{\cancel{200}}}{1 \times \underset{3}{\cancel{300}} \times 1} = \frac{32 \text{ mx}}{3} = 10.67 \text{ mx}$$

3. Factors: 6 g = 4 ml; 250 mg/l. Conversion factor: 1 g = 1000 mg

$$ml = \frac{4 \text{ ml} \times 1 \text{ g} \times 250 \text{ mg}}{6 \text{ g} \times 1000 \text{ mg} \times 1} = \frac{\overset{1}{\cancel{4}} \text{ ml} \times 1 \times \overset{1}{\cancel{250}}}{6 \times \underset{\underset{1}{\cancel{250}}}{\cancel{1000}} \times 1} = \frac{1 \text{ ml}}{6} = 0.167 \text{ ml} = 0.17 \text{ ml}$$

4. Factors: 600,000 U = 2 ml; 900,000 U/l

$$ml = \frac{2 \text{ ml} \times 900,000 \text{ U}}{600,000 \text{ U} \times 1} = \frac{2 \text{ ml} \times \overset{3}{\cancel{900,000}}}{\underset{2}{\cancel{600,000}} \times 1} = \frac{6 \text{ ml}}{2} = 3 \text{ ml}$$

5. Factors: 100 U = 1 ml; 36 U/l

$$ml = \frac{1 \text{ ml} \times 36 \text{ U}}{100 \text{ U} \times 1} = \frac{1 \text{ ml} \times 36}{100 \times 1} = \frac{36 \text{ ml}}{100} = 0.36 \text{ ml}$$

6. Factors: 1 mg = 1000 mcg; 0.6 mg/l.

$$mcg = \frac{1000 \text{ mcg} \times 0.6 \text{ mg}}{1 \text{ mg} \times 1} = \frac{1000 \text{ mcg} \times 0.6}{1 \text{ mg} \times 1} = \frac{600 \text{ mcg}}{1} = 600 \text{ mcg}$$

Because 0.6 mg = 600 mcg, Amp C, 600 mcg/ml, is the appropriate amp to choose.

7. Factors: 100 U = 1 ml; 68 U/l

$$ml = \frac{1 \text{ ml} \times 68 \text{ U}}{100 \text{ U} \times 1} = \frac{1 \text{ ml} \times 68}{100 \times 1} = \frac{68 \text{ ml}}{100} = 0.68 \text{ ml}$$

8. 10,000 U = 1 ml; 7500 U/l

$$ml = \frac{1 \text{ ml} \times 7500 \text{ U}}{10,000 \text{ U} \times 1} = \frac{1 \text{ ml} \times \overset{75}{\cancel{7500}}}{\underset{100}{\cancel{10,000}} \times 1} = \frac{75 \text{ ml}}{100} = 0.75 \text{ ml}$$

9. Factors: 400 mcg = 1 ml; 1/200 gr. Conversion factors: 1 gr = 60 mg; 1 mg = 1000 mcg

$$ml = \frac{1 \text{ ml} \times 1000 \text{ mcg} \times 60 \text{ mg} \times \text{gr } 1/200}{400 \text{ mcg} \times 1 \text{ mg} \times 1 \text{ gr} \times 1} = \frac{1 \text{ ml} \times \overset{1}{\cancel{1000}} \times \overset{3}{\cancel{60}} \times 1}{\underset{2}{\cancel{400}} \times 1 \times 1 \times \underset{10}{\cancel{200}}} = \frac{3 \text{ ml}}{4} = 0.75 \text{ ml}$$

10. Factors: 100 mg = 1 ml; gr 1.5/1 Conversion factor: 15 gr = 1000 mg

$$ml = \frac{1 \text{ ml} \times 1000 \text{ mg} \times \text{gr } 1.5}{100 \text{ mg} \times 15 \text{ gr} \times 1} = \frac{1 \text{ ml} \times \overset{10}{\cancel{1000}} \times \overset{0.1}{\cancel{1.5}}}{\underset{1}{\cancel{100}} \times \underset{1}{\cancel{15}} \times 1} = \frac{1 \text{ ml}}{1} = 1 \text{ ml}$$

11. Factors: 130 mg = 2 ml; 1/4 gr/1 Conversion factor: gr 1 = 60 mg

$$ml = \frac{2 \text{ ml} \times 60 \text{ mg} \times \text{gr } 1/4}{130 \text{ mg} \times 1 \text{ gr} \times 1} = \frac{\overset{1}{\cancel{2}} \text{ ml} \times \overset{3}{\cancel{60}} \times 1}{\underset{13}{\cancel{130}} \times 1 \times \underset{\underset{1}{\cancel{2}}}{\cancel{4}}} = \frac{3 \text{ ml}}{13} = 0.23 \text{ ml}$$

12. Factors: 500 mg = 1 ml; 0.5 g/1 Conversion factor: 1 g = 1000 ml

$$ml = \frac{1 \text{ ml} \times 1000 \text{ mg} \times 0.5 \text{ g}}{500 \text{ mg} \times 1 \text{ g} \times 1} = \frac{1 \text{ ml} \times \overset{2}{\cancel{1000}} \times 0.5}{\underset{1}{\cancel{500}} \times 1 \times 1} = \frac{1 \text{ ml}}{1} = 1 \text{ ml}$$

13. Factors: 250 mcg = 1 ml; 0.125 mg/1 Conversion factor: 1 mg = 1000 mcg

$$ml = \frac{1 \text{ ml} \times 1000 \text{ mcg} \times 0.125 \text{ mg}}{250 \text{ mcg} \times 1 \text{ mg} \times 1} = \frac{1 \text{ ml} \times \overset{4}{\cancel{1000}} \times 0.125}{\underset{1}{\cancel{250}} \times 1 \times 1} = \frac{0.5 \text{ ml}}{1} = 0.5 \text{ ml}$$

14. Factors: 1 g = 1 ml; 600 mg/1 Conversion factor: 1 g = 1000 mg

$$ml = \frac{1 \text{ ml} \times 1 \text{ g} \times 600 \text{ mg}}{1 \text{ g} \times 1000 \text{ mg} \times 1} = \frac{1 \text{ ml} \times 1 \times \overset{6}{\cancel{600}}}{1 \times \underset{10}{\cancel{1000}} \times 1} = \frac{6 \text{ ml}}{10} = 0.6 \text{ ml}$$

15. Factors: 25 mcg = 1 ml; 0.05 mg/l. Conversion factor: 1 mg = 1000 mcg

$$ml = \frac{1 \ ml \ \times \ 1000 \ mcg \ \times \ 0.05 \ mg}{25 \ mcg \ \times \ 1 \ mg \ \times \ 1} = \frac{1 \ ml \ \times \ \overset{40}{\cancel{1000}} \ \times \ 0.05}{\underset{1}{\cancel{25}} \ \times \ 1 \ \times \ 1} = \frac{2 \ ml}{1} = 2 \ ml$$

16. Factors: 1 g = 5 ml; gr 3/1. Conversion factor: 15 gr = 1000 mg

$$ml = \frac{5 \ ml \ \times \ 1 \ g \ \times \ 3 \ gr}{1 \ g \ \times \ 15 \ gr \ \times \ 1} = \frac{\overset{1}{\cancel{5}} \ ml \ \times \ 1 \ \times \ \overset{1}{\cancel{3}}}{1 \ \times \ \underset{\underset{1}{3}}{\cancel{15}} \ \times \ 1} = \frac{1 \ ml}{1} = 1 \ ml$$

17. Factors: 60 mg = 1 ml; 30 mg/1

$$ml = \frac{1 \ ml \ \times \ 30 \ mg}{60 \ mg \ \times \ 1} = \frac{1 \ ml \ \times \ \overset{1}{\cancel{30}}}{\underset{2}{\cancel{60}} \ \times \ 1} = \frac{1 \ ml}{2} = 0.5 \ ml$$

18. Factors: 20,000 U = 1 ml; 10,000 U/1

$$ml = \frac{1 \ ml \ \times \ 10,000 \ U}{20,000 \ U \ \times \ 1} = \frac{1 \ ml \ \times \ \overset{1}{\cancel{10,000}}}{\underset{2}{\cancel{20,000}} \ \times \ 1} = \frac{1 \ ml}{2} = 0.5 \ ml$$

19. Factors: 1 g × 2 ml; 125 mg/1 Conversion factor: 1 g = 1000 mg

$$ml = \frac{2 \ ml \ \times \ 1 \ g \ \times \ 125 \ mg}{1 \ g \ \times \ 1000 \ mg \ \times \ 1} = \frac{\overset{1}{\cancel{2}} \ ml \ \times \ 1 \ \times \ \overset{1}{\cancel{125}}}{1 \ \times \ \underset{\underset{4}{500}}{\cancel{1000}} \ \times \ 1} = \frac{1 \ ml}{4} = 0.25 \ ml$$

20. Factors: 1 g = 1 ml; 800 mg/1 Conversion factor: 1 g = 1000 mg

$$ml = \frac{1 \ ml \ \times \ 1 \ g \ \times \ 800 \ mg}{1 \ g \ \times \ 1000 \ mg \ \times \ 1} = \frac{1 \ ml \ \times \ 1 \ \times \ \overset{8}{\cancel{800}}}{1 \ \times \ \underset{10}{\cancel{1000}} \ \times \ 1} = \frac{8 \ ml}{10} = 0.8 \ ml$$

UNIT V: CALCULATIONS BASED ON BODY WEIGHT

Chapter 13: Dosages Based On Client Weight

1. Factors: 0.7 mcg = 1 lb; 1 kg = 2.2 lb; 45 kg/1

$$mcg = \frac{0.7 \ mcg \ \times \ 2.2 \ lb \ \times \ 45 \ kg}{1 \ lb \ \times \ 1 \ kg \ \times \ 1} = \frac{0.7 \ mcg \ \times \ 2.2 \ \times \ 45}{1 \ \times \ 1 \ \times \ 1} = \frac{69.3 \ mcg}{1} = 69.3 \ mcg$$

2. Factors: 30 mcg = 1 kg; 1 kg = 2.2 lb; 132 lb/1

$$mcg = \frac{30 \ mcg \ \times \ 1 \ kg \ \times \ 132 \ lb}{1 \ kg \ \times \ 2.2 \ lb \ \times \ 1} = \frac{30 \ mcg \ \times \ 1 \ \times \ \overset{60}{\cancel{132}}}{1 \ \times \ \underset{1}{\cancel{2.2}} \ \times \ 1} = \frac{1800 \ mcg}{1} = 1800 \ mcg \ (/d)$$

Factors: 2 doses = 1 d; 1800 mcg = 1 d

$$\frac{mcg}{dose} = \frac{1800 \ mcg \ \times \ 1 \ d}{1 \ d \ \times \ 2 \ doses} = \frac{\overset{900}{\cancel{1800}} \ mcg \ \times \ 1}{1 \ \times \ \underset{1}{\cancel{2}} \ doses} = \frac{900 \ mcg}{1 \ dose} = 900 \ mcg/dose$$

3. Factors: Recommended: up to 30 mg = 1 kg; 1 kg = 2.2 lb; 209 lb/1

$$mg = \frac{30 \ mg \ \times \ 1 \ kg \ \times \ 209 \ lb}{1 \ kg \ \times \ 2.2 \ lb \ \times \ 1} = \frac{30 \ mg \ \times \ 1 \ \times \ \overset{95}{\cancel{209}}}{1 \ \times \ \underset{1}{\cancel{2.2}} \ \times \ 1} = \frac{2850 \ mg}{1} = 2850 \ mg$$

Factors: Ordered: 400 mg = (q) 4 h; 24 h = 1 d

$$mg = \frac{400 \ mg \ \times \ 24 \ h}{4 \ h \ \times \ 1 \ d} = \frac{400 \ mg \ \times \ \overset{6}{\cancel{24}}}{\underset{1}{\cancel{4}} \ \times \ 1 \ d} = \frac{2400 \ mg}{1 \ d} = 2400 \ mg/d$$

The ordered dosage is within the recommended range.

4. Factors: 1 tab = 250 mg; 25 mg = 1 kg; 1 kg = 2.2 lb; 110 lb/1

$$tab = \frac{1 \ tab \ \times \ 25 \ mg \ \times \ 1 \ kg \ \times \ 110 \ lb}{250 \ mg \ \times \ 1 \ kg \ \times \ 2.2 \ lb \ \times \ 1} = \frac{1 \ tab \ \times \ \overset{1}{\cancel{25}} \ \times \ 1 \ \times \ \overset{\overset{5}{\cancel{50}}}{\cancel{110}}}{\underset{\underset{1}{10}}{\cancel{250}} \ \times \ 1 \ \times \ \underset{1}{\cancel{2.2}} \ \times \ 1} = \frac{5 \ tabs}{1} = 5 \ tabs$$

5. Factors: 0.5 mg = 1 lb; 150 lb/1

$$mg = \frac{0.5 \ mg \ \times \ 150 \ lb}{1 \ lb \ \times \ 1} = \frac{0.5 \ mg \ \times \ 150}{1 \ \times \ 1} = \frac{75 \ mg}{1} = 75 \ mg \ (/d)$$

Factors: 1 tab = 25 mg; 75 mg = 1 day; 3 doses = 1 day

$$\frac{tab}{dose} = \frac{1 \ tab \ \times \ 75 \ mg \ \times \ 1 \ d}{25 \ mg \ \times \ 1 \ d \ \times \ 3 \ doses} = \frac{1 \ tab \ \times \ \overset{3}{\cancel{75}} \ \times \ 1}{\underset{1}{\cancel{25}} \ \times \ 1 \ \times \ \underset{1}{\cancel{3}} \ doses} = \frac{1 \ tab}{1} = 1 \ tab$$

6. Factors: 1 ml = 1000 U; 20 U = 1 kg; 1 kg = 2.2 lb; 189 lb/1

$$ml = \frac{1 \ ml \ \times \ 20 \ U \ \times \ 1 \ kg \ \times \ 189 \ lb}{1000 \ U \ \times \ 1 \ kg \ \times \ 2.2 \ lb \ \times \ 1} = \frac{1 \ ml \ \times \ \overset{1}{\cancel{20}} \ \times \ 1 \ \times \ 189}{\underset{50}{\cancel{1000}} \ \times \ 1 \ \times \ 2.2 \ \times \ 1} = \frac{189 \ ml}{110} = 1.718 \ ml$$

7. Factors: 1.5 mcg = 1 kg; 1 kg = 2.2 lb; 220 lb/1

$$mcg = \frac{1.5 \ mcg \ \times \ 1 \ kg \ \times \ 220 \ lb}{1 \ kg \ \times \ 2.2 \ lb \ \times \ 1} = \frac{1.5 \ mcg \ \times \ 1 \ \times \ \overset{100}{\cancel{220}}}{1 \ \times \ \underset{1}{\cancel{2.2}} \ \times \ 1} = \frac{150 \ mcg}{1} = 150 \ mcg \ (/d)$$

8. Factors: Recommended minimum: 20 mg = 1 kg; 1 kg = 2.2 lb; 132 lb/1

$$mg = \frac{20 \ mg \ \times \ 1 \ kg \ \times \ 132 \ lb}{1 \ kg \ \times \ 2.2 \ lb \ \times \ 1} = \frac{20 \ mg \ \times \ 1 \ \times \ \overset{60}{\cancel{132}}}{1 \ \times \ \underset{1}{\cancel{2.2}} \ \times \ 1} = \frac{1200 \ mg}{1} = 1200 \ mg$$

Factors: Recommended maximum: 30 mg = 1 kg; 1 kg = 2.2 lb; 132 lb/1

$$mg = \frac{30 \ mg \ \times \ 1 \ kg \ \times \ 132 \ lb}{1 \ kg \ \times \ 2.2 \ lb \ \times \ 1} = \frac{30 \ mg \ \times \ 1 \ \times \ \overset{60}{\cancel{132}}}{1 \ \times \ \underset{1}{\cancel{2.2}} \ \times \ 1} = \frac{1800 \ mg}{1} = 1800 \ mg$$

Factors: Ordered: 500 mg = 1 dose; 3 doses = 1 day

$$mg = \frac{500 \ mg \ \times \ 3 \ doses}{1 \ dose \ \times \ 1 \ d} = \frac{500 \ mg \ \times \ 3}{1 \ \times \ 1 \ d} = \frac{1500 \ mg}{1 \ d} = 1500 \ mg/d$$

The ordered dosage is within the recommended range.

9. Factors: 0.004 ml = 1 lb; 185 lb/1

$$ml = \frac{0.004 \ ml \ \times \ 185 \ lb}{1 \ lb \ \times \ 1} = \frac{0.004 \ ml \ \times \ 185}{1 \ \times \ 1} = \frac{0.74 \ ml}{1} = 0.74 \ ml$$

10. Factors: 1 mg = 1 kg; 71 kg/1

$$mg = \frac{1 \ mg \ \times \ 71 \ kg}{1 \ kg \ \times \ 1} = \frac{1 \ mg \ \times \ 71}{1 \ \times \ 1} = \frac{71 \ mg}{1} = 71 \ mg$$

(If 1 mg = 1 kg, then 71 kg = 71 mg)

UNIT VI: SOLUTIONS

Chapter 14: Calculation Of Solutes And Solvents

1. Factors: 1 tsp = 5 ml; 500 ml = 100%; 0.9%/1

$$tsp = \frac{1 \ tsp \ \times \ 500 \ ml \ \times \ 0.9\%}{5 \ ml \ \times \ 100\% \ \times \ 1} = \frac{1 \ tsp \ \times \ \overset{1}{\cancel{500}} \ \times \ 0.9}{\underset{1}{\cancel{5}} \ \times \ \underset{1}{\cancel{100}} \ \times \ 1} = \frac{0.9 \ tsp}{1} = 0.9 \ (1) \ tsp$$

2. Factors: 4 Cal = 1 g; 1000 ml (g) = 100%; 10%/1

$$Cal = \frac{4 \ Cal \ \times \ 1000 \ g \ \times \ 10\%}{1 \ g \ \times \ 100\% \ \times \ 1} = \frac{4 \ Cal \ \times \ \overset{10}{\cancel{1000}} \ \times \ 10}{1 \ \times \ \underset{1}{\cancel{100}} \ \times \ 1} = \frac{400 \ Cal}{1} = 400 \ Cal$$

3. Factors: 200 ml = 100%; 5%/1

$$ml = \frac{200 \ ml \ \times \ 5\%}{100\% \ \times \ 1} = \frac{\overset{2}{\cancel{200}} \ ml \ \times \ 5}{\underset{1}{\cancel{100}} \ \times \ 1} = \frac{10 \ ml}{1} = 10 \ ml$$

4. Factors: 1 tsp = 5 ml; 1000 ml = 100%; 0.45%/1

$$tsp = \frac{1 \ tsp \ \times \ 1000 \ ml \ \times \ 0.45\%}{5 \ ml \ \times \ 100\% \ \times \ 1} = \frac{1 \ tsp \ \times \ \overset{2}{\cancel{1000}} \ \times \ 0.45}{\underset{1}{\cancel{5}} \ \times \ \underset{1}{\cancel{100}} \ \times \ 1} = \frac{0.9 \ tsp}{1} = 0.9 \ (1) \ tsp \ salt$$

1000 ml − 1 tsp (5 ml) = 995 ml water or q.s. to 1000 ml.

5. Factors: 1 g = 1000 mg; 1 g = 1000 ml (1 ml (1 g) medication in 1000 ml solution)

$$\text{mg} = \frac{1000 \text{ mg} \times 1 \text{ g}}{1 \text{ g} \times 1000 \text{ ml}} = \frac{\overset{1}{\cancel{1000}} \text{ mg} \times 1}{1 \times \cancel{1000} \text{ ml}} = \frac{1 \text{ mg}}{1 \text{ ml}} = 1 \text{ mg/ml}$$

6. Factors: 500 ml = 100%; 0.45%/1

$$\text{ml} = \frac{500 \text{ ml} \times 0.45\%}{100\% \times 1} = \frac{\overset{5}{\cancel{500}} \text{ ml} \times 0.45}{\underset{1}{\cancel{100}} \times 1} = \frac{2.25 \text{ ml}}{1} = 2.25 \text{ ml}$$

7. Factors: 500 ml = 60%; 15%/1

$$\text{ml} = \frac{500 \text{ ml} \times 15\%}{60\% \times 1} = \frac{\overset{25}{\cancel{500}} \text{ ml} \times \overset{5}{\cancel{15}}}{\underset{\underset{1}{\cancel{6}}}{\cancel{60}} \times 1} = \frac{125 \text{ ml}}{1} = 125 \text{ ml}$$

8. Factors: 1 L = 1000 ml; 1 L = 1/50; 1 = 100%; 1%/1

$$\text{ml} = \frac{1000 \text{ ml} \times 1 \text{ L} \times 1 \times 1\%}{1 \text{ L} \times 1/50 \times 100\% \times 1} = \frac{\cancel{1000} \text{ ml} \times 50 \times 1 \times \overset{10}{1} \times 1}{1 \times 1 \times \cancel{100} \times 1} = \frac{500 \text{ ml}}{1} = 500 \text{ ml}$$

9. Factors: dextrose: 500 ml (g) = 100%; 2.5%/1

$$\text{g} = \frac{500 \text{ g} \times 2.5\%}{100\% \times 1} = \frac{\overset{5}{\cancel{500}} \text{ g} \times 2.5}{\underset{1}{\cancel{100}} \times 1} = \frac{12.5 \text{ g}}{1} = 12.5 \text{ g dextrose}$$

Factors: salt: 500 g = 100%; 0.9%/1

$$\text{g} = \frac{500 \text{ g} \times 0.9\%}{100\% \times 1} = \frac{\overset{5}{\cancel{500}} \text{ g} \times 0.9}{\underset{1}{\cancel{100}} \times 1} = \frac{4.5 \text{ g}}{1} = 4.5 \text{ g salt}$$

10. Factors: 250 ml = 10%; 1/1000

$$\text{ml} = \frac{250 \text{ ml} \times 100\% \times 1}{10\% \times 1 \times 1000} = \frac{\overset{25}{\cancel{250}} \text{ ml} \times \overset{1}{\cancel{100}} \times 1}{\underset{1}{\cancel{10}} \times 1 \times \underset{10}{\cancel{1000}}} = \frac{25 \text{ ml}}{10} = 2.5 \text{ ml}$$

UNIT VII: INTRAVENOUS FLUID ADMINISTRATION

Chapter 15: Calculations Associated With Intravenous Fluid Administration

1. Factors: 1000 ml = 10 h; 15 gtt = 1 ml; 1 h = 60 min

$$\frac{\text{gtt}}{\text{min}} = \frac{15 \text{ gtt} \times 1000 \text{ ml} \times 1 \text{ h}}{1 \text{ ml} \times 10 \text{ h} \times 60 \text{ min}} = \frac{\overset{1}{\cancel{15}} \text{ gtt} \times \overset{\overset{25}{\cancel{100}}}{\cancel{1000}} \times 1}{1 \times \underset{1}{\cancel{10}} \times \underset{\underset{1}{\cancel{4}}}{\cancel{60}} \text{ min}} = \frac{25 \text{ gtt}}{1 \text{ min}} = 25 \text{ gtt/min}$$

2. Factors: Volume/h: 500 ml = 6 h

$$\frac{\text{ml}}{\text{h}} = \frac{500 \text{ ml}}{6 \text{ h}} = \frac{\overset{250}{\cancel{500}} \text{ ml}}{\underset{3}{\cancel{6}} \text{ h}} = \frac{250 \text{ ml}}{3 \text{ h}} = 83.3 \text{ ml/h}$$

Factors: Volume/3 h: 500 ml = 6 h (83.3 ml = 1 h); 3 h = 1

$$\text{ml} = \frac{500 \text{ ml} \times 3 \text{ h}}{6 \text{ h} \times 1} = \frac{\overset{250}{\cancel{500}} \text{ ml} \times \overset{1}{\cancel{3}}}{\underset{\underset{1}{\cancel{3}}}{\cancel{6}} \times 1} = \frac{250 \text{ ml}}{1} = 250 \text{ ml}$$

3. Factors: Drip rate: 1000 ml = 12 h; 60 gtt = 1 ml; 1 h = 60 min

$$\frac{\text{gtt}}{\text{min}} = \frac{60 \text{ gtt} \times 1000 \text{ ml} \times 1 \text{ h}}{1 \text{ ml} \times 12 \text{ h} \times 60 \text{ min}} = \frac{\overset{1}{\cancel{60}} \text{ gtt} \times \overset{250}{\cancel{1000}} \times 1}{1 \times \underset{3}{\cancel{12}} \times \underset{1}{\cancel{60}} \text{ min}} = \frac{250 \text{ gtt}}{3 \text{ min}} = 83.3 \text{ (83) gtt/min}$$

Factors: Infusion time: Expected: 1000 ml = 12 h; 5 h = 1; Actual: 500 ml

$$\text{ml} = \frac{1000 \text{ ml} \times 5 \text{ h}}{12 \text{ h} \times 1} = \frac{\overset{250}{\cancel{1000}} \text{ ml} \times 5}{\underset{3}{\cancel{12}} \times 1} = \frac{1250 \text{ ml}}{3} = 416.6 \text{ ml} \pm 25 = 392 \text{ to } 441 \text{ ml}$$

500 ml > 416 ml (392 to 441). Therefore, IV is infusing too rapidly.

Factors: Recalculation: 500 ml = 7 h; 60 gtt = 1 ml; 60 min = 1 h

$$\frac{gtt}{min} = \frac{60\ gtt \times 500\ ml \times 1\ h}{1\ ml \times 7\ h \times 60\ min} = \frac{\overset{1}{\cancel{60}}\ gtt \times 500 \times 1}{1 \times 7 \times \cancel{60}\ min} = \frac{500\ gtt}{7\ min} = 71.4\ (71)\ gtt/min$$

4. Factors: 500 ml = 3 h; 10 gtt = 1 ml; 1 h = 60 min

$$\frac{gtt}{min} = \frac{10\ gtt \times 500\ ml \times 1\ h}{1\ ml \times 3\ h \times 60\ min} = \frac{\overset{1}{\cancel{10}}\ gtt \times \overset{250}{\cancel{500}} \times 1}{1 \times 3 \times \underset{3}{\underset{\cancel{6}}{\cancel{60}}}\ min} = \frac{250\ gtt}{9\ min} = 27.7(28)gtt/min$$

5. Factors: 3 L = 24 h; 1 l = 1000 ml; 20 gtt = 1 ml; 1 h = 60 min

$$\frac{gtt}{min} = \frac{20\ gtt \times 1000\ ml \times 3\ L \times 1\ h}{1\ ml \times 1\ L \times 24\ h \times 60\ min} = \frac{\overset{1}{\cancel{20}}\ gtt \times \overset{125}{\cancel{1000}} \times \overset{1}{\cancel{3}} \times 1}{1 \times 1 \times \underset{\underset{1}{8}}{\cancel{24}} \times \underset{3}{\cancel{60}}\ min} = \frac{125\ gtt}{3\ min} = 41.6\ (42)\ gtt/min$$

6. Factors: 250 ml = 8 h; 60 gtt = 1 ml; 1 h = 60 min

$$\frac{gtt}{min} = \frac{60\ gtt \times 250\ ml \times 1\ h}{1\ ml \times 8\ h \times 60\ min} = \frac{\overset{1}{\cancel{60}}\ gtt \times \overset{125}{\cancel{250}} \times 1}{1 \times \underset{4}{\cancel{8}} \times \underset{1}{\cancel{60}}\ min} = \frac{125\ gtt}{4\ min} = 31.25\ (32)\ gtts/min$$

7. Factors: 250 ml = 4 h; 10 gtt = 1 ml; 1 h = 60 min

$$\frac{gtt}{min} = \frac{10\ gtt \times 250\ ml \times 1\ h}{1\ ml \times 4\ h \times 60\ min} = \frac{\overset{1}{\cancel{10}}\ gtt \times \overset{125}{\cancel{250}} \times 1}{1 \times \underset{2}{\cancel{4}} \times \underset{6}{\cancel{60}}\ min} = \frac{125\ gtt}{12\ min} = 10.4\ (10)\ gtt/min$$

8. Factors: Volume/h: 500 ml = 8 h

$$\frac{ml}{h} = \frac{500\ ml}{8\ h} = \frac{\overset{125}{\cancel{500}}\ ml}{\underset{2}{\cancel{8}}\ h} = \frac{125\ ml}{2\ h} = 62.5\ ml/h$$

Factors: Drip rate: 500 ml = 8 h; 15 gtt = 1 ml; 1 h = 60 min

$$\frac{gtt}{min} = \frac{15\ gtt \times 500\ ml \times 1\ h}{1\ ml \times 8\ h \times 60\ min} = \frac{\overset{1}{\cancel{15}}\ gtt \times \overset{125}{\cancel{500}} \times 1}{1 \times \underset{2}{\cancel{8}} \times \underset{4}{\cancel{60}}\ min} = \frac{125\ gtt}{8\ min} = 15.6\ (16)\ gtt/min$$

Factors: Infusion time: Expected; 500 ml = 8 h; 4 h/1. Actual; 250 ml

Half the time has elapsed, so half the solution, 250 ml, should have infused. The IV is on time.

9. Factors: 50 ml = 30 min; 20 gtt = 1 ml

$$\frac{gtt}{min} = \frac{20\ gtt \times 50\ ml}{1\ ml \times 30\ min} = \frac{\overset{2}{\cancel{20}}\ gtt \times 50}{1 \times \underset{3}{\cancel{30}}\ min} = \frac{100\ gtt}{3\ min} = 33.3\ (33)\ gtt/min$$

10. Factors: 1000 ml = 8 h; 15 gtt = 1 ml; 1 h = 60 min

$$\frac{gtt}{min} = \frac{15\ gtt \times 1000\ ml \times 1\ h}{1\ ml \times 8\ h \times 60\ min} = \frac{\overset{1}{\cancel{15}}\ gtt \times \overset{125}{\cancel{1000}} \times 1}{1 \times \underset{1}{\cancel{8}} \times \underset{4}{\cancel{60}}\ min} = \frac{125\ gtt}{4\ min} = 31.25\ (31)\ gtt/min$$

UNIT VIII: INTRAVENOUS MEDICATIONS

Chapter 16: Piggyback, Bolus And Titrated Medications

1. Factors: 100 ml = 30 min; 20 gtt = 1 ml

$$\frac{gtt}{min} = \frac{20\ gtt \times 100\ ml}{1\ ml \times 30\ min} = \frac{\overset{2}{\cancel{20}}\ gtt \times 100}{1 \times \underset{3}{\cancel{30}}\ min} = \frac{200\ gtt}{3\ min} = 66.6\ (67)\ gtt/min$$

2. Factors: 1 mg = 1 ml; 10 mg/1; 1 ml available

$$ml = \left(\frac{1\ ml \times 10\ mg}{1\ mg \times 1}\right) - 1\ ml = \left(\frac{1\ ml \times 10}{1 \times 1}\right) - 1\ ml = 10\ ml - 1\ ml = 9\ ml$$

3.a. Factors: mcg/ml: 1 g = 500 ml; 1 g = 1000 mg; 1 mg = 1000 mcg

$$\frac{mcg}{ml} = \frac{1000\ mcg \times 1000\ mg \times 1\ g}{1\ mg \times 1\ g \times 500\ ml} = \frac{\cancel{1000}\ mcg \times 1000 \times 1}{1 \times 1 \times \underset{1}{\cancel{500}}\ ml} \overset{2}{=} \frac{2000\ mcg}{1\ ml}$$

= 2000 mcg/ml (2000 mcg/ml = 2 mg/ml = 0.002 g/ml)

b. Factors: mcg/min: 20 mcg = 1 kg × 1 min; 1 kg = 2.2 lb; 154 lb/1

$$\frac{mcg}{min} = \frac{20\ mcg}{1\ kg} \times \frac{1\ kg}{1\ min} \times \frac{154\ lb}{2.2\ lb} \times \frac{1}{1} = \frac{20\ mcg}{1} \times \frac{1}{1\ min} \times \frac{1 \times \overset{70}{\cancel{154}}}{\cancel{2.2} \times 1} = \frac{1400\ mcg}{1\ min}$$

$$= 1400\ mcg/min$$

c. Factors: Drip rate: 60 gtt = 1 ml; 1 ml = 2000 mcg; 1400 mcg = 1 min

$$\frac{gtt}{min} = \frac{60\ gtt}{1\ ml} \times \frac{1\ ml}{2000\ mg} \times \frac{1400\ mcg}{1\ min} = \frac{\overset{3}{\cancel{60}}\ gtt \times 1 \times \overset{14}{\cancel{1400}}}{1 \times \underset{\underset{1}{100}}{\cancel{2000}} \times 1\ min} = \frac{42\ gtt}{1\ min} = 42\ gtt/min$$

d. Factors: ml/h: 1 ml = 2000 mcg; 1400 mcg = 1 min; 1 h = 60 min

$$\frac{ml}{h} = \frac{1\ ml}{2000\ mcg} \times \frac{1400\ mcg}{1\ min} \times \frac{60\ min}{1\ h} = \frac{1\ ml \times \overset{14}{\cancel{1400}} \times \overset{3}{\cancel{60}}}{\underset{\underset{1}{100}}{\cancel{2000}} \times 1 \times 1\ h} = \frac{42\ ml}{1\ h} = 42\ ml/h$$

4. a. Factors: Maximum mcg/min: 50 mcg = 1 kg × 1 min; 1 kg = 2.2 lb; 154 lb/1

$$\frac{gtt}{min} = \frac{50\ mcg}{1\ kg} \times \frac{1\ kg}{1\ min} \times \frac{154\ lb}{2.2\ lb} \times \frac{1}{1} = \frac{50\ mcg}{1} \times \frac{1}{1\ min} \times \frac{1 \times \overset{70}{\cancel{154}}}{\cancel{2.2} \times 1} = \frac{3500\ mcg}{1\ min}$$

$$= 3500\ mcg/min\ (3500 mcg/min = 3.5 mg/min)$$

b. Factors: Maximum drip rate: 3500 mcg = 1 min; 60 gtt = 1 ml; 2000 mcg = 1 ml

$$\frac{gtt}{min} = \frac{60\ gtt}{1\ ml} \times \frac{1\ ml}{2000\ mcg} \times \frac{3500\ mcg}{1 min} = \frac{\overset{15}{\cancel{60}}\ gtt \times 1 \times \overset{7}{\cancel{3500}}}{1 \times \underset{\underset{1}{\cancel{4}}}{\cancel{2000}} \times 1\ min} = \frac{105\ gtt}{1\ min} = 105\ gtt/min$$

5. Factors: 100 ml = 20 min; 15 gtt = 1 ml

$$\frac{gtt}{min} = \frac{15\ gtt \times 100\ ml}{1\ ml \times 20\ min} = \frac{\overset{3}{\cancel{15}}\ gtt \times \overset{25}{\cancel{100}}}{1 \times \underset{\underset{1}{\cancel{4}}}{\cancel{20}}\ min} = \frac{75\ gtt}{1\ min} = 75\ gtt/min$$

6. a. Factors: mcg/min: 50 mg = 500 ml; 1 mg = 1000 mcg; 60 gtt = 1 ml; 18 gtt = 1 min

$$\frac{mcg}{min} = \frac{1000\ mcg \times 50\ mg \times 1\ ml \times 18\ gtt}{1\ mg \times 500\ ml \times 60\ gtt \times 1\ min} = \frac{\cancel{1000}\ mcg \times \overset{2}{\underset{1}{\cancel{50}}} \times 1 \times \overset{3}{\cancel{18}}}{1 \times \underset{\underset{1}{\cancel{500}}}{5} \times \underset{\underset{1}{\cancel{60}}}{6} \times 1\ min} = \frac{30\ mcg}{1\ min} = 30\ mcg/min$$

b. Factors: mcg/kg/min: 30 mcg/min = 180 lb; 2.2 lb = 1 kg

$$\frac{mcg}{kg(/min)} = \frac{30\ mcg/min \times 2.2\ lb}{180\ lb \times 1\ kg} = \frac{\overset{1}{\cancel{30}}\ mcg \times 2.2}{1\ min \times \underset{6}{\cancel{180}} \times 1\ kg} = \frac{2.2\ mcg}{min \times 6\ kg} = 0.366\ mcg/kg/min$$

7. Factors: 250 ml = 250 mg; 1 mg = 1000 mcg; 150 mcg = 1 min; 1 h = 60 min

$$\frac{ml}{h} = \frac{250\ ml \times 1\ mg \times 150\ mcg \times 60\ min}{250\ mg \times 1000\ mcg \times 1\ min \times 1\ h} = \frac{\overset{1}{\cancel{250}}\ ml \times 1 \times \overset{3}{\cancel{150}} \times \overset{3}{\cancel{60}}}{\underset{1}{\cancel{250}} \times \underset{\underset{1}{\cancel{20}}}{\cancel{1000}} \times 1 \times 1\ h} = \frac{9\ ml}{1\ h} = 9\ ml/h$$

8. a. Factors: 1 U = 1000 mU; 10 U = 1 L; 1 L = 1000 ml; 60 gtt = 1 ml; 26 gtt = 1 min

$$\frac{mU}{min} = \frac{1000\ mU \times 10\ U \times 1\ L \times 1\ ml \times 26\ gtt}{1\ U \times 1\ L \times 1000\ ml \times 60\ gtt \times 1\ min} = \frac{\overset{1}{\cancel{1000}}\ mU \times \overset{1}{\cancel{10}} \times 1 \times 1 \times 26}{1 \times 1 \times \underset{1}{\cancel{1000}} \times \underset{6}{\cancel{60}} \times 1\ min}$$

$$= \frac{26\ mU}{6\ min} = 4.3\ mU/min$$

b. Factors: Infusion: 4.3 mU/min; Maximum recommended: 20 mU/min

Because 4.3 mU < maximum dosage of 20 mU/min, this infusion is within recommended dosage.

9. Factors: 60 gtt = 1 ml; 500 ml = 500 mg; 1 mg = 1000 mcg; 12 mcg = 1 kg × 1 min; 70 kg/1

$$\frac{gtt}{min} = \frac{60\ gtt \times 500\ ml \times 1\ mg \times 12\ mcg \times 70\ kg}{1\ ml \times 500\ mg \times 1000\ mcg \times 1\ kg \times 1\ min \times 1} = \frac{\overset{3}{\cancel{60}}\ gtt \times \overset{1}{\cancel{500}} \times 1 \times 12 \times \overset{7}{\cancel{70}}}{1 \times \underset{\underset{5}{50}}{\cancel{500}} \times \cancel{1000} \times 1 \times 1\ min \times 1}$$

$$= \frac{252\ gtt}{5\ min} = 50.4\ (50)\ gtt/min$$

10. Factors: 60 gtt = 1 ml; 250 ml = 400 mg; 1 mg = 1000 mcg; 2 mcg = 1 kg × 1 min; 1 kg = 2.2 lb; 154 lb/1

$$\frac{gtt}{min} = \frac{60\ gtt \times 250\ ml \times 1\ mg \times 2\ mcg \times 1\ kg \times 154\ lb}{1\ ml \times 400\ mg \times 1000\ mcg \times 1\ kg \times 1\ min \times 2.2\ lb \times 1}$$

$$= \frac{\overset{3}{\cancel{60}}\ gtt \times \overset{1}{\cancel{250}} \times 1 \times \overset{1}{\cancel{2}} \times 1 \times \overset{\overset{7}{\cancel{70}}}{\cancel{154}}}{1 \times \underset{\underset{\underset{1}{\cancel{10}}}{\cancel{20}}}{\cancel{400}} \times \underset{4}{\cancel{1000}} \times 1 \times 1\ min \times 2.2 \times 1} = \frac{21\ gtt}{4\ min} = 5.25\ gtt/min$$

UNIT IX: PEDIATRIC CALCULATIONS

Chapter 17: Pediatric Medications And Intravenous Fluids

1. Factors: 5 ml = 250 mg; 225 mg/1

$$ml = \frac{5\ ml \times 225\ mg}{250\ mg \times 1} = \frac{\overset{1}{\cancel{5}}\ ml \times \overset{9}{\cancel{225}}}{\underset{\underset{2}{50}}{\cancel{250}} \times 1} = \frac{9\ ml}{2} = 4.5\ ml$$

2. Factors: 225 mg = (q) 8 h; 24 h = 1 d

$$\frac{mg}{d} = \frac{225\ mg \times 24\ h}{(q)8\ h \times 1\ d} = \frac{225\ mg \times \overset{3}{\cancel{24}}}{\underset{1}{\cancel{8}} \times 1\ d} = \frac{675\ mg}{1\ d} = 675\ mg/d$$

3. Factors: 50 mg = 1 kg; 1 kg = 2.2 lb; 30 lb/1

$$mg(/d) = \frac{50\ mg \times 1\ kg \times 30\ lb}{1\ kg \times 2.2\ lb \times 1} = \frac{\overset{25}{\cancel{50}}\ mg \times 1 \times 30}{1 \times \underset{1.1}{\cancel{2.2}} \times 1} = \frac{750\ mg}{1.1} = 681.81\ mg$$

4. Child's BSA is 0.9 square meters.

5. Factors: 1 ml = 25 mg; 30 mg/1

$$ml = \frac{1\ ml \times 30\ mg}{25\ mg \times 1} = \frac{1\ ml \times \overset{6}{\cancel{30}}}{\underset{5}{\cancel{25}} \times 1} = \frac{6\ ml}{5} = 1.2\ ml$$

6. Factors: 30 mg = 1 m²; 0.9 m²/1

$$mg = \frac{30\ mg \times 0.9\ m^2}{1\ m^2 \times 1} = \frac{30\ mg \times 0.9}{1 \times 1} = \frac{27\ mg}{1} = 27\ mg$$

7. Factors: 100,000 U = 1 ml; 200,000 U/1

$$ml = \frac{1\ ml \times 200,000\ U}{100,000\ U \times 1} = \frac{1\ ml \times \overset{2}{\cancel{200,000}}}{\underset{1}{\cancel{100,000}} \times 1} = \frac{2\ ml}{1} = 2\ ml$$

8. Clark's rule = c. Based on body weight
9. Fried's rule = b. Based on age in months
10. Young's rule = d. Based on age in years
11. Factors: 25 mg = 1 kg; 1 kg = 2.2 lb; 16 lb 4 oz (16 1/4 or 16.25 lb)/1

$$mg = \frac{25\ mg \times 1\ kg \times 16.25\ lb}{1\ kg \times 2.2\ lb \times 1} = \frac{25\ mg \times 1 \times 16.25}{1 \times 2.2 \times 1} = \frac{406.25\ mg}{2.2} = 184.659\ mg$$

12. Factors: 90 mcg = 1 dose; 2 doses = 1 d

$$\frac{mcg}{d} = \frac{90\ mcg \times 2\ doses}{1\ dose \times 1\ d} = \frac{90\ mcg \times 2}{1 \times 1\ d} = \frac{180\ mcg}{1\ d} = 180\ mcg/d$$

13. Factors: 1 mg = 1 ml; 1 mg = 1000 mcg; 90 mcg/1

$$ml = \frac{1\ ml \times 1\ mg \times 90\ mcg}{1\ mg \times 1000\ mcg \times 1} = \frac{1\ ml \times 1 \times \overset{9}{\cancel{90}}}{1 \times \underset{100}{\cancel{1000}} \times 1} = \frac{9\ ml}{100} = 0.09\ ml$$

14. Factors: 5 ml = 125 mg; 100 mg/1

$$ml = \frac{5 \text{ ml} \times 100 \text{ mg}}{125 \text{ mg} \times 1} = \frac{\overset{1}{\cancel{5}} \text{ ml} \times \overset{4}{\cancel{100}}}{\underset{\underset{1}{\cancel{5}}}{\cancel{125}} \times 1} = \frac{4 \text{ ml}}{1} = 4 \text{ ml}$$

15. Factors: 5 ml = 200,000 U; 100,000 U/1

$$ml = \frac{5 \text{ ml} \times 100,000 \text{ U}}{200,000 \text{ U} \times 1} = \frac{5 \text{ ml} \times \overset{1}{\cancel{100,000}}}{\underset{2}{\cancel{200,000}} \times 1} = \frac{5 \text{ ml}}{2} = 2.5 \text{ ml}$$

16. Factors: 2 mg = 1 m²; 0.8 m²/1

$$mg = \frac{2 \text{ mg} \times 0.8 \text{ m}^2}{1 \text{ m}^2 \times 1} = \frac{2 \text{ mg} \times 0.8}{1 \times 1} = \frac{1.6 \text{ mg}}{1} = 1.6 \text{ mg}$$

17. Factors: 1 mg = 1 ml; 1.6 mg/1

$$ml = \frac{1 \text{ ml} \times 1.6 \text{ mg}}{1 \text{ mg} \times 1} = \frac{1 \text{ ml} \times 1.6}{1 \times 1} = \frac{1.6 \text{ ml}}{1} = 1.6 \text{ ml}$$

18. Factors: 100 mg = 1 kg; 1 kg = 2.2 lb; 6 lb 10 oz (6 $\frac{5}{8}$ lb)/1

$$mg = \frac{100 \text{ mg} \times 1 \text{ kg} \times 6\frac{5}{8} \text{ lb}}{1 \text{ kg} \times 2.2 \text{ lb} \times 1} = \frac{100 \text{ mg} \times 1 \times 53}{1 \times 2.2 \times 8} = \frac{5300 \text{ mg}}{17.6} = 301.136 \text{ mg}$$

19. Factors: 75 mg = (q) 6 h; 24 h = 1 d

$$\frac{mg}{d} = \frac{75 \text{ mg} \times 24 \text{ h}}{(q)6h \times 1 \text{ d}} = \frac{75 \text{ mg} \times \overset{4}{\cancel{24}}}{\underset{1}{\cancel{6}} \times 1 \text{ d}} = \frac{300 \text{ mg}}{1 \text{ d}} = 300 \text{ mg/d}$$

20. Factors: 5 ml = 125 mg; 75 mg/1

$$ml = \frac{5 \text{ ml} \times 75 \text{ mg}}{125 \text{ mg} \times 1} = \frac{\overset{1}{\cancel{5}} \text{ ml} \times \overset{3}{\cancel{75}}}{\underset{\underset{1}{\cancel{5}}}{\cancel{125}} \times 1} = \frac{3 \text{ ml}}{1} = 3 \text{ ml}$$

21. Factors: 60 gtt = 1 ml; 35 ml = 1 h; 1 h = 60 min

$$\frac{gtt}{min} = \frac{60 \text{ gtt} \times 35 \text{ ml} \times 1 \text{ h}}{1 \text{ ml} \times 1 \text{ h} \times 60 \text{ min}} = \frac{\overset{1}{\cancel{60}} \text{ gtt} \times 35 \times 1}{1 \times 1 \times \underset{1}{\cancel{60}} \text{ min}} = \frac{35 \text{ gtt}}{1 \text{ min}} = 35 \text{ gtt/min}$$

22. Factors: 35 ml = 1 h; 1 h = 60 min; 30 min/1

$$ml = \frac{35 \text{ ml} \times 1 \text{ h} \times 30 \text{ min}}{1 \text{ h} \times 60 \text{ min} \times 1} = \frac{35 \text{ ml} \times 1 \times \overset{1}{\cancel{30}}}{1 \times \underset{2}{\cancel{60}} \times 1} = \frac{35 \text{ ml}}{2} = 17.5 \text{ ml}$$

23. Factors: 300 mg = 1 ml; 60 mg/1

$$ml = \frac{1 \text{ ml} \times 60 \text{ mg}}{300 \text{ mg} \times 1} = \frac{1 \text{ ml} \times \overset{1}{\cancel{60}}}{\underset{5}{\cancel{300}} \times 1} = \frac{1 \text{ ml}}{5} = 0.2 \text{ ml}$$

24. Factors: recommended dosage/dose: 15 mg = 1 kg × 1 day; 1 kg = 2.2 lb; 44 lb/1; 4 doses = 1 day

$$\frac{mg}{dose} = \frac{15 \text{ mg} \times 1 \text{ kg} \times 44 \text{ lb} \times 1 \text{ d}}{1 \text{ kg} \times 1 \text{ d} \times 2.2 \text{ lb} \times 1 \times 4 \text{ doses}} = \frac{15 \text{ mg} \times 1 \times \overset{\overset{5}{\cancel{20}}}{\cancel{44}} \times 1}{1 \times 1 \times \underset{1}{\cancel{2.2}} \times 1 \times \underset{1}{\cancel{4}} \text{ doses}}$$

$$= \frac{75 \text{ mg}}{1 \text{ dose}} = 75 \text{ mg/dose}$$

25. Factors: 150 mg = 5 ml; 75 mg/1

$$ml = \frac{5 \text{ ml} \times 75 \text{ mg}}{150 \text{ mg} \times 1} = \frac{5 \text{ ml} \times \overset{1}{\cancel{75}}}{\underset{2}{\cancel{150}} \times 1} = \frac{5 \text{ ml}}{2} = 2.5 \text{ ml}$$

UNIT POSTTEST ANSWERS

UNIT III: CONVERSIONS WITHIN AND AMONG MEASUREMENT SYSTEMS

Unit III Posttest A

1. Factors: 1 gr = 60 mg; 1 mg = 1000 mcg; 1/300 gr/1

$$\text{mcg} = \frac{1000\,\text{mcg} \times 60\,\text{mg} \times \text{gr} \quad 1/300}{1\,\text{mg} \times 1\,\text{gr} \times \quad 1} = \frac{\overset{10}{\cancel{1000}}\,\text{mcg} \times \overset{20}{\cancel{60}} \times 1}{1 \times 1 \times \underset{\underset{1}{\cancel{5}}}{\cancel{300}}} = \frac{200\,\text{mcg}}{1} = 200\,\text{mcg}$$

2. Factors: 1 in = 2.5 cm; 1 cm = 10 mm; 200 mm/1

$$\text{in} = \frac{1\,\text{in} \times 1\,\text{cm} \times 200\,\text{mm}}{2.5\,\text{cm} \times 10\,\text{mm} \times 1} = \frac{1\,\text{in} \times 1 \times \overset{\overset{8}{\cancel{20}}}{\cancel{200}}}{\underset{1}{\cancel{2.5}} \times \underset{1}{\cancel{10}} \times 1} = \frac{8\,\text{in}}{1} = 8\,\text{in}$$

3. Factors: 1 lb = 16 oz; 1 kg = 2.2 lb; 7 lb 12 oz = 7 $^3/_4$ (31/4) lb/1

$$\text{kg} = \frac{1\,\text{kg} \times 7^3/_4\,\text{lb}}{2.2\,\text{lb} \times 1} = \frac{1\,\text{kg} \times 31}{2.2 \times 4} = \frac{31\,\text{kg}}{8.8} = 3.5227\,\text{kg}$$

4. Factors: 1 g = 1000 mg; 0.03 g/1

$$\text{mg} = \frac{1000\,\text{mg} \times 0.03\,\text{g}}{1\,\text{g} \times 1} = \frac{1000\,\text{mg} \times 0.03}{1 \times 1} = \frac{30\,\text{mg}}{1} = 30\,\text{mg}$$

5. Factors: 1 ml = 15 (16) mx; 12 mx/1

$$\text{ml} = \frac{1\,\text{ml} \times 12\,\text{mx}}{15\,\text{mx} \times} = \frac{1\,\text{ml} \times \overset{4}{\cancel{12}}}{\underset{5}{\cancel{15}} \times 1} = \frac{4\,\text{ml}}{5} = 0.8\,\text{ml}$$
$$\text{ml} = \frac{1\,\text{ml} \times 12\,\text{mx}}{16\,\text{mx} \times 1} = \frac{1\,\text{ml} \times \overset{3}{\cancel{12}}}{\underset{4}{\cancel{16}} \times 1} = \frac{3\,\text{ml}}{4} = 0.75\,\text{ml}$$

6. Factors: 1 mg = 1000 mcg; 4 mcg/1

$$\text{mg} = \frac{1\,\text{mg} \times 4\,\text{mcg}}{1000\,\text{mcg} \times 1} = \frac{1\,\text{mg} \times 4}{1000 \times 1} = \frac{4\,\text{mg}}{1000} = 0.004\,\text{mg}$$

7. Factors: 1 gr = 60 mg (15 gr = 1000 mg); 15 mg/1

$$\text{gr} = \frac{1\,\text{gr} \times 15\,\text{mg}}{60\,\text{mg} \times 1} = \frac{1\,\text{gr} \times \overset{1}{\cancel{15}}}{\underset{4}{\cancel{60}} \times 1} = \frac{1\,\text{gr}}{4} = \text{gr}\,1/4$$
$$\text{gr} = \frac{15\,\text{gr} \times 15\,\text{mg}}{1000\,\text{mg} \times 1} = \frac{\overset{3}{\cancel{15}}\,\text{gr} \times \overset{3}{\cancel{15}}}{\underset{\underset{40}{\cancel{200}}}{\cancel{1000}} \times 1} = \frac{9\,\text{gr}}{40} = \text{gr}\,9/40$$

8. Factors: 1 tsp = 1 dram; 7 dr/1. If 1 tsp = 1 dram, then 7 drams = 7 tsp.

9. Factors: 1 gr = 60 mg (15 gr = 1000 mg); 1/200 gr/1

$$\text{mg} = \frac{60\,\text{mg} \times \text{gr} \quad 1/200}{1\,\text{gr} \times \quad 1} = \frac{\overset{3}{\cancel{60}}\,\text{mg} \times 1}{1 \times \underset{10}{\cancel{200}}}$$
$$= \frac{3\,\text{mg}}{10} = 0.3\,\text{mg}$$

$$\text{mg} = \frac{1000\,\text{mg} \times \text{gr} \quad 1/200}{15\,\text{gr} \times \quad 1} = \frac{\overset{\overset{1}{\cancel{5}}}{\cancel{1000}}\,\text{mg} \times 1}{\underset{3}{\cancel{15}} \times \underset{1}{\cancel{200}}}$$
$$= \frac{1\,\text{mg}}{3} = 0.33\,\text{mg}$$

10. Factors: 1 ml = 15 (16) mx; 0.3 ml/1

$$\text{mx} = \frac{15\,\text{mx} \times 0.3\,\text{ml}}{1\,\text{ml} \times 1} = \frac{15\,\text{mx} \times 0.3}{1 \times 1} = 4.5\,\text{mx}$$
$$\text{mx} = \frac{16\,\text{mx} \times 0.3\,\text{ml}}{1\,\text{ml} \times 1} = \frac{16\,\text{mx} \times 0.3}{1 \times 1} = 4.8\,\text{mx}$$

11. Factors: 2 Tbsp = 1oz; 1 $^1/_2$ oz/1

$$\text{Tbsp} = \frac{2\,\text{Tbsp} \times 1^1/_2\,\text{oz}}{1\,\text{oz} \times 1} = \frac{\overset{1}{\cancel{2}}\,\text{Tbsp} \times 3}{1 \times \underset{1}{\cancel{2}}} = \frac{3\,\text{Tbsp}}{1} = 3\,\text{Tbsp}$$

12. Factors: 1 mg = 1000 mcg; 2.5 mcg/1

$$\text{mg} = \frac{1\,\text{mg} \times 2.5\,\text{mcg}}{1000\,\text{mcg} \times 1} = \frac{1\,\text{mg} \times 2.5}{1000 \times 1} = \frac{2.5\,\text{mg}}{1000} = 0.0025\,\text{mg}$$

13. Factors: 1 cc = 1 ml; 8 cc/1. If 1 cc = 1 ml, then 8 cc = 8 ml

14. 1 kg = 2.2 lb; 1 kg = 1000 g; 6 lb 13 oz = 6 $^{13}/_{16}$ (109/16) lb/1

$$g = \frac{1000\,g \times 1\,\text{kg} \times 6^{13}/_{16}\,\text{lb}}{1\,\text{kg} \times 2.2\,\text{lb} \times 1\,\text{lb}} = \frac{\overset{125}{\cancel{1000}}\,g \times 1 \times 109}{1 \times 2.2 \times \underset{2}{\cancel{16}}} = \frac{13625\,g}{4.4} = 3096.59\,g$$

15. Factors: 1 in = 2.5 cm; 12 cm/1

$$\text{in} = \frac{1\,\text{in} \times 12\,\text{cm}}{2.5\,\text{cm} \times 1} = \frac{1\,\text{in} \times 12}{2.5 \times 1} = \frac{12\,\text{in}}{2.5} = 4.8\,\text{in} = 4^4/_5\,\text{in}$$

16. Factors: 1 g = 1000 mg; 1 mg = 1000 mcg; 0.03 g/1

$$\text{mcg} = \frac{1000\text{ mcg} \times 1000\text{ mg} \times 0.03\text{ g}}{1\text{ mg} \times 1\text{ g} \times 1} = \frac{1000\text{ mcg} \times 1000 \times 0.03}{1 \times 1 \times 1} = \frac{30,000\text{ mcg}}{1} = 30,000\text{ mcg}$$

17. Factors: 1 kg = 2.2 lb; 77 kg/1

$$\text{lb} = \frac{2.2\text{ kg} \times 77\text{ kg}}{1\text{ kg} \times 1} = \frac{2.2\text{ lb} \times 77}{1 \times 1} = \frac{169.4\text{ lb}}{1} = 169^2/_5\text{ lb}$$

18. Factors: 1 qt = 1000 ml; 1 ½ qt/1

$$\text{ml} = \frac{1000\text{ ml} \times 1.5\text{ qt}}{1\text{ qt} \times 1} = \frac{1000\text{ ml} \times 1.5}{1 \times 1} = \frac{1500\text{ ml}}{1} = 1500\text{ ml}$$

19. Factors: 1 gr = 60 mg (15 gr = 1000 mg); 1 mg = 100 mcg; 600 mcg/1

$$\text{gr} = \frac{1\text{ gr} \times 1\text{ mg} \times 600\text{ mcg}}{60\text{ mg} \times 1000\text{ mcg} \times 1} = \frac{1\text{ gr} \times 1 \times \overset{\overset{1}{\cancel{10}}}{\cancel{600}}}{\underset{1}{\cancel{60}} \times \cancel{1000} \times \underset{100}{1}}$$

$$= \frac{1\text{ gr}}{100} = \text{gr } 1/100$$

$$\text{gr} = \frac{15\text{ gr} \times 1\text{ mg} \times 600\text{ mcg}}{1000\text{ mg} \times 1000\text{ mcg} \times 1}$$

$$= \frac{\overset{3}{\cancel{15}}\text{ gr} \times 1 \times \overset{3}{\cancel{600}}}{\underset{\underset{1}{\cancel{5}}}{\cancel{1000}} \times 1000 \times 1} = \frac{9\text{ gr}}{1000} = \text{gr } 9/1000$$

20. Factors: 1 tsp = 5 ml; 9 tsp/1

$$\text{ml} = \frac{5\text{ ml} \times 9\text{ tsp}}{1\text{ tsp} \times 1} = \frac{5\text{ ml} \times 9}{1 \times 1} = \frac{45\text{ ml}}{1} = 45\text{ ml}$$

21. Factors: 1 qt = 1000 cc; 750 cc/1

$$\text{qt} = \frac{1\text{ qt} \times 750\text{ cc}}{1000\text{ cc} \times 1} = \frac{1\text{ qt} \times \overset{3}{\cancel{750}}}{\underset{4}{\cancel{1000}} \times 1} = \frac{3\text{ qt}}{4} = 3/4\text{ qt}$$

22-25. Factors: 1 Tbsp = 15 ml; 1 C = 8 oz; 1 C = 250 ml; 1 oz = 30 ml

1/2 C fresh fruit: not fluid intake

10 Tbsp cream soup:

$$\text{ml} = \frac{15\text{ ml} \times 10\text{ Tbsp}}{1\text{ Tbsp} \times 1} = \frac{15\text{ ml} \times 10}{1 \times 1} = \qquad 150\text{ ml} \qquad\qquad\qquad 150\text{ ml}$$

1/2 tuna salad sandwich: not fluid intake

3/4 C grapefruit juice:

$$\text{ml} = \frac{30\text{ ml} \times 8\text{ oz} \times 3/4\text{ C}}{1\text{ oz} \times 1\text{ C} \times 1} = \frac{30\text{ ml} \times \overset{2}{\cancel{8}} \times 3}{1 \times 1 \times \underset{1}{\cancel{4}}} = 180\text{ ml}$$

$$\text{ml} = \frac{250\text{ ml} \times 3/4\text{ C}}{1\text{ C} \times 1} = \frac{\overset{125}{\cancel{250}}\text{ ml} \times 3}{1 \times \underset{2}{\cancel{4}}} = \frac{375\text{ ml}}{1} = 187.5\text{ ml}$$

4 oz slice chocolate cake: not fluid intake

10 oz Pepsi:

$$\text{ml} = \frac{30\text{ ml} \times 10\text{ oz}}{1\text{ oz} \times 1} = \frac{30\text{ ml} \times 10}{1 \times 1} = \qquad 300\text{ ml} \qquad\qquad\qquad 300\text{ ml}$$

Total   630 ml   637.5 ml

Unit III Posttest B

1. Factors: gr 1 = 60 mg (15 gr = 1000 mg); 1 mg = 1000 mcg; 1/400 gr/1

$$\text{mcg} = \frac{1000\text{ mcg} \times 60\text{ mg} \times \text{gr } 1/400}{1\text{ mg} \times 1\text{ gr} \times 1}$$

$$\text{mcg} = \frac{1000\text{ mcg} \times 1000\text{ mg} \times \text{gr } 1/400}{1\text{ mg} \times 15\text{ gr} \times 1}$$

$$= \frac{1000\text{ mcg} \times \overset{\overset{5}{\cancel{30}}}{\cancel{60}} \times 1}{1 \times 1 \times \underset{1}{\cancel{400}}} = \frac{150\text{ mcg}}{1} = 150\text{ mcg}$$

$$= \frac{\overset{1}{\cancel{1000}}\text{ mcg} \times \overset{500}{\cancel{1000}} \times 1}{1 \times \underset{3}{\cancel{15}} \times \underset{\underset{1}{\cancel{2}}}{\cancel{400}}} = \frac{500\text{ mcg}}{3} = 166.67\text{ mcg}$$

2. Factors: 1 in = 2.5 cm; 1 cm = 10 mm; 100 mm/1

$$\text{in} = \frac{1\text{ in} \times 1\text{ cm} \times 100\text{ mm}}{2.5\text{ cm} \times 10\text{ mm} \times 1} = \frac{1\text{ in} \times 1 \times \overset{10}{\cancel{100}}}{2.5 \times \underset{1}{\cancel{10}} \times 1} = \frac{10\text{ in}}{2.5} = 4\text{ in}$$

3. Factors: 1 kg = 2.2 lb; 1 lb = 16 oz; 9 lb 10 oz = 9⅝ (77/8) lb/1

$$\text{kg} = \frac{1\text{ kg} \times 9\tfrac{5}{8}\text{ lb}}{2.2\text{ lb} \times 1} = \frac{1\text{ kg} \times \overset{7}{\cancel{77}}}{\underset{0.2}{\cancel{2.2}} \times 8} = \frac{7\text{ kg}}{1.6} = 4.375\text{ kg}$$

4. Factors: 1 g = 1000 mg; 0.05 g/1

$$\text{mg} = \frac{1000\text{ mg} \times 0.05\text{ g}}{1\text{ g} \times 1} = \frac{1000\text{ mg} \times 0.05}{1 \times 1} = \frac{50\text{ mg}}{1} = 50\text{ mg}$$

5. Factors: 1 ml = 15 (16) mx; 20 mx/1

$$ml = \frac{1\,ml \times 20\,mx}{15\,mx \times 1} = \frac{1\,ml \times \overset{4}{\cancel{20}}}{\underset{3}{\cancel{15}} \times 1} = \frac{4\,mx}{3} = 1.33\,ml \qquad\qquad ml = \frac{1\,ml \times 20\,mx}{16\,mx \times 1} = \frac{1\,ml \times \overset{5}{\cancel{20}}}{\underset{4}{\cancel{16}} \times 1} = \frac{5\,ml}{4} = 1.25\,ml$$

6. Factors: 1 mg = 1000 mcg; 12 mcg/1

$$mg = \frac{1\,mg \times 12\,mcg}{1000\,mcg \times 1} = \frac{1\,mg \times 12}{1000 \times 1} = \frac{12\,mg}{1000} = 0.012\,mg$$

7. Factors: 1 gr = 60 mg (15 gr = 1000 mg); 30 mg/1

$$gr = \frac{1\,gr \times 30\,mg}{60\,mg \times 1} = \frac{1\,gr \times \overset{1}{\cancel{30}}}{\underset{2}{\cancel{60}} \times 1} = \frac{1\,gr}{2} = gr\ 1/2 \qquad\qquad gr = \frac{15\,gr \times 30\,mg}{1000\,mg \times 1} = \frac{\overset{3}{\cancel{15}}\,gr \times \overset{3}{\cancel{30}}}{\underset{\underset{20}{\cancel{100}}}{\cancel{1000}} \times 1} = \frac{9\,gr}{20} = gr\ 9/20$$

8. Factors: 1 dram = 1 tsp; 9 dr/1. If 1 dr = 1 tsp, then 9 dr = 9 tsp

9. Factors: 1 gr = 60 mg (15 gr = 1000 mg); 1/150 gr/1

$$mg = \frac{60\,mg \times gr\ 1/150}{1\,gr \times 1} = \frac{\overset{2}{\cancel{60}}\,mg \times 1}{1 \times \underset{5}{\cancel{150}}} = \frac{2\,mg}{5}$$
$$= 0.4\,mg$$

$$mg = \frac{1000\,mg \times gr\ 1/150}{15\,gr \times 1} = \frac{\overset{200}{\cancel{\overset{4}{\cancel{1000}}}}\,mg \times 1}{\underset{3}{\cancel{15}} \times \underset{3}{\cancel{150}}} = \frac{4\,mg}{9}$$
$$= 0.444\,mg$$

10. Factors: 1 ml = 15 (16) mx; 0.6 ml/1

$$mx = \frac{15\,mx \times 0.6\,ml}{1\,ml \times 1} = \frac{15\,mx \times 0.6}{1 \times 1} = \frac{9\,mx}{1} = 9\,mx \qquad\qquad mx = \frac{16\,mx \times 0.6\,ml}{1\,ml \times 1} = \frac{16\,mx \times 0.6}{1 \times 1} = \frac{9.6\,mx}{1} = 9.6\,mx$$

11. Factors: 1 oz = 2 Tbsp; 5 oz/1

$$Tbsp = \frac{2\,Tbsp \times 5\,oz}{1\,oz \times 1} = \frac{2\,Tbsp \times 5}{1 \times 1} = \frac{10\,Tbsp}{1} = 10\,Tbsp$$

12. Factors: 1 mg = 1000 mcg; 150 mcg/1

$$mg = \frac{1\,mg \times 150\,mcg}{1000\,mcg \times 1} = \frac{1\,mg \times \overset{15}{\cancel{150}}}{\underset{100}{\cancel{1000}} \times 1} = \frac{15\,mg}{100} = 0.15\,mg$$

13. Factors: 1 cc = 1 ml; 10 cc/1. If 1 cc = 1 ml, then 10 cc = 10 ml.

14. Factors: 1 lb = 16 oz; 1 kg = 2.2 lb; 1 kg = 1000 g; 4 lb 2 oz = 4 1/8 (33/8) lb/1

$$g = \frac{1000\,g \times 1\,kg \times 4\,1/8\,lb}{1\,kg \times 2.2\,lb \times 1} = \frac{\overset{125}{\cancel{1000}}\,g \times 1 \times \overset{3}{\cancel{33}}}{1 \times \underset{0.2}{\cancel{2.2}} \times \underset{1}{\cancel{8}}} = \frac{375\,g}{0.2} = 1875\,g$$

15. Factors: 1 in = 2.5 cm; 6 cm/1

$$in = \frac{1\,in \times 6\,cm}{2.5\,cm \times 1} = \frac{1\,in \times 6}{2.5 \times 1} = \frac{6\,in}{2.5} = 2^{2/5}\ (2.4)\,in$$

16. Factors: 1 g = 1000 mg; 1 mg = 1000 mcg; 0.007 g/1

$$mcg = \frac{1000\,mcg \times 1000\,mg \times 0.007\,g}{1\,mg \times 1\,g \times 1} = \frac{1000\,mcg \times 1000 \times 0.007}{1 \times 1 \times 1} = \frac{7000\,mcg}{1} = 7000\,mcg$$

17. Factors: 1 kg = 2.2 lb; 99 kg/1

$$lb = \frac{2.2\,lb \times 99\,kg}{1\,kg \times 1} = \frac{2.2\,lb \times 99}{1 \times 1} = \frac{217.8\,lb}{1} = 217^{4/5}\,lb$$

18. Factors: 1 qt = 1000 ml; 1.75 qt/1

$$ml = \frac{1000\,ml \times 1.75\,qt}{1\,qt \times 1} = \frac{1000\,ml \times 1.75}{1 \times 1} = \frac{1750\,ml}{1} = 1750\,ml$$

19. Factors: 1 gr = 60 mg; 1 mg = 1000 mcg; 200 mcg/1

$$gr = \frac{1\,gr \times 1\,mg \times 200\,mcg}{60\,mg \times 1000\,mcg \times 1}$$
$$= \frac{1\,gr \times 1 \times \overset{1}{\cancel{200}}}{60 \times \underset{5}{\cancel{1000}} \times 1} = \frac{1\,gr}{300} = gr\ 1/300$$

$$gr = \frac{15\,gr \times 1\,mg \times 200\,mcg}{1000\,mg \times 1000\,mcg \times 1}$$
$$= \frac{\overset{3}{\cancel{15}}\,gr \times 1 \times \overset{1}{\cancel{200}}}{1000 \times \underset{\underset{1}{5}}{\cancel{1000}} \times 1} = \frac{3\,gr}{1000} = gr\ 3/1000$$

20. Factors: 1 tsp = 5 ml; 7 tsp/1

$$ml = \frac{5\,ml \times 7\,tsp}{1\,tsp \times 1} = \frac{5\,ml \times 7}{1 \times 1} = \frac{35\,ml}{1} = 35\,ml$$

21. Factors: 1 qt = 1000 cc; 1250 cc/1

$$qt = \frac{1\,qt \times 1250\,cc}{1000\,cc \times 1} = \frac{1\,qt \times \overset{125}{\cancel{1250}}}{\underset{100}{\cancel{1000}} \times 1} = \frac{125\,qt}{100} = 1^{1/4}\,qt$$

22-25. Factors: 1 Tbsp = 15 ml; 1 C = 8 oz; 1 C = 250 ml; 1 oz = 20 ml

1/2 peach: not fluid intake

8 Tbsp chicken broth:

$$ml = \frac{15\ ml \quad \times 8\ Tbsp}{1\ Tbsp \times 1} = \frac{15\ ml \quad \times 8}{1 \quad \times 1} = \qquad 120\ ml \qquad\qquad\qquad 120\ ml$$

1 C tossed green salad: not fluid intake   2 C Koolade:

$$ml = \frac{30\ ml \times 8\ oz \times 2\ C}{1\ oz \times 1\ C \times 1\ C} = \frac{30\ ml \times 8 \times 2}{1 \times 1 \times 1} = \quad 480ml \qquad\qquad ml = \frac{250\ ml \times 2\ C}{1\ C \times 1} = \frac{250\ ml \times 2}{1 \times 1} = 500\ ml$$

3 oz broiled chicken: not fluid intake

1/2 C milk:

$$ml = \frac{30\ ml \times 8\ oz \times 1/2\ C}{1\ oz \times 1\ C \times 2\ C} = \frac{30\ ml \times \overset{4}{\cancel{8}} \times 1}{1 \times 1 \times \underset{1}{\cancel{2}}} = 120\ ml \qquad\qquad ml = \frac{250\ ml \times 1/2\ C}{1\ C \times 1} = \frac{\overset{125}{\cancel{250}}\ ml \times 1}{1 \times \underset{1}{\cancel{2}}} = 125\ ml$$

Total   720 ml   745 ml

Unit III Posttest C

1. Factors: 1 gr = 60 mg (15 gr = 1000 mg); 1 mg = 1000 mcg; 1/600 gr/1

$$mcg = \frac{1000\ mcg \times 60\ mg \quad \times gr \quad 1/600}{1\ mg \quad \times 1\ gr \quad \times \quad 1} \qquad\qquad mcg = \frac{1000\ mcg \times 1000\ mg \quad \times gr \quad 1/600}{1\ mg \quad \times \quad 15\ gr \quad \times \quad 1}$$

$$= \frac{\overset{10}{\cancel{1000}}\ mcg \times \overset{10}{\cancel{60}} \times 1}{1 \quad \times 1 \times \underset{\underset{1}{\cancel{6}}}{\cancel{600}}} = \frac{100\ mcg}{1} = 100\ mcg \qquad = \frac{1000\ mcg \times \overset{1}{\cancel{1000}} \times 1}{1 \quad \times \underset{3}{\cancel{15}} \times \underset{3}{\cancel{600}}} = \frac{1000\ mcg}{g} = 11.1\ mcg$$

2. Factors: 1 in = 2.5 cm; 1 cm = 10 mm; 50 mm/1

$$in = \frac{1\ in \quad \times \quad 1\ cm \times 50\ mm}{2.5\ cm \quad \times 10\ mm \times \quad 1} = \frac{1\ in \quad \times \quad 1 \times \overset{2}{\cancel{50}}}{\underset{1}{\cancel{2.5}} \quad \times \underset{1}{\cancel{10}} \times \quad 1} = \frac{2\ in}{1} = 2\ in$$

3. Factors: 1 kg = 2.2 lb; 1 lb = 16 oz; 8 lb 4 oz = 8 ¹/₄ (33/4) lb/1

$$kg = \frac{1\ kg \times 8^{1/4}\ lb}{2.2\ lb \times \quad 1} = \frac{1\ kg \times \overset{3}{\cancel{33}}}{\underset{0.2}{\cancel{2.2}} \times 4} = \frac{3\ kg}{0.8} = 3.75\ kg$$

4. Factors: 1 g = 1000 mg; 0.07 g/1

$$mg = \frac{1000\ mg \times 0.07\ g}{1\ g \quad \times \quad 1} = \frac{1000\ mg \times 0.07}{1 \quad \times \quad 1} = \frac{70\ mg}{1} = 70\ mg$$

5. Factors: 1 ml = 15 (16) mx; 4 mx/1

$$ml = \frac{1\ ml \times 4\ mx}{15\ mx \times 1} = \frac{1\ ml \times 4}{15 \quad \times 1} = \frac{4\ ml}{15} = 0.267\ ml \qquad\qquad ml = \frac{1\ ml \times 4\ mx}{16\ mx \times 1} = \frac{1\ ml \times \overset{1}{\cancel{4}}}{\underset{4}{\cancel{16}} \times 1} = \frac{1\ ml}{4} = 0.25\ ml$$

6. Factors: 1 mg = 1000 mcg; 8 mcg/1

$$mg = \frac{1\ mg \quad \times 8\ mcg}{1000\ mcg \times 1} = \frac{1\ mg \quad \times 8}{1000 \quad \times 1} = \frac{8\ mg}{1000} = 0.008\ mg$$

7. Factors: 1 gr = 60 mg (15 gr = 1000 mg); 45 mg/1

$$gr = \frac{1\ gr \quad \times 45\ mg}{60\ mg \times \quad 1} = \frac{1\ gr \times \overset{3}{\cancel{45}}}{\underset{4}{\cancel{60}} \times 1} = \frac{3\ gr}{4} = gr\ 3/4 \qquad\qquad gr = \frac{15\ gr \quad \times 45\ mg}{1000\ mg \times \quad 1} = \frac{\overset{3}{\cancel{15}}gr \times \overset{9}{\cancel{45}}}{\underset{\underset{40}{\cancel{200}}}{\cancel{1000}} \times \quad 1} = \frac{27\ gr}{40} = gr\ 27/40$$

8. Factors: 1 tsp = 1 dram; 11 dr/1. If 1 tsp = 1 dr, then 11 dr = 11 tsp.

9. Factors: 1 gr = 60 mg (15 gr = 1000 mg); gr 1/400/1

$$mg = \frac{60\ mg \times gr \quad 1/400}{1\ gr \times \quad 1} = \frac{\overset{3}{\cancel{60}}\ mg \times \quad 1}{1 \quad \times \underset{20}{\cancel{400}}} \qquad\qquad mg = \frac{1000\ mg \times gr \quad 1/400}{15\ gr \times \quad 1} = \frac{\overset{1}{\cancel{1000}}\ mg \times \quad 1}{\underset{3}{\cancel{15}} \quad \times \underset{2}{\cancel{400}}}$$

$$= \frac{3\ mg}{20} = 0.15\ mg \qquad\qquad\qquad\qquad = \frac{1\ mg}{6} = 0.167\ mg$$

10. Factors: 1 ml = 15 (16) mx; 0.9 ml/1

$$mx = \frac{15\ mx \times 0.9\ ml}{1\ ml \times \quad 1} = \frac{15\ mx \times 0.9}{1 \quad \times \quad 1} = \frac{13.5\ mx}{1} = 13.5\ mx \qquad mx = \frac{16\ mx \times 0.9\ ml}{1\ ml \times \quad 1} = \frac{16\ mx \times 0.9}{1 \quad \times \quad 1} = \frac{14.4\ mx}{1} = 14.4\ mx$$

11. Factors: 1 oz = 2 Tbsp; 7.5 oz/1

$$= \frac{2\ Tbsp \times 7.5\ oz}{1\ oz \quad \times \quad 1} = \frac{2\ Tbsp \times 7.5}{1 \quad \times \quad 1} = \frac{15\ Tbsp}{1} = 15\ Tbsp$$

12. Factors: 1 mg = 1000 mcg; 25 mcg/1

$$mg = \frac{1\,mg \times 25\,mcg}{1000\,mcg \times 1} = \frac{1\,mg \times \overset{1}{\cancel{25}}}{\underset{40}{\cancel{1000}} \times 1} = \frac{1\,ml}{40} = 0.025\,mg$$

13. Factors: 1 ml = 1 cc; 6 cc/1. If 1 ml = 1 cc, then 6 cc = 6 ml.
14. Factors: 1 kg = 1000 g; 1 kg = 2.2 lb; 1 lb = 16 oz; 5 lb 8 oz = 5.5 lb/1

$$g = \frac{1000\,g \times 1\,kg \times 5.5\,lb}{1\,kg \times 2.2\,lb \times 1} = \frac{\overset{500}{\cancel{1000}}\,g \times 1 \times \overset{5}{\cancel{5.5}}}{1 \times \underset{\underset{1}{\cancel{2}}}{\cancel{2.2}} \times 1} = \frac{2500\,g}{1} = 2500\,g$$

15. Factors: 1 in = 2.5 cm; 15 cm/1

$$in = \frac{1\,in \times 15\,cm}{2.5\,cm \times 1} = \frac{1\,in \times \overset{6}{\cancel{15}}}{\underset{1}{\cancel{2.5}} \times 1} = \frac{6\,in}{1} = 6\,in$$

16. Factors: 1 g = 1000 mg; 1 mg = 1000 mcg; 0.06 g/1

$$mcg = \frac{1000\,mcg \times 1000\,mcg \times 0.06\,g}{1\,mg \times 1\,g \times 1} = \frac{1000\,mcg \times 1000 \times 0.06}{1 \times 1 \times 1} = \frac{60000\,mcg}{1} = 60,000\,mcg$$

17. Factors: 1 kg = 2.2 lb; 110 kg/1

$$lb = \frac{2.2\,lb \times 110\,kg}{1\,kg \times 1} = \frac{2.2\,lb \times 110}{1 \times 1} = \frac{242\,lb}{1} = 242\,lb$$

18. Factors: 1 qt = 1000 ml; 3/4 qt/1

$$ml = \frac{1000\,ml \times 3/4\,qt}{1\,qt \times 1} = \frac{\overset{250}{\cancel{1000}}\,ml \times 3}{1 \times \underset{1}{\cancel{4}}} = \frac{750\,ml}{1} = 750\,ml$$

19. Factors: 1 gr = 60 mg (15 gr = 1000 mg); 1 mg = 1000 mcg; 300 mcg/1

$$gr = \frac{1\,gr \times 1\,mg \times 300\,mcg}{60\,mg \times 1000\,mcg \times 1} = \frac{1\,gr \times 1 \times \overset{\overset{1}{\cancel{3}}}{\cancel{300}}}{\underset{1}{\cancel{60}} \times \underset{200}{\cancel{1000}} \times 1} \qquad gr = \frac{15\,gr \times 1\,mg \times 300\,mcg}{1000\,mg \times 1000\,mcg \times 1}$$

$$= \frac{1\,gr}{200} = gr\ 1/200 \qquad\qquad = \frac{\overset{3}{\cancel{15}}\,gr \times 1 \times \overset{3}{\cancel{300}}}{\underset{200}{\cancel{1000}}\ \underset{10}{\cancel{1000}} \times 1} = \frac{9\,gr}{2000} = gr\ 9/2000$$

20. Factors: 1 tsp = 5 ml; 5 tsp/1

$$ml = \frac{5\,ml \times 5\,tsp}{1\,tsp \times 1} = \frac{5\,ml \times 5}{1 \times 1} = \frac{25\,ml}{1} = 25\,ml$$

21. Factors: 1 qt = 1000 cc; 400 cc/1

$$qt = \frac{1\,qt \times 400\,cc}{1000\,cc \times 1} = \frac{1\,qt \times \overset{2}{\cancel{400}}}{\underset{5}{\cancel{1000}} \times 1} = \frac{2\,qt}{5} = 2/5\,qt$$

22-25. Factors: 1 Tbsp = 15 ml; 1 oz = 30 ml

    1 orange: not fluid intake

    5 Tbsp tomato soup: $ml = \dfrac{15\,ml \times 5\,Tbsp}{1\,Tbsp \times 1} = \dfrac{15\,ml \times 5}{1 \times 1} = \dfrac{75\,ml}{1} =$ 75 ml

    1 C chicken salad: not fluid intake

    12 oz Coke: $ml = \dfrac{30\,ml \times 12\,oz}{1\,oz \times 1} = \dfrac{30\,ml \times 12}{1 \times 1} = \dfrac{360\,ml}{1} =$ 360 ml

    4 cookies: not fluid intake

    4 oz ice cream: $ml = \dfrac{30\,ml \times 4\,oz}{1\,oz \times 1} = \dfrac{30\,ml \times 4}{1 \times 1} = \dfrac{120\,ml}{1} =$ 120 ml

    Total   555 ml

UNIT IV: DOSAGE CONVERSIONS AND CALCULATIONS

Unit IV Posttest A

1. Bicillin CR 1,200,000 U IM stat. = Bicillin CR 1,200,000 units intramuscularly immediately.
2. Oretic 50 mg PO b.i.d. = Oretic 50 milligrams by mouth twice a day.
3. Lanoxin 0.5 mg PO stat., then 0.125 mg q.d. = Lanoxin 0.5 milligrams by mouth immediately, then 0.125 milligrams daily.
4. Factors: 100 U = 1 ml; 45 U/1

$$ml = \frac{1\,ml \times 45\,U}{100\,U \times 1} = \frac{1\,ml \times 45}{100 \times 1} = \frac{45\,ml}{100} = 0.45\,ml$$

5. Factors: 3 mg = 1 ml; 1/60 gr/1; 1 gr = 60 mg

$$ml = \frac{1\ ml\ \times 60\ mg \times gr\ \ 1/60}{3\ mg \times\ 1\ gr\ \times\ \ \ 1} = \frac{1\ ml\ \times \overset{1}{\cancel{60}} \times\ 1}{3\ \ \ \times\ 1 \times \cancel{60}} = \frac{1\ ml}{3} = 0.33\ ml$$

6. Factor: 500 mcg = 5 ml; 0.2 mg/1; 1 mg = 1000 mcg

$$ml = \frac{5\ ml\ \ \times 1000\ mcg \times 0.2\ mg}{500\ mcg \times\ \ \ 1\ mg\ \ \times\ 1} = \frac{5\ ml\ \ \ \times \overset{2}{\cancel{1000}} \times 0.2}{\underset{1}{\cancel{500}}\ \ \ \ \times\ 1 \times\ 1} = \frac{2\ ml}{1} = 2\ ml$$

7. Factors: 0.5 g = 5 ml; 200 mg/1; 1 g = 1000 mg

$$ml = \frac{5\ ml\ \times\ \ \ 1\ g\ \ \ \times 200\ mg}{0.5\ g\ \ \times 1000\ mg \times\ \ 1} = \frac{\overset{1}{\cancel{5}}\ ml\ \times\ \ \ 1 \times \overset{1}{\cancel{200}}}{0.5\ \ \ \times \underset{\cancel{5}}{\cancel{1000}} \times\ 1} = \frac{1\ ml}{0.5} = 2\ ml$$

8. Factors: 300 mg = 5 ml (1 tsp); gr 10/1; 15 gr = 1000 mg

$$tsp = \frac{1\ tsp \times 1000\ mg \times 10\ gr}{300\ mg \times\ \ 15\ gr\ \times\ 1} = \frac{1\ tsp \times \overset{10}{\underset{3}{\cancel{1000}}} \times \overset{2}{\underset{3}{\cancel{10}}}}{\cancel{300}\ \ \ \times \cancel{15} \times\ 1}$$

$$tsp = \frac{1\ tsp \times 60\ mg \times 10\ gr}{300\ mg \times\ 1\ gr\ \times\ 1} = \frac{1\ tsp \times \overset{1}{\cancel{60}} \times \overset{2}{\cancel{10}}}{\underset{1}{\cancel{300}}\ \ \times\ 1 \times\ 1}$$

$$= \frac{20\ tsp}{9} = 2\ ^{2/9}\ tsp \qquad\qquad = \frac{2\ tsp}{1} = 2\ tsp$$

9. Factors: 250 mg = 1 ml; 0.5 g/1; 1 g = 1000 mg

$$ml = \frac{1\ ml\ \times 1000\ mg \times 0.5\ g}{250\ mg \times\ \ 1\ g\ \ \times\ 1} = \frac{1\ ml\ \times \overset{4}{\cancel{1000}} \times 0.5}{\underset{1}{\cancel{250}} \times\ \ 1\ \times\ 1} = \frac{2\ ml}{1} = 2\ ml$$

10. Factors: 0.1 g = 1 ml; 1/2 gr/1; 1 g = 15 gr

$$ml = \frac{1\ ml \times\ 1\ g\ \ \times gr\ \ 1/2}{0.1\ g\ \times 15\ gr \times\ \ \ 1} = \frac{1\ ml \times\ 1 \times\ 1}{0.1\ \ \ \times 15 \times 2} = \frac{1\ ml}{3} = 0.33\ ml$$

11. Factors: 600 mcg = 1 tab; 1/200 gr/1; 1 mg = 1000 mcg; 1 gr = 60 mg

$$tab = \frac{1\ tab\ \ \times 1000\ mcg \times 60\ mg\ \ \times gr\ \ 1/200}{600\ mcg \times\ \ \ \ 1\ mg\ \ \times 1\ gr\ \ \times\ \ \ \ \ 1} = \frac{1\ tab\ \ \times \overset{\cancel{100}}{\underset{\cancel{10}}{\cancel{1000}}} \times \overset{1}{\cancel{60}} \times\ \ \overset{1}{\ } \ 1}{\underset{1}{\underset{\cancel{10}}{\cancel{600}}}\ \ \ \times\ 1 \times 1 \times \underset{2}{\cancel{200}}} = \frac{1\ tab}{2} = 1/2\ tab$$

12. Factors: 250 mg = 2.5 ml; 500 ml/1

$$ml = \frac{2.5\ ml\ \times 500\ mg}{250\ mg \times\ \ 1} = \frac{2.5\ ml\ \times \overset{2}{\cancel{500}}}{\underset{1}{\cancel{250}}\ \ \times\ 1} = \frac{5\ ml}{1} = 5\ ml\ total\ medication\ solution$$

5 ml − 2.8 ml = 2.2 ml dry powder

13. Factors: 2.5 g = 5 ml; 250 mg/1; 1 g = 1000 mg

$$ml = \frac{5\ ml\ \times\ \ \ 1\ g\ \ \ \times 250\ mg}{2.5\ g\ \ \times 1000\ mg \times\ \ 1} = \frac{\overset{2}{\cancel{5}}\ ml\ \times\ \ \ 1 \times \overset{1}{\cancel{250}}}{\underset{1}{\cancel{2.5}}\ \ \ \times \underset{4}{\cancel{1000}} \times\ 1} = \frac{2\ ml}{4} = 0.5\ mg$$

14. Factors: 1 mg = 2 ml; 100 mcg/1; 1 mg = 1000 mcg

$$ml = \frac{2\ ml\ \ \times\ \ \ 1\ mg\ \ \times 100\ mcg}{1\ mg\ \ \times 1000\ mcg \times\ \ 1} = \frac{\overset{1}{\cancel{2}}\ ml\ \ \times\ \ \ 1 \times \overset{1}{\cancel{100}}}{1\ \ \ \ \times \underset{5}{\underset{\cancel{10}}{\cancel{1000}}} \times\ 1} = \frac{1\ ml}{5} = 0.2\ ml$$

15. Factors: 1 tab = 0.325 g; 15gr/1; 1 g = 15 gr

$$tab = \frac{1\ tab \times\ 1\ g\ \ \times 15\ gr}{0.325\ g\ \ \times 15\ gr \times\ 1} = \frac{1\ tab \times\ 1 \times \overset{1}{\cancel{15}}}{0.325\ \ \times \cancel{15} \times\ 1} = \frac{1\ tab}{0.325} = 3.076\ (3)\ tab$$

16. Factors: 1 tab = 50 mcg; 0.2 mg/1; 1 mg = 1000 mcg

$$ml = \frac{1\ tab\ \ \times 1000\ mcg \times 0.2\ mg}{50\ mcg \times\ \ \ 1\ mg\ \ \times\ 1} = \frac{1\ tab\ \ \times \overset{20}{\cancel{1000}} \times 0.2}{\underset{1}{\cancel{50}}\ \ \times\ \ 1\ \times\ 1} = \frac{4\ tab}{1} = 4\ tab$$

17. Factors: 0.4 mg = 1 ml; 200 mcg/1; 1 mg = 1000 mcg; 15 (16) mx = 1 ml

$$mx = \frac{15\ mx \times 1\ ml \times 1\ mg \times 200\ mcg}{1\ ml \times 0.4\ mg \times 1000\ mcg \times 1}$$

$$= \frac{\overset{3}{\cancel{15}}\ mx \times 1 \times 1 \times \cancel{200}}{1 \times 0.4 \times \underset{\underset{1}{\cancel{5}}}{\cancel{1000}} \times 1} = \frac{3\ mx}{0.4} = 7.5\ mx$$

$$mx = \frac{16\ mx \times 1\ ml \times 1\ mg \times 200\ mcg}{1\ ml \times 0.4\ mg \times 1000\ mcg \times 1}$$

$$= \frac{\overset{4}{\cancel{16}}\ mx \times 1 \times 1 \times \cancel{200}}{1 \times \underset{0.1}{\cancel{0.4}} \times \underset{5}{\cancel{1000}} \times 1} = \frac{4\ mx}{0.5} = 8\ mx$$

18. Factors: 1 tab = 200 mcg; 0.6 mg/1; 1 mg = 1000 mcg

$$tab = \frac{1\ tab \times 1000\ mcg \times 0.6\ mg}{200\ mcg \times 1\ mg \times 1} = \frac{1\ tab \times \overset{5}{\cancel{1000}} \times 0.6}{\underset{1}{\cancel{200}} \times 1 \times 1} = \frac{3\ tab}{1} = 3\ tab$$

19. Factors: 5 mg = 5 ml; 1/30 gr/1; 1 gr = 60mg

$$ml = \frac{5\ ml \times 60\ mg \times gr\ 1/30}{5\ mg \times 1\ gr \times 1} = \frac{\overset{1}{\cancel{5}}\ ml \times \overset{2}{\cancel{60}} \times 1}{\underset{1}{\cancel{5}} \times 1 \times \underset{1}{\cancel{30}}} = \frac{2\ ml}{1} = 2\ ml$$

20. Factors: 500 mg = 5 ml (1 tsp); 250 mg/1

$$tsp = \frac{1\ tsp \times 250\ mg}{500\ mg \times 1} = \frac{1\ tsp \times \overset{1}{\cancel{250}}}{\underset{2}{\cancel{500}} \times 1} = \frac{1\ tsp}{2} = 1/2\ tsp$$

21. Factors: 1/60 gr; 1 gr = 60 mg

$$mg = \frac{60\ mg \times gr\ 1/60}{1\ gr \times 1} = \frac{\overset{1}{\cancel{60}}\ mg \times 1}{1 \times \underset{1}{\cancel{60}}} = \frac{1\ mg}{1} = 1\ mg$$

Tablet A, 1 mg, is the appropriate tab.

22. Factors: 250 mg = 1 tab; 0.5 g/1; 1 g = 1000 mg

$$tab = \frac{1\ tab \times 1000\ mg \times 0.5\ g}{250\ mg \times 1\ g \times 1} = \frac{1\ tab \times \overset{4}{\cancel{1000}} \times 0.5}{\underset{1}{\cancel{250}} \times 1 \times 1} = \frac{2\ tab}{1} = 2\ tab$$

23. Factors: 20 mcg/1; 1 mg = 1000 mcg

$$mg = \frac{1\ mg \times 20\ mcg}{1000\ mcg \times 1} = \frac{1\ mg \times \overset{1}{\cancel{20}}}{\underset{50}{\cancel{1000}} \times 1} = \frac{1\ mg}{50} = 0.02\ mg$$

Amp C is the appropriate ampule.

24. Factors: 1 tab = 500 mg; 1.5 g/1; 1 g = 1000 mg

$$tab = \frac{1\ tab \times 1000\ mg \times 1.5\ g}{500\ mg \times 1\ g \times 1} = \frac{1\ tab \times \overset{2}{\cancel{1000}} \times 1.5}{\underset{1}{\cancel{500}} \times 1 \times 1} = \frac{3\ tab}{1} = 3\ tab$$

25. Factors: 100 mg = 1 ml; 75 mg/1

$$ml = \frac{1\ ml \times 75\ mg}{100\ mg \times 1} = \frac{1\ ml \times 75}{100 \times 1} = \frac{75\ ml}{100} = 0.75\ mg$$

Unit IV Posttest B

1. Epinephrine 0.3 mg s.c. stat. = epinephrine 0.3 milligrams subcutaneously immediately.
2. Seconal gr iss PO h.s. PRN = Seconal grains 1 1/2 by mouth at bedtime as needed.
3. Lanoxin 0.125 mg PO q.o.d. = Lanoxin 0.125 milligrams by mouth every other day.
4. Factors: 100 U = 1 ml; 35 U/1

$$ml = \frac{1\ ml \times 35\ U}{100\ U \times 1} = \frac{1\ ml \times 35}{100 \times 1} = \frac{35\ ml}{100} = 0.35\ ml$$

5. Factors: 3 mg = 1 ml; 1/100 gr/1; 1 gr = 60 mg

$$ml = \frac{1\ ml \times 60\ mg \times gr\ 1/100}{3\ mg \times 1\ gr \times 1} = \frac{1\ ml \times \overset{\overset{2}{\cancel{20}}}{\cancel{60}} \times 1}{\underset{1}{\cancel{3}} \times 1 \times \underset{10}{\cancel{100}}} = \frac{2\ ml}{10} = 0.2\ ml$$

6. Factors: 200 mcg = 1 ml; 0.3 mg/1; 1 mg = 1000 mcg

$$ml = \frac{1\ ml \times 1000\ mcg \times 0.3\ mg}{200\ mcg \times 1\ mg \times 1\ mg} = \frac{1\ ml \times \overset{5}{\cancel{1000}} \times 0.3}{\underset{1}{\cancel{200}} \times 1 \times 1} = \frac{1.5\ ml}{1} = 1.5\ ml$$

7. Factors: 0.5 g = 5 ml; 150 mg/1; 1 g = 1000 mg

$$ml = \frac{5\,ml \times 1\,g \times 150\,mg}{0.5\,g \times 1000\,mg \times 1} = \frac{\overset{1}{\cancel{5}}\,ml \times 1 \times \overset{15}{\cancel{150}}}{\underset{0.1}{\cancel{0.5}} \times \underset{100}{\cancel{1000}} \times 1} = \frac{15\,ml}{10} = 1.5\,ml$$

8. Factors: 500 mg = 5 ml (1 tsp); gr 15/1; 15 gr = 1000 mg

$$tsp = \frac{1\,tsp \times 1000\,mg \times gr\ 15}{500\,mg \times 15\,gr \times 1} = \frac{1\,tsp \times \overset{2}{\cancel{1000}} \times \overset{1}{\cancel{15}}}{\underset{1}{\cancel{500}} \times \underset{1}{\cancel{15}} \times 1} = \frac{2\,tsp}{1} = 2\,tsp$$

9. Factors: 500 mg = 1 ml; 0.25 g/1; 1 g = 1000 mg

$$ml = \frac{1\,ml \times 1000\,mg \times 0.25\,g}{500\,mg \times 1\,g \times 1\,g} = \frac{1\,ml \times \overset{2}{\cancel{1000}} \times 0.25}{\underset{1}{\cancel{500}} \times 1 \times 1} = \frac{0.5\,ml}{1} = 0.5\,ml$$

10. Factors: 0.1 g = 1 ml; gr 1.5/1; 1 g = 15 gr

$$ml = \frac{1\,ml \times 1\,g \times gr\ 1.5}{0.1\,g \times 15\,gr \times 1} = \frac{1\,ml \times 1 \times \overset{0.1}{\cancel{1.5}}}{0.1 \times \underset{1}{\cancel{15}} \times 1} = \frac{0.1\,ml}{0.1} = 1\,ml$$

11. Factors: 1 tab = 100 mcg; 1/300 gr/1; 1 mg = 1000 mcg; 1 gr = 60 mg

$$tab = \frac{1\,tab \times 1000\,mcg \times 60\,mg \times gr\ 1/300}{100\,mcg \times 1\,mg \times 1\,gr \times 1} = \frac{1\,tab \times \overset{2}{\cancel{1000}} \times 60 \times 1}{\underset{1}{\cancel{100}} \times 1 \times 1 \times \cancel{300}} = \frac{2\,tab}{1} = 2\,tab$$

12. Factors: 250 mg = 1 ml; 2 g/1; 1 g = 1000 mg

$$ml = \frac{1\,ml \times 1000\,mg \times 2\,g}{250\,mg \times 1\,g \times 1} = \frac{1\,ml \times \overset{4}{\cancel{1000}} \times 2}{\underset{1}{\cancel{250}} \times 1 \times 1} = \frac{8\,ml}{1} = 8\,ml\ \text{total medication solution}$$

8 ml − 4.8 ml = 3.2 ml dry powder

13. Factors: 2 g = 5 ml; 300 mg/1; 1 g = 1000 mg

$$ml = \frac{5\,ml \times 1\,g \times 300\,mg}{2\,g \times 1000\,mg \times 1} = \frac{\overset{1}{\cancel{5}}\,ml \times 1 \times \overset{3}{\cancel{300}}}{2 \times \underset{2}{\cancel{1000}} \times 1} = \frac{3\,ml}{4} = 0.75\,mg$$

14. Factors: 1 mg = 2 ml; 300 mcg/1; 1 mg = 1000 mcg

$$ml = \frac{2\,ml \times 1\,mg \times 300\,mcg}{1\,mg \times 1000\,mcg \times 1} = \frac{2\,ml \times 1 \times \overset{3}{\cancel{300}}}{1 \times \underset{10}{\cancel{1000}} \times 1} = \frac{6\,ml}{10} = 0.6\,ml$$

15. Factors: 1 tab = 0.325 g; 20 gr/1; 1 g = 15 gr

$$tab = \frac{1\,tab \times 1\,g \times 20\,gr}{0.325\,g \times 15\,gr \times 1} = \frac{1\,tab \times 1 \times \overset{4}{\cancel{20}}}{0.325 \times \underset{3}{\cancel{15}} \times 1} = \frac{4\,tab}{0.975} = 4.1\ \text{or}\ 4\,tab$$

16. Factors: 25 mcg = 1 tab; 0.1 mg/1; 1 mg = 1000 mcg

$$tab = \frac{1\,tab \times 1000\,mcg \times 0.1\,mg}{25\,mcg \times 1\,mg \times 1} = \frac{1\,tab \times \overset{40}{\cancel{1000}} \times 0.1}{\underset{1}{\cancel{25}} \times 1 \times 1} = \frac{4\,tab}{1} = 4\,tab$$

17. Factors: 0.4 mg = 1 ml; 400 mcg/1; 1 mg = 1000 mcg; 15 (16) mx = 1 ml

$$mx = \frac{15\,mx \times 1\,ml \times 1\,mg \times 400\,mcg}{1\,ml \times 0.4\,mg \times 1000\,mcg \times 1}$$

$$= \frac{\overset{3}{\cancel{15}}\,mx \times 1 \times 1 \times \overset{4}{\cancel{400}}}{1 \times \underset{0.1}{\cancel{0.4}} \times \underset{2}{\cancel{1000}} \times 1} = \frac{3\,mx}{0.2} = 15\,mx$$

$$mx = \frac{16\,mx \times 1\,ml \times 1\,mg \times 400\,mg}{1\,ml \times 0.4\,mg \times 1000\,mcg \times 1}$$

$$= \frac{\overset{4}{\cancel{16}}\,mx \times 1 \times 1 \times \overset{2}{\cancel{400}}}{1 \times \underset{0.1}{\cancel{0.4}} \times \underset{5}{\cancel{1000}} \times 1} = \frac{8\,mx}{0.5} = 16\,mx$$

18. Factors: 200 mcg = 1 tab; 0.5 mg/1; 1 mg = 1000 mcg

$$tab = \frac{1\,tab \times 1000\,mcg \times 0.5\,mg}{200\,mcg \times 1\,mg \times 1} = \frac{1\,tab \times \overset{5}{\cancel{1000}} \times 0.5}{\underset{1}{\cancel{200}} \times 1 \times 1} = \frac{2.5\,tab}{1} = 2.5\,tab$$

19. Factors: 5 mg = 5 ml; 1/3 gr/1; 1 gr = 60 mg

$$\text{ml} = \frac{5\text{ ml}\times 60\text{ mg}\times 1/3\text{ gr}}{5\text{ mg}\times 1\text{ gr}\times 1} = \frac{\cancel{5}\text{ ml}\times\cancel{60}\overset{20}{\times} 1}{\cancel{5}\text{ mg}\times 1\times\cancel{3}\underset{1}{}} = \frac{20\text{ ml}}{1} = 20\text{ ml}$$

20. Factors: 500 mg = 5 ml (1 tsp); 750 mg/1

$$\text{tsp} = \frac{1\text{ tsp}\times 750\text{ mg}}{500\text{ mg}\times 1} = \frac{1\text{ tsp}\times\overset{3}{\cancel{750}}}{\underset{2}{\cancel{500}}\times 1} = \frac{3\text{ tsp}}{2} = 1^{1/2}\text{ tsp}$$

21. Factors: 1 gr = 60 mg; 1/2 gr/1

$$\text{mg} = \frac{60\text{ mg}\times\text{gr }1/2}{1\text{ gr}\times 1} = \frac{\overset{30}{\cancel{60}}\text{ mg}\times 1}{1\times\underset{1}{\cancel{2}}} = \frac{30\text{ mg}}{1} = 30\text{ mg}$$

The appropriate tablet is tab B.

22. Factors: 500 mg = 1 tab; 0.25 g/1; 1 g = 1000 mg

$$\text{tab} = \frac{1\text{ tab}\times 1000\text{ mg}\times 0.25\text{ g}}{500\text{ mg}\times 1\text{ g}\times 1} = \frac{1\text{ tab}\times\overset{2}{\cancel{1000}}\times 0.25}{\underset{1}{\cancel{500}}\times 1\times 1} = \frac{0.5\text{ tab}}{1} = 0.5\text{ tab}$$

23. Factors: 1000 mcg = 1 mg; 400 mcg/1

$$\text{mg} = \frac{1\text{ mg}\times 400\text{ mcg}}{1000\text{ mcg}\times 1} = \frac{1\text{ mg}\times\overset{4}{\cancel{400}}}{\underset{10}{\cancel{1000}}\times 1} = \frac{4\text{ mg}}{10} = 0.4\text{ mg}$$

Ampule B, 0.4 mg/ml is appropriate

24. Factors: 250 mg = 1 tab; 0.5 g/1; 1 g = 1000 mg

$$\text{tab} = \frac{1\text{ tab}\times 1000\text{ mg}\times 0.5\text{ g}}{250\text{ mg}\times 1\text{ g}\times 1} = \frac{1\text{ tab}\times\overset{4}{\cancel{1000}}\times 0.5}{\underset{1}{\cancel{250}}\times 1\times 1} = \frac{2\text{ tab}}{1} = 2\text{ tab}$$

25. Factors: 100 mg = 1 ml; 60 mg/1

$$\text{ml} = \frac{1\text{ ml}\times 60\text{ mg}}{100\text{ mg}\times 1} = \frac{1\text{ ml}\times\overset{6}{\cancel{60}}}{\underset{10}{\cancel{100}}\times 1} = \frac{6\text{ ml}}{10} = 0.6\text{ ml}$$

Unit IV Posttest C

1. Keflin 1 g IV PB stat., then 500 mg IV PB q.6h. = Keflin 1 gram intravenously piggyback immediately, then 500 milligrams intravenously piggyback every 6 hours.
2. Dilantin 100 mg PO t.i.d. = Dilantin 100 milligrams by mouth three times a day
3. Benadryl elix 12.5 mg PO q.4h. PRN = Benadryl elixer 12.5 milligrams by mouth every 4 hours as needed.
4. Factors: 100 U = 1 ml; 28 U/1

$$\text{ml} = \frac{1\text{ ml}\times 28\text{ U}}{100\text{ U}\times 1} = \frac{1\text{ ml}\times 28}{100\times 1} = \frac{28\text{ ml}}{100} = 0.28\text{ ml}$$

5. Factors: 3 mg = 2 ml; 1/30 gr/1; 1 gr = 60 mg

$$\text{ml} = \frac{2\text{ ml}\times 60\text{ mg}\times\text{gr }1/30}{3\text{ mg}\times 1\text{ gr}\times 1} = \frac{2\text{ ml}\times\overset{2}{\cancel{60}}\times 1}{3\times 1\times\underset{1}{\cancel{30}}} = \frac{4\text{ ml}}{3} = 1.3\text{ ml}$$

6. Factors: 500 mcg = 1 ml; 0.4 mg/1; 1 mg = 1000 mcg

$$\text{ml} = \frac{1\text{ ml}\times 1000\text{ mcg}\times 0.4\text{ mg}}{500\text{ mcg}\times 1\text{ mg}\times 1} = \frac{1\text{ ml}\times\overset{2}{\cancel{1000}}\times 0.4}{\underset{1}{\cancel{500}}\times 1\times 1} = \frac{0.8\text{ ml}}{1} = 0.8\text{ ml}$$

7. Factors: 0.5 g = 5 ml; 300 mg/1; 1 g = 1000 mcg

$$\text{ml} = \frac{5\text{ ml}\times 1\text{ g}\times 300\text{ mg}}{0.5\text{ g}\times 1000\text{ mg}\times 1} = \frac{\overset{1}{\cancel{5}}\text{ ml}\times 1\times\overset{3}{\cancel{300}}}{\underset{0.1}{\cancel{0.5}}\times\underset{10}{\cancel{1000}}\times 1} = \frac{3\text{ ml}}{1} = 3\text{ ml}$$

8. Factors: 500 mg = 5 ml (1 tsp); gr 7.5/1; 15 gr = 1000 mg

$$\text{tsp} = \frac{1\text{ tsp}\times 1000\text{ mg}\times\text{gr }7.5}{500\text{ mg}\times 15\text{ gr}\times 1} = \frac{1\text{ tsp}\times\overset{2}{\cancel{1000}}\times\overset{0.5}{\cancel{7.5}}}{\underset{1}{\cancel{500}}\times\underset{1}{\cancel{15}}\times 1} = \frac{1\text{ tsp}}{1} = 1\text{ tsp}$$

9. Factors: 500 mg = 1 ml; 0.25 g/1; 1 g = 1000 mg

$$\text{ml} = \frac{1\text{ ml}\times 1000\text{ mg}\times 0.25\text{ g}}{500\text{ mg}\times 1\text{ g}\times 1} = \frac{1\text{ ml}\times\overset{2}{\cancel{1000}}\times 0.25}{\underset{1}{\cancel{500}}\times 1\times 1} = \frac{0.5\text{ ml}}{1} = 0.5\text{ ml}$$

10. Factors: 0.5 g = 5 ml; gr 1.5/1; 15 gr = 1 g

$$ml = \frac{5\,ml \times 1\,g \times 1.5\,gr}{0.5\,gr \times 15\,gr \times 1} = \frac{5\,ml \times 1 \times \overset{0.1}{\cancel{1.5}}}{0.5 \times \cancel{15} \times 1} = \frac{0.5\,ml}{0.5} = 1\,ml$$

11. Factors: 200 mcg = 1 tab; 1/150 gr/1; 1 mg = 1000 mcg; 1 gr = 60 mg

$$tab = \frac{1\,tab \times 1000\,mcg \times 60\,mg \times gr\ 1/150}{200\,mcg \times 1\,mg \times 1\,gr \times 1} = \frac{1\,tab \times \cancel{1000} \times \overset{2}{\cancel{60}} \times 1}{\cancel{200} \times 1 \times 1 \times \cancel{150}} = \frac{2\,tab}{1} = 2\,tab$$

12. Factors: 250 mg = 2.5 ml; 1 g/1; 1 g = 1000 mg

$$ml = \frac{2.5\,ml \times 1000\,mg \times 1\,g}{250\,mg \times 1\,g \times 1} = \frac{2.5\,ml \times \overset{4}{\cancel{1000}} \times 1}{\cancel{250} \times 1 \times 1} = \frac{10\,ml}{1} = 10\,ml\ total\ medication\ solution$$

10 ml − 7.3 ml = 2.7 ml dry powder

13. Factors: 2 g = 5 ml; 400 mg/1; 1 g = 1000 mg

$$ml = \frac{5\,ml \times 1\,g \times 400\,mg}{2\,g \times 1000\,mg \times 1} = \frac{\cancel{5}\,ml \times 1 \times \cancel{400}}{\cancel{2} \times \cancel{1000} \times 1} = \frac{1\,ml}{1} = 1\,ml$$

14. Factors: 1 mg = 2 ml; 200 mcg/1; 1 mg = 1000 mcg

$$ml = \frac{2\,ml \times 1\,mg \times 200\,mcg}{1\,mg \times 1000\,mcg \times 1} = \frac{2\,ml \times 1 \times \cancel{200}}{1 \times \cancel{1000} \times 1} = \frac{2\,ml}{5} = 0.4\,ml$$

15. Factors: 0.5 g = 1 tab; gr 15/1; 1 g = 15 gr

$$tab = \frac{1\,tab \times 1\,g \times gr\ 15}{0.5\,g \times 15\,gr \times 1} = \frac{1\,tab \times 1 \times \cancel{15}}{0.5 \times \cancel{15} \times 1} = \frac{1\,tab}{0.5} = 2\,tab$$

16. Factors: 50 mcg = 1 tab; 0.15 mg/1; 1 mg = 1000 mcg

$$tab = \frac{1\,tab \times 1000\,mcg \times 0.15\,mg}{50\,mcg \times 1\,mg \times en1} = \frac{1\,tab \times \overset{20}{\cancel{1000}} \times 0.15}{\cancel{50} \times 1 \times 1} = \frac{3\,tab}{1} = 3\,tab$$

17. Factors: 0.4 mg = 1 ml; 300 mcg/1; 1 mg = 1000 mcg; 15 (16) mx = 1 ml

$$mx = \frac{15\,mx \times 1\,ml \times 1\,mg \times 300\,mcg}{1\,ml \times 0.4\,mg \times 1000\,mcg \times 1}$$
$$= \frac{\overset{3}{\cancel{15}}\,mx \times 1 \times 1 \times \cancel{300}}{1 \times 0.4 \times \cancel{1000} \times 1} = \frac{9\,mx}{0.8} = 11.25\,mx$$

$$mx = \frac{16\,mx \times 1\,ml \times 1\,mg \times 300\,mcg}{1\,ml \times 0.4\,mg \times 1000\,mcg \times 1}$$
$$= \frac{\overset{4}{\cancel{16}}\,mx \times 1 \times 1 \times \cancel{300}}{1 \times \cancel{0.4} \times \cancel{1000} \times 1} = \frac{12\,mx}{1} = 12\,mx$$

18. Factors: 200 mcg = 1 tab; 0.5 mg/1; 1 mg = 1000 mcg

$$tab = \frac{1\,tab \times 1000\,mcg \times 0.5\,mg}{200\,mcg \times 1\,mg \times 1} = \frac{1\,tab \times \overset{5}{\cancel{1000}} \times 0.5}{\cancel{200} \times 1 \times 1} = \frac{2.5\,tab}{1} = 2.5\,tab$$

19. Factors: 5 mg = 5 ml; 1/4 gr/1; gr 1 = 60 mg

$$ml = \frac{5\,ml \times 60\,mg \times gr\ 1/4}{5\,mg \times 1\,gr \times 1} = \frac{\cancel{5}\,ml \times \cancel{60} \times 1}{\cancel{5} \times 1 \times \cancel{4}} = \frac{15\,ml}{1} = 15\,ml$$

20. Factors: 5 ml (1 tsp) = 100 mg; 250 mg

$$tsp = \frac{1\,tsp \times 250\,mg}{100\,mg \times 1} = \frac{1\,tsp \times \overset{25}{\cancel{250}}}{\underset{10}{\cancel{100}} \times 1} = \frac{25\,tsp}{10} = 2.5\,tsp$$

21. Factors: 1 gr = 60 mg; 1/3 gr/1

$$mg = \frac{60\,mg \times gr\ 1/3}{1\,gr \times 1} = \frac{\overset{20}{\cancel{60}}\,mg \times 1}{1 \times \cancel{3}} = \frac{20\,mg}{1} = 20\,mg$$

Tab A is the appropriate tab.

22. Factors: 250 mg = 1 tab; 0.125 g/1; 1 g = 1000 mg

$$\text{tab} = \frac{1\text{ tab} \times 1000\text{ mg} \times 0.125\text{ g}}{250\text{ mg} \times 1\text{ g} \times 1} = \frac{1\text{ tab} \times \overset{4}{\cancel{1000}} \times 0.125}{\underset{1}{\cancel{250}} \times 1 \times 1} = \frac{0.5\text{ tab}}{1} = 0.5\text{ tab}$$

23. Factors: 1 mg = 1000 mcg; 30 mcg/1

$$\text{mg} = \frac{1\text{ mg} \times 30\text{ mcg}}{1000\text{ mcg} \times 1} = \frac{1\text{ mg} \times \overset{3}{\cancel{30}}}{\underset{100}{\cancel{1000}} \times 1} = \frac{3\text{ mg}}{100} = 0.03\text{ mg}$$

Amp C is the appropriate amp.

24. Factors: 500 mg = 1 tab; 0.25 g/1; 1 g = 1000 mg

$$\text{tab} = \frac{1\text{ tab} \times 1000\text{ mg} \times 0.25\text{ g}}{500\text{ mg} \times 1\text{ g} \times 1} = \frac{1\text{ tab} \times \overset{2}{\cancel{1000}} \times 0.25}{\underset{1}{\cancel{500}} \times 1 \times 1} = \frac{0.5\text{ tab}}{1} = 0.5\text{ tab}$$

25. Factors: 100 mg = 1 ml; 40 mg/1

$$\text{ml} = \frac{1\text{ ml} \times 40\text{ mg}}{100\text{ mg} \times 1} = \frac{1\text{ ml} \times \overset{4}{\cancel{40}}}{\underset{10}{\cancel{100}} \times 1} = \frac{4\text{ ml}}{10} = 0.4\text{ ml}$$

UNIT V: CALCULATIONS BASED ON BODY WEIGHT

Unit V Test A

1. Factors: 1 mg = 1 lb; 1 kg = 2.2 lb; 50 kg/1

$$\text{mg} = \frac{1\text{ mg} \times 2.2\text{ lb} \times 50\text{ kg}}{1\text{ lb} \times 1\text{ kg} \times 1} = \frac{1\text{ mg} \times 2.2 \times 50}{1 \times 1 \times 1} = \frac{110\text{ mg}}{1} = 110\text{ mg}$$

2. Factors: 50 mcg = 1 kg; 1 kg = 2.2 lb; 176 lb/1; 2 doses = 1 d

$$\text{mcg} = \frac{50\text{ mcg} \times 1\text{ kg} \times 176\text{ lb}}{1\text{ kg} \times 2.2\text{ lb} \times 1\text{ lb}} = \frac{50\text{ mcg} \times 1 \times \overset{80}{\cancel{176}}}{1 \times \underset{1}{\cancel{2.2}} \times 1} = \frac{4000\text{ mcg}}{1} = 4000\text{ mcg (/d)}$$

$$\frac{\text{mcg}}{\text{dose}} = \frac{4000\text{ mcg} \times 1\text{ d}}{1\text{ d} \times 2\text{ doses}} = \frac{\overset{2000}{\cancel{4000}}\text{ mcg} \times 1}{1 \times \underset{1}{\cancel{2}}\text{ doses}} = \frac{2000\text{ mcg}}{1\text{ dose}} = 2000\text{ mcg/dose}$$

3. Factors: recommended: (up to) 35 mg = 1 kg; 1 kg = 2.2 lb; 198 lb/1

$$\text{mg} = \frac{35\text{ mg} \times 1\text{ kg} \times 198\text{ lb}}{1\text{ kg} \times 2.2\text{ lb} \times 1} = \frac{35\text{ mg} \times 1 \times \overset{90}{\cancel{198}}}{1 \times \underset{1}{\cancel{2.2}} \times 1} = \frac{3150\text{ mg}}{1\text{ mg}} = 3150\text{ mg (/d)}$$

Factors: 500 mg = (q) 4 h; 24 h = 1 d

$$\text{mg} = \frac{500\text{ mg} \times 24\text{ h}}{(q)\ 4\text{h} \times 1\text{ d}} = \frac{500\text{ mg} \times \overset{6}{\cancel{24}}}{\underset{1}{\cancel{4}} \times 1} = \frac{3000\text{ mg}}{1\text{ d}} = 3000\text{ mg/d}$$

The ordered dosage is within the recommended range.

4. Factors: 1 tab = 500 mg; 30 mg = 1 kg; 1 kg = 2.2 lb; 110 lb/1

$$\text{tab} = \frac{1\text{ tab} \times 30\text{ mg} \times 1\text{ kg} \times 110\text{ lb}}{500\text{ mg} \times 1\text{ kg} \times 2.2\text{ lb} \times 1} = \frac{1\text{ tab} \times \overset{3}{\cancel{30}} \times 1 \times \overset{\overset{1}{\cancel{50}}}{\cancel{110}}}{\underset{\underset{1}{\cancel{50}}}{\cancel{500}} \times 1 \times \underset{1}{\cancel{2.2}} \times 1} = \frac{3\text{ tabs}}{1} = 3\text{ tabs}$$

5. Factors: 0.5 mg = 1 lb; 120 lb/1

$$\text{mg} = \frac{0.5\text{ mg} \times 120\text{ lb}}{1\text{ lb} \times 1} = \frac{0.5\text{ mg} \times 120}{1 \times 1} = \frac{60\text{ mg}}{1} = 60\text{ mg}$$

6. Factors: 20 U = 1 kg; 1 kg = 2.2 lb; 189 lb/1

$$\text{U} = \frac{20\text{ U} \times 1\text{ kg} \times 189\text{ lb}}{1\text{ kg} \times 2.2\text{ lb} \times 1} = \frac{\overset{10}{\cancel{20}}\text{ U} \times 1 \times 189}{1 \times \underset{1.1}{\cancel{2.2}} \times 1} = \frac{1890\text{ U}}{1.1} = 1718.18\text{ U}$$

7. Factors: 1.5 mcg = 1 kg; 1 kg = 2.2 lb; 88 lb/1

$$\text{mcg} = \frac{1.5\text{ mcg} \times 1\text{ kg} \times 88\text{ lb}}{1\text{ kg} \times 2.2\text{ lb} \times 1} = \frac{1.5\text{ mcg} \times 1 \times \overset{40}{\cancel{88}}}{1 \times \underset{1}{\cancel{2.2}} \times 1} = \frac{60\text{ mcg}}{1} = 60\text{ mcg}$$

8. Factors: Recommended minimum: 20 mg = 1 kg; 1 kg = 2.2 lb; 132 lb/1

$$mg = \frac{20\ mg \times 1\ kg \times \overset{60}{\cancel{132\ lb}}}{1\ kg \times \cancel{2.2}\ lb \times 1\ lb} = \frac{1200\ mg}{1} = 1200\ mg\ (/d)$$

Factors: Recommended maximum: 50 mg = 1 kg; 1 kg = 2.2 lb; 132 lb/1

$$mg = \frac{50\ mg \times 1\ kg \times 132\ lb}{1\ kg \times 2.2\ lb \times 1} = \frac{50\ mg \times 1 \times \overset{60}{\cancel{132}}}{1\ kg \times \underset{1}{\cancel{2.2}} \times 1} = \frac{3000\ mg}{1} = 3000\ mg\ (/d)$$

Factors: 500 mg = (q) 4 h; 24 h = 1 d

$$mg = \frac{500\ mg \times 24\ h}{(q)\ 4h \times 1\ d} = \frac{500\ mg \times \overset{6}{\cancel{24}}}{\underset{1}{\cancel{4}} \times 1\ d} = \frac{3000\ mg}{1} = 3000\ mg/d$$

The ordered dosage is within the recommended range.

9. Factors: 0.01 ml = 1 kg; 1 kg = 2.2 lb; 121 lb/1

$$ml = \frac{0.01\ ml \times 1\ kg \times 121\ lb}{1\ kg \times 2.2\ lb \times 1} = \frac{0.01\ ml \times 1 \times \overset{55}{\cancel{121}}}{1 \times \underset{1}{\cancel{2.2}} \times 1} = \frac{0.55\ ml}{1} = 0.55\ ml$$

10. Factors: 10 mcg = 1 kg; 68 kg/1

$$mcg = \frac{10\ mcg \times 68\ kg}{1\ kg \times 1} = \frac{10\ mcg \times 68}{1 \times 1} = \frac{680\ mcg}{1} = 680\ mcg\ (/d)$$

Unit V Test B

1. Factors: 2 mg = 1 lb; 1 kg = 2.2 lb; 50 kg/1

$$mg = \frac{2\ mg \times 2.2\ lb \times 50\ kg}{1\ lb \times 1\ kg \times 1} = \frac{2\ mg \times 2.2 \times 50}{1 \times 1 \times 1} = \frac{220\ mg}{1} = 220\ mg$$

2. Factors: 100 mcg = 1 kg; 1 kg = 2.2 lb; 176 lb/1; 2 doses = 1 d

$$mcg = \frac{100\ mcg \times 1\ kg \times 176\ lb}{1\ kg \times 2.2\ lb \times 1} = \frac{100\ mcg \times 1 \times \overset{80}{\cancel{176}}}{1 \times \underset{1}{\cancel{2.2}} \times 1} = \frac{8000\ mcg}{1} = 8000\ mcg\ (/d)$$

$$\frac{mcg}{dose} = \frac{8000\ mcg \times 1\ d}{1\ d \times 2\ doses} = \frac{\overset{4000}{\cancel{8000}}\ mcg \times 1}{1 \times \underset{1}{\cancel{2}}\ doses} = \frac{4000\ mcg}{1\ dose} = 4000\ mcg/dose$$

3. Factors: Recommended: (up to) 50 mg = 1 kg; 1 kg = 2.2 lb; 198 lb/1

$$mg = \frac{50\ mg \times 1\ kg \times 198\ lb}{1\ kg \times 2.2\ lb \times 1} = \frac{50\ mg \times 1 \times \overset{90}{\cancel{198}}}{1 \times \underset{1}{\cancel{2.2}} \times 1} = \frac{4500\ mg}{1} = 4500\ mg\ (/d)$$

Factors: Ordered: 750 mg = (q) 4 h; 24 h = 1 d

$$\frac{mg}{d} = \frac{750\ mg \times 24\ h}{(q)\ 4h \times 1\ d} = \frac{750\ mg \times \overset{6}{\cancel{24}}}{\underset{1}{\cancel{4}} \times 1} = \frac{4500\ mg}{1} = 4500\ mg/d$$

The ordered dosage is within the recommended range.

4. Factors: 1 tab = 500 mg; 40 mg = 1 kg; 1 kg = 2.2 lb; 110 lb/1

$$tab = \frac{1\ tab \times 40\ mg \times 1\ kg \times 110\ lb}{500\ mg \times 1\ kg \times 2.2\ lb \times 1} = \frac{1\ tab \times \overset{4}{\cancel{40}} \times 1 \times \overset{\overset{1}{\cancel{50}}}{\cancel{110}}}{\underset{\underset{1}{\cancel{50}}}{\cancel{500}} \times 1 \times \underset{1}{\cancel{2.2}} \times 1} = \frac{4\ tabs}{1} = 4\ tabs$$

5. Factors: 0.05 mg = 1 lb; 120 lb/1

$$mg = \frac{0.05\ mg \times 120\ lb}{1\ lb \times 1} = \frac{0.05\ mg \times 120}{1 \times 1} = \frac{6\ mg}{1} = 6\ mg$$

6. Factors: 30 U = 1 kg; 1 kg = 2.2 lb; 189 lb/1

$$U = \frac{30\ U \times 1\ kg \times 189\ lb}{1\ kg \times 2.2\ lb \times 1} = \frac{30\ U \times 1 \times 189}{1 \times 2.2 \times 1} = \frac{5670\ U}{2.2} = 2577.27\ U$$

7. Factors: 1.8 mcg = 1 kg; 1 kg = 2.2 lb; 88 lb

$$mcg = \frac{1.8\ mcg \times 1\ kg \times 88\ lb}{1\ kg \times 2.2\ lb \times 1} = \frac{1.8\ mcg \times 1 \times \overset{40}{\cancel{88}}}{1 \times \underset{1}{\cancel{2.2}} \times 1} = \frac{72\ mcg}{1} = 72\ mcg$$

8. Factors: Recommended minimum: 20 mg = 1 kg; 1 kg = 2.2 lb; 132 lb/1

$$mg = \frac{20\,mg \times\ 1\,kg\ \times 132\,lb}{1\,kg\ \times 2.2\,lb\ \times\ \ 1} = \frac{20\,mg \times\ 1 \times \overset{60}{\cancel{132}}}{1\ \ \times \cancel{2.2} \times\ 1} = \frac{1200\,mg}{1} = 1200\,mg\ (/d)$$

Factors: Recommended maximum: 50 mg = 1 kg; 1 kg = 2.2 lb; 132 lb/1

$$mg = \frac{50\,mg \times\ 1\,kg\ \times 132\,lb}{1\,kg\ \times 2.2\,lb\ \times\ \ 1} = \frac{50\,mg \times\ 1 \times \overset{60}{\cancel{132}}}{1\ \ \times \cancel{2.2} \times\ 1} = \frac{3000\,mg}{1} = 3000\,mg\ (/d)$$

Factors: Ordered: 250 mg = (q) 4 h; 24 h = 1 d

$$\frac{mg}{d} = \frac{250\,mg \times 24\,h}{(q)\ 4h\ \times\ 1\,d} = \frac{250\,mg \times \overset{6}{\cancel{24}}}{\cancel{4}\ \ \times\ 1\,d} = \frac{1500\,mg}{1\,d} = 1500\,mg/d$$

The ordered dosage is within the recommended range.

9. Factors: 0.05 ml = 1 kg; 1 kg = 2.2 lb; 121 lb/1

$$1\,ml = \frac{0.05\,ml \times\ \ 1\,kg \times 121\,lb}{1\,kg \times 2.2\,lb\ \times\ \ 1} = \frac{0.05\,mg \times\ \ 1 \times \overset{55}{\cancel{121}}}{1\ \ \times \cancel{2.2}\ \times\ 1} = \frac{2.75\,ml}{1} = 2.75\,ml$$

10. Factors: 10 mcg = 1 kg; 78 kg/1

$$mcg = \frac{10\,mcg \times 78\,kg}{1\,kg\ \ \times\ 1} = \frac{10\,mcg \times 78}{1\ \ \times\ 1} = \frac{780\,mcg}{1} = 780\,mcg$$

Unit V Test C

1. Factors: 8 mg = 1 lb; 1 kg = 2.2 lb; 50 kg/1

$$mg = \frac{8\,mg \times 2.2\,lb\ \times 50\,kg}{1\,lb\ \times\ 1\,kg \times\ 1} = \frac{8\,mg \times 2.2 \times 50}{1\ \ \times\ 1 \times 1} = \frac{880\,mg}{1} = 880\,mg$$

2. Factors: 25 mcg = 1 kg; 1 kg = 2.2 lb; 176 lb; 2 doses = 1 d

$$mcg = \frac{25\,mcg \times\ \ 1\,kg\ \ \times 176\,lb}{1\,kg\ \ \times 2.2\,lb\ \times\ \ 1} = \frac{25\,mcg \times\ 1 \times \overset{80}{\cancel{176}}}{1\ \ \times \cancel{2.2} \times\ 1} = \frac{2000\,mcg}{1} = 2000\,mcg(/d)$$

$$\frac{mcg}{dose} = \frac{2000\,mcg\ \ \times 1\,day}{1\,day\ \ \times 2\,doses} = \frac{\overset{1000}{\cancel{2000}}\,mcg\ \ \times 1}{1\ \ \times \cancel{2}\,doses} = \frac{1000\,mcg}{1\,dose} = 1000\,mcg/dose$$

3. Factors: Recommended: (up to) 25 mg = 1 kg; 1 kg = 2.2 lb; 198 lb/1

$$mg = \frac{25\,mg \times\ \ 1\,kg\ \times 198\,lb}{1\,kg\ \times 2.2\,lb\ \times\ \ 1} = \frac{25\,mg \times\ 1 \times \overset{90}{\cancel{198}}}{1\ \ \times \cancel{2.2} \times\ 1} = \frac{2250\,mg}{1} = 2250\ (/d)$$

Factors: Ordered: 250 mg = (q) 4 h; 24 h = 1 d

$$\frac{mg}{d} = \frac{250\,mg \times 24\,h}{(q)\ 4h\ \times\ 1} = \frac{250\,mg \times \overset{6}{\cancel{24}}}{\cancel{4}\ \ \times\ 1} = \frac{1500\,mg}{1\,d} = 1500\,mg/d$$

The ordered dosage is within the recommended dosage.

4. Factors: 500 mg = 1 tab; 35 mg = 1 kg; 1 kg = 2.2 lb; 110 lb/1

$$tab = \frac{1\,tab \times 35\,mg \times\ \ 1\,kg\ \ \times 110\,lb}{500\,mg \times\ \ 1\,kg\ \times 2.2\,lb\ \times\ \ 1} = \frac{1\,tab \times \overset{7}{\cancel{35}} \times\ \ 1 \times \overset{\overset{1}{\cancel{50}}}{\cancel{110}}}{\underset{\underset{2}{\cancel{100}}}{\cancel{500}}\ \ \times\ \ 1 \times \cancel{2.2}\ \ \times\ 1} = \frac{7\,tabs}{2} = 3.5\,tabs$$

5. Factors: 0.005 mg = 1 lb; 120 lb/1

$$mg = \frac{0.005\,mg \times 120\,lb}{1\,lb\ \ \times\ 1} = \frac{0.005\,mg \times 120}{1\ \ \times\ 1} = \frac{0.6\,mg}{1} - 0.6\,mg$$

6. Factors: 15 U = 1 kg; 1 kg = 2.2 lb; 189 lb/1

$$U = \frac{15\,U\ \times\ 1\,kg \times 189\,lb}{1\,kg \times 2.2\,lb\ \times\ 1\,lb} = \frac{15\,U\ \times\ \ 1 \times 189}{1\ \ \times\ 2.2 \times\ 1} = \frac{2835\,U}{2.2} = 1288.6\,U$$

7. Factors: 2.2 mcg = 1 kg; 1 kg = 2.2 lb; 88 lb/1

$$mcg = \frac{2.5\,mcg \times\ \ 1\,kg\ \ \times 88\,lb}{1\,kg\ \ \times 2.2\,lb\ \times\ \ 1} = \frac{2.5\,mcg \times\ \ 1 \times \overset{40}{\cancel{88}}}{1\,mcg \times \cancel{2.2} \times\ 1} = \frac{100\,mcg}{1} = 100\,mcg\ (/d)$$

8. Factors: Recommended minimum: 20 mg = 1 kg; 1 kg = 2.2 lb; 198 lb/1

$$mg = \frac{20\,mg \times\ 1\,kg\ \times 198\,lb}{1\,kg\ \times 2.2\,lb\ \times\ 1} = \frac{20\,mg \times\ 1 \times \overset{90}{\cancel{198}}}{1\ \times \cancel{2.2} \times\ 1} = \frac{1800\,mg}{1} = 1800\,mg\ (/d)$$

Factors: Recommended maximum: 50 mg = 1 kg; 1 kg = 2.2 lb; 198 lb/1

$$mg = \frac{50\,mg \times\ 1\,kg\ \times 198\,lb}{1\,kg\ \times 2.2\,lb\ \times\ 1} = \frac{50\,mg \times\ 1 \times \overset{90}{\cancel{198}}}{1\ \times \cancel{2.2} \times\ 1} = \frac{4500\,mg}{1} = 4500\,mg\ (/d)$$

Factors: Ordered: 1 g = 1000 mg; 1 g = (q) 4 h; 24 h = 1 d

$$mg = \frac{1000\,mg \times\ 1\,g\ \times 24\,h}{1\,g\ \times (q)4h\ \times\ 1\,d} = \frac{1000\,mg \times 1 \times \overset{6}{\cancel{24}}}{1\ \times \cancel{4} \times\ 1\,d} = \frac{6000\,mg}{1d} = 6000\,mg/d$$

Ordered dosage exceeds recommended dosage.

9. Factors: 0.02 ml = 1 kg; 1 kg = 2.2 lb; 121 lb/1

$$ml = \frac{0.02\,ml \times\ 1\,kg \times 121\,lb}{1\,kg \times 2.2\,lb \times\ 1} = \frac{0.02\,ml \times\ 1 \times \overset{55}{\cancel{121}}}{1\ \times \cancel{2.2} \times\ 1} = \frac{1.1\,ml}{1} = 1.1\,ml$$

10. Factors: 10 mcg = 1 kg; 98 kg/1

$$mcg = \frac{10\,mcg \times 98\,kg}{1\,kg\ \times\ 1} = \frac{10\,mcg \times 98}{1\ \times\ 1} = \frac{980\,mcg}{1} = 980\,mcg\ (/d)$$

UNIT VI: SOLUTIONS

Unit VI Posttest A

1. Factors: 1 g = 1000 mg; 1 g = 500 ml (1:500 = 1 ml (g) medication in 500 ml solution)

$$\frac{mg}{ml} = \frac{1000\,mg \times\ 1\,g}{1\,g\ \times 500\,ml} = \frac{\overset{2}{\cancel{1000}}\,mg \times\ 1}{1\ \times \cancel{500}\,ml} = \frac{2\,mg}{1\,ml} = 2\,mg/ml$$

2. Factors: 1 L = 1000 ml; 2 L = 100%; 0.9%/1

$$ml = \frac{1000\,ml \times\ 2\,L\ \times 0.9\%}{1\,L\ \times 100\%\ \times\ 1} = \frac{\cancel{1000}\,ml \times\ 2 \times 0.9}{1\,ml \times \overset{10}{\cancel{100}} \times\ 1} = \frac{18\,ml}{1} = 18\,ml$$

3. Factors: 1 oz = 30 ml; 150 ml = 50%; 20%/1

$$oz = \frac{1\,oz \times 150\,ml \times 20\%}{30\,ml \times\ 50\% \times\ 1} = \frac{1\,oz \times \overset{1}{\cancel{150}} \times \overset{2}{\cancel{20}}}{\cancel{30} \times\ \cancel{50} \times\ 1} = \frac{2\,oz}{1} = 2\,oz$$

4. Factors: 200 ml = 1/10; 1 = 100%; 5%/1

$$ml = \frac{200\,ml \times\ 1\ \times 5\%}{1/10\ \times 100\% \times 1} = \frac{10 \times \overset{2}{\cancel{200}}\,ml \times\ 1 \times 5}{1\ \times \cancel{100} \times 1} = \frac{100\,ml}{1} = 100\,ml$$

5. Factors: 1 g = 4 Cal; 50 ml (g) = 100%; 50%/1

$$Cal = \frac{4\,Cal \times\ 50\,g\ \times 50\%}{1\,g\ \times 100\% \times\ 1} = \frac{\overset{1}{\cancel{4}}\,Cal \times \overset{2}{\cancel{50}} \times 50}{1\ \times \underset{25}{\cancel{100}} \times 50} = \frac{100\,Cal}{1} = 100\,Cal$$

6. Factors: 50 ml = 100%; 5%/1

$$ml = \frac{50\,ml \times 5\%}{100\% \times 1} = \frac{\cancel{50}\,ml \times 5}{\underset{2}{\cancel{100}} \times 1} = \frac{5\,ml}{2} = 2.5\,ml$$

7. Factors: 1 tsp = 5 ml; 1000 ml = 1 L; 2 L = 100%; 0.45%/1

$$tsp = \frac{1\,tsp \times 1000\,ml \times\ 2\,L\ \times 0.45\%}{5\,ml \times\ 1\,L \times 100\% \times\ 1} = \frac{1\,tsp \times \overset{\overset{2}{\cancel{10}}}{\cancel{1000}} \times\ 2 \times 0.45}{\cancel{5} \times\ 1 \times \cancel{100} \times\ 1} = \frac{1.8\,tsp}{1} = 1.8\,tsp$$

8. Factors: 250 ml = 30%; 15%/1

$$ml = \frac{250\ ml \times 15\%}{30\% \times 1} = \frac{\overset{125}{\cancel{250}}\ ml \times \overset{1}{\cancel{15}}}{\underset{\underset{1}{2}}{\cancel{30}} \times 1} = \frac{125\ ml}{1} = 125\ ml$$

9. Factors: 1 L = 1000 ml (g); 1 L = 100%; 5%/1

$$g = \frac{1000\ g \times\ 1\ L \times 5\%}{1\ L \times 100\% \times 1} = \frac{\overset{10}{\cancel{1000}}\ g \times\ 1 \times 5}{1\ \times \underset{1}{\cancel{100}} \times 1} = \frac{50\ g}{1} = 50\ g$$

10. Factors: 1 L = 1000 ml; 1 L = 5%; 1/1000; 1 = 100 %

$$ml = \frac{1000\ ml \times 1\ L\ \times 100\% \times\ 1}{1\ L\ \times 5\%\ \times\ 1\ \times 1000} = \frac{\overset{1}{\cancel{1000}}\ ml \times 1 \times \overset{20}{\cancel{100}} \times\ 1}{1\ \times \underset{1}{\cancel{5}} \times\ 1 \times \underset{1}{\cancel{1000}}} = \frac{20\ ml}{1} = 20\ ml$$

Unit VI Posttest B

1. Factors: 1 g = 1000 mg; 1 g = 40 ml (1:40 = 1 ml (g) medication in 40 ml solution)

$$\frac{mg}{ml} = \frac{1000\ mg \times\ 1\ g}{1\ g\ \times 40\ ml} = \frac{\overset{25}{\cancel{1000}}\ mg \times\ 1}{1\ \times \underset{1}{\cancel{40}}\ ml} = \frac{25\ mg}{1\ ml} = 25\ mg/ml$$

2. Factors: 1 L = 1000 ml; 1.5 L = 100%; 0.9%

$$ml = \frac{1000\ ml \times\ 1.5\ L\ \times 0.9\%}{1\ L\ \times 100\%\ \times\ 1} = \frac{\overset{10}{\cancel{1000}}\ ml \times\ 1.5 \times 0.9}{1\ \times \underset{1}{\cancel{100}} \times\ 1} = \frac{13.5\ ml}{1} = 13.5\ ml$$

3. Factors: 1 oz = 30 ml; 100 ml = 40%; 20%/1

$$oz = \frac{1\ oz \times 100\ ml \times 20\%}{30\ ml \times\ 40\%\ \times\ 1} = \frac{1\ oz \times \overset{\overset{5}{\cancel{10}}}{\cancel{100}} \times \overset{1}{\cancel{20}}}{\underset{3}{\cancel{30}}\ \times \underset{\underset{1}{2}}{\cancel{40}} \times\ 1} = \frac{5\ oz}{3} = 1\ ^2/_3\ oz$$

4. Factors: 100 ml = 1/10; 1 = 100%; 2.5%1

$$ml = \frac{100\ ml \times\ 1\ \times 2.5\%}{1/10\ \times 100\%\ \times\ 1} = \frac{10 \times \overset{1}{\cancel{100}}\ ml \times\ 1 \times 2.5}{1\ \times \underset{1}{\cancel{100}} \times\ 1} = \frac{25\ ml}{1} = 25\ ml$$

5. Factors: 1 g = 4 Cal; 100 ml (g) = 100%; 50%/1

$$Cal = \frac{4\ Cal \times 100\ g\ \times 50\%}{1\ g\ \times 100\%\ \times\ 1} = \frac{4\ Cal \times \overset{1}{\cancel{100}} \times 50}{1\ \times \underset{1}{\cancel{100}} \times\ 1} = \frac{200\ Cal}{1} = 200\ Cal$$

6. Factors: 500 ml = 100%; 5%/1

$$ml = \frac{500\ ml \times 5\%}{100\% \times 1} = \frac{\overset{5}{\cancel{500}}\ ml \times 5}{\underset{1}{\cancel{100}}\ \times 1} = \frac{25\ ml}{1} = 25\ ml$$

7. Factors: 1 tsp = 5 ml; 1 L = 1000 ml; 1 L = 100%; 0.45%/1

$$tsp = \frac{1\ tsp \times 1000\ ml \times\ 1\ L\ \times 0.45\%}{5\ ml \times\ 1\ L\ \times 100\%\ \times\ 1} = \frac{1\ tsp \times \overset{\overset{2}{\cancel{10}}}{\cancel{1000}} \times\ 1 \times 0.45}{\underset{1}{\cancel{5}}\ \times\ 1 \times \underset{1}{\cancel{100}} \times\ 1} = \frac{0.9\ tsp}{1} = 0.9\ (1)\ tsp$$

8. Factors: 250 ml = 30%; 10%/1

$$ml = \frac{250\ ml \times 10\%}{30\% \times\ 1} = \frac{250\ ml \times \overset{1}{\cancel{10}}}{\underset{3}{\cancel{30}}\ \times 1} = \frac{250\ ml}{3} = 83.3\ ml$$

9. Factors: 1000 ml (g) = 1 L; 0.5 L = 100%; 5%/1

$$g = \frac{1000\ g\ \times\ 0.5\ L \times 5\%}{L \times 100\% \times 1} = \frac{\overset{10}{\cancel{1000}}\ g\ \times\ 0.5 \times 5}{1\ \times \underset{1}{\cancel{100}} \times 1} = \frac{25\ g}{1} = 25\ g$$

10. Factors: 500 ml = 5%; 1 = 100%; 1/1000

$$\text{ml} = \frac{500\,\text{ml} \times 100\% \times 1}{5\% \times 1 \times 1000} = \frac{\cancel{500}\,\text{ml} \times \cancel{100} \times 1}{\cancel{5} \times 1 \times \cancel{1000}} = \frac{10\,\text{ml}}{1} = 10\,\text{ml}$$

Unit VI Posttest C

1. Factors: 1 g = 1000 mg; 1 g = 100 ml (1:100 = 1 ml (g) medication in 100 ml solution)

$$\frac{\text{mg}}{\text{ml}} = \frac{1000\,\text{mg} \times 1\,\text{g}}{1\,\text{g} \times 100\,\text{ml}} = \frac{\cancel{1000}\,\text{mg} \times 1}{1 \times \cancel{100}\,\text{ml}} = \frac{10\,\text{mg}}{1\,\text{ml}} = 10\,\text{mg/ml}$$

2. Factors: 1 L = 1000 ml; 1 L = 100%; 0.9%/1

$$\text{ml} = \frac{1000\,\text{ml} \times 1\,\text{L} \times 0.9\%}{1\,\text{L} \times 100\% \times 1} = \frac{\cancel{1000}\,\text{ml} \times 1 \times 0.9}{1 \times \cancel{100} \times 1} = \frac{9\,\text{ml}}{1} = 9\,\text{ml}$$

3. Factors: 1 oz = 30 ml; 200 ml = 50%; 25%/1

$$\text{oz} = \frac{1\,\text{oz} \times 200\,\text{ml} \times 25\%}{30\,\text{ml} \times 50\% \times 1} = \frac{1\,\text{oz} \times \cancel{200} \times \cancel{25}}{\cancel{30} \times \cancel{50} \times 1} = \frac{10\,\text{oz}}{3} = 3\,^{1}/_{3}\,\text{oz}$$

4. Factors: 200 ml = 1/5; 1 = 100%; 10%/1

$$\text{ml} = \frac{200\,\text{ml} \times 1 \times 10\%}{1/5 \times 100\% \times 1} = \frac{5 \times \cancel{200}\,\text{ml} \times 1 \times 10}{1 \times \cancel{100} \times 1} = \frac{100\,\text{ml}}{1} = 100\,\text{ml}$$

5. Factors: 4 Cal = 1 g; 250 ml (g) = 100%; 10%/1

$$\text{Cal} = \frac{4\,\text{Cal} \times 250\,\text{g} \times 10\%}{1\,\text{g} \times 100\% \times 1} = \frac{\cancel{4}\,\text{Cal} \times \cancel{250} \times 10}{1 \times \cancel{100} \times 1} = \frac{100\,\text{Cal}}{1} = 100\,\text{Cal}$$

6. Factors: 150 ml = 100%; 5%/1

$$\text{ml} = \frac{150\,\text{ml} \times 5\%}{100\% \times 1} = \frac{\cancel{150}\,\text{ml} \times \cancel{5}}{\cancel{100} \times 1} = \frac{15\,\text{ml}}{2} = 7.5\,\text{ml}$$

7. Factors: 1 tsp = 5 ml; 1 L = 1000 ml; 1.5 L = 100%; 0.45%

$$\text{tsp} = \frac{1\,\text{tsp} \times 1000\,\text{ml} \times 1.5\,\text{L} \times 0.45\%}{5\,\text{ml} \times 1\,\text{L} \times 100\% \times 1} = \frac{1\,\text{tsp} \times \cancel{1000} \times \cancel{1.5} \times 0.45}{\cancel{5} \times 1 \times \cancel{100} \times 1} = \frac{1.35\,\text{tsp}}{1} = 1.35\,\text{tsp}$$

8. Factors: 500 ml = 50%; 15%/1

$$\text{ml} = \frac{500\,\text{ml} \times 15\%}{50\% \times 1} = \frac{\cancel{500}\,\text{ml} \times 15}{\cancel{50}\,\text{ml} \times 1} = \frac{150\,\text{ml}}{1} = 150\,\text{ml}$$

9. Factors: 1 L = 1000 ml (g); 0.5 L = 100%; 0.9%

$$\text{g} = \frac{1000\,\text{g} \times 0.5\,\text{L} \times 0.9\%}{1\,\text{L} \times 100\% \times 1} = \frac{\cancel{1000}\,\text{g} \times 0.5 \times 0.9}{1 \times \cancel{100} \times 1} = \frac{4.5\,\text{g}}{1} = 4.5\,\text{g}$$

10. Factors: 1 L = 1000 ml; 1 L = 10%; 100% = 1; 1/1000

$$\text{ml} = \frac{1000\,\text{ml} \times 1\,\text{L} \times 100\% \times 1}{1\,\text{L} \times 10\% \times 1 \times 1000} = \frac{\cancel{1000}\,\text{ml} \times 1 \times \cancel{100} \times 1}{1 \times \cancel{10} \times 1 \times \cancel{1000}} = \frac{10\,\text{ml}}{1} = 10\,\text{ml}$$

UNIT VII: INTRAVENOUS FLUID ADMINISTRATION

Unit VII Posttest A

1. Factors: Volume/h: 1000 ml = 6 h

$$\frac{\text{ml}}{\text{h}} = \frac{1000\,\text{ml}}{6\,\text{h}} = 166.6\,\text{ml/h}$$

Factors: Volume/3 h: 1000 ml = 6 h; 3 h/1

$$ml = \frac{1000\,ml \times 3\,h}{6\,h \times 1} = \frac{\overset{500}{\cancel{1000\,ml}} \times \overset{1}{\cancel{3}}}{\underset{\underset{1}{2}}{\cancel{6}} \times 1} = \frac{500\,ml}{1} = 500\,ml$$

If half the time has elapsed, half the solution should have infused.

2. Factors: 1000 ml = 12 h; 15 gtt = 1 ml; 1 h = 60 min

$$\frac{gtt}{min} = \frac{15\,gtt}{1\,ml} \times \frac{1000\,ml}{12\,h} \times \frac{1\,h}{60\,min} = \frac{\overset{1}{\cancel{15\,gtt}} \times \overset{125}{\cancel{\overset{250}{\cancel{1000}}}} \times 1}{1 \times \underset{3}{\cancel{12}} \times \underset{2}{\cancel{60}}\,min} = \frac{125\,gtt}{6\,min} = 20.8\,(21)\,gtt/min$$

3. Factors: Drip rate: 1000 ml = 24 h; 60 gtt = 1 ml; 1 h = 60 min

$$\frac{gtt}{min} = \frac{60\,gtt}{1\,ml} \times \frac{1000\,ml}{24\,h} \times \frac{1\,h}{60\,min} = \frac{\overset{1}{\cancel{60\,gtt}} \times \overset{125}{\cancel{1000}} \times 1}{1 \times \underset{3}{\cancel{24}} \times \underset{1}{\cancel{60}}\,min} = \frac{125\,gtt}{3\,min} = 41.6\,(42)\,gtt/min$$

Factors: Infusion time: Expected: 1000 ml = 24 h; 10 h/1; Actual: 500 ml

$$ml = \frac{1000\,ml \times 10\,h}{24\,h \times 1} = \frac{\overset{125}{\cancel{1000}}\,ml \times 10}{\underset{3}{\cancel{24}} \times 1} = \frac{1250\,ml}{3} = 416.6 \pm 25 = 391\,to\,441$$

500 ml > 416 (391 to 441). Therefore, IV is infusing too rapidly.

Factors: Recalculation: 500 ml = 14 h; 60 gtt = 1 ml; 1 h = 60 min

$$\frac{gtt}{min} = \frac{60\,gtt}{1\,ml} \times \frac{500\,ml}{14\,h} \times \frac{1\,h}{60\,min} = \frac{\overset{1}{\cancel{60\,gtt}} \times \overset{250}{\cancel{500}} \times 1}{1 \times \underset{7}{\cancel{14}} \times \underset{1}{\cancel{60}}\,min} = \frac{250\,gtt}{7\,min} = 35.7\,(36)\,gtt/min$$

4. Factors: 500 ml = 6 h; 10 gtt = 1 ml; 1 h = 60 min

$$\frac{gtt}{min} = \frac{10\,gtt}{1\,ml} \times \frac{500\,ml}{6\,h} \times \frac{1\,h}{60\,min} = \frac{\overset{1}{\cancel{10\,gtt}} \times \overset{125}{\cancel{\overset{250}{\cancel{500}}}} \times 1}{1 \times \underset{3}{\cancel{6}} \times \underset{\underset{3}{6}}{\cancel{60}}\,min} = \frac{125\,gtt}{9\,min} = 13.8\,(14)\,gtt/min$$

5. Factors: 100 ml = 1/2 (0.5) h; 20 gtt = 1 ml; 1 h = 60 min

$$\frac{gtt}{min} = \frac{20\,gtt}{1\,ml} \times \frac{100\,ml}{0.5\,h} \times \frac{1\,h}{60\,min} = \frac{\overset{1}{\cancel{20\,gtt}} \times \overset{20}{\cancel{100}} \times 1}{1 \times \underset{0.1}{\cancel{0.5}} \times \underset{3}{\cancel{60}}\,min} = \frac{20\,gtt}{0.3\,min} = 66.6\,(67)\,gtt/min$$

6. Factors: 50 ml = 1 h; 60 gtt = 1 ml; 1 h = 60 min

$$\frac{gtt}{min} = \frac{60\,gtt}{1\,ml} \times \frac{50\,ml}{1\,h} \times \frac{1\,h}{60\,min} = \frac{\overset{1}{\cancel{60\,gtt}} \times 50 \times 1}{1 \times 1 \times \underset{1}{\cancel{60}}\,min} = \frac{50\,gtt}{1\,min} = 50\,gtt/min$$

7. Factors: 250 ml = 2 h; 10 gtt = 1 ml; 1 h = 60 min

$$\frac{gtt}{min} = \frac{10\,gtt}{1\,ml} \times \frac{250\,ml}{2\,h} \times \frac{1\,h}{60\,min} = \frac{\overset{1}{\cancel{10\,gtt}} \times \overset{125}{\cancel{250}} \times 1}{1 \times \underset{1}{\cancel{2}} \times \underset{6}{\cancel{60}}\,min} = \frac{125\,gtt}{6\,min} = 20.8\,(21)\,gtt/min$$

8. Factors: Volume/h: 1000 ml = 4 h

$$\frac{ml}{h} = \frac{1000\,ml}{4\,h} = \frac{\overset{250}{\cancel{1000}}\,ml}{\underset{1}{\cancel{4}}\,h} = \frac{250\,ml}{1\,h} = 250\,ml/h$$

Factors: Drip rate: 1000 ml = 4 h; 10 gtt = 1 ml; 1 h = 60 min

$$\frac{gtt}{min} = \frac{10\,gtt}{1\,ml} \times \frac{1000\,ml}{4\,h} \times \frac{1\,h}{60\,min} = \frac{\overset{1}{\cancel{10\,gtt}} \times \overset{250}{\cancel{1000}} \times 1}{1 \times \underset{1}{\cancel{4}} \times \underset{6}{\cancel{60}}\,min} = \frac{250\,gtt}{6\,min} = 41.6\,(42)\,gtt/min$$

Factors: Infusion time: Expected: 250 ml = 1 h (1000 ml = 4 h); 1.5 h/1:
Actual: 1000 ml − 350 ml = 650 ml

$$ml = \frac{250\,ml \times 1.5\,h}{1\,h \times 1} = \frac{250\,ml \times 1.5}{1 \times 1} = \frac{375\,ml}{1} = 375\,ml \pm 25 = 350\,to\,400\,ml$$

650 > 375 ml (350 to 400 ml). IV infusing too rapidly.

Factors: Recalculation: 350 ml = 2.5 h (4h − 1.5 h); 10 gtt = 1 ml; 1 h = 60 min

$$\frac{gtt}{min} = \frac{10\ gtt}{1\ ml} \times \frac{350\ ml}{2.5\ h} \times \frac{1\ h}{60\ min} = \frac{\overset{1}{\cancel{10\ gtt}} \times \overset{14}{\cancel{350}} \times 1}{1 \times \underset{0.1}{\cancel{2.5}} \times \underset{6}{\cancel{60}}\ min} = \frac{14\ gtt}{0.6\ min} = 23.3\ (24)\ gtt/min$$

9. Factors: 1000 ml = 6 h; 15 gtt = 1 ml; 1 h = 60 min

$$\frac{gtt}{min} = \frac{15\ gtt}{1\ ml} \times \frac{1000\ ml}{6\ h} \times \frac{1\ h}{60\ min} = \frac{\overset{1}{\cancel{15\ gtt}} \times \overset{\overset{125}{\cancel{250}}}{\cancel{1000}} \times 1}{1 \times \underset{3}{\cancel{6}} \times \underset{\underset{1}{\cancel{4}}}{\cancel{60}}\ min} = \frac{125\ gtt}{3\ min} = 41.6\ (42)\ gtt/min$$

10. Factors: 500 ml = 8 h; 15 gtt = 1 ml; 1 h = 60 min

$$\frac{gtt}{min} = \frac{15\ gtt}{1\ ml} \times \frac{500\ ml}{8\ h} \times \frac{1\ h}{60\ min} = \frac{\overset{1}{\cancel{15\ gtt}} \times \overset{125}{\cancel{500}} \times 1}{1 \times \underset{2}{\cancel{8}} \times \underset{4}{\cancel{60}}\ min} = \frac{125\ gtt}{8\ min} = 15.6\ (16)\ gtt/min$$

Unit VII Posttest B

1. Factors: Volume/h: 1000 ml = 8 h

$$\frac{ml}{h} = \frac{1000\ ml}{8\ h} = \frac{\overset{125}{\cancel{1000}}\ ml}{\underset{1}{\cancel{8}}\ h} = \frac{125\ ml}{1\ h} = 125\ ml/h$$

Factors: Volume/3h: 125 ml = 1 h (1000 ml = 8 h); 3 h/1

$$ml = \frac{125\ ml \times 3\ h}{1\ h \times 1} = \frac{125\ ml \times 3}{1 \times 1} = \frac{375\ ml}{1} = 375\ ml$$

2. Factors: 1000 ml = 10 h; 20 gtt = 1 ml; 1 h = 60 min

$$\frac{gtt}{min} = \frac{20\ gtt}{1\ ml} \times \frac{1000\ ml}{10\ h} \times \frac{1\ h}{60\ min} = \frac{\overset{1}{\cancel{20\ gtt}} \times \overset{100}{\cancel{1000}} \times 1}{1 \times \underset{1}{\cancel{10}} \times \underset{3}{\cancel{60}}\ gtt} = \frac{100\ gtt}{3\ min} = 33.3\ gtt/min$$

3. Factors: Drip rate: 1000 ml = 12 h; 60 gtt = 1 ml; 1 h = 60 min

$$\frac{gtt}{min} = \frac{60\ gtt}{1\ ml} \times \frac{1000\ ml}{12\ h} \times \frac{1\ h}{60\ min} = \frac{\overset{1}{\cancel{60\ gtt}} \times \overset{250}{\cancel{1000}} \times 1}{1 \times \underset{3}{\cancel{12}} \times \underset{1}{\cancel{60}}\ min} = \frac{250\ gtt}{3\ min} = 83.3\ gtt/min$$

Factors: Infusion time: Expected: 1000 ml = 12 h; 8 h/1; Actual: 500 ml

$$ml = \frac{1000\ ml \times 8\ h}{12\ h \times 1} = \frac{\overset{250}{\cancel{1000}}\ ml \times 8}{\underset{3}{\cancel{12}} \times 1} = \frac{2000\ ml}{3} = 666.6\ ml \pm 25 = 641\ to\ 691$$

500 ml < 666 ml (641 to 691)ml. IV is infusing too slowly.

Factors: Recalculation: 500 ml = 4 h (12 − 8 h); 60 gtt = 1 ml; 1 h = 60 min

$$\frac{gtt}{min} = \frac{60\ gtt}{1\ ml} \times \frac{500\ ml}{4\ h} \times \frac{1\ h}{60\ min} = \frac{\overset{1}{\cancel{60\ gtt}} \times \overset{125}{\cancel{500}} \times 1}{1 \times \underset{1}{\cancel{4}} \times \underset{1}{\cancel{60}}\ min} = \frac{125\ gtt}{1\ min} = 125\ gtt/min$$

4. Factors: 500 ml = 4 h; 10 gtt = 1 ml; 1 h = 60 min

$$\frac{gtt}{min} = \frac{10\ gtt}{1\ ml} \times \frac{500\ ml}{4\ h} \times \frac{1\ h}{60\ min} = \frac{\overset{1}{\cancel{10\ gtt}} \times \overset{125}{\cancel{500}} \times 1}{1 \times \underset{1}{\cancel{4}} \times \underset{6}{\cancel{60}}\ min} = \frac{125\ gtt}{6\ min} = 20.8\ (21)\ gtt/min$$

5. Factors: 100 ml = 1/3 h; 15 gtt = 1 ml; 1 h = 60 min

$$\frac{gtt}{min} = \frac{15\ gtt}{1\ ml} \times \frac{100\ ml}{1/3\ h} \times \frac{1\ h}{60\ min} = \frac{\overset{1}{\cancel{15\ gtt}} \times 3 \times \overset{25}{\cancel{100}} \times 1}{1 \times 1 \times \underset{\underset{1}{\cancel{4}}}{\cancel{60}}\ min} = \frac{75\ gtt}{1\ min} = 75\ gtt/min$$

6. Factors: 80 ml = 1 h; 60 gtt = 1 ml; 1 h = 60 min

$$\frac{gtt}{min} = \frac{60\ gtt}{1\ ml} \times \frac{80\ ml}{1\ h} \times \frac{1\ h}{60\ min} = \frac{\overset{1}{\cancel{60\ gtt}} \times 80 \times 1}{1 \times 1 \times \underset{1}{\cancel{60}}\ min} = \frac{80\ gtt}{1\ min} = 80\ gtt/min$$

7. Factors: 250 ml = 3 h; 10 gtt = 1 ml; 1 h = 60 min

$$\frac{gtt}{min} = \frac{10\ gtt}{1\ ml} \times \frac{250\ ml}{3\ h} \times \frac{1\ h}{60\ min} = \frac{\overset{1}{\cancel{10\ gtt}} \times \overset{125}{\cancel{250}} \times 1}{1 \times 3 \times \underset{\underset{3}{\cancel{6}}}{\cancel{60}}\ min} = \frac{125\ gtt}{9\ min} = 13.8\ (14)\ gtt/min$$

8. Factors: Volume/h: 1000 ml = 2 h

$$\frac{ml}{h} = \frac{1000\ ml}{2\ h} = \frac{\overset{500}{\cancel{1000}}\ ml}{\underset{1}{\cancel{2}\ h}} = \frac{500\ ml}{1\ h} = 500\ ml/h$$

Factors: Drip rate: 1000 ml = 2 h; 10 gtt = 1 ml; 1h = 60 min

$$\frac{gtt}{min} = \frac{10\ gtt}{1\ ml} \times \frac{1000\ ml}{2\ h} \times \frac{1\ h}{60\ min} = \frac{\overset{1}{\cancel{10}\ gtt} \times \overset{\overset{250}{\cancel{500}}}{\cancel{1000}} \times 1}{1 \times \underset{1}{\cancel{2}} \times \underset{\underset{3}{\cancel{6}}}{\cancel{60}\ min}} = \frac{250\ gtt}{3\ min} = 83.3\ gtt/min$$

Factors: Infusion time: Expected: 500 ml = 1 h (1000 ml = 2 h); 1.5 h/1;
Actual: 1000 ml − 350 ml = 650 ml

$$ml = \frac{500\ ml \times 1.5\ h}{1\ h \times 1} = \frac{500\ ml \times 1.5}{1 \times 1} = \frac{750\ ml}{1} = 750\ ml \pm 25 = 725\ to\ 775\ ml$$

650 ml < 750 ml (725 to 775 ml). IV is infusing too slowly.

Factors: 350 ml = 0.5 h (2 − 1.5 h); 10 gtt = 1 ml; 1 h = 60 min

$$\frac{gtt}{min} = \frac{10\ gtt}{1\ ml} \times \frac{350\ ml}{0.5\ h} \times \frac{1\ h}{60\ min} = \frac{\overset{1}{\cancel{10}\ gtt} \times \overset{70}{\cancel{350}} \times 1}{1 \times \underset{0.1}{\cancel{0.5}} \times \underset{6}{\cancel{60}\ min}} = \frac{70\ gtt}{0.6\ min} = 116.6\ (117)\ gtt/min$$

9. Factors: 1000 ml = 6 h; 20 gtt = 1 ml; 1 h = 60 min

$$\frac{gtt}{min} = \frac{20\ gtt}{1\ ml} \times \frac{1000\ ml}{6\ h} \times \frac{1\ h}{60\ min} = \frac{\overset{1}{\cancel{20}\ gtt} \times \overset{500}{\cancel{1000}} \times 1}{1 \times \underset{3}{\cancel{6}} \times \underset{3}{\cancel{60}\ min}} = \frac{500\ gtt}{9\ min} = 55.5\ (56)\ gtt/min$$

10. Factors: 500 ml = 10 h; 20 gtt = 1 ml; 1 h = 60 min

$$\frac{gtt}{min} = \frac{20\ gtt}{1\ ml} \times \frac{500\ ml}{10\ h} \times \frac{1\ h}{60\ min} = \frac{\overset{1}{\cancel{20}\ gtt} \times \overset{50}{\cancel{500}} \times 1}{1 \times \underset{1}{\cancel{10}} \times \underset{3}{\cancel{60}\ min}} = \frac{50\ gtt}{3\ min} = 16.6\ (17)\ gtt/min$$

Unit VII Posttest C

1. Factors: 1000 ml = 10 h

$$\frac{ml}{h} = \frac{1000\ ml}{10\ h} = \frac{\overset{100}{\cancel{1000}}\ ml}{\underset{1}{\cancel{10}\ h}} = \frac{100\ ml}{1\ h} = 100\ ml/h$$

Factors: 100 ml = 1 h (1000 ml = 10 h); 3 h/1

$$ml = \frac{100\ ml \times 3\ h}{1\ h \times 1} = \frac{100\ ml \times 3}{1 \times 1} = \frac{300\ ml}{1} = 300\ ml$$

2. Factors: 1000 ml = 8 h; 15 gtt = 1 ml; 1 h = 60 min

$$\frac{gtt}{min} = \frac{15\ gtt}{1\ ml} \times \frac{1000\ ml}{8\ h} \times \frac{1\ h}{60\ min} = \frac{\overset{1}{\cancel{15}\ gtt} \times \overset{125}{\cancel{1000}} \times 1}{1 \times \underset{1}{\cancel{8}} \times \underset{4}{\cancel{60}\ min}} = \frac{125\ gtt}{4\ min} = 31.25\ gtt/min$$

3. Factors: Drip rate: 1000 ml = 10 h; 60 gtt = 1 ml; 1 h = 60 min

$$\frac{gtt}{min} = \frac{60\ gtt}{1\ ml} \times \frac{1000\ ml}{10\ h} \times \frac{1\ h}{60\ min} = \frac{\overset{1}{\cancel{60}\ gtt} \times \overset{100}{\cancel{1000}} \times 1}{1 \times \underset{1}{\cancel{10}} \times \underset{1}{\cancel{60}\ min}} = \frac{100\ gtt}{1\ min} = 100\ gtt/min$$

Factors: Infusion time: Expected: 1000 ml = 10 h; 7 h/1; Actual: 500 ml

$$ml = \frac{1000\ ml \times 7\ h}{10\ h \times 1\ h} = \frac{\overset{100}{\cancel{1000}}\ ml \times 7}{\underset{1}{\cancel{10}} \times 1} = \frac{700\ ml}{1} = 700\ ml \pm 25 = 675\ to\ 725\ ml$$

500 ml < 700 ml (675 to 725 ml). IV is infusing too slowly.

Factors: Recalculation: 500 ml = 3 h (10 − 7 h); 60 gtt = 1 ml; 1 h = 60 min

$$\frac{gtt}{min} = \frac{60\ gtt}{1\ ml} \times \frac{500\ ml}{3\ h} \times \frac{1\ h}{60\ min} = \frac{\overset{1}{\cancel{60}\ gtt} \times 500 \times 1}{1 \times 3 \times \underset{1}{\cancel{60}\ min}} = \frac{500\ gtt}{3\ min} = 166.6\ (167)\ gtt/min$$

4. Factors: 500 ml = 3 h; 10 gtt = 1 ml; 1 h = 60 min

$$\frac{gtt}{min} = \frac{10\ gtt}{1\ ml} \times \frac{500\ ml}{3\ h} \times \frac{1\ h}{60\ min} = \frac{\overset{1}{\cancel{10}\ gtt} \times \overset{250}{\cancel{500}} \times 1}{1 \times 3 \times \underset{\underset{3}{\cancel{6}}}{\cancel{60}\ min}} = \frac{250\ gtt}{9\ min} = 27.7\ (28)\ gtt/min$$

5. Factors: 100 ml = 30 min; 20 gtt = 1 ml

$$\frac{gtt}{min} = \frac{20\,gtt}{1\,ml} \times \frac{100\,ml}{30\,min} = \frac{20\,gtt \times 100}{1} \times \frac{1}{\overset{2}{\underset{3}{\cancel{30}}}\,min} = \frac{200\,gtt}{3\,min} = 66.6\,(67)\,gtt/min$$

6. Factors: 100 ml = 1 h; 60 gtt = 1 ml; 1 h = 60 min

$$\frac{gtt}{min} = \frac{60\,gtt}{1\,ml} \times \frac{100\,ml}{1\,h} \times \frac{1\,h}{60\,min} = \frac{\cancel{60}\,gtt \times 100 \times \overset{1}{1}}{1 \times 1 \times \underset{1}{\cancel{60}}\,min} = \frac{100\,gtt}{1\,min} = 100\,gtt/min$$

7. Factors: 250 ml = 4 h; 10 gtt = 1 ml; 1 h = 60 min

$$\frac{gtt}{min} = \frac{10\,gtt}{1\,ml} \times \frac{250\,ml}{4\,h} \times \frac{1\,h}{60\,min} = \frac{\overset{1}{\cancel{10}}\,gtt \times \overset{125}{\cancel{250}} \times 1}{1 \times \underset{2}{\cancel{4}} \times \underset{6}{\cancel{60}}\,min} = \frac{125\,gtt}{12\,min} = 10.4\,(10)\,gtt/min$$

8. Factors: Volume/h: 1000 ml = 5 h

$$\frac{ml}{h} = \frac{1000\,ml}{5\,h} = \frac{\overset{200}{\cancel{1000}}\,ml}{\underset{1}{\cancel{5}}\,h} = \frac{200\,ml}{1\,h} = 200\,ml/h$$

Factors: Drip rate: 1000 ml = 5 h; 20 gtt = 1 ml; 1 h = 60 min

$$\frac{gtt}{min} = \frac{20\,gtt}{1} \times \frac{1000\,ml}{5\,h} \times \frac{1\,h}{60\,min} = \frac{\overset{1}{\cancel{20}}\,gtt \times \overset{200}{\cancel{1000}} \times 1}{1 \times \underset{1}{\cancel{5}} \times \underset{3}{\cancel{60}}\,min} = \frac{200\,gtt}{3\,min} = 66.6\,(67)gtt/min$$

Factors: Infusion time: Expected: 200 ml = 1 h (1000 ml = 5 h); 2.5 h/1; Actual: 1000 ml − 350 ml = 650 ml.

$$ml = \frac{200\,ml \times 2.5\,h}{1\,h \times 1} = \frac{200\,ml \times 2.5}{1 \times 1} = \frac{500\,ml}{1} = 500\,ml \pm 25 = 475\,to\,525ml$$

650 ml > 500 ml (475 to 515 ml). The IV is infusing too rapidly.
Factors: Recalculation: 350 ml = 2.5 h (5 − 2.5 h); 20 gtt = 1 ml; 1 h = 60 min

$$\frac{gtt}{min} = \frac{20\,gtt}{1\,ml} \times \frac{350\,ml}{2.5\,h} \times \frac{1\,h}{60\,min} = \frac{\overset{1}{\cancel{20}}\,gtt \times \overset{14}{\cancel{350}} \times 1}{1\,ml \times \underset{0.1}{\cancel{2.5}} \times \underset{3}{\cancel{60}}\,min} = \frac{14\,gtt}{0.3\,min} = 46.6\,(47)\,gtt/min$$

9. Factors: 1000 ml = 8 h; 15 gtt = 1 ml; 1 h = 60 min

$$\frac{gtt}{min} = \frac{15\,gtt}{1\,ml} \times \frac{1000\,ml}{8\,h} \times \frac{1\,h}{60\,min} = \frac{\overset{1}{\cancel{15}}\,gtt \times \overset{125}{\cancel{1000}} \times 1}{1 \times \underset{1}{\cancel{8}} \times \underset{4}{\cancel{60}}\,min} = \frac{125\,gtt}{4\,min} = 31.25\,(31)\,gtt/min$$

10. Factors: 500 ml = 12 h; 15 gtt = 1 ml; 1 h = 60 min

$$\frac{gtt}{min} = \frac{15\,gtt}{1\,ml} \times \frac{500\,ml}{12\,h} \times \frac{1\,h}{60\,min} = \frac{\overset{1}{\cancel{15}}\,gtt \times \overset{125}{\cancel{500}} \times 1}{1 \times \underset{3}{\cancel{12}} \times \underset{4}{\cancel{60}}\,min} = \frac{125\,gtt}{12\,min} = 10.4\,(10)\,gtt/min$$

UNIT VIII INTRAVENOUS MEDICATIONS

Unit VIII Posttest

1. Factors: 20 mg = 500 ml; 1 mg = 1000 mcg

$$\frac{mcg}{ml} = \frac{1000\,ml \times 20\,mg}{1\,mg \times 500\,ml} = \frac{\overset{2}{\cancel{1000}}\,mcg \times 20}{1 \times \underset{1}{\cancel{500}}\,ml} = \frac{40\,mcg}{1\,ml} = 40\,mcg/ml$$

2. Factors: 60 gtt = 1 ml; 1 U = 1000 mU; 10 U = 1000 ml; 28 gtt = 1 min

$$\frac{mU}{in} = \frac{1000\,mU \times 10\,U \times 1\,ml \times 28\,gtt}{1\,U \times 1000\,ml \times 60\,gtt \times 1\,min} = \frac{\cancel{1000}\,mU \times \overset{1}{\cancel{10}} \times 1 \times \overset{14}{\cancel{28}}}{1 \times \underset{1}{\cancel{1000}} \times \underset{\underset{3}{6}}{\cancel{60}} \times 1\,min} = \frac{14\,mU}{3\,min} = 4.67\,mU/min$$

3. Factors: 60 gtt = 1 ml; 1 g = 500 ml; 1 g = 1000 mg; 1 mg = 1000 mcg; 50 mcg = 1 kg × 1 min; 1 kg = 2.2 lb; 176 lb/1

$$\frac{gtt}{min} = \frac{60\,gtt \times 500\,ml \times 1\,g \times 1\,mg \times 50\,mcg \times 1\,kg \times 176\,lb}{1\,ml \times 1\,g \times 1000\,mg \times 1000\,mcg \times 1\,kg \times 1\,min \times 2.2\,lb \times 1}$$

$$= \frac{\overset{3}{\cancel{60}}\,gtt \times \overset{1}{\cancel{500}} \times 1 \times \overset{1}{\cancel{1}} \times \underset{1}{\overset{1}{\cancel{50}}} \times 1 \times \overset{40}{\cancel{176}}}{1 \times 1 \times \underset{2}{\cancel{1000}} \times \underset{1}{\overset{1}{\cancel{50}}} \times 1 \times 1\,min \times \underset{1}{\cancel{2.2}} \times 1} = \frac{120\,gtt}{1\,min} = 120\,gtt/min$$

4. Factors: 1000 mcg = 1 mg; 1000 mg = 1 g; 500 ml = 1 g; 1 ml = 60 gtt; 120 gtt = 1 min

$$\frac{mcg}{min} = \frac{1000\ mcg \times 1000\ mg \times 1\ g \times 1\ ml \times 120\ gtt}{1\ mg \times 1\ g \times 500\ ml \times 60\ gtt \times 1\ min}$$

$$= \frac{1000\ mcg \times 1000 \times 1 \times 1 \times 120}{1 \times 1 \times 500 \times 60 \times 1\ min} = \frac{4000\ mcg}{1\ min} = 4000\ mcg/min$$

5. Factors: 1000 mcg = 1 mg; 1000 mg = 1 g; 1 g = 500 ml

$$\frac{mcg}{ml} = \frac{1000\ mcg \times 1000\ mg \times 1\ g}{1\ mg \times 1\ g \times 500\ ml} = \frac{1000\ mcg \times 1000 \times 1}{1 \times 1 \times 500\ ml} = \frac{2000\ mcg}{1\ ml} = 2000\ mcg/ml$$

6. Factors: 50 ml = 30 min; 15 gtt = 1 ml

$$\frac{gtt}{min} = \frac{15\ gtt \times 50\ ml}{1\ ml \times 30\ min} = \frac{15\ gtt \times 50}{1 \times 30\ min} = \frac{25\ gtt}{1\ min} = 25\ gtt/min$$

7. Factors: 1000 mcg = 1 mg; 200 mg = 1000 ml; 60 gtt = 1 ml; 20 gtt = 1 min

$$\frac{mcg}{min} = \frac{1000\ mcg \times 200\ mg \times 1\ ml \times 20\ gtt}{1\ mg \times 1000\ ml \times 60\ gtt \times 1\ min} = \frac{1000\ mcg \times 200 \times 1 \times 20}{1 \times 1000 \times 60 \times 1\ min} = \frac{200\ mcg}{3\ min} = 66.67\ (67)\ mcg/min$$

8. Factors: 67 mcg = 1 min × 67 kg

$$\frac{mcg}{kg(/min)} = \frac{67\ mcg}{1\ min \times 67\ kg} = 1\ mcg/kg/min$$

9. Factors: Maximum: 3 mcg/kg/min Infusion: 1 mcg/kg/min
   Infusion is within recommended dosage range.

10. Factors: 1000 mcg = 1 mg; 50 mg = 500 ml

$$\frac{mcg}{ml} = \frac{1000\ mcg \times 50\ mg}{1\ mg \times 500\ ml} = \frac{1000\ mcg \times 50}{1 \times 500\ ml} = \frac{100\ mcg}{1\ ml} = 100\ mcg/ml$$

11. Factors: 1000 mcg = 1 mg; 50 mg = 500 ml; 60 gtt = 1 ml; 18 gtt = 1 min

$$\frac{mcg}{min} = \frac{1000\ mcg \times 50\ mg \times 1\ ml \times 18\ gtt}{1\ mg \times 500\ ml \times 60\ gtt \times 1\ min} = \frac{1000\ mcg \times 50 \times 1 \times 18}{1 \times 500 \times 60 \times 1\ min} = 30\ mcg/min$$

12. Factors: Maximum: 10 mcg/kg/min; Infusion: 30 mcg = 1 min × 187 lb; 1 kg = 2.2 lb

$$\frac{mcg}{kg\ (/min)} = \frac{30\ mcg \times 2.2\ lb}{1\ min \times 187\ lb \times 1\ kg} = \frac{30\ mcg \times 2.2}{1\ min \times 187 \times 1\ kg} = \frac{30\ mcg}{min \times 85\ kg} = 0.35\ mcg/kg/min$$

   Infusion is wihin recommended range.

13. Factors: 1000 mcg = 1 mg; 500 ml = 5 mg; 24 gtt = 1 min; 60 gtt = 1 ml

$$\frac{mcg}{min} = \frac{1000\ mcg \times 5\ mg \times 1\ ml \times 24\ gtt}{1\ mg \times 500\ ml \times 60\ gtt \times 1\ min} = \frac{1000\ mcg \times 5 \times 1 \times 24}{1 \times 500 \times 60 \times 1\ min} = \frac{4\ mcg}{1\ min} = 4\ mcg/min$$

14. Factors: 0.08 mcg = 1 kg × 1 min; 1 kg = 2.2 lb; 121 lb/1

$$\frac{mcg}{min} = \frac{0.08\ mcg \times 1\ kg \times 121\ lb}{1\ kg \times 1\ min \times 2.2\ lb \times 1} = \frac{0.08\ mcg \times 1 \times 121}{1 \times 1\ min \times 2.2 \times 1} = \frac{4.4\ mcg}{1\ min} = 4.4\ mcg/min$$

15. Factors: 4.4 mcg = 1 min; 60 gtt = 1 ml; 500 ml = 5 mg; 1000 mcg = 1 mg

$$\frac{gtt}{min} = \frac{60\ gtt \times 500\ ml \times 1\ mg \times 4.4\ mcg}{1\ ml \times 5\ mg \times 1000\ mcg \times 1\ min} = \frac{60\ gtt \times 500 \times 1 \times 4.4}{1 \times 5 \times 1000 \times 1\ min} = \frac{26.4\ gtt}{1\ min} = 26.4\ (26)\ gtt/min$$

16. Factors: 500 ml = 10 mg; 1 mg = 1000 mcg; 0.2 mcg = 1 kg × 1 min; 1 kg = 2.2 lb; 132 lb/1; 60 min = 1 h

$$\frac{500\ ml\ \times\ \ 1\ mg\ \times\ 0.2\ mcg\ \times\ 1\ kg\ \ \ \ \ \ \ \ 132\ lb\ \ \ 60\ min}{10\ mg\ \times\ 1000\ mcg\ \times\ \ \ 1\ kg\ \ \ \times\ 1\ min\ \times\ 2.2\ lb\ \times\ \ \ 1\ \ \ \times\ \ \ \ 1\ h}$$

$$=\frac{\cancel{500}\ ml\ \times\ \ \ 1\ \times\ \cancel{0.2}\ \ \ \ \ \ \times\ 1\ \times\ \cancel{132}\ \times\ 60}{\cancel{10}\ \ \ \times\ \cancel{1000}\times\ 1\ \times\ 1\ min\ \times\ \cancel{2.2}\ \times\ \ 1\ \times\ 1\ h}=\frac{36\ ml}{1\ h}=36\ ml/h$$

17. Factors: 60 gtt = 1 ml; 60 mg = 500 ml; 1 mg = 1000 mcg; 0.4 mcg = 1 kg × 1 min; 1 kg = 2.2 lb; 110 lb/1

$$\frac{gtt}{min}=\frac{60\ gtt\ \times 500\ ml\ \times\ \ \ \ 1\ mg\ \times\ 0.4\ mcg\ \ \ \ \ \ \ \times\ 1\ kg\ \ \times 110\ lb}{1\ ml\ \times\ 60\ mg\ \times 1000\ mcg\times\ 1\ kg\ \ \times\ 1\ min\times 2.2\ lb\ \times\ \ \ 1}$$

$$=\frac{\cancel{60}\ gtt\ \times \cancel{500}\times\ \ \ 1\times\cancel{0.4}\ \ \ \ \ \ \times\ 1\times\cancel{110}}{1\ \ \ \times\ \cancel{60}\times\cancel{1000}\times\ 1\times 1\ min\times\cancel{2.2}\times\ \ 1}=\frac{10\ gtt}{1\ min}=10\ gtt/min$$

18. Factors: 500 ml = 500 mg; 1 mg = 1000 mcg; 12 mcg = 1 kg × 1 min; 70 kg/1; 1 h = 60 min

$$\frac{ml}{h}=\frac{500\ ml\ \times\ \ \ 1\ mg\ \times\ 12\ mcg\ \ \ \ \ \ \ \times\ 70\ kg\ \ \times\ 60\ min}{500\ mg\ \times 1000\ mcg\times\ 1\ kg\ \ \times\ 1\ min\times\ \ 1\ \ \ \ \times\ \ 1\ h}$$

$$=\frac{\cancel{500}\ ml\times\ \ \ 1\ \times\ 12\ \ \ \ \ \times\cancel{70}\times\cancel{60}}{\cancel{500}\ \ \ \times\cancel{1000}\times\ 1\ \times 1\ \times\ \ 1\ \times\ 1\ h}=\frac{252\ ml}{5}=50.4\ ml/h$$

19. Factors: 1000 mcg = 1 mg; 100 mg = 250 ml; 60 gtt = 1 ml; 46 gtt = 1 min

$$\frac{mcg}{min}=\frac{1000\ mcg\times 100\ mg\ \times\ \ 1\ ml\ \times\ 46\ gtt}{1\ mg\ \times 250\ ml\ \times 60\ gtt\ \times\ \ 1\ min}=\frac{\cancel{1000}\ mcg\times\cancel{100}\times\ 1\times 46}{1\ \ \ \ \times\cancel{250}\times\cancel{60}\times\ 1\ min}=\frac{920\ mcg}{3\ min}=306.6\ mcg/min$$

20. Factors: mcg/min: 1000 mcg = 1 mg; 250 mg = 500 ml; 1 ml = 60 gtt; 22 gtt = 1 min

$$\frac{mcg}{min}=\frac{1000\ mcg\times 250\ mg\ \times\ \ 1\ ml\ \times\ 22\ gtt}{1\ mg\ \times 500\ ml\ \times 60\ gtt\ \times\ \ 1\ min}=\frac{\cancel{1000}\ mcg\times\cancel{250}\times\ 1\times\cancel{22}}{1\ \ \ \ \times\cancel{500}\times\cancel{60}\times\ 1\ min}=\frac{550\ mcg}{3\ min}=183.3\ mcg/min$$

Factors: 183.3 mcg = 1 min × 66 kg

$$\frac{mcg}{kg\times min}=\frac{183.3\ mcg}{1\ min\ \times 66\ kg}=2.777\ mcg/kg/min$$

UNIT IX: PEDIATRIC CALCULATIONS

Unit IX Posttest

1. Factors: 250 mg = 5 ml; 60 mg/1

$$ml=\frac{5\ ml\ \times 60\ mg}{250\ mg\times\ 1}=\frac{\cancel{5}\ ml\ \times\cancel{60}}{\cancel{250}\ \ \ \times\ 1}=\frac{6\ ml}{5}=1.2\ ml$$

2. Factors: 60 mg = (q) 4 h; 24 h = 1 d

$$\frac{mg}{d}=\frac{60\ mg\times 24\ h}{(q)4h\ \times\ 1\ d}=\frac{60\ mg\times\cancel{24}}{\cancel{4}\ \ \ \times\ 1\ d}=\frac{360\ mg}{1\ d}=360\ mg/d$$

3. Factors: 50 mg = 1 kg; 1 kg = 2.2 lb; 15 lb 2 oz (15 1/8 lb)/1

$$mg\ (/d)=\frac{50\ mg\times\ \ \ 1\ kg\ \times 15\ 1/8\ lb}{1\ kg\ \times 2.2\ lb\ \times\ \ \ 1}=\frac{50\ mg\times\ \ \ 1\times\cancel{121}}{1\ \ \ \ \times\cancel{2.2}\times\ 8}=\frac{2750\ mg}{8}=343.75\ mg$$

4. Factors: 7.5 mg = 1 kg; 1 kg = 2.2 lb; 33 lb/1

$$mg=\frac{7.5\ mg\times\ \ \ 1\ kg\ \times 33\ lb}{1\ kg\ \times 2.2\ lb\ \times\ \ 1}=\frac{7.5\ mg\times\ \ 1\times\cancel{33}}{1\ \ \ \ \times\cancel{2.2}\times\ 1}=\frac{22.5\ mg}{0.2}=112.5\ mg$$

5. Factors: 6 mg = 1 kg; 1 kg = 2.2 lb; 33 lb/1

$$mg=\frac{6\ mg\times\ \ \ 1\ kg\ \times 33\ lb}{1\ kg\ \times 2.2\ lb\ \times\ \ 1}=\frac{6\ mg\times\ \ 1\times\cancel{33}}{1\ \ \ \ \times\cancel{2.2}\times\ 1}=\frac{18\ mg}{0.2}=90\ mg$$

6. Factors: Georgie's dosage: 30 mg = (q) 8 h; 24 h = 1 d

$$\frac{mg}{d} = \frac{30\ mg \times 24\ h}{(q)\ 8h \times 1\ d} = \frac{30\ mg \times \overset{3}{\cancel{24}}}{\cancel{8} \times 1\ d} = \frac{90\ mg}{1\ d} = 90\ mg/d$$

$$\underset{1}{}$$

Ordered dosage is within the recommended range.

7. Factors: 60 ml = 1 h; 1 h = 60 min; 30 min/1

$$\frac{ml}{} = \frac{60\ ml \times 1\ h \times 30\ min}{1\ h \times 60\ min \times 1} = \frac{\cancel{60}\ ml \times \overset{1}{} \times 30}{1 \times \cancel{60} \times 1} = \frac{30\ ml}{1} = 30\ ml$$

8. Factors: 10 mg = 1 ml; 30 mg/1

$$ml = \frac{1\ ml \times 30\ mg}{10\ mg \times 1} = \frac{1\ ml \times \overset{3}{\cancel{30}}}{\cancel{10} \times 1} = \frac{3\ ml}{1} = 3\ ml$$

9. Factors: 20 mg = 1 m²; 0.74 m²/1

$$mg = \frac{20\ mg \times 0.74\ m^2}{1\ m^2 \times 1} = \frac{20\ mg \times 0.74}{1 \times 1} = \frac{14.8\ mg}{1} = 14.8\ mg$$

10. Factors: 5 mg = 1 kg; 1 kg = 2.2 lb; 33 lb/1

$$mg = \frac{5\ mg \times 1\ kg \times 33\ lb}{1\ kg \times 2.2\ lb \times 1} = \frac{5\ mg \times 1 \times \overset{3}{\cancel{33}}}{1 \times \underset{0.2}{\cancel{2.2}} \times 1} = \frac{15\ mg}{0.2} = 75\ mg$$

11. Factors: 7 mg = 1 kg; 1 kg = 2.2 lb; 33 lb/1

$$mg = \frac{7\ mg \times 1\ kg \times 33\ lb}{1\ kg \times 2.2\ lb \times 1} = \frac{7\ mg \times 1 \times \overset{3}{\cancel{33}}}{1 \times \underset{0.2}{\cancel{2.2}} \times 1} = \frac{21\ mg}{0.2} = 105\ mg$$

12. Factors: 25 mg = (q) 6 h; 24 h = 1 d

$$mg = \frac{25\ mg \times 24\ h}{(q)\ 6h \times 1\ d} = \frac{25\ mg \times \overset{4}{\cancel{24}}}{\underset{1}{\cancel{6}} \times 1\ d} = \frac{100\ mg}{1\ d} = 100\ mg/d$$

Ordered dosage is within the recommended range.

13. Factors: 60 gtt = 1 ml; 50 ml = 1 h; 1 h = 60 min

$$\frac{gtt}{min} = \frac{60\ gtt \times 50\ ml \times 1\ h}{1\ ml \times 1\ h \times 60\ min} = \frac{\cancel{60}\ gtt \times 50 \times 1}{1 \times 1 \times \underset{1}{\cancel{60}}\ min} = \frac{50\ gtt}{1\ min} = 50\ gtt/min$$

14. Factors: 200 mcg = 1 kg; 1 kg = 2.2 lb; 10 lb 5 oz (10 ⁵/₁₆ lb)/1

$$mcg = \frac{200\ mcg \times 1\ kg \times 10^{5/16}\ lb}{1\ kg \times 2.2\ lb \times 1} = \frac{\overset{25}{\cancel{200}}\ mcg \times 1 \times \overset{75}{\cancel{165}}}{1 \times \underset{1}{\cancel{2.2}} \times \underset{2}{\cancel{16}}} = \frac{1875\ mcg}{2} = 937.5\ mcg$$

15. Factors: 937.5 mcg = 1 d; 3 doses = 1 d

$$mcg = \frac{937.5\ mcg \times 1\ d}{1\ d \times 3\ doses} = \frac{937.5\ mcg \times 1}{1 \times 3\ doses} = \frac{937.5\ mcg}{3\ doses} = 312.5\ mcg/dose$$

16. Factors: 8 mg = 1 kg; 1 kg = 2.2 lb; 13 lb 12 oz (13³/₄ or 13.75 lb)/1

$$mg = \frac{8\ mg \times 1\ kg \times 13^{3/4}\ lb}{1\ kg \times 2.2\ lb \times 1\ lb} = \frac{\overset{2}{\cancel{8}}\ mg \times 1 \times \overset{5}{\cancel{55}}}{1 \times \underset{0.2}{\cancel{2.2}} \times \underset{1}{\cancel{4}}} = \frac{10\ mg}{0.2} = 50\ mg$$

17. Factors: 7 mg = 1 kg; 1 kg = 2.2 lb; 13 lb 12 oz (13 ³/₄ or 13.75 lb)/1

$$mg = \frac{7\ mg \times 1\ kg \times 13^{3/4}\ lb}{1\ kg \times 2.2\ lb \times 1\ lb} = \frac{7\ mg \times 1 \times \overset{5}{\cancel{55}}}{1 \times \underset{0.2}{\cancel{2.2}} \times 4} = \frac{35\ mg}{0.8} = 43.75\ mg$$

18. Factors: 12.5 mg = (q) 6h; 24 h = 1 d

$$\frac{mg}{d} = \frac{12.5\ mg \times 24\ h}{(q)\ 6h \times 1\ d} = \frac{12.5\ mg \times \overset{4}{\cancel{24}}}{\underset{1}{\cancel{6}} \times 1\ d} = \frac{50\ mg}{1\ d} = 50\ mg/d$$

19. Yes, 50 mg/d is within the range of 43.75 to 50 mg/d.

20. Factors: 25 ml = 1 h; 60 gtt = 1 ml; 60 min = 1 h

$$\frac{gtt}{min} = \frac{60\ gtt \times 25\ ml \times 1\ h}{1\ ml \times 1\ h \times 60\ min} = \frac{\cancel{60}\ gtt \times 25 \times 1}{1 \times 1 \times \underset{1}{\cancel{60}}\ min} = \frac{25\ gtt}{1\ min} = 25\ gtt/min$$